A Pictorial Treatise on Gall Bladder Cancer

Vinay K. Kapoor
Editor

A Pictorial Treatise on Gall Bladder Cancer

Springer

Editor
Vinay K. Kapoor
Medical Sciences
Sanjay Gandhi Post Graduate Institute of Medical Sciences
Lucknow, Uttar Pradesh
India

ISBN 978-981-15-5288-5 ISBN 978-981-15-5289-2 (eBook)
https://doi.org/10.1007/978-981-15-5289-2

This Springer imprint is published by the registered company Springer Nature Singapore Pte Ltd.
The registered company address is: 152 Beach Road, #21-01/04 Gateway East, Singapore 189721, Singapore

To

Prof Anil K. Agarwal
Chief of Gastrointestinal Surgery
GB Pant Hospital (GBPH) New Delhi

Prof (Mrs) Anu Behari
Professor of Surgical Gastroenterology
Sanjay Gandhi Post-Graduate Institute of Medical Sciences (SGPGIMS) Lucknow

Prof Vinod K. Shukla
Professor of Surgery
Institute of Medical Sciences (IMS) Varanasi

three of my contemporary surgical colleagues in India, who have made invaluable contributions to the science of "chole-cysto-oncology" (gall bladder cancer).

Foreword by Yuji Nimura

Gallbladder cancer (GBC) is more lethal cancer than other biliary tract carcinomas: distal, perihilar, and intrahepatic cholangiocarcinomas. Incidence of GBC is high in India (especially upstream areas of the Ganges River), South America (Chile), and east Asia (Japan and Korea). This may be one of the reasons why the Author (VKK) (Fig. 1) succeeded in establishing his own treatment strategy, made the study of this disease his life work and publishes this book. He has written this unique book to include widely arranged chapters related to GBC: loco-regional anatomy, pathophysiology, etiological epidemiology, pathology, modern diagnostic technology, advanced surgical treatments, and adjuvant therapy, which are followed by invited commentaries by internationally recognized specialists on various aspects of GBC. This idea to invite global experts could moderate his personally biased statements and offer the readers a balanced view on each subject. As written in the Preface, it is certain that this effort will provide the reader with a globally agreed viewpoint on how to manage GBC, a bad cancer with a dismal prognosis.

Although recent advance of diagnostic modalities in the GBC patients provides precise information about the stage of the disease, most of them have been diagnosed at an advanced stage leading to a poor prognosis. Furthermore, treatment strategy for advanced GBC has not been standardized internationally. As shown in the Chap. 9, there are different approaches to advanced GBC in the world, which range from Japanese aggressive approach at one end and to the western pessimistic nihilism (inappropriate management of even early disease) at the other. The Author (VKK) advocates an Indian "Buddhist" middle path, i.e., aggressive surgical approach toward early (and incidental) GBC and non-surgical palliation for advanced GBC. He also emphasizes that aggressive Japanese strategy for advanced stage IV GBC conveys high morbidity, mortality, and small number of long-term survivors and should not be recommended as an appropriate treatment of choice. As has been done for each chapter in this book, a Japanese "Buddhist" comment can be made on the Author's (VKK) opinion. If the Author (VKK) recommends the Indian "Buddhist" approach and likes to criticize the Japanese aggressive approach to advanced stage IV GBC, all postoperative morbidity, 90 days mortality, and survival should be compared between Japanese aggressive resectional approach and Indian non-surgical palliation which usually develops cholangitis with or without sepsis, gastrointestinal bleeding, and/or obstruction with or without abdominal pain during the course of treatment. Are the morbidity and 90 days mortality really lower in the conservative treatments? Is the postoperative survival time really shorter in the aggressive approach than the other? The real advantages in postoperative results should carefully be evaluated between resectional and non-resectional approaches. We HPB surgeons, gastroenterologists, endoscopists, radiologists, and clinical oncologists need to ponder over the above questions again from the patients' perspective after obtaining written informed consent from them. Readers of this book can understand the real advantages of these different approaches and interests of GBC patients.

In addition, the following sentence should be carefully reconsidered. "Most of GBCs in India are infiltrating type while in Japan, papillary tumors are more common. This may be one of the reasons for better outcome in GBC in Japan." It is well known that papillary carcinoma in any organ shows a mild behavior than other histological type of carcinomas. More common type of resected Japanese GBC is not papillary adenocarcinoma but well or moderately differentiated adenocarcinoma which shows nodular and/or infiltrating type tumor.

Finally, I would propose a sentence: "What is borderline resectable GBC?" as pancreatic cancer specialists have succeeded in establishing a diagnostic and therapeutic guideline for borderline resectable pancreatic cancer with perioperative multidisciplinary approach and improving the postoperative results.

I hope that above important issues will be discussed in the next version of this book.

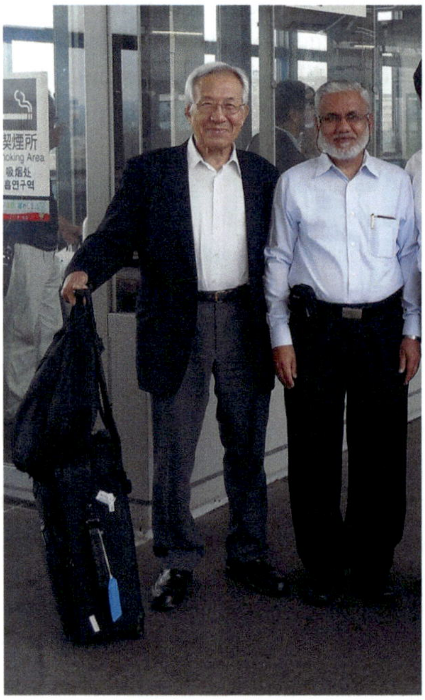

Fig. 1 The Author (VKK) with Prof Yuji Nimura (Left) in Niigata July 2014

Yuji Nimura, MD, PhD
Nagoya University Graduate School of Medicine
Nagoya, Japan
Aichi Cancer Center
Nagoya, Japan

Foreword by Masaru Miyazaki

Prof Vinay Kumar Kapoor (Fig. 2) is one of the greatest HPB surgeons in the world. He has been especially involved in surgical treatment of gallbladder cancer for a long time at the Department of Surgical Gastroenterology, Sanjay Gandhi Post-Graduate Institute of Medical Sciences, Lucknow, India. He has been achieving and publishing many excellent clinical and research papers on gallbladder cancer, not only about surgical management but also about epidemiologic, diagnostic, and non-surgical treatments. Based on these clinical and nonclinical researches, he has been involved for long periods, he could always offer new opinions and has continued to give clinically effective impacts in the fields of management of gallbladder cancer to HPB surgeons in the world until the present time. I have continuously kept communicating with him academically for a long time. I also visited his institution, Sanjay Gandhi Post-Graduate Institute of Medical Sciences in Lucknow, in 2005, as a visiting professor of his institution. At that time, I was so impressed about the remarkable intelligent passion for academism of Prof Kapoor's surgical team at the Grand Rounds. Since then, I have always recognized him as a respectable academic HPB surgeon. Herein he published and offered an excellent book entitled as "*A Treatise on Gall Bladder Cancer*."

Gallbladder cancer still remains a highly aggressive malignancy with a poor prognosis. Because laparoscopic cholecystectomy is nowadays performed more commonly for patients with suspicious gallbladder polyp or tumor, gallbladder cancer is now more usually identified at an earlier stage. However, some type of gallbladder cancer is still difficult to be diagnosed until late advanced stage. Patients with these advanced-staged gallbladder cancers have very dismal prognosis despite of aggressive treatments of surgery and nonsurgical therapies. Therefore, various issues remain to be resolved in clinical practice on the treatment of gallbladder cancer. For example, staging of T2a and T2b such as peritoneal-side or hepatic-side, targeted chemotherapy, and basic genomic research, these important new issues should be clarified by effective clinical and basic researches in near future. In this book, Prof Kapoor has also proposed his very meaningful consideration on these future issues.

I would like to really appreciate Prof Kapoor for giving me this honorable opportunity to write a "*Foreword*" of this book.

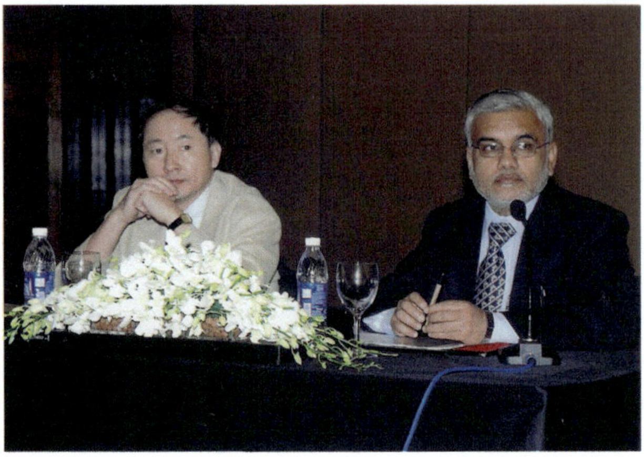

Fig. 2 The Author (VKK) with Prof Masaru Miyazaki (Left) at the International Hepato-pancreato-biliary Association (IHPBA) World Congress Mumbai India 2008

Masaru Miyazaki, MD, PhD
Department of General Surgery
Chiba University
Chiba, Japan
International University of Health & Welfare
Tokyo, Japan

Foreword by Masato Nagino

Despite recent advances in imaging modalities, refinement of surgical techniques, and revision of perioperative management, gallbladder cancer, especially advanced cancer, is the most difficult to treat and a highly fatal malignancy. One reason behind the intractability of gallbladder cancer is that the majority of patients with this disease are diagnosed with advanced disease at initial presentation, due to a lack of specific symptoms. In 2010, a famous randomized controlled study, ABC-02 trial, showed survival benefit of gemcitabine and cisplatin in patients with relapsed or unresectable biliary tract cancer. Thereafter, this combination regimen has been widely used as the first-choice-standard therapy in patients with unresectable gallbladder cancer. Unfortunately, its clinical value is extremely limited because almost all patients died within 30 months. Thus, development of more effective regimen is an urgent task.

Over the past decades, hepatobiliary surgeons have substantially contributed to improve surgical outcome of biliary tract cancer with decreased morbidity and mortality. In addition, hepatobiliary surgeons, mainly from the East, have aggressively challenged extended procedures, including major hepatectomy with vascular resection or major hepatectomy combined with pancreato-duodenectomy (hepato-pancreato-duodenectomy HPD), to treat locally advanced gallbladder cancer previously regarded as unresectable. However, morbidity and mortality associated with such extended surgery is still high, and improvement in survival after resection is small, not as expected. Previously, we at Nagoya University (Fig. 3) actively performed HPD in patients with locally advanced gallbladder cancer but have revised its indication due to poor surgical outcome.

Overall, there are many issues to be resolved in the treatment of gallbladder cancer. In such difficult status, Dr. Kapoor, an experienced hepatobiliary surgeon, has timely published this remarkable comprehensive text book, "*A Pictorial Treatise on Gallbladder Cancer*." For all doctors involved in the treatment of gallbladder cancer, surgeons, oncologists, radiologists, and endoscopists, this textbook will be an outstanding tool to enhance knowledge and guide clinical practice. Dr. Kapoor should be congratulated for gathering and editing a wealth of knowledge in a treatise that updates the fascinating field regarding gallbladder cancer.

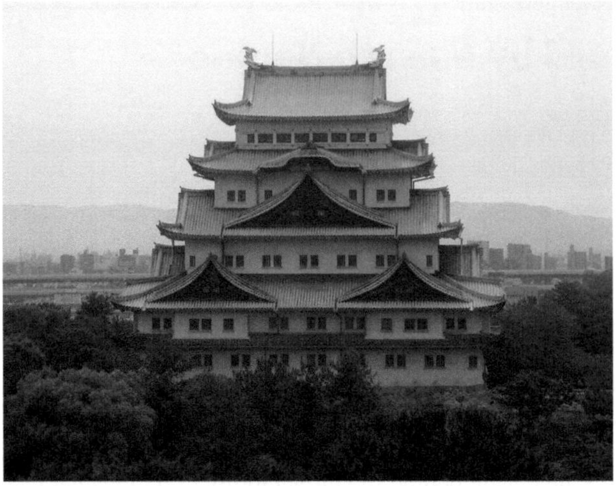

Fig. 3 The Nagoya Castle—the Author's institution, Sanjay Gandhi Post-Graduate Institute of Medical Sciences (SGPGIMS), Lucknow, India—had a collaborative exchange program with the Nagoya University Graduate School of Medicine under the auspices of Japan International Cooperation Agency (JICA)

Masato Nagino, MD
Nagoya University Graduate School of Medicine
Nagoya, Japan

Also by the Author

Kapoor VK, editor. Post-cholecystectomy bile duct injury (*Forewords by Henri Bismuth, John L. Cameron and Steven M. Strasberg*). New York: Springer; 2020. p. 1–244. ISBN 978-981-15-1235-3. Contributions from Australia, Austria, Brazil, France, Italy, Mexico, Netherlands, New Zealand, Portugal, South Africa, Sweden, UK and USA.

Preface

Way back in 1986, Prof. Leslie H. Blumgart—the doyen of biliary surgery—was to visit the Department of Surgery at my *janmabhoomi* (place of "birth"—the alma mater) the All India Institute of Medical Sciences (AIIMS), New Delhi (Fig. 4). The departmental faculty was discussing and debating as to what to present to him. Everyone felt that talking about our experience with any aspect of biliary surgery will be like "lighting a candle in front of the sun." As a young faculty member, I gathered courage and suggested that it may be worthwhile presenting our experience with a biliary disease which he may not see very often so that (at least in numbers) we have more to show than him—gall bladder cancer (GBC). It was their fondness for me which probably made my seniors accept my suggestion. Two of us, Dr. Arvind Kumar (currently Thoracic and Robotic Surgeon, Sir Ganga Ram Hospital SGRH, New Delhi) and myself, were asked to collect the retrospective data, and my teacher and mentor Dr. TK Chattopadhyay (currently Professor of Hepato-Biliary Surgery, Institute of Liver and Biliary Sciences ILBS, New Delhi) was assigned the task of supervising us and presenting the data to Prof. Blumgart. The experience, though a very dismal one, was later published in the Postgraduate Medical Journal (1988;64:593–5)—one of the few publications from the Department of Surgery at the AIIMS, with names of the heads of all four units in the Department.

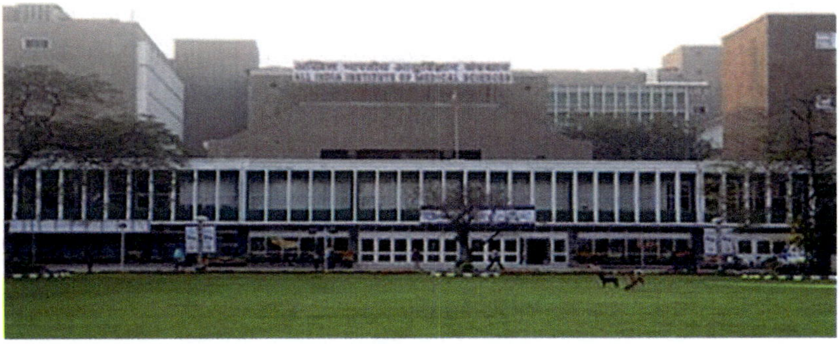

Fig. 4 The All India Institute of Medical Sciences (AIIMS), New Delhi, India—the Author's (VKK) *janmabhoomi* (place of "birth"—the alma mater)

In 1989, when I moved over to the Sanjay Gandhi Post-Graduate Institute of Medical Sciences (SGPGIMS) at Lucknow, in the very few first weeks I observed that GBC was probably more common in Lucknow than it was in New Delhi. I asked my Senior Resident (Fellow) Dr. Sandeep Awasthi (currently Consultant GI Surgeon, Globe Medicare, Lucknow) to prospectively start collecting data about patients with GBC. And rest, as they said it, is history.

GBC was first described in two autopsy specimens by Maximillian de Stoll, an Austrian physician in Vienna in 1777. GBC is a numerically rare but highly lethal disease. Its nonspecific symptoms, especially in the early stages, delay the diagnosis which is usually made in advanced stages of the disease. Management of GBC is an astronomical therapeutic challenge. Surgical resection is the treatment of choice but resectability rates are low, surgical resection may involve important adjacent structures and recurrence rates, even after complete surgical resection, are high. The aggressive biology of the disease results in rapid progression with a dismal prognosis and poor outcome. Overall median survival is dismally short, and long-term (even 5 year) survivals are anecdotal.

GBC, being a "non-western" cancer, has not received much attention either from the clinicians or from the scientists nor adequate support of funding agencies, not even as much as its less common "cousin" cholangiocarcinoma and rarer but "western" tumors, e.g., gastrointestinal stromal tumors (GIST), cystic neoplasms of the pancreas (CNP), and neuro-endocrine tumors (NET). GBC is an "orphan" cancer with no randomized trials, scarcity of publications (and that too single institution and retrospective), very little (and that too low level) evidence and very few management guidelines.

GBC is one of the biliary tract cancers (BTC) which also include bile duct cancer or cholangiocarcinoma—intrahepatic and extrahepatic. Though clubbed with other BTCs, GBC is "*different*." There are several texts and book on BTC, but very few cover GBC alone. This book is an attempt in that direction.

We live (and practice medicine) in the era of evidence-based medicine (EBM). But off late, the evidence itself is being questioned. Evidence is coming up to show that the methodology of generation of the evidence, its authenticity and reliability, and the value of the evidence may not be as much and as high as it is believed to be. In any case, very little, and that too of not very good or high quality, evidence is available for GBC. While I have tried my best to include most of the historical, large, and recent evidence on GBC, many of the opinions expressed and statements made by me in various chapters of this book are, obviously so, heavily biased with the sheer weight of the fairly large experience of more than 1000 resections (and many more operations and patients) for GBC performed over the last three decades (1989–2019) at my *karmabhoomi* (the place of work), the SGPGIMS, Lucknow, India (Fig. 5), than the nimble and feeble "evidence" on GBC available in the published literature. Obviously, some of the statements may appear to be too didactic. In order to remove that opinion bias and to give the reader a bal-

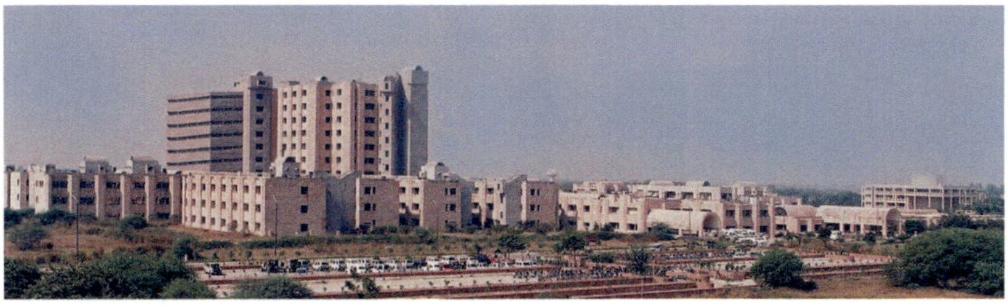

Fig. 5 The Sanjay Gandhi Post-Graduate Institute of Medical Sciences (SGPGIMS), Lucknow, India—the Author's (VKK) *karmabhoomi* (the place of work)

anced view on the subject, I have invited (and they very kindly agreed) global experts on various aspects of GBC from all over the world to write an invited commentary on each chapter so that these personally "biased" statements are moderated and a balanced view is offered to the reader. Debate or comments, if any, are most welcome so that they could be addressed/included in the next edition.

There is no uniformity about the name and spelling of the organ itself—whether "gallbladder" or "gall bladder" (I prefer and have used the latter, abbreviated as GB)—what to talk of the management of its cancer! We have come a long way from AA Blalock, Johns Hopkins Hospital Bulletin 1924 "*No operation should be performed* (in patients with GBC) *as it will only shorten patient life*." I sincerely hope that this effort of mine, strongly supported by the valuable inputs of the invited commenters, will provide the reader with a globally agreed viewpoint on how to manage GBC, *a bad cancer per se*.

Lucknow, India

Vinay K. Kapoor
vkkapoor.india@gmail.com

Acknowledgments

I am deeply indebted to Yuji Nimura, Masaru Miyazaki, and Masato Nagino—three globally renowned and acclaimed stalwarts of hepatobiliary surgery from Japan, for agreeing to write the Forewords for this book.

I would like to thank the contributors of invited commentaries from all continents of the globe for accepting my request to write invited commentaries on the chapters written by me.

I am grateful to the MCh students/fellows (Sandeep Awasthi, Rebala Pradeep, Sanjiv P. Haribhakti, Rajendra N. Sonawane, Anu Behari, Gajanan D. Wagholikar, Shaleen Agarwal, D.K.V. Prasad, Ram Daga, Biju Pottakkat, Jitendra Agrawal, and Gaurav Singh) in the Department of Surgical Gastroenterology at the Sanjay Gandhi Post-Graduate Institute of Medical Sciences (SGPGIMS), Lucknow, India, who have prospectively collected, maintained, and analyzed the computerized database of patients with gall bladder cancer (GBC). Acknowledgments are also due to generations of fellows and residents (List on page xxv) of my department who have looked after these patients in the last three decades. I would also like to thank research students (Mila Ghosh, Mahendra K. Singh, T. Padma Priya, Kumudesh Mishra, Pooja Shukla, Ruchira Vishwakarma, Ratnakar Shukla, O.B. Ijare, Madhulika Srivastava, K. Jayalakshmi, Kanchan Sonkar, Santosh K. Bharti, Raj K. Sharma, and Adnan Siddiqui) who have conducted various research projects related to GBC.

I am thankful to my teachers and trainers (Late) Atm Prakash, Lalit K. Sharma, Tushar K. Chattopadhyay, and Mahesh C. Misra at the All India Institute of Medical Sciences (AIIMS), New Delhi, India.

I am thankful to my faculty colleagues at the SGPGIMS, Lucknow—in the Departments of Surgical Gastroenterology (Satyendra P. Kaushik, Rajan Saxena, Sadiq S. Sikora, Ashok Kumar I, Richa Lal, Sujoy Pal, Anu Behari, Rajneesh K. Singh, Anand Prakash, Biju Pottakkat, Ashok Kumar II, Supriya Sharma, Ashish Singh, and Rahul Rai) who have contributed patients and images (some of which have been used in this book) to the departmental database of GBC, Medical Gastroenterology (Late SR Naik, G Choudhuri, VA Saraswat, Rakesh Aggarwal, UC Ghoshal, Samir Mohindra, Praveer Rai, Abhai Verma, Gaurav Pandey and Amit Goel who provided endoscopic images), Radiology (RK Gupta, SS Baijal, Sheo Kumar, Hira Lal and Rajnikant Yadav who provided radiological images), Medical Genetics (Suraksha Agarwal, who introduced me to basic sciences, and Balraj Mittal), Pathology (Narendra Krishnani, Vinita Agrawal, and Niraj Kumari who also provided the microphotographs), and Radiotherapy (Shaleen Kumar, Punita Lal, and Neeraj Rastogi). Special word of thanks to Anand, Supriya and Rahul and Usha Dutta (PGIMER Chandigarh) for reading the final drafts of chapters and making valuable corrections/suggestions.

The Department of Biotechnology (DBT), Government of India provided grants for research into various aspects of GBC. The Indian Council of Medical Research (ICMR) awarded an International Fellowship for discussions for research collaboration. I am thankful to my coresearchers in India—C.L. Khetrapal, Raja Roy, G.A. Nagangowda, Neeraj Sinha (Centre for Biomedical Research CBMR, Lucknow), and Preeti Bajpai (Mahatma Gandhi Central University, Motihari, Bihar).

I am thankful to my international research collaborators in

- Germany: Justo Lorenzo Bermejo, Institute of Medical Biometry and Informatics (IMBI), University of Heidelberg, Heidelberg
- Japan: Masanao Miwa, Nagahama Institute of Bio-Science and Technology, Nagahama, Shiga; Yasuo Tsuchiya and Kazutoshi Nakamura, Division of Preventive Medicine, Kazuo Endoh, Department of Health and Nutrition, Takao Asai, Department of Clinical Engineering and Medical Technology, Niigata University of Health & Welfare, Niigata; Toshikazu Ikoma, Hokuriku University, Kanazawa
- United Kingdom (UK): Anthony J. McMichael, Epidemiology Unit, London School of Hygiene and Tropical Medicine, London; Irving S. Benjamin, Department of Surgery, King's College School of Medicine, London
- United States of America (USA): Christopher Corless, Department of Pathology, Oregon Health & Science University (OHSU), Portland OR; Milind Javle, Department of Gastrointestinal Medical Oncology, MD Anderson Cancer Center, Houston TX

Acknowledgments are also due to (Late) Ashish Agnihotri (database management), Anil Verma (follow up), Pankaj Srivastava and Shraddha Srivastava (secretarial assistance) and Mithilesh K. Dwivedi and Ram Sanehi (scanning the images).

The typed manuscripts for this book could not have been produced but for the hard work put in by my secretarial assistants Ajay Srivastava and K.K. Srivastava (Fig. 6) who could read (and transcribe) my almost illegible micro-sized hand-written scripts (which sometimes even I myself found difficult to decipher) (Fig. 7).

The final shape has been given to this book by colleagues at Springer by Beauty Christobel Gunasekaran, Gobalakrishnan Venkataraman, Naren Aggarwal, and Teena Bedi.

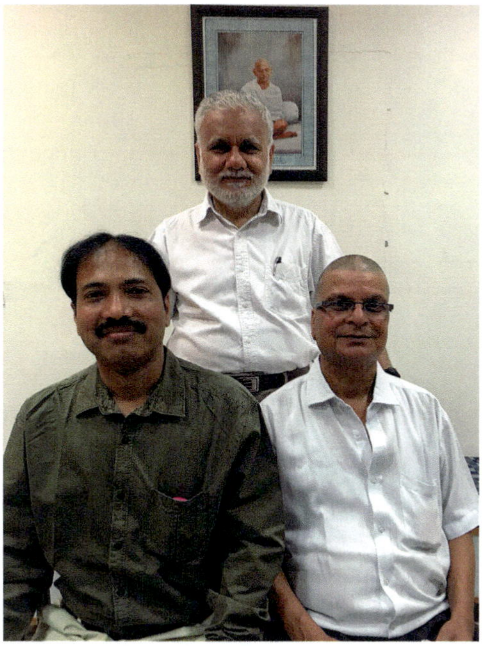

Fig. 6 Ajay Srivastava (Left) and K.K. Srivastava (Right) could read (and transcribe) my almost illegible micro-sized hand-written scripts (in the background is a portrait of Mahatma Gandhi)

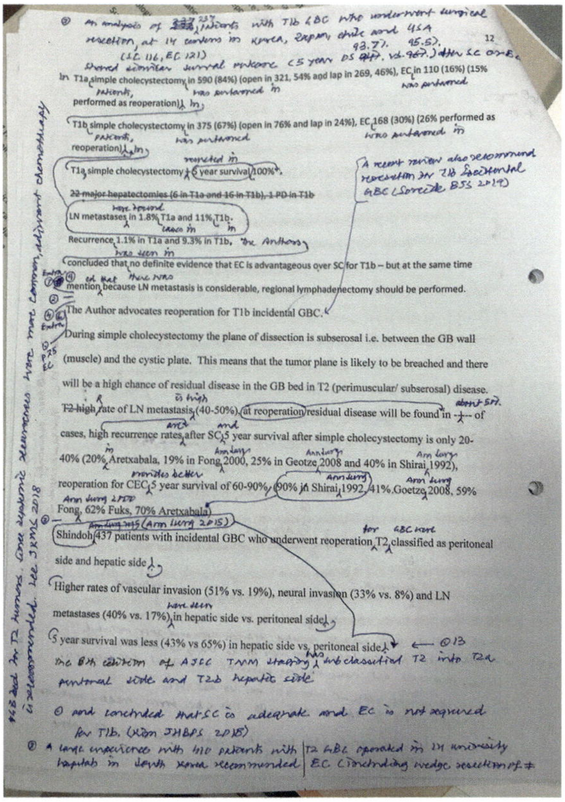

12

In T1a simple cholecystectomy in 590 (84%) (open in 321, 54% and lap in 269, 46%), EC in 110 (16%) (15% performed as reoperation)

T1b simple cholecystectomy in 375 (67%) (open in 76% and lap in 24%), EC 168 (30%) (26% performed as reoperation)

T1a simple cholecystectomy 5 year survival 100%.

~~22 major hepatectomies (6 in T1a and 16 in T1b), 1 PD in T1b~~

LN metastases in 1.8% T1a and 11% T1b.

Recurrence 1.1% in T1a and 9.3% in T1b.

concluded that no definite evidence that EC is advantageous over SC for T1b – but at the same time mention because LN metastasis is considerable, regional lymphadenectomy should be performed.

The Author advocates reoperation for T1b incidental GBC.

During simple cholecystectomy the plane of dissection is subserosal i.e. between the GB wall (muscle) and the cystic plate. This means that the tumor plane is likely to be breached and there will be a high chance of residual disease in the GB bed in T2 (perimuscular/ subserosal) disease.

~~T2 high~~ rate of LN metastasis (40-50%), at reoperation residual disease will be found in of cases, high recurrence rates after SC 5 year survival after simple cholecystectomy is only 20-40% (20% Aretxabala, 19% in Fong 2000, 25% in Geotze 2008 and 40% in Shirai 1992), reoperation for CEC 5 year survival of 60-90% (90% in Shirai 1992, 41% Goetze 2008, 59% Fong, 62% Fuks, 70% Aretxabala)

Shindoh 437 patients with incidental GBC who underwent reoperation T2 classified as peritoneal side and hepatic side

Higher rates of vascular invasion (51% vs. 19%), neural invasion (33% vs. 8%) and LN metastases (40% vs. 17%) in hepatic side vs. peritoneal side

5 year survival was less (43% vs 65%) in hepatic side vs peritoneal side

Fig. 7 Hand-written manuscripts transcribed by Ajay Srivastava and K.K. Srivastava

Fellows and Residents

of
the Department of Surgical Gastroenterology at
the Sanjay Gandhi Post-Graduate Institute of Medical Sciences
(SGPGIMS)
Lucknow Uttar Pradesh India

Since 1989

- A. Lakshmaiah, Abhijit Chandra, Abhimanyu Kapoor, Abhinav A. Sonkar, Abishek Rajan, Ajay Sharma, Ajit K. Mishra, Alister J. Victor, Amit Rastogi, Anand Prakash, Anshuman Pandey, Anu Behari, Anuj Sarkari, Arpit Verma, Arun Kumar M.L., Ashish K. Bansal, Ashish Singh, Ashok Kumar, Ashwini Kudari, Avinash Singh, Avinash Tank
- B. Satyasree, Bappaditya Har, Biju Pottakkat, B.N. Sreedhar Murty, Brijendra Singh
- Ch Srinath, Chandan Chatterjee, Chirag Makkar
- Dasari Mukteshwar, Debashish Banerjee, Deepti Agdur, Devendra Choudhary, Devendra K. Khare, Devendra Naik, Disha Sood Syal, D.K.V. Prasad
- G. Srikanth, Gaurav Singh, Gajanan D. Wagholikar, Gogireddy N. Teja, Gurana K. Rao, G.V. Rajgopal
- Hemant Jain, Hirdaya H. Nag, Himanshu Yadav, H.M. Lokesha
- Jayanth Reddy, Jitendra Agrawal, Joy Abraham, Joseph George
- Kailash C. Kurdia, Kanwal Jeet Singh, Kaushal Anand, Kadiyala V. Ravindra, Kiran Nath A.V., K. Raj Prasad, Kulbhushan Haldeniya, Kushal Mittal
- Luv K. Kacker
- M. Mallappa, M. Manisegaran, M. Ramakrishna Rao, Magnus Jarasand, Mahendra Narwaria, Mahesh Sundaram, Mahesh Thombare, Manas Aggarwal, Manish Srivastava, Manoj Kumar, Mayank Gupta, Mayank Jain, Mohammad Ibrarullah
- N. Murugappan, Nalini Kant Ghosh, Naresh V. Gabani, Neha Bhatt, Nikhil Agrawal, Nikunj Gupta, Nisar H. Hamdani, Nishant K. Malviya, Nihar R. Dash

- Palat Balachandran Menon, Paari Vijayaragavan, Pankaj Sihag, Parthasarathy G., Parvinder Singh, Peeyush Varshney, Prakash K. Sasmal, Prasad Kavatekar, Prasad Babu T.L.V.D., Pratul R. Gupta, Preeti Kimothi, Puneet Gupta, Puneet Puri
- Rachapoodivenkata Raghavendra Rao, Raghuram S. Reddy, Rajendra Desai, Rajendra N. Sonawane, Rajesh Kapoor, Rakesh Shivhare, Rakesh Singh, Ram Daga, Ranjit Vijayahari, Ravindra Budhwani, Ravula Phani Krishna, Rebala Pradeep, Ritu Khare, Rohit Dhawan
- S. Raju, S. Roy Choudhary, S. Shridhar, Sachin Arora, Sadiq S. Sikora, Sajeesh Sahadevan, Sandeep Awasthi, Sandeep Verma, Sanjai Srivastava, Sanjay S. Negi, Sanjiv P. Haribhakti, Satish T.M., Saurabh Galodha, Selvakumar Balakrishnan, Senthil Ganesan, Shabi Ahmad, Shakeel Masood, Shaleen Agarwal, Shivendra Singh, Sidharth Jain, Somanath Malage, Sourav Choudhury, Sunil T.
- T. Ravindranath, Tapas Mishra, Thakur D. Yadav
- Utpal Anand
- V. Vishwanath Reddy, Vijay K. Sharma, Vijay Ramachandran, Vikas Kumar, Vineet Gautam, Vinod Singhal, Vipin K. Sharma, Vivek Singh
- Wasif Ali
- Y. Raghavendra Babu, Yash V. Sinha

- Special thanks to Abhimanyu Kapoor, Ajay Sharma, Ashish Bansal, Gajanan D. Wagholikar, Hirdaya H. Nag, Mahesh Thombare, N. Murugappan, Neha Bhatt, Prakash K. Sasmal, Selvakumar Balakrishnan, Senthil Ganesan, Sourav Choudhury, Supriya Sharma for reading the final drafts of chapters and making valuable corrections/suggestions.

- Special thanks to Ajit K. Mishra, Avinash Singh, Avinash Tank, Bappaditya Har, Dasari Mukteshwar, Gajanan D. Wagholikar, Joy Abraham, Kailash C. Kurdia, Kulbhushan Haldeniya, Mahesh Thombare, Manas Aggarwal, N Murugappan, Nalini Kant Ghosh, Nihar R Dash, Nisar H. Hamdani, Prakash K. Sasmal, Peeyush Varshney, Rohit Dhawan, Saurabh Galodha, Selvakumar Balakrishnan, Shaleen Agarwal, Somanath Malage, Sourav Choudhury, Thakur D Yadav, V Vishwanath Reddy, for reading the proofs.

About the Book

This book covers various aspects of gall bladder cancer, viz. epidemiology, etiology, pathology, clinical presentation, diagnosis, investigations, staging, management, and prevention. Gall bladder cancer is the commonest biliary tract cancer worldwide. Its incidence has peculiar geographical variations, while it is an uncommon cancer in the developed west (north America and western Europe), high incidence rates are reported from central and south America, central and eastern Europe, east Asia (Japan and Korea), and northern India. The book addresses complicated and difficult issues including thick-walled gall bladder, gall bladder cancer with surgical obstructive jaundice, incidental gall bladder cancer, role and place of common bile duct excision, the Japanese philosophy of aggressive surgical approach, management of asymptomatic gall stones, etc.

The text is useful to physicians in high incidence areas who manage patients with gall bladder cancer on a frequent basis as well as to physicians in low incidence areas who see patients with gall bladder cancer infrequently. In addition, chapters include large number of illustrations and photographs including radiographs (US, CT, MRI, etc.), and operative and specimen photos.

This authoritative book provides detailed insight to the readers into various aspects of gall bladder cancer and helps them to manage such patients.

Contents

About the Editor

Vinay K. Kapoor is Professor of Surgical Gastroenterology at the Sanjay Gandhi Post-Graduate Institute of Medical Sciences (SGPGIMS), Lucknow, India. Prof Kapoor has been a Visiting Professor to the Oregon Health and Science University (OHSU), Portland, OR, USA; the King's College Hospital (KCH), London, UK, and the International Medical University (IMU), Kuala Lumpur, Malaysia, and a Visiting Consultant Surgeon to the Zayed Military Hospital (ZMH), Abu Dhabi, UAE. He is an examiner for the Intercollegiate MRCS at the Royal Colleges of Surgeons of England, Edinburgh, and Glasgow UK and has been an examiner at the University Kebangsan Malaysia (UKM), Kuala Lumpur Malaysia; Anna Medical College, Mauritius; BP Koirala Institute of Health Sciences (BPKIHS), Dharan Nepal and the Health Authority of Abu Dhabi (HAAD), UAE. Dr. Kapoor has been awarded with Fulbright Fellowship, Commonwealth Fellowship, Scholarship of the International College of Surgeons, Clinical Oncology Fellowship of the UICC, and Fellowship of the German Academic Exchange Service (DAAD). He has also been awarded Dr. BC Roy Award (Medical Council of India), International Fellowship of the Indian Council of Medical Research (ICMR) and Overseas Associateship of the Department of Biotechnology (DBT). Prof Kapoor has been an invited speaker at international conferences and at institutions in Australia, Austria, Bangladesh, Bhutan, Chile, China, Czech Republic, Dominican Republic, Egypt, France, Germany, Hong Kong, Hungary, Japan, Malaysia, Mauritius, Nepal, Oman, Pakistan, Peru, Poland, Russia, Singapore, South Korea, Sri Lanka, Switzerland, Thailand, Turkey, UAE, UK, and USA. Prof Kapoor was the only surgeon from India figuring in the list of top 2% scientists in Surgery compiled by the Stanford University CA USA and published in PLoS Biology in October 2020. Prof Kapoor has launched an online education portal Prashna India, http://prashna-india.weebly.com/, which answers questions asked by surgical students. In addition to having published books on clinical surgery, safe cholecystectomy, gall bladder cancer, acute pancreatitis, and venous thrombo-embolism, Prof Kapoor has authored a quiz book on Mahatma Gandhi also.

Contributors of Invited Commentaries

Thomas A. Aloia Institute for Cancer Care Innovation, University of Texas MD Anderson Cancer Center, Houston, TX, USA

Christopher T. Aquina Department of Surgery, Wexner Medical Center, The Ohio State University, Columbus, OH, USA

Xabier de Aretxabala Department of Surgery, Clínica Alemana de Santiago, Santiago, Chile

Jean Michel Butte Department of Surgery, Instituto Oncológico Fundación Arturo López Pérez, Santiago, Chile

Isidoro Di Carlo University of Catania, Catania, Italy

Yuman Fong Department of Surgery, City of Hope Medical Center, Duarte, CA, USA

Pradeep Ghimire Department of Surgery, Manipal Teaching Hospital, Pokhara, Nepal

Thorsten Oliver Goetze UCT - University Cancer Center, Frankfurt, Germany

Kiyoshi Hasegawa Hepato-Biliary-Pancreatic Surgery Division, Department of Surgery, Graduate School of Medicine, University of Tokyo, Tokyo, Japan

Ryota Higuchi Department of Surgery, Institute of Gastroenterology, Tokyo Women's Medical University, Tokyo, Japan

Jin-Young Jang Division of Hepatobiliary and Pancreatic Surgery, Department of Surgery, Seoul National University Hospital and Seoul National University College of Medicine, Seoul, South Korea

Nicolas Jarufe Clinica Las Condes, Santiago, Chile

Milind Javle MD Anderson Cancer Center, Houston, TX, USA

Junichi Kaneko Hepato-Biliary-Pancreatic Surgery Division, Department of Surgery, Graduate School of Medicine, University of Tokyo, Tokyo, Japan

Hyeong Seok Kim Division of Hepatobiliary and Pancreatic Surgery, Department of Surgery, Seoul National University Hospital and Seoul National University College of Medicine, Seoul, South Korea

Jonathan Koea Waitemata District Health Board, Auckland, New Zealand

Shishir K. Maithel Emory Liver and Pancreas Center, Winship Cancer Institute, Emory University, Atlanta, GA, USA

Mannino Maurizio University of Catania, Catania, Italy

Prasoon Pankaj Division of Digestive and General Surgery, Niigata University Graduate School of Medical and Dental Sciences, Niigata, Japan

Timothy M. Pawlik Department of Surgery, Wexner Medical Center, The Ohio State University, Columbus, OH, USA

Juan Carlos Roa Department of Pathology, School of Medicine, Pontificia Universidad Católica de Chile, Santiago, Chile

Hiroaki Shimizu Department of Surgery, Teikyo University Chiba Medical Center, Chiba, Japan

Prabin Bikram Thapa Department of Surgery, Kathmandu Medical College, Kathmandu, Nepal

Toshifumi Wakai Division of Digestive and General Surgery, Niigata University Graduate School of Medical and Dental Sciences, Niigata, Japan

Masakazu Yamamoto Department of Surgery, Institute of Gastroenterology, Tokyo Women's Medical University, Tokyo, Japan

Yoo-Seok Yoon Seoul National University Bundang Hospital, Seoul, South Korea

Abbreviations

AEC	Anticipatory extended cholecystectomy
AHC	Atrophy hypertrophy complex
AJCC	American Joint Committee on Cancer
ALP	Alkaline phosphatase
ALPSS	Associating liver partition and portal vein ligation for staged hepatectomy
ALT	Alanine transaminase
APBDJ	Anomalous pancreatic-bile duct junction
APBDU	Anomalous pancreatic-bile duct union
aPTT	Activated partial thromboplastin time
ASR	Age-standardized rate
AST	Aspartate transaminase
BDC	Bile duct cancer (cholangiocarcinoma)
BEA	Biliary-enteric anastomosis
BTC	Biliary tract cancers
CA 19.9	Carbohydrate antigen 19.9
CBD	Common bile duct
CC	Chronic cholecystitis; cholangiocacinoma
CE CT	Contrast enhanced computed tomography
CEA	Carcino-embryonic antigen
CEC	Completion extended cholecystectomy
CHA	Common hepatic artery
CHD	Common hepatic duct
CLD	Chronic liver disease
CR	Complete response (to neodajuvant therapy)
CT	Computed tomography
CTA	Computed tomographic angiography
CTAP	Computed tomographic arterio-portography
DFS	Disease free survival
DSS	Disease specific survival
EBD	Endoscopic biliary drainage
EBS	Endoscopic biliary stenting
EC	Extended cholecystectomy
EHBDR	Extrahepatic bile duct resection
ENBD	Endoscopic naso-biliary drainage
ERC	Endoscopic retrograde cholangiography
ERCP	Endoscopic retrograde cholangio-pancreatography

ERH	Extended right hepatectomy
ES	Endoscopic stenting
EUS	Endoscopic ultrasonography
FNAC	Fine needle aspiration cytology
GB	Gall bladder
GBC	Gall bladder cancer
GI	Gastrointestinal
GJ	Gastro-jejunostomy
GOO	Gastric outlet obstruction
GS	Gall stone
GSD	Gall stone disease
HA	Hepatic artery
HDL	Hepato-duodenal ligament
HPD	Hepato-pancreatico-duodenectomy
ICMR	Indian Council of Medical Research
IHBRD	Intra-hepatic biliary radicle dilatation
IVC	Inferior vena cava
JSBS	Japanese Society of Biliary Surgery
LC	Laparoscopic cholecystectomy
LHA	Left hepatic artery
LHD	Left hepatic duct
LHV	Left hepatic vein
LN	Lymph node
LPV	Left portal vein
LVI	Lymphovascular invasion
MHV	Middle hepatic vein
MPV	Main portal vein
MRA	Magnetic resonance angiography
MRC	Magnetic resonance cholangiography
MRCP	Magnetic resonance cholangio-pancreatography
MRI	Magnetic resonance imaging
MRPV	Magnetic resonance porto-venography
NACRT	Neoadjuvant chemo-radiotherapy
NACT	Neoadjuvant chemotherapy
NAT	Neoadjuvant therapy
NCCN	National Comprehensive Cancer Network
NCD	National Clinical Database (Japan)
NCDB	National Cancer Database (USA)
OC	Open cholecystectomy
OR	Odds ratio
OS	Overall survival
PBD	Preoperative biliary drainage
PBM	Pancreato-biliary malunion (maljunction)
PCI	Pericapsular invasion (in the lymph node)
PD	Pancreato-duodenectomy
PD	Progressive disease
PET	Positron emission tomography
PET CT	Positron emission tomography–computed tomography

PFS	Progression-free survival
PHA	Proper hepatic artery
PNI	Perineural invasion
PR	Partial response (to neodajuvant therapy)
PSE	Port site excision
PSM	Port site metastasis
PTBD	Percutaneous transhepatic biliary drainage
PTC	Percutaneous transhepatic cholangiography
PV	Portal vein
RFS	Recurrence (relapse) free survival
RHA	Right hepatic artery
RHV	Right hepatic vein
RPV	Right portal vein
RR	Relative risk or risk ratio
RT	Radiotherapy
SEER	Surveillance, Epidemiology, and End Results (USA)
SMA	Superior mesenteric artery
SMV	Superior mesenteric vein
SOJ	Surgical obstructive jaundice
SOL	Space occupying lesion
SV	Splenic vein
TWGB	Thick-walled gall bladder
UGIE	Upper gastrointestinal endoscopy
UICC	Union for International Cancer Control
US	Ultrasonography
XGC	Xantho-granulomatous cholecystitis

Surgical Anatomy of the Hepatobiliary System

1

Vinay K. Kapoor

1.1 Gall Bladder

Gall bladder (GB) lies on the undersurface of the liver between segment IV to its left and segment V to its right (Fig. 1.1); that is why any surgical resection for gall bladder cancer (GBC) has to include parts of both segments IV and V. GB is a pyriform organ having fundus (part which protrudes beyond the liver), body, infundibulum, and neck. An outpouching of the infundibulum, Hartmann's pouch, is sometimes present. In a patient with obstructive jaundice if the GB is distended (mucocele) it is more likely to be malignant obstruction at the lower end of the common bile duct, e.g., pancreatic head or periampullary cancer versus stone disease where the GB is usually fibrotic, contracted and shrunken due to chronic inflammation (and does not distend). In GBC, the GB is palpable as a firm to hard lump. As an exception, the GB may be distended in GBC at neck, causing cystic duct obstruction (Fig. 1.2). In hilar cholangiocarcinoma, GB is not palpable. On computed tomography (CT), the GB neck is seen in higher cuts than the body and fundus.

Please also see an Invited Commentary on Surgical Anatomy of the Hepatobiliary System by Mannino Maurizio and Isidoro Di Carlo (pp **–**)

V. K. Kapoor (✉)
Department of Surgical Gastroenterology, Sanjay Gandhi Post-Graduate Institute of Medical Sciences (SGPGIMS), Lucknow, Uttar Pradesh, India
e-mail: vkkapoor.india@gmail.com

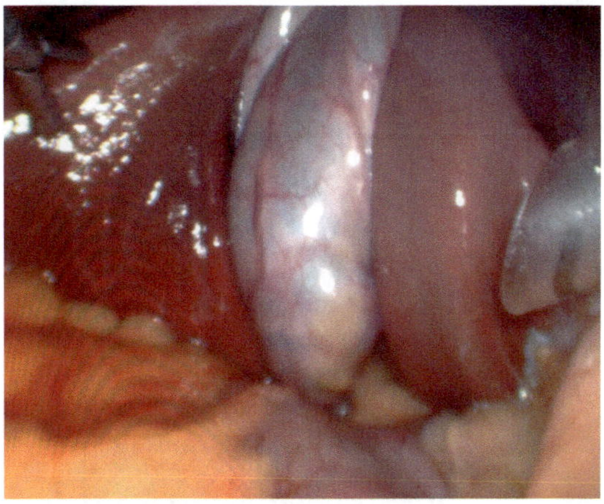

Fig. 1.1 Gall bladder lies on the undersurface of the liver between segment IV to its left and segment V to its right; any surgical resection for gall bladder cancer has, therefore, to include parts of both segments IV and V

GB wall is very thin (<3 mm), making it very easy for a GBC to infiltrate through the GB wall into the adjacent organs/structures. GB is an anatomically "busy" organ with liver, hepatic hilum (porta hepatis), hepatoduodenal ligament (containing the common bile duct CBD, proper hepatic artery PHA, and main portal vein MPV), duodenum (Fig. 1.3), pancreas, and colon (Fig. 1.4) lying very close to it; this means early involvement of these organs in advanced GBC which necessitates their resection to achieve R0 resection status.

In the mucosal layer, the lamina propria (mucosa of tall columnar epithelium) of the GB

V. K. Kapoor (ed.), *A Pictorial Treatise on Gall Bladder Cancer*,
https://doi.org/10.1007/978-981-15-5289-2_1

is thin and has no muscularis mucosa; in addition, outpouchings of the mucosa, the Rokitansky Aschoff (RA) sinuses, extend through the muscularis propria into the perimuscular (subserosal) adventitia, and lie very close to the serosa. GB wall is peculiar in the sense that it has no submucosa, so that a mucosal cancer very easily and quickly infiltrates into the muscularis propria which is a single muscle layer of loosely arranged crisscrossing longitudinal, circular, and oblique fibers. Involvement of RA sinus in T1a (mucosal) and T1b (muscularis) cancer was associated with lower survival (de Aretxabala et al. 2009). The peritoneal surface of the GB is covered with serosa (visceral peritoneum), but there is no serosa on the hepatic side so that a GBC easily infiltrates into the liver parenchyma. A condensation of fibroareolar tissue, the cystic (cholecytsic) plate (Fig. 1.5), lies between the GB wall and liver parenchyma; the cystic plate continues as the hilar plate in the hepatic hilum. In the recent (eighth) edition of the AJCC-UICC classification (AJCC-UICC classification 2017), T2 (perimuscular connective tissue) GBC has been subclassified as T2a (peritoneal side) and T2b (hepatic side) (Fig. 1.6).

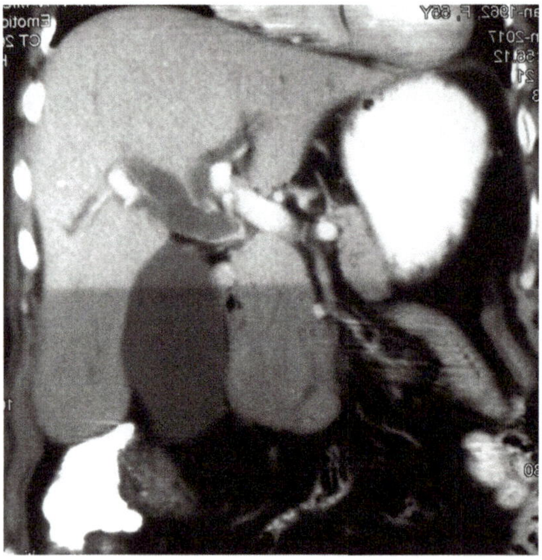

Fig. 1.2 CT showing distended gall bladder (mucocele) in a patient with gall bladder cancer at neck causing cystic duct obstruction; the common hepatic duct is also dilated as a result of mid common bile duct obstruction

GB is supplied by the cystic artery—a branch of the right hepatic artery. Cystic artery lies in the hepato-cystic triangle (commonly called the Calot's triangle) bound by the inferior surface of the liver, common hepatic duct (CHD), and cystic duct and is easily identified running close to the cystic lymph node.

Multiple (2–20) small cholecysto-hepatic veins (Fig. 1.7) drain from the GB into the branches of the portal vein primarily in segments IVB and V and secondarily into segments I, VI, and VII of liver. Tumor spread through these veins is responsible for multiple liver metastases. In some cases, a prominent but small cholecystic vein (Fig. 1.8) is present in the Calot's triangle;

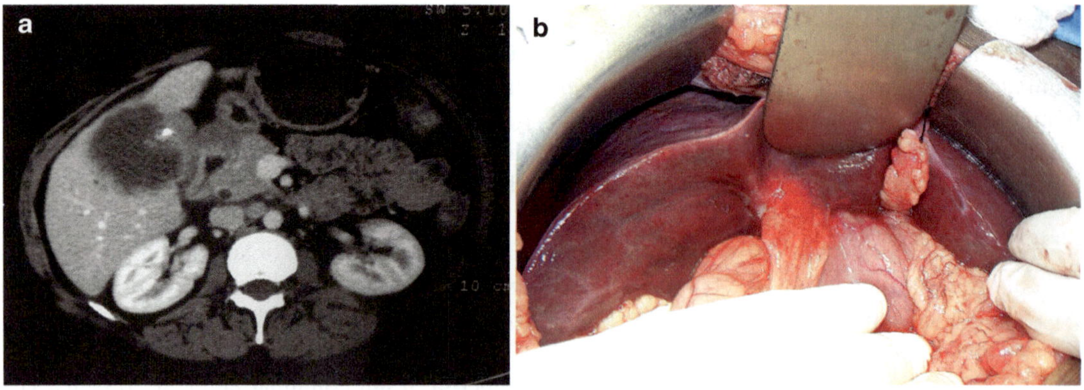

Fig. 1.3 (**a**) The first and second parts of the duodenum lie very close to the gall bladder and can be infiltrated by gall bladder cancer. (**b**) Gall bladder cancer infiltrating the duodenum

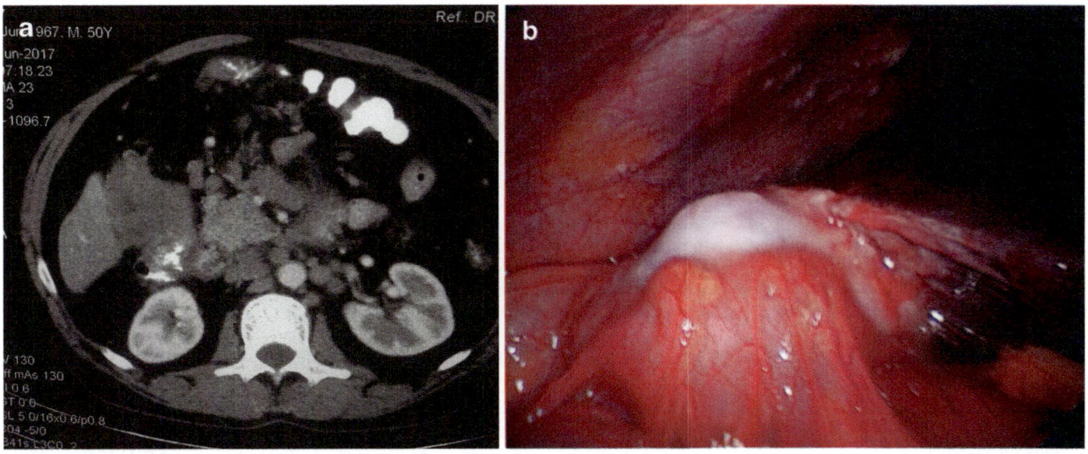

Fig. 1.4 (**a**) Transverse colon and hepatic flexure lie very close to the gall bladder; CT showing gall bladder cancer infiltrating the hepatic flexure of the colon. (**b**) Gall bladder cancer infiltrating the colon

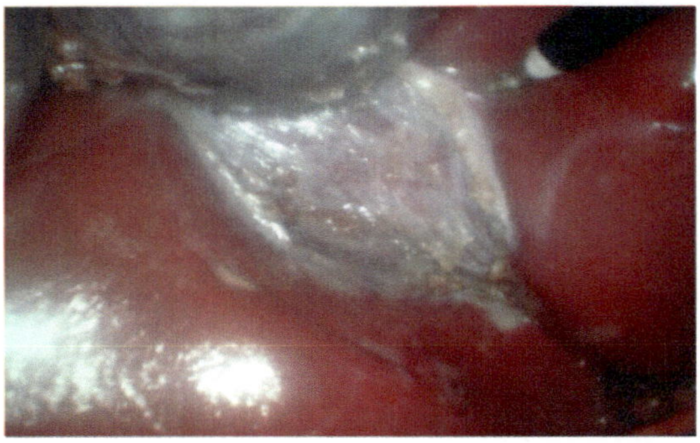

Fig. 1.5 Cystic plate, a condensation of fibro-areolor tissue, seen on the liver parenchyma after the gall bladder has been removed (simple cholecystectomy for gall stones)

it drains from the GB into the MPV, right portal vein (RPV), or right anterior portal vein (RAPV).

Muscularis propria of the GB is rich in lymphatics. That is why even an early, i.e., T1b (muscularis propria) lesion has a significant risk of lymph node (LN) involvement. Lymphatics lie in the entire thickness of the GB wall but are more prominent and are larger in the perimuscular subserosal layer between the muscularis propria and the liver parenchyma on the hepatic side, thus explaining the higher incidence of LN metastasis in T2 lesions, especially those located on the hepatic side, i.e., T2b (Nagahashi et al. 2007). Once the tumor penetrates the muscle, it reaches the perimuscular (subserosal) connective tissue and is liable to lymphatic and vascular spread; once it penetrates the serosa, it can spill into the peritoneal cavity. Lymphatics from the medial (left) wall of the GB drain first into the cystic LN, but those from the right (lateral) wall of the GB may drain directly into the pericholedochal LNs skipping the cystic LN. There are three prominent lymphatic pathways from the GB.

1. Cholecysto-retropancreatic pathway, i.e., cystic (12c) LN—hepatoduodenal (Fig. 1.9), i.e., pericholedochal (12b), hepatic arterial (12a), periportal and retroportal (12p)—retroduodenal/retropancreatic (13a) LN (Fig. 1.10); this is the principal pathway present in large majority of cases. Retroduodenal/retropancreatic LNs are a matter of debate between the AJCC-UICC (AJCC-UICC classification 2017) (which considers them as distant LNs) and the JSBS (2004) (which considers them as regional LNs) classifications.
2. Cholecysto-celiac pathway, i.e., cystic LN—common hepatic artery (CHA) LN—celiac LNs (through the gastro-hepatic ligament).
3. Cholecysto-mesenteric pathway, i.e., preportal LNs—LNs at the root (origin) of the superior mesenteric artery (SMA).

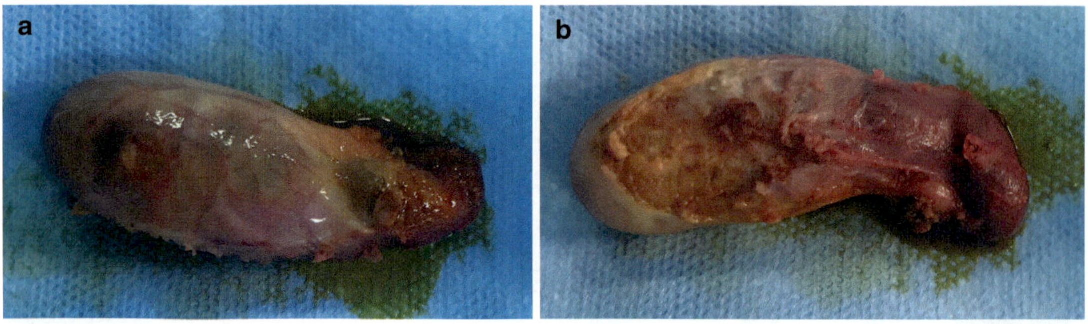

Fig. 1.6 (**a**) Peritoneal surface of the gall bladder is covered with serosa (visceral peritoneum). (**b**) Bare hepatic surface of the gall bladder

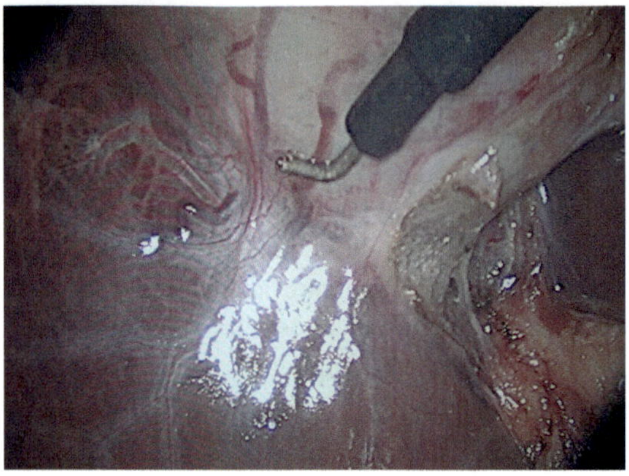

Fig. 1.7 Multiple cholecysto-hepatic veins drain from the gall bladder into the branches of the portal vein in segments IV and V of liver; these are responsible for metastases in these segments of the liver

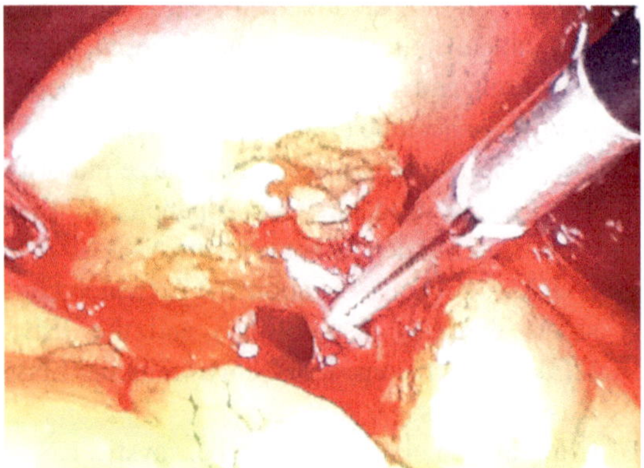

Fig. 1.8 A thin-walled small length cholecystic vein is often present in the Calot's triangle—it drains the gall bladder directly into the portal vein, resulting in multiple metastases in the liver

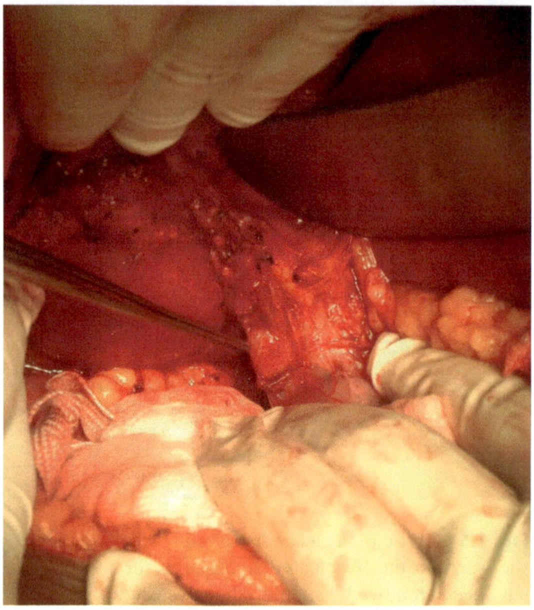

Fig. 1.9 Lymph nodes in the hepatoduodenal ligament, e.g., pericholedochal, hepatic arterial, and periportal are frequently involved in gall bladder cancer

These three pathways finally converge to the aorto-caval LNs (Fig. 1.11). The lymph node stations are classified as first echelon (cystic and pericholedochal), second echelon (periportal, hepatic artery, and pancreato-duodenal), and distant (celiac, superior mesenteric, and aorto-caval). There is, however, no consistent lymphatic drainage of the GB and lymphatic spread is erratic in that distant LNs may be involved in the absence of involvement of the intermediate LNs. Cystic LN is not a sentinel LN for the GB, i.e., other LNs can be involved even if the cystic LN is negative.

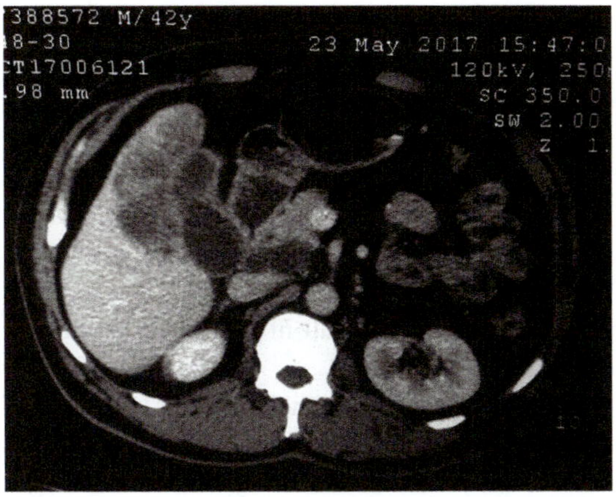

Fig. 1.10 Retropancreatic (and retroduodenal) lymph nodes are a matter of debate between the AJCC–UICC and JSBS classifications of gall bladder cancer; AJCC–UICC considers them to be distant nodes while JSBS considers them to be regional nodes

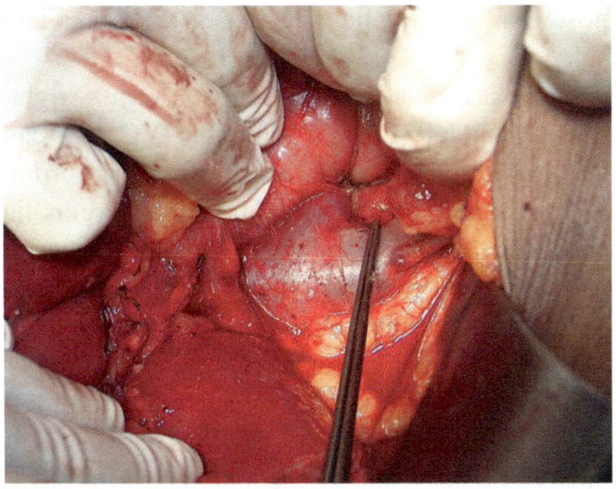

Fig. 1.11 All three lymphatic pathways from the gall bladder viz. cholecysto-retropancreatic, cholecysto-celiac, and cholecysto-mesenteric finally drain into the aorto-caval lymph nodes

1.2 Liver

The normal span of the liver in an average-sized adult is 12–16 cm; it may be increased (hepatomegaly) due to cholestasis of biliary obstruction in patients with jaundice. The liver has superior, anterior, posterior, and right surfaces which are continuous with each other. The anterior (inferior) border separates the anterior surface from the inferior surface; it usually is sharp (leafy) but can get rounded in fatty liver, cholestasis and cirrhosis. The posterosuperior surface of the liver is attached to the undersurface of the diaphragm by right and left coronary ligaments—reflections of the parietal peritoneum on to the capsule of the liver. Between the anterior and posterior layers of the coronary ligaments lies the bare (extraperitoneal) area of the liver. The coronary ligaments fuse to form the triangular ligaments, left more prominent than right. The anterosuperior surface of the liver is attached to the anterior abdominal wall by the falciform ligament, the free edge of which is ligamentum teres (round ligament)—containing the obliterated umbilical vein. The undersurface of the liver attaches to the stomach (hepatogastric ligament) and the first part of the duodenum (hepatoduodenal ligament) by the lesser omentum; the free edge of the lesser omentum is the hepatoduodenal ligament. The hepatoduodenal ligament is formed by two peritoneal layers of the lesser (gastro-hepatic) omentum; it contains the CBD in front, PHA to the left, and MPV behind. The hollow space behind the hepatoduodenal ligament in front of the inferior vena cava (IVC) is the foramen of Winslow which leads to the lesser sac. The structures in the free edge of the hepatoduodenal ligament, especially the PHA and MPV can be temporarily compressed with a finger in the foramen of Winslow and the thumb in front to control brisk bleeding during liver parenchymal transection.

Porta hepatis (hepatic hilum) is a transverse slit (fissure) on the inferior surface of the liver bounded by segment IV (quadrate lobe) in front and segment I (caudate lobe) behind.

The liver has dual blood supply from the portal vein and the hepatic artery—portal vein contributing to about 75% of the total blood flow of about 1.0–1.5 L/min. It is supplied by the proper hepatic artery (PHA), the continuation of the common hepatic artery (CHA), a branch of the celiac axis (Fig. 1.12). PHA lies in the hepatoduodenal ligament to the left of the CBD. It divides in a Y-shaped manner in the hepatic hilum into right and left hepatic arteries. Unlike the branches of the portal vein, right hepatic artery (RHA) has a longer extrahepatic course than the left hepatic artery (LHA); RHA crosses in front of the CBD (Fig. 1.13). A middle hepatic artery (MHA) supplying the segment IV is also sometimes present.

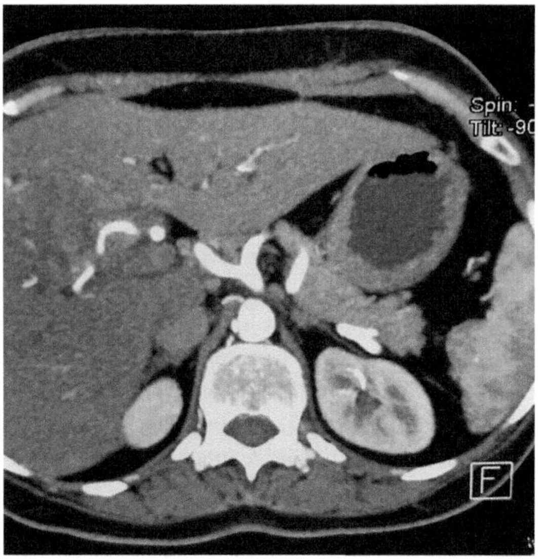

Fig. 1.12 CT showing the celiac axis, the common hepatic artery, and the right hepatic artery (splenic artery is also seen behind the pancreas)

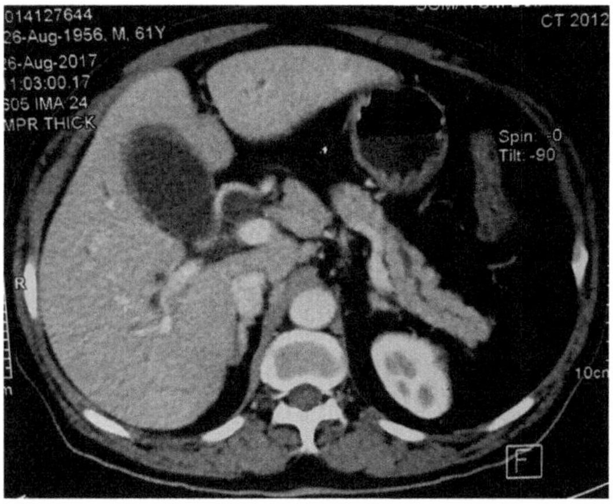

Fig. 1.13 CT showing the right hepatic artery in front of the common bile duct

RHA can be aberrant (accessory or replaced) from the SMA and lie to the right of the CBD (Fig. 1.14a) in the hepatoduodenal ligament and LHA can be aberrant (accessory or replaced) from the left gastric artery (LGA) (Fig. 1.14b). An aberrant hepatic artery is useful during hepatectomy.

Portal vein, formed by the union of the superior mesenteric vein (SMV) and splenic vein behind the neck of the pancreas runs in the hepatoduodenal ligament behind the CBD. It divides in a T-shaped manner in the hepatic hilum into a wider shorter right and a narrower longer left portal vein. The left portal vein gives off branches to the segment IV (Fig. 1.15)—there may be separate branches to subsegment B (which are divided for a segment IVB + V resection) and subsegment A, still sometimes they may be shared and their division may result in inadvertent ischemia of segment IVA also.

The right portal pedicle lies at a depth of 2–9 mm from the GB bed. A GBC neck that infiltrates the liver can easily involve the right portal pedicle thus requiring an extended right hepatectomy (ERH) necessitating the sacrifice of a large volume of normal liver parenchyma. The right anterior sectoral pedicle lies in the GB bed (where it can be injured if care is not exercised during liver wedge resection), while the right posterior sectoral pedicle lies in the Rouviere sulcus.

Liver is drained by three hepatic veins—right, middle, and left (Fig. 1.16) into the IVC. IVC can be dissected and controlled above the insertion of the three hepatic veins. The hepatic veins lie within the liver parenchyma near the posterior surface of the liver; they have a very short extrahepatic course thus making their control difficult. The middle hepatic vein (MHV) lies in the major interlobar fissure, i.e., it separates right from left lobe. The terminal part of MHV lies between segments IV and V and is encountered during liver wedge resection or segment IVB + V resection. Right hepatic vein (RHV) lies between right anteromedial (segments V and VIII) and right posterolateral (segments VI and VII) sectors of the liver. Left hepatic vein (LHV) lies between the left anterior and posterior sectors. MHV and LHV may unite to form a common trunk (Fig. 1.17) which then drains into the IVC; this may make an extended right hepatectomy technically difficult. Caudate lobe (segment I) drains directly into the IVC by few small veins.

Anatomical division of the liver into a large right and small left lobe by the falciform ligament (Fig. 1.18) is not followed by the surgeons. From a surgical point of view, liver is divided into a slightly larger (60%) right and smaller

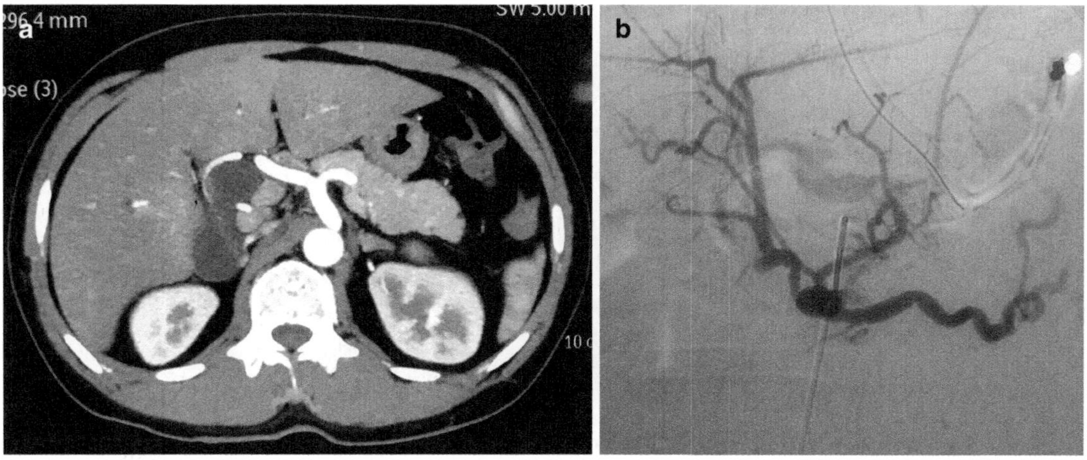

Fig. 1.14 (**a**) Aberrant (accessory) right hepatic artery, arising from the superior mesenteric artery, running behind the common bile duct along its right border (normally placed right hepatic artery is also seen anterior to the common bile duct). (**b**) Aberrant left hepatic artery arising from the left gastric artery

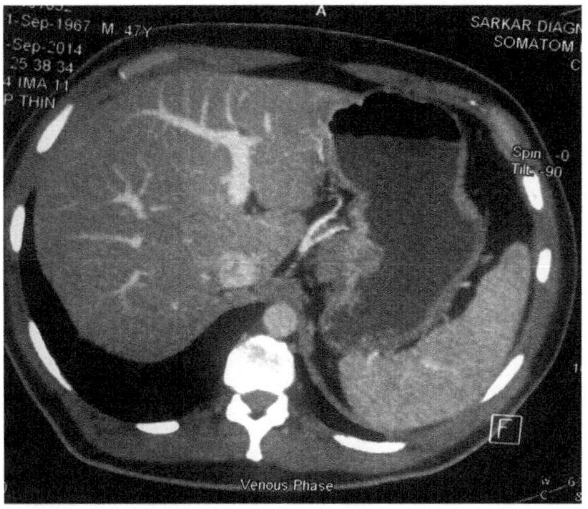

Fig. 1.15 Branches arising from the right superior surface of the left portal vein (LPV) supplying segment IV of the liver

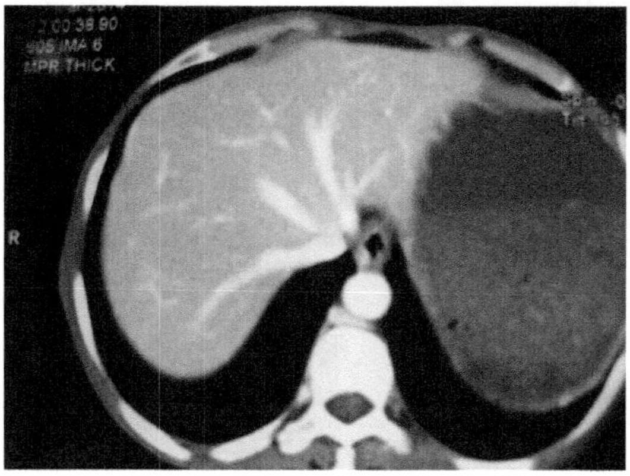

Fig. 1.16 Three hepatic veins (right, middle, and left) divide the liver into four sectors—right posterolateral (segments VI and VII), right anteromedial (segments V and VIII), left medial (segment IV), and left lateral (segments II and III)

(40%) left lobes by the major fissure (Cantlie's line) between the GB fossa anteriorly and the IVC fossa posteriorly, based on its arterial and portal venous blood supply, the bile ducts follow.

IHPBA Brisbane 2000 guidelines (Strasberg 2005) define the following parts of liver:

1. Section—second-order division based on the branches of the hepatic artery and the bile duct.
2. Sector—another second-order division based on the hepatic veins.
3. Eight Couinaud segments.

The right lobe of the liver is divided by the RHV into right anteromedial sector containing superior segment VIII and inferior segment V and posterolateral sector containing superior segment VII and inferior segment VI; the left lobe is divided by the LHV into medial sector containing segment IV (quadrate lobe) and

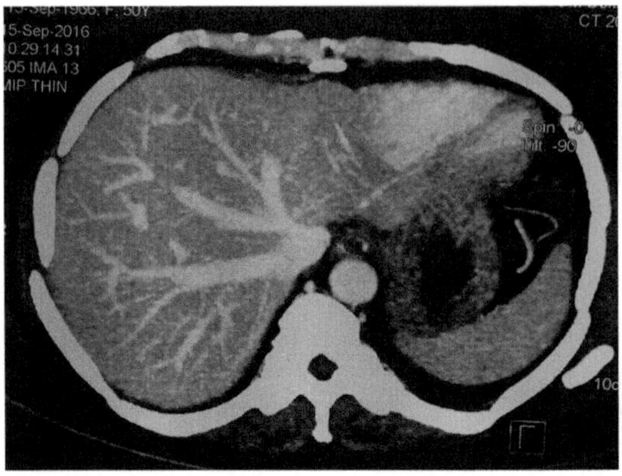

Fig. 1.17 Left hepatic vein and middle hepatic vein may sometimes join to form a common trunk which opens into the inferior vena cava

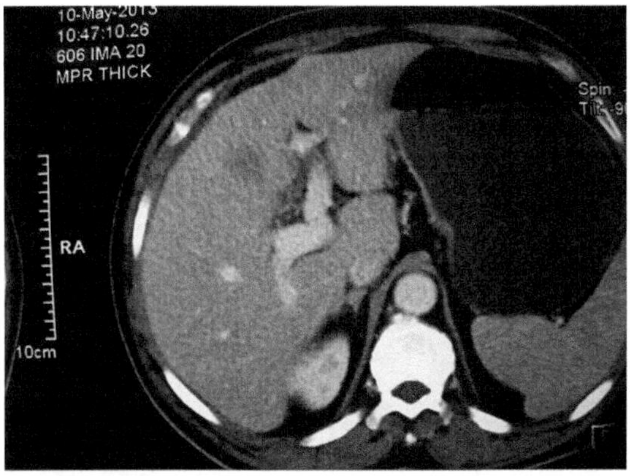

Fig. 1.19 On CT, portal vein bifurcation into the right portal vein and left portal vein divides the liver into a cranial (segments VII, VIII, IVA, and II) and a caudal (segments VI, V, IVB, and III) half

lateral sector containing segments II (superior) and III (inferior). Segment IV (quadrate lobe) is arbitrarily subdivided into a superior (cranial) subsegment A and inferior (caudal) subsegment B (NOTE: The Japanese, for some reasons, call the superior (cranial) subsegment B and inferior (caudal) subsegment A). On CT, portal vein bifurcation (Fig. 1.19) and the right portal vein (RPV) and the left portal vein (LPV) divide the right and left lobes of the liver into superior (cranial) segments VII, VIII, IVA, and II and inferior (caudal) segments VI, V, IVB, and III from right to left.

The segment I (caudate lobe) lies on the undersurface of the liver between the IVC on the

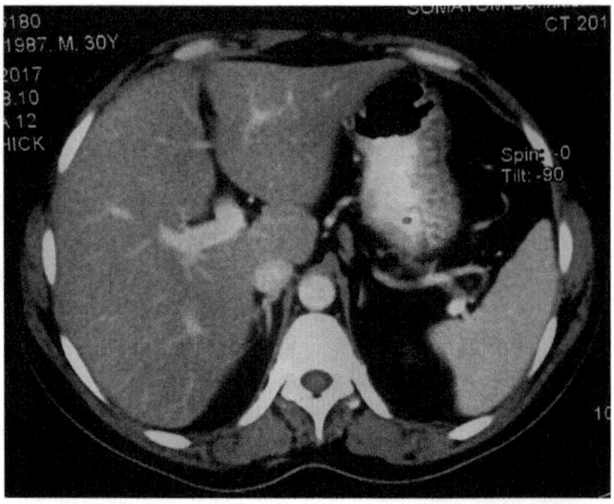

Fig. 1.18 Anatomically speaking, the falciform ligament divides the liver into a large right and a small left lobe; this division is, however, not followed by the surgeons

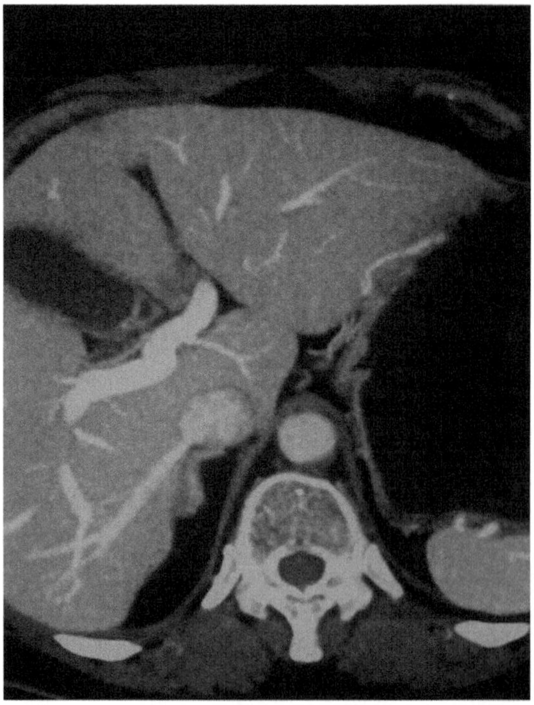

Fig. 1.20 The caudate lobe (segment I) receives small direct branches from the portal vein bifurcation and the left portal vein

right, the ligamentum venosum on the left, and the porta hepatis in front. The caudate lobe continues into the right lobe through the caudate process. It received blood supply from both right and left hepatic arteries and portal veins (Fig. 1.20) and drains directly into the IVC through multiple small veins. While caudate lobe is usually resected along with either right or the left lobe of the liver in a hilar cholangiocarcinoma, this is not required in GBC.

1.3 Bile Ducts

Intrahepatic bile ducts drain the liver parenchyma into right and left hepatic ducts. While the left hepatic duct (LHD) has a long extrahepatic course at the base of segment IV, right hepatic duct (RHD) has a short extrahepatic length. RHD and LHD join to form the CHD which is joined by the cystic duct and continues as the CBD in the hepatoduodenal ligament to the right of the proper hepatic artery and in front of the main portal vein. The CBD is joined by the pancreatic duct inside the pancreatic parenchyma to form a common channel—the ampulla of Vater, which runs through the duodenal wall to open on the medial wall of the second part of the duodenum at the papilla of Vater. Anomalous pancreatico-biliary ductal union (APBDU) (also called anomalous pancreatico-biliary ductal maljunction APBDJ or pancreatico-biliary maljunction PBM), is a rare anatomic congenital variation in which there is abnormal union of the CBD and the pancreatic duct outside the duodenal wall with a long (>8 or 10 mm) common channel of the CBD and pancreatic duct. There is no sphincter in the part of the common channel outside the duodenal wall leading to persistent reflux of the pancreatic juice into the biliary system (including the GB) which predisposes to carcinogenesis in the biliary system including the GB.

1.4 Liver Resections

Liver resections can be lobar, sectoral, or segmental, i.e., lobectomy, sectorectomy, or segmentectomy. Common liver resections in GBC range from a nonanatomical wedge (2–3 cm) around the GB bed in segments IVB and V, formal anatomical resection of segments IVB + V and right hepatectomy (lobectomy) with segment IVB (extended right hepatectomy (ERH) also called right trisegmentectomy). The vascular structures in the hepatoduodenal ligament, i.e., PHA and MPV can be compressed by a clamp (vascular clamp or even soft non-crushing intestinal clamp) to stop/reduce the inflow with an aim to reduce blood loss during liver parenchymal transection—Pringle maneuver.

Surgical anatomy around the gall bladder is like a jungle—danger lurks in every corner!

Invited Commentary on Surgical Anatomy of the Hepatobiliary System

Mannino Maurizio and Isidoro Di Carlo

A full knowledge of the anatomy of the gall bladder, as reported in this chapter, is mandatory to explain the pathophysiology and the behavior of malignancies occurring in this organ; furthermore, an intimate knowledge of the morphological, functional, and real anatomy is a necessary prerequisite to obtain optimal results in the complex surgery of gall bladder cancer (GBC).

Although cholecystectomy is one of the most commonly performed surgical operation nowadays and the anatomy of the Calot's triangle is theoretically simple and familiar to almost every general surgeon, the great variability in anatomy both of the extrahepatic biliary tract and the arterial supply of this organ can lead to major complications. It is fundamental for a surgeon to know the possibility of these anatomical variations in order to perform a safe surgery both for benign as well as malignant conditions.

Liver anatomy has a major importance for surgeons. The Couinaud classification represented the first step to arrive, as reported in this chapter, to the 2000 Brisbane Classification which describes the internationally accepted nomenclature which has come to be known to be the best for planning any type of liver surgery. The Brisbane classification discriminates first-order division (two hemi-livers separated by a plane intersecting the gall bladder fossa and the fossa for the inferior vena cava (IVC)), second-order division based on bile ducts and hepatic artery, third-order division based on intersegmental planes and second alternative order, based on portal vein distribution. As well reported in this chapter, liver resection in case of GBC can range between various possibilities. Although the most frequent possibility is represented by a wedge nonanatomical resection around the gall bladder bed, a surgeon approaching this condition has to know and master the landmarks (and the terms) which can permit him to discriminate the various possible resections.

In addition to liver resections, the lymphatic flow of the gall bladder is also well described in the chapter. This is a fundamental step to select the patients in which a surgical procedure for GBC can be curative and those with positive lymph nodes between the aorta and the inferior vena cava in whom it becomes palliative.

References

AJCC-UICC classification. 2017. www.cancerstaging.org.

de Aretxabala X, Roa I, Hepp J, Maluenda F, Mordojovich G, Leon J, Roa JC. Early gallbladder cancer: is further treatment necessary? J Surg Oncol. 2009;100(7):589–93. https://doi.org/10.1002/jso.21389.

Japanese Society of Biliary Surgery (JSBS). Classification of biliary tract carcinomas. 2nd ed. Tokyo: Kanehara; 2004.

Nagahashi M, Shirai Y, Wakai T, Sakata J, Ajioka Y, Hatakeyama K. Perimuscular connective tissue contains more and larger lymphatic vessels than the shallower layers in human gallbladders. World J Gastroenterol. 2007;13(33):4480–3.

Strasberg SM. Nomenclature of hepatic anatomy and resections: a review of the Brisbane 2000 system. J Hepatobiliary Pancreat Surg. 2005;12(5):351–5.

2 Pathophysiology of Obstructive Jaundice

Vinay K. Kapoor

Gall bladder cancer (GBC) can cause biliary obstruction by

1. Direct infiltration of the common bile duct (CBD) from a GBC neck/cystic duct tumor causing mid-CBD obstruction (Fig. 2.1).
2. GBC neck tumor infiltrating the hepatic hilum (biliary ductal confluence) causing a high (hilar) biliary obstruction (Fig. 2.2).
3. GBC neck tumor infiltrating the liver parenchyma in the gall bladder (GB) bed and obstructing the right portal pedicle which lies in the GB bed causing an intrahepatic biliary obstruction (Fig. 2.3).
4. Metastatic enlarged lymph nodes (LNs) in the porta hepatis, hepatoduodenal ligament, and periduodenal and peripancreatic region, causing CBD obstruction at various levels (Fig. 2.4).
5. Tumor embolus in the CBD from a papillary tumor in the GB (Fig. 2.5).
6. CBD stones secondary to associated gall stones (Fig. 2.6).

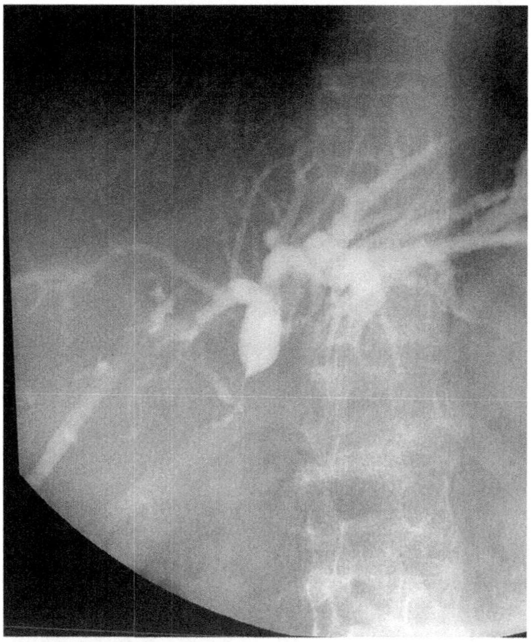

Fig. 2.1 Gall bladder cancer at the neck can directly infiltrate the common bile duct (CBD) to cause mid-CBD obstruction

2.1 Cholestasis

Biliary obstruction leads to cholestasis, i.e., retention of bile (bilirubin and bile salts), reflux of these substances into the blood stream causing jaundice (icterus) (Fig. 2.7), pruritus, and bradycardia. Serum bilirubin level rises; soluble

Please also see an Invited Commentary on Pathophysiology of Obstructive Jaundice by Jin-Young Jang and Hyeong Seok Kim (pp **–**)

V. K. Kapoor (✉)
Department of Surgical Gastroenterology, Sanjay Gandhi Post-Graduate Institute of Medical Sciences (SGPGIMS), Lucknow, Uttar Pradesh, India

V. K. Kapoor (ed.), *A Pictorial Treatise on Gall Bladder Cancer*,
https://doi.org/10.1007/978-981-15-5289-2_2

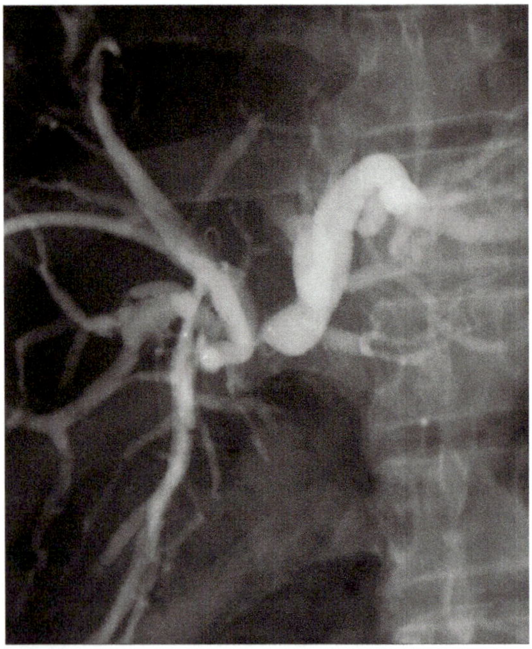

Fig. 2.2 Gall bladder cancer at the neck can directly infiltrate the hepatic hilum to cause high (hilar) biliary obstruction

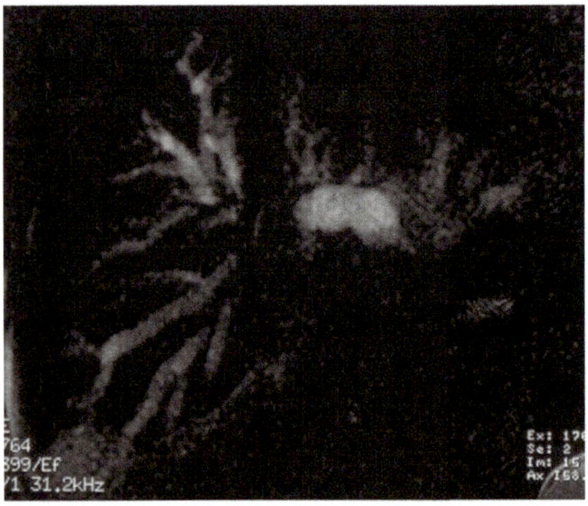

Fig. 2.3 Gall bladder cancer at the neck can directly infiltrate the liver parenchyma near the hepatic hilum to cause intrahepatic biliary obstruction

conjugated bilirubin passes into the urine, causing the characteristic high-colored urine (Fig. 2.8); the absence of bilirubin in the stool results in pale clay-colored stools.

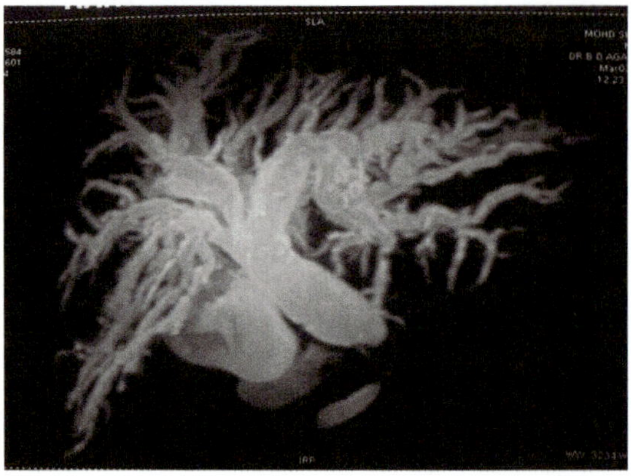

Fig. 2.4 Metastatic lymph nodes in the periduodenal/peripancreatic region can cause low biliary obstruction in gall bladder cancer

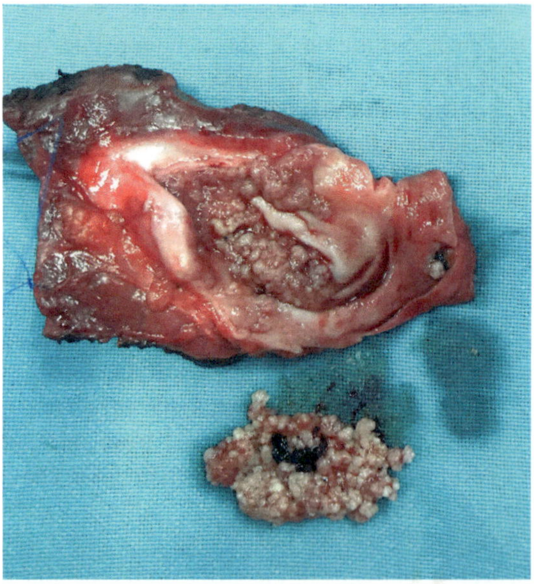

Fig. 2.5 Tissue fragments from a papillary tumor in the gall bladder can "embolize" to the common bile duct and cause biliary obstruction

2.1.1 Pruritus

Pruritus due to extrahepatic biliary obstruction does not respond to oral administration of bile acids and bile salts (cf. pruritus due to intrahepatic cholestasis, e.g., in hepatitis, which does). The pruritus can sometimes be severe enough to interfere with sleep and quality of life. Scratch

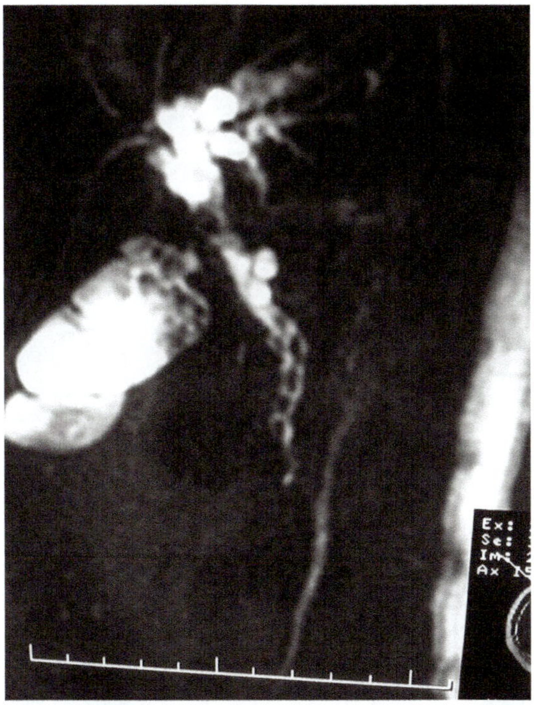

Fig. 2.6 Gall bladder cancer with obstructive jaundice due to associated common bile duct stones is a favorable situation to treat

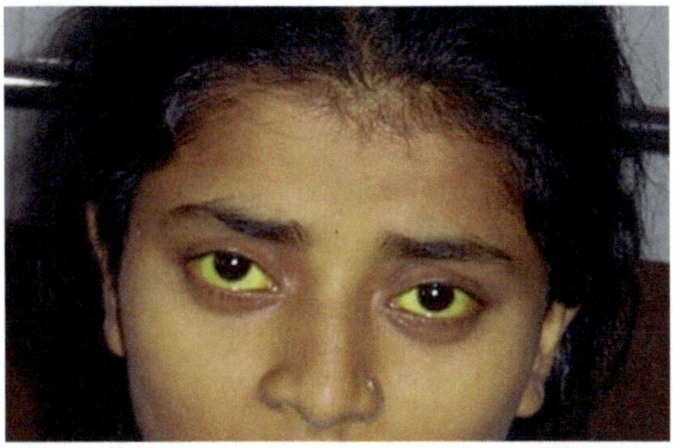

Fig. 2.7 Patients with advanced gall bladder cancer can have obstructive jaundice presenting as yellow eyes (icterus)

marks of severe pruritus may get infected with Gram-positive organisms. Pruritus gets relieved only after the biliary obstruction is taken care of by endoscopic, percutaneous, or surgical methods.

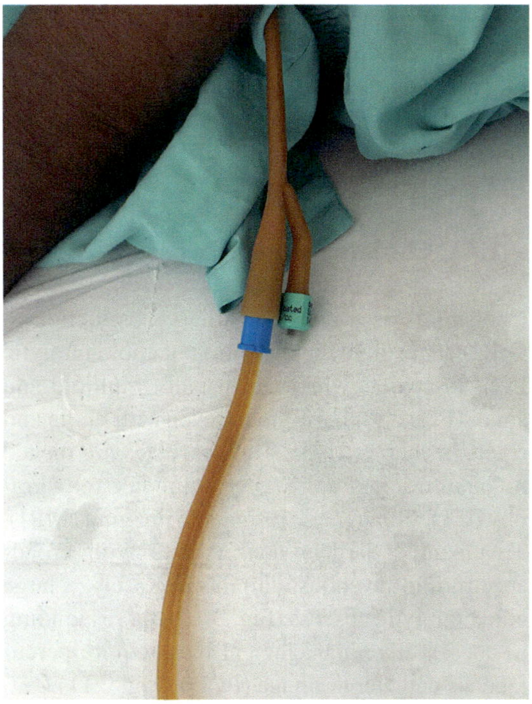

Fig. 2.8 Conjugated bilirubin is water-soluble—it is excreted in the urine to cause high-colored urine

2.1.2 Liver Function Tests (LFT)

Elevated levels of alkaline phosphatase (ALP) and gamma-glutamyl transpeptidase (GGTP) suggest biliary obstruction. Liver enzymes, i.e., alanine transaminase (ALT) and aspartate transaminase (AST) are elevated in presence of cholangitis due to biliary obstruction. Tests of synthetic functions of liver, i.e., serum albumin and prothrombin time (PT), are more important for the evaluation of liver function.

2.1.3 Cholangitis

Patients with GBC may have recurrent attacks of cholangitis secondary to biliary obstruction. Total leukocyte counts (TLC) and differential leukocyte counts (DLC) must be obtained in all patients with GBC (even if there is no fever) to diagnose subclinical cholangitis. Cholangitis, if present, needs treatment with appropriate broad-spectrum antibiotics; uncontrolled cholangitis (not responding to parenteral antibiotics in 24–48 h) may require biliary drainage—this may be endoscopic or percutaneous.

2.1.4 Cholangiolytic Abscess

Cholangitis as a result of biliary obstruction in GBC can result in the formation of cholangiolytic liver abscesses, which are usually multiple and small (Fig. 2.9); high-grade fever with chills and rigors is characteristic. The abscesses are picked up on ultrasonography (US), computed tomography (CT), or magnetic resonance imaging (MRI). Treatment is largely conservative with broad-spectrum intravenous antibiotics. Rarely, a large cholangiolytic abscess (Fig. 2.10) not responding to conservative management may require percutaneous catheter drainage (PCD) (Fig. 2.11).

2.2 Malnutrition

Patients with advanced GBC, more so those with jaundice, are nutritionally depleted (Fig. 2.12) because of the anorexia of cancer and poor intake due to gastric outlet obstruction and/or gastroparesis. Presence of bile is required in the intestine for absorption of many nutrients—absence

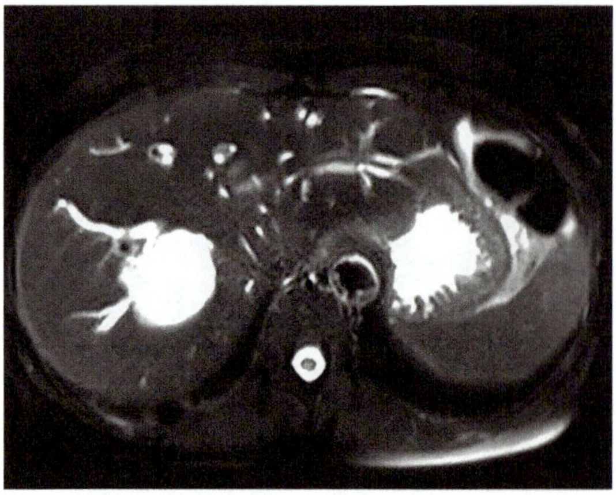

Fig. 2.10 MRI showing a large cholangiolytic abscess

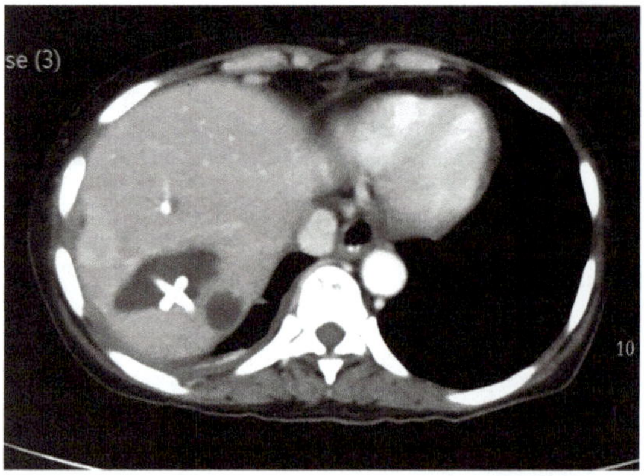

Fig. 2.11 A large cholangiolytic abscess treated with percutaneous catheter drainage (PCD)

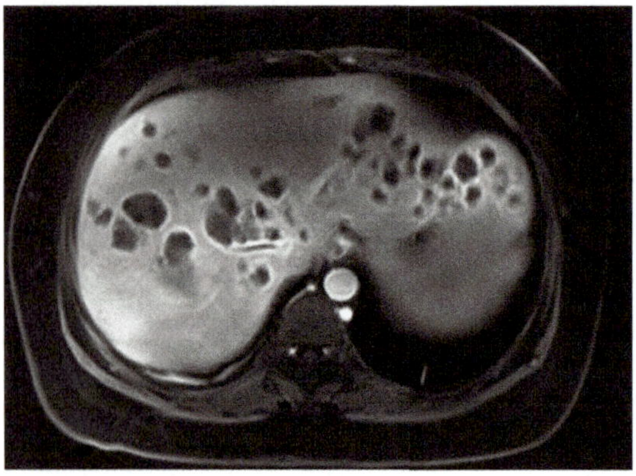

Fig. 2.9 Cholangiolytic abscesses secondary to cholangitis caused by a biliary obstruction are usually multiple and small

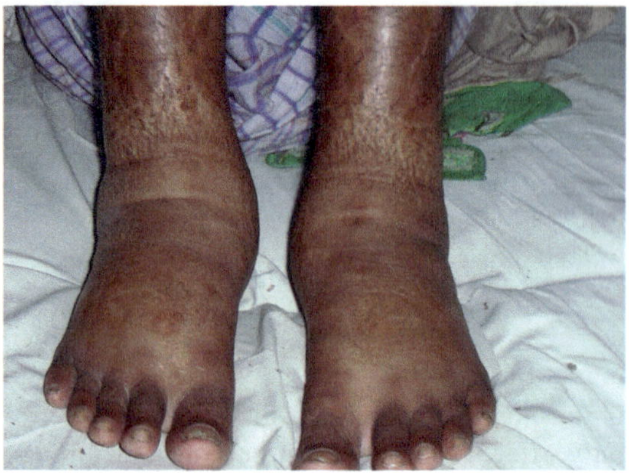

Fig. 2.12 Pedal edema due to hypoalbuminemia caused by malnutrition in gall bladder cancer

of bile in the intestines causes fat malabsorption resulting in protein–calorie malnutrition (PCM) and deficiency of fat-soluble vitamins, i.e., A, D, E, and K. These patients may be in a catabolic phase because of the combined effects of cancer, malnutrition, and sepsis. They may require nutritional support before they are operated. They should be given proper advice regarding nutrition—adequate calorie and protein intake with vitamins so that they return to an anabolic phase. The coagulopathy as a result of vitamin K deficiency manifests as a deranged coagulation profile. Complete coagulation profile, i.e., bleeding time (BT), clotting time (CT), prothrombin time (PT), international normalized ratio (INR), and activated partial thomboplastin time (aPTT), should be obtained in all patients with GBC and jaundice. Endoscopic and percutaneous interventions and surgery are contraindicated in the presence of uncorrected coagulopathy. All patients with GBC and jaundice who are scheduled to undergo an operation or even a nonsurgical, e.g., endoscopic or percutaneous, intervention should receive 3–5 days of vitamin K 10 mg IM daily. The coagulopathy as a result of vitamin K deficiency usually responds to the administration of vitamin K cf. coagulopathy of liver dysfunction which requires administration of fresh frozen plasma (FFP) for correction.

2.3 Other Disturbances

Bile is an important vehicle for the excretion of several products of normal metabolism and many toxic substances. Accumulation of these substances in the bloodstream may cause renal dysfunction. Cholestasis because of biliary obstruction results in impaired hepatocyte mitochondrial function. Patients with biliary obstruction have impaired immune status and are more prone to infective complications. The absence of bile in the intestines due to the biliary obstruction disrupts the gut mucosal barrier and increases the susceptibility to endotoxemia. The jaundiced liver has poor tolerance to ischemia, e.g., if the Pringle maneuver is used during liver resection.

2.4 Preoperative Biliary Drainage (PBD)

Some of the pathophysiological effects of biliary obstruction and jaundice can be reversed, to some extent at least, by preoperative biliary drainage (PBD). PBD to relieve biliary obstruction can be endoscopic or percutaneous transhepatic. Percutaneous PBD is associated with bile leak, which can cause peritoneal dissemination of the disease and carries the risk of needle tract implantation of the tumor. There has been a change in strategy in Japan from percutaneous transhepatic biliary drainage (PTBD) (Fig. 2.13) to endoscopic biliary drainage (EBD) as the method of choice for PBD in GBC. EBD in the form of an endoscopic biliary stent (EBS) (Fig. 2.14) provides internal (enteral) drainage of bile but is prone to get blocked; endoscopic nasobiliary drainage (ENBD) (Fig. 2.15) drains the bile externally but has the advantage that it can be flushed to prevent block. Prolonged total (high volume) external bile loss, e.g., after PTBD or ENBD may cause chronic dehydration and electrolyte imbalance in the form of hyponatremia and hypokalemia, and hypochloremic metabolic acidosis. The patient may feel weak, tired, and lethargic. Decreased plasma volume (hypovolemia) may lead to low output acute renal failure and hyperkalemia. The ill effects of prolonged external bile loss may be reduced by refeeding the bile (Kamiya et al. 2004) but this should be

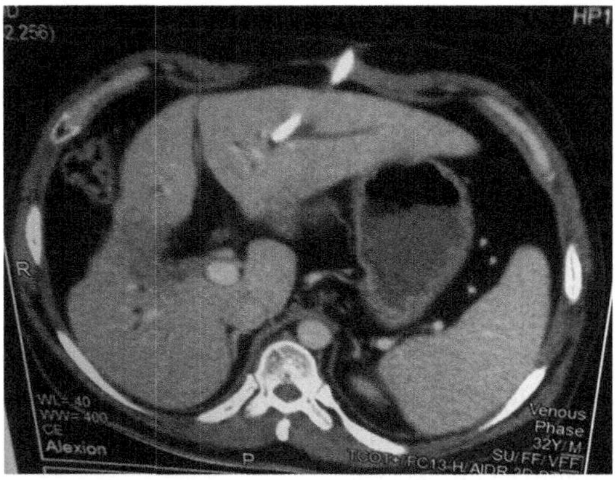

Fig. 2.13 Percutaneous transhepatic biliary drain (PTBD) in situ in the left lateral segment of the liver

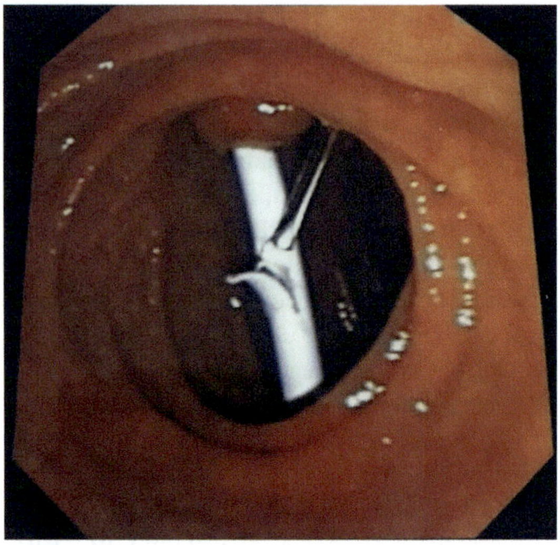

Fig. 2.14 Endoscopic biliary stent in situ seen on endoscopy

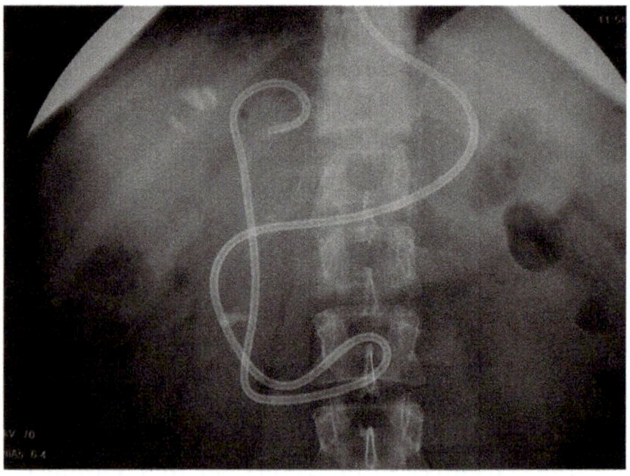

Fig. 2.15 Endoscopic naso-biliary drain (ENBD) in situ

done only if it is clear (not muddy) and sterile (on culture). Bile refeed should be encouraged; bile, however, is very sour and bitter in taste and is highly unpalatable. Small amounts of bile may be taken mixed with food or a sweet syrup, e.g., honey or a fizzy drink. Many patients, however, do not like the idea and are reluctant and hesitant to take bile because of aesthetic reasons. Bile refeeding, even in small amounts, may also restore the intestinal mucosal barrier function (Kamiya et al. 2004).

Indications for PBD in GBC include

1. Cholangitis not controlled with parenteral antibiotics. Biliary obstruction in GBC usually involves the primary biliary ductal confluence and bilateral drainage is required for control of cholangitis; multiple (right anterior and right posterior) drains may be required on the right side in case the secondary biliary ductal confluence is also blocked.
2. Before portal vein embolization (PVE)—because less hypertrophy occurs following PVE in the presence of jaundice.
3. Before neoadjuvant therapy (NAT).
4. Before a major liver resection to bring the serum bilirubin down to near normal (<3 mg/dL). The left hepatic duct should be drained before an extended right hepatectomy (ERH); right hepatic duct may also require to be drained if the serum bilirubin does not fall after left drainage.

The duration of biliary drainage depends on the indication for PBD.

2.5 Portal Vein Embolization (PVE)

Some patients with advanced GBC may require a major liver resection, e.g., extended right hepatectomy (ERH). This leaves a small remnant liver volume (RLV) in the form of the left lateral segment (segments II and III) (Fig. 2.16), which can result in postoperative liver failure. The commonest cause of postoperative mortality after a major liver resection, e.g., ERH, is a hepatic failure because of an inadequate functional liver remnant (FLR).

Preoperative estimation of RLV/FLR with CT, MRI, or isotope scintigraphy is essential before a major hepatectomy. Indo-cyanine green (ICG) is a fluorescent dye with a short (3–4 min) half-life. It binds to the plasma proteins and is then excreted in bile. Patients with normal liver excrete most of the ICG (i.e., no/very little reten-

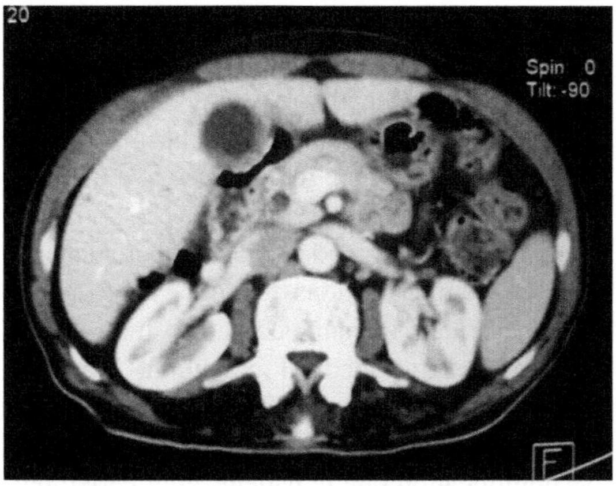

Fig. 2.16 Remnant liver volume (RLV) in the form of the left lateral segment after extended right hepatectomy is usually small—less than the desired 20%

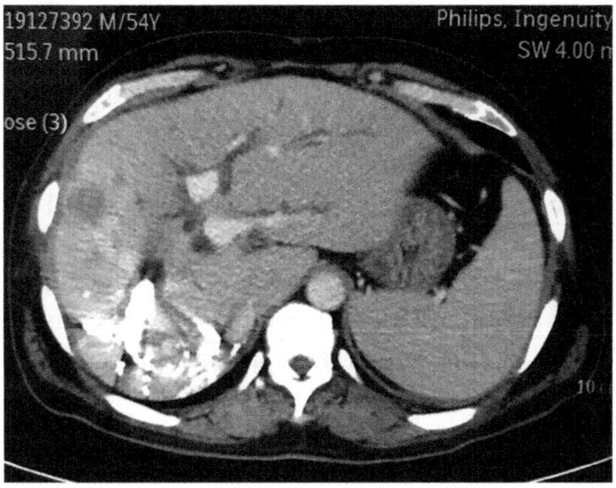

Fig. 2.17 Coils of portal vein embolization (PVE) in the right lobe; the left lateral segment has hypertrophied following the PVE

tion) by 15 min. ICG retention of >30% at 15 min suggests poor liver function. Indocyanine green (ICG) plasma clearance rate of the FLR is a good predictor of the surgical outcome of a major hepatectomy (Yokoyama et al. 2010).

The liver has immense regenerative capacity. This phenomenon is utilized by the intervention of portal vein embolization (PVE) to induce atrophy of the ipsilateral (right) lobe and compensatory hypertrophy of the contralateral (left) lobe of liver (Fig. 2.17) to increase the RLV (Ebata et al. 2012). The regenerative capacity of the jaundiced liver in response to PVE is poor—PBD should, therefore, be performed before PVE is done. If an ERH is anticipated and the RLV is less than 30%, which is usually the case, preoperative PVE should be performed. This is done with ipsilateral transhepatic approach using fibrin glue or steel coils with absolute alcohol. In addition to the right portal vein (RPV), the segment IV branch of the left portal vein (LPV) also needs to be embolized—otherwise segment IV will also hypertrophy and make ERH technically difficult. Atrophy hypertrophy, however, takes 4–6 weeks to occur and the disease may progress during this waiting phase.

FLR takes into account the RLV as well as the quality of the liver. Safe RLV is 20% for normal liver, 30% in the presence of jaundice or chemotherapy-associated steato-hepatitis (CASH) and 40% in patient with chronic liver disease (CLD) e.g. cirrhosis. Patients with nonmetastatic loco-regionally advanced possibly unresectable GBC may be candidates for neoadjuvant therapy (NAT); chemotherapy-associated steato-hepatitis (CASH), steatosis, and sinusoidal dilatation also induce less hypertrophy following PVE.

Associating liver partition with portal vein ligation for staged hepatectomy (ALPPS) has been described as an alternative to PVE to increase the FLR in patients requiring major/multiple liver resections for colorectal liver metastases (CRLM). Liver parenchymal division in ALPPS causes quicker and greater hypertrophy than PVE. The second stage surgery (hepatectomy) can be performed after 1–2 weeks of the first stage. Access to the hilum of the liver may, however, be technically challenging in patients with GBC neck with hilar involvement—the very patients in whom a major liver resection is usually required (Tsui et al. 2016).

2.6 Atrophy Hypertrophy

Biliary obstruction, when combined with portal vein occlusion, can result in ipsilateral atrophy. These patients will often not be candidates for surgical resection, the exception being an involvement of the right portal pedicle only and the main portal vein being free where ERH may be performed.

2.7 Secondary Biliary Cirrhosis (SBC)

Unlike in benign biliary obstruction, e.g., due to post-cholecystectomy biliary stricture and choledochal cyst, secondary biliary cirrhosis (SBC) is hardly ever seen even in untreated patients with GBC who have obstructive jaundice and recurrent cholangitis because of their short (usually less than 6 months) life span which does not allow enough time for SBC to develop.

Malignant surgical obstructive jaundice is a pathophysiological high tide—the fisherman (surgeon) should set to sail (perform major hepatectomy) after it has settled (with PBD and PVE).

Invited Commentary on Pathophysiology of Obstructive Jaundice

Jin-Young Jang and Hyeong Seok Kim

Gallbladder cancer (GBC) is a rare but aggressive cancer; its incidence varies around the world. Recently, with the widespread use of high-resolution imaging techniques and laparoscopic cholecystectomy for benign gallbladder disease, early GBC is being detected increasingly. However, advanced GBC still accounts for a large proportion of disease and it has a dismal prognosis. Obstructive jaundice, which is one of the representative symptoms of locally advanced GBC, has been traditionally considered not to be surgically explored (Hawkins et al. 2004). It is helpful to understand the clinical significance of jaundice and important to divide patients with jaundice into subgroups who will potentially benefit from aggressive surgical resection or not. It will offer some patients potentially curable treatment options, or save some patients from unnecessary operation and hospitalization, thereby focusing on palliation and quality of life.

In this chapter, pathophysiology and management of obstructive jaundice have been addressed by Dr. Kapoor. Among the preoperative management, preoperative biliary drainage (PBD) is usually performed, by endoscopic or percutaneous transhepatic interventions, to reduce the local and systemic effects of jaundice and to improve the patients' general medical condition. However, the role and benefits of PBD are controversial. A study conducted in Korea showed that postoperative complication rate in patients with periampullary cancer was higher in patients with PBD than those without PBD (46.4% vs. 38.2%, $P = 0.027$) (Lee et al. 2018). A multicenter study from the United States also showed that patients with PBD had more complications than those without PBD (67.9% vs. 45.5%, $P = 0.005$) and there was no difference in 5-year survival rate between patients with PBD and those without PBD (32.4% vs. 36.4%, $P = 0.344$) (Zhang et al. 2018). Meanwhile, there are many studies for the optimal method for the PBD, however, outcomes varied according to the studies. In Japan, trend for the PBD in patients with perihilar cholangiocarcinoma has changed from percutaneous transhepatic biliary drainage (PTBD) to endoscopic biliary drainage (EBD) for the risk of peritoneal dissemination along the tract of the PTBD catheter and shorter postoperative survival (Komaya et al. 2017). In this study, 5-year survival rate of PTBD patients was shorter than that of EBD (37.0% vs. 44.3%, $P = 0.019$) and PTBD was associated with seeding metastasis (HR 2.18, 95% CI 1.26–3.77, $P = 0.005$). Therefore, they recommended EBD as the initial preoperative procedure for the biliary drainage. However, the above-mentioned study conducted in Korea (Lee et al. 2018) showed that complication rate after EBD was higher than after PTBD in patients with periampullary cancers (HR 1.927, 95% CI 1.452–2.556, $P < 0.001$). Moreover, in a recently published meta-analysis, EBD was associated with higher overall procedure-related morbidity (OR 2.23, 95% CI 1.39–3.57) including pancreatitis and cholangitis, and similar postoperative morbidity and mortality (Al Mahjoub et al. 2017). The above-mentioned multicenter study in the United States also demonstrated comparable long-term oncologic outcome including disease-specific survival (43.7 vs. 36.9 months, $P = 0.802$) and relapse-free survival (26.7 vs. 24.0 months, $P = 0.571$) between PTBD and EBD with no difference in the site of tumor recurrence ($P = 0.669$) (Zhang et al. 2018). Further research is required to evaluate and verify the clear indication for the PBD and which method of PBD is best. Moreover, weighing the pros and cons, surgeons should choose the best method for an individual patient considering the circumstance of the institution and the proficiency of the interventionists.

In conclusion, although jaundice in patients with GBC indicates locally advanced disease, surgeons should not simply exclude these patients from surgical indication. Patients should be evaluated and selected cautiously for the surgical indication, then managed with preoperative management in centers with hepatobiliary–pancreatic specialists. In a small subset of patients, radical resection can be performed and long-term survival can be achieved.

References

Chapter References

Ebata T, Yokoyama Y, Igami T, Sugawara G, Takahashi Y, Nagino M. Portal vein embolization before extended hepatectomy for biliary cancer: current technique and review of 494 consecutive embolizations. Dig Surg. 2012;29(1):23–9. https://doi.org/10.1159/000335718. Epub 2012 Mar 15.

Kamiya S, Nagino M, Kanazawa H, Komatsu S, Mayumi T, Takagi K, Asahara T, Nomoto K, Tanaka R, Nimura Y. The value of bile replacement during external biliary drainage: an analysis of intestinal permeability, integrity, and microflora. Ann Surg. 2004;239(4):510–7.

Tsui TY, Heumann A, Vashist YK, Izbicki JR. How we do it: double in situ split for staged mesohepatectomy in patients with advanced gall bladder cancer and marginal future liver remnant. Langenbecks Arch Surg. 2016;401(4):565–71. https://doi.org/10.1007/s00423-016-1410-7. Epub 2016 Mar 30.

Yokoyama Y, Nishio H, Ebata T, Igami T, Sugawara G, Nagino M. Value of indocyanine green clearance of the future liver remnant in predicting outcome after resection for biliary cancer. Br J Surg. 2010;97(8):1260–8. https://doi.org/10.1002/bjs.7084.

References for Commentary Notes

Al Mahjoub A, Menahem B, Fohlen A, et al. Preoperative biliary drainage in patients with resectable perihilar cholangiocarcinoma: is percutaneous transhepatic biliary drainage safer and more effective than endoscopic biliary drainage? A meta-analysis. J Vasc Interv Radiol. 2017;28(4): 576–82. https://doi.org/10.1016/j.jvir.2016.12.1218. Review.

Hawkins WG, et al. Jaundice predicts advanced disease and early mortality in patients with gallbladder cancer. Ann Surg Oncol. 2004;11(3):310–5.

Komaya K, Ebata T, Yokoyama Y, et al. Verification of the oncologic inferiority of percutaneous biliary drainage to endoscopic drainage: a propensity score matching analysis of resectable perihilar cholangiocarcinoma. Surgery. 2017;161(2):394–404. https://doi.org/10.1016/j.surg.2016.08.008. Epub 2016 Oct 4.

Lee H, et al. Preoperative biliary drainage adversely affects surgical outcomes in periampullary cancer: a retrospective and propensity score-matched analysis. J Hepatobiliary Pancreat Sci. 2018;25(3):206–13. https://doi.org/10.1002/jhbp.529. Epub 2018 Jan 21.

Zhang XF, Beal EW, Merath K, et al. Oncologic effects of preoperative biliary drainage in resectable hilar cholangiocarcinoma: percutaneous biliary drainage has no adverse effects on survival. J Surg Oncol. 2018;117(6):1267–77. https://doi.org/10.1002/jso.24945. Epub 2017 Dec 4.

Epidemiology of Gall Bladder Cancer

3

Vinay K. Kapoor

Gall bladder cancer (GBC) is a relatively rare (overall age-adjusted incidence being about 2–3 per 100,000 per year Shaffer 2008), yet the most common (more common than cholangiocarcinoma which, for some reasons, has received much more attention) biliary tract cancer (BTC) worldwide. According to the International Classification of Diseases (ICD) 10th Revision, GBC is ranked as 20th in incidence and 17th in mortality worldwide. Prevalence of GBC has peculiar geographic and ethnic/racial distribution with wide variations in the incidence rates in different areas of the globe and various ethnic/racial groups.

3.1 Incidence Variations

3.1.1 Geographic Variations

GBC is a "non-Western" disease. Incidence rates of GBC are low (<1 per 100,000 per year in women) in the Western developed world including North America (United States and Canada), United Kingdom and western Europe, and the Pacific (Australia and New Zealand), reported incidences being United States 1.8, Canada 2.1, United Kingdom 1.1, Denmark 1.4, and Norway 0.9. On the other hand, high incidence rates have been reported from certain geographical pockets, e.g., central and South America CSA (Bolivia, Chile (Fig. 3.1), Colombia and Ecuador), Eastern Europe (Czech Republic, Germany, Hungary (Fig. 3.2), Poland, and Slovakia), east Asia (Japan (Fig. 3.3), Korea (Fig. 3.4), China (Fig. 3.5), and India. Data from WHO's cancer mortality database revealed that age-standardized death rates from GBC in women vary from as low as 0.8 deaths per 100,000 population in South Africa to as high as 21.2 in Chile (Torre et al. 2018). A descriptive epidemiological study (1965–1989) from 25 European countries showed highest mortality rates (3.9 in men and 7.4 in women) in Hungary followed by Austria, Czechoslovakia, and Poland (Zatonskí et al. 1993). Table 3.1 shows some high incidence areas of GBC in the world.

The less-developed regions of the World account for the majority of the global burden of GBC; the highest burden of GBC is in the Western Pacific region (based on the six regions of WHO) or in Asia (based on continents) or in India, Chile, and China (based on countries) (Are et al. 2017). Some areas in Chile and India have "near epidemic" incidence rates of GBC. There is no single factor to explain these peculiarities. These variations *may* have some

Please also see an Invited Commentary on Epidemiology of Gall Bladder Cancer by Jonathan Koea (pp **–**)

V. K. Kapoor (✉)
Department of Surgical Gastroenterology, Sanjay Gandhi Post-Graduate Institute of Medical Sciences (SGPGIMS), Lucknow, Uttar Pradesh, India
e-mail: vkkapoor.india@gmail.com

V. K. Kapoor (ed.), *A Pictorial Treatise on Gall Bladder Cancer*,
https://doi.org/10.1007/978-981-15-5289-2_3

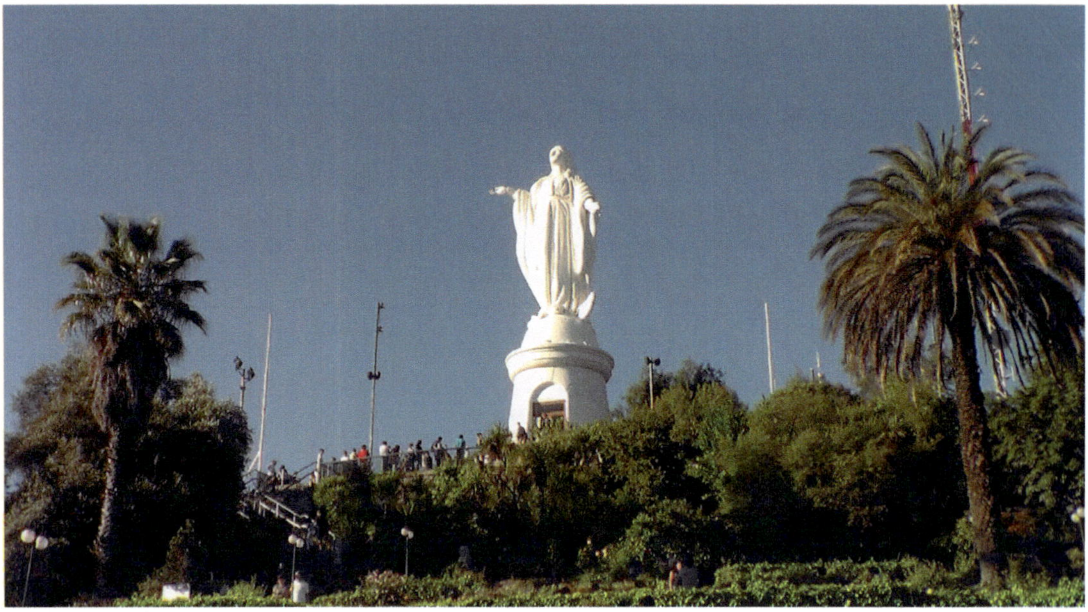

Fig. 3.1 Cerra San Cristobel in Santiago Chile—gall bladder cancer is very common in countries of central and south America (CSA), e.g., Bolivia, Chile, Colombia, and Ecuador

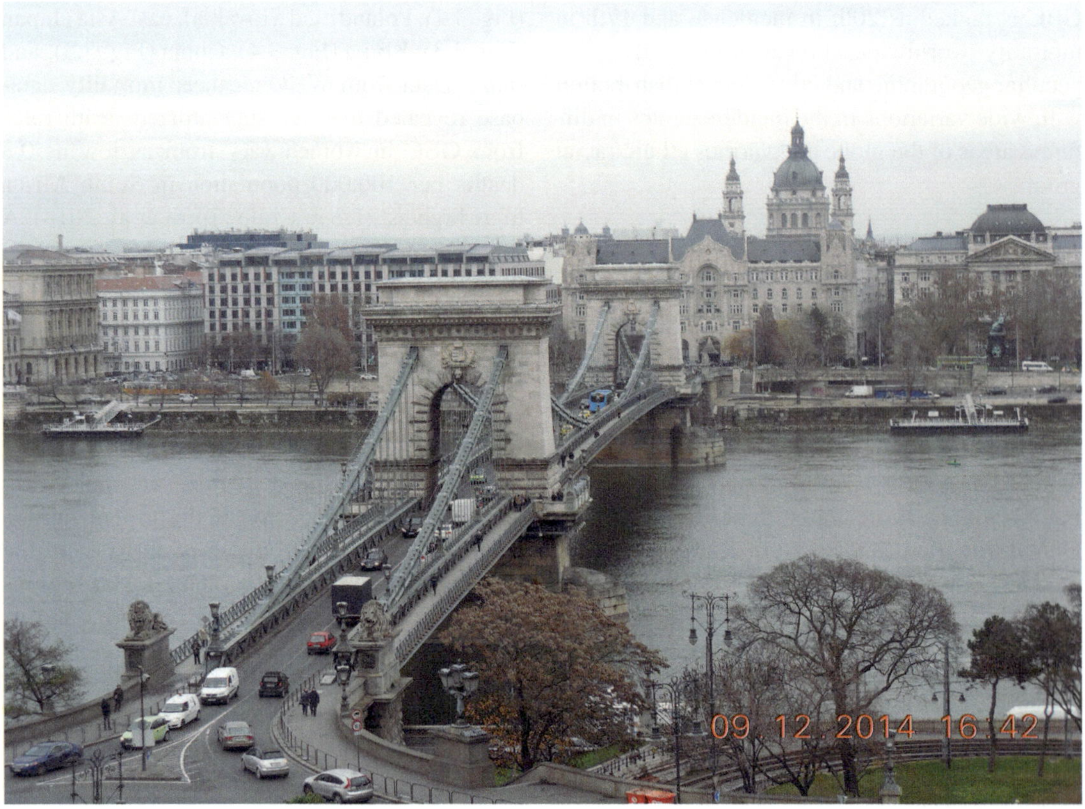

Fig. 3.2 Chain Bridge in Budapest Hungary—gall bladder cancer is common in countries of eastern Europe, e.g., Czech Republic, Germany, Hungary, Poland, and Slovakia

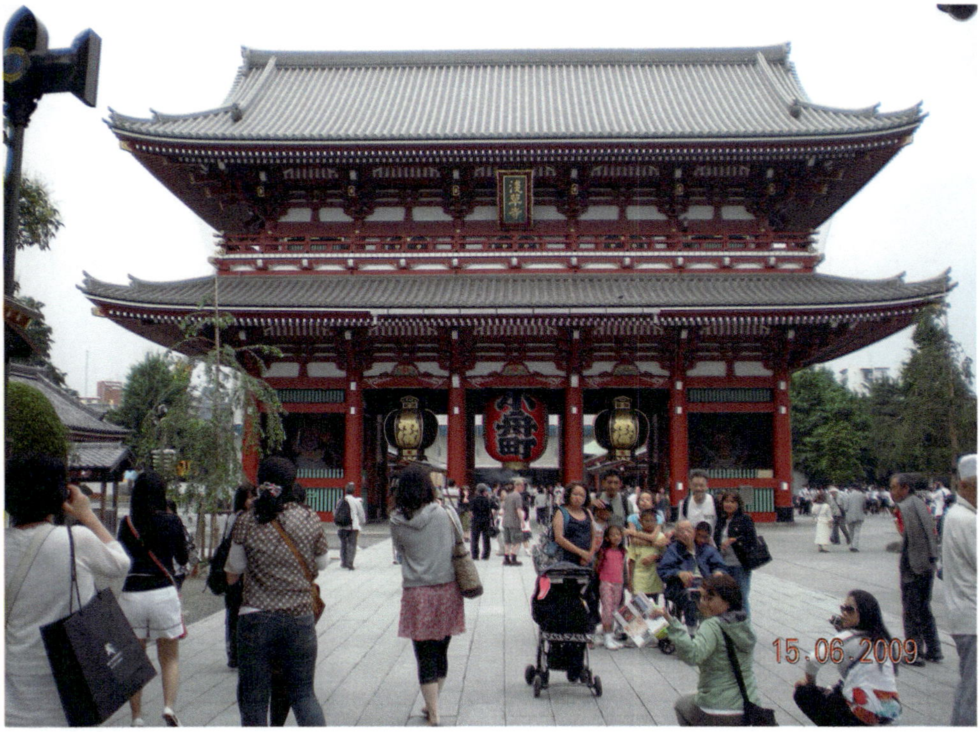

Fig. 3.3 Sensoji temple in Tokyo Japan—gall bladder cancer is common in countries of east Asia, e.g., Japan, Korea, and China

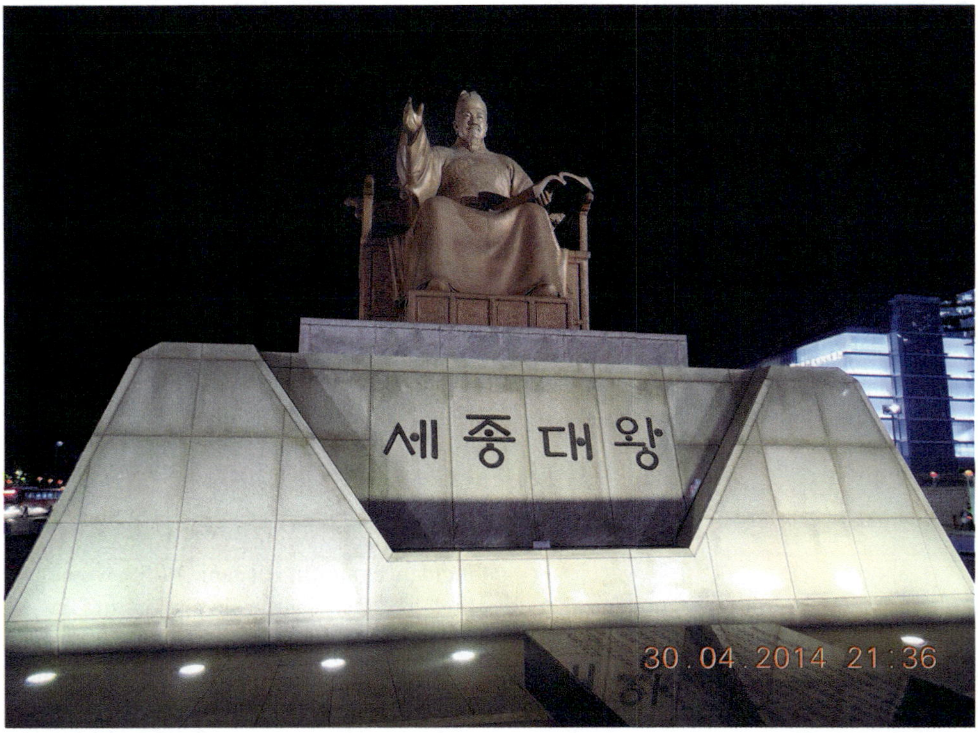

Fig. 3.4 Statue of Sejong the Great in Seoul South Korea—gall bladder cancer is common in countries of east Asia, e.g., Korea, Japan, and China

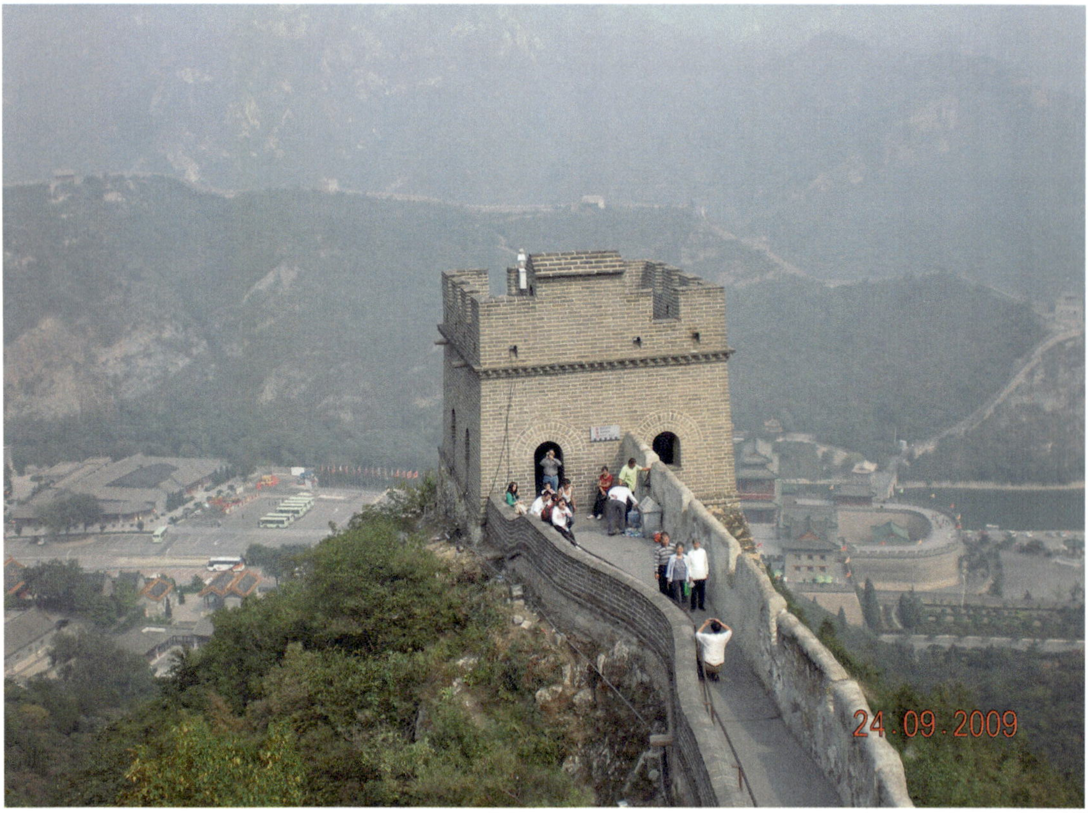

Fig. 3.5 The Great Wall of China—gall bladder cancer is common in countries of east Asia, e.g., China, Japan, and Korea

Table 3.1 Some high (rates per 100,000 per year in women) incidence areas of GBC in the world

Mapuche Indians in Chile (27.3) (Hundal and Shaffer 2014)
Delhi India 21.5, South Karachi Pakistan 13.8, Quito Ecuador 12.9, Native American Indians in New Mexico 8.9 (Randi et al. 2006)
Truji Peru (11.0), Busan Korea (10.5) (Eslick 2010)
Bolivia 14, Busan Korea 10.5, Slovakia 10.2, Lower Silesia Poland 10.2, Czech Republic 10.0, Cali Colombia 9.5, Chile 9.3, Nagasaki Japan 7.6, Thailand 7.4, Nepal 6.7, Montevideo Uruguay 6.2, Shanghai China 5.5, Bangladesh 5.1 (Incidence in five continents Arroyo 7.)
Korea 3 (Wi et al. 2018)

links to the human migration from central Asia to South Asia and to the Americas through the Bering Strait during the last glacial era (Carey and Paigen 2002).

3.1.2 Ethnic Variations

GBC shows wide variations in its incidence rates in various ethnic groups, even within the same country. GBC is very common in the Native American (Fig. 3.6) people of North, Central, and South Americas. In the United States, incidence rate of GBC is three times higher in Native American Indians, Mexican Americans and Hispanic Americans (Morris et al. 1978; Wiggins et al. 1993), Asia Pacific Islanders, and Alaska Natives including Inuits (3.3 vs. 1.0 Lemrow et al. 2008; 2.3 vs. 0.6 Alberts et al. 2012) versus non-Hispanic Whites (NHW) and Blacks. The incidence rates in Hispanic White women were as high as 8.2 in California and 5.4 in New Mexico in the United States (Randi et al. 2006). The incidence rates of GBC were 4.1 in men and 8.1 in women in Native American Indians versus 1.1 and 2.1 in Hispanics and 0.8% and 1.0% in NHW

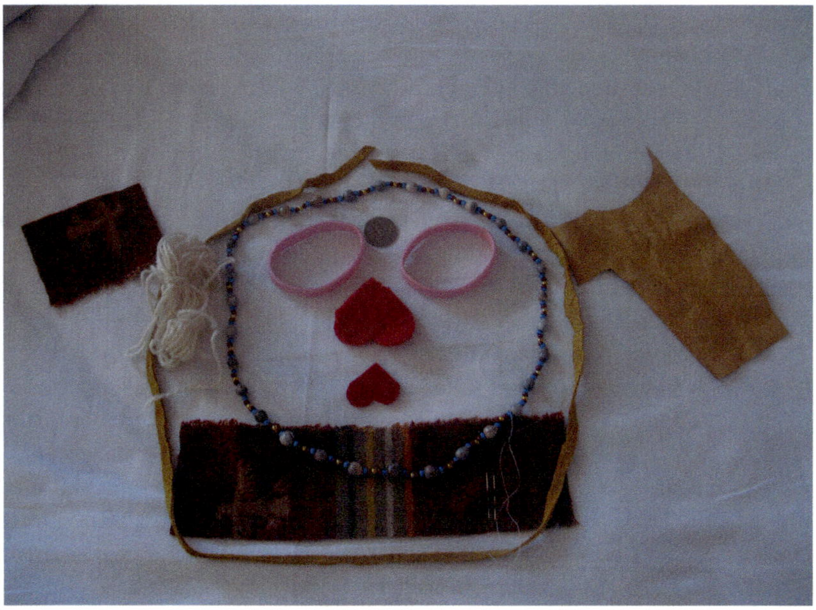

Fig. 3.6 Native American giveaways. (Image Courtesy Carol June Strickland, PhD, RN. Associate Professor, University of Washington School of Nursing, Seattle WA USA—a member of the Cherokee Nation)

in New Mexico (Nir et al. 2012). Incidence and death rates were three times higher in American Indians and Alaska Natives than NHW (Henley et al. 2015). Age-adjusted incidence of GBC was 6.5, 2.2, and 1.0 per 100,000 in Native American, Hispanic, and Caucasian women, respectively in New Mexico (Nemunaitis et al. 2018). An analysis of 7769 cases found in 18 registries of the Surveillance, Epidemiology, and End Results (SEER) program of the National Cancer Institute (NCI) (2001–2012) revealed three times higher incidence rates in Hispanics than in NHW (Jaruvongvanich et al. 2019). In Canada, the First Nations women had higher incidence of GBC than non-aboriginal women (Mazereeuw et al. 2018). An international collaborative study (1969–1988) of cancer in circumpolar Inuits in Alaska, Canada, Greenland, and Russia showed 3255 cancers in about 85,000–110,000 people—excess risk of GBC was seen as compared to the non-Inuit population (Nielsen et al. 1996). In Chile, a high incidence area for GBC, Mapuche ancestry was found to be associated with even higher risk of GBC (Lorenzo Bermejo et al. 2017; Villanueva 2016). The New Zealand Cancer Registry registered 608 GBCs between 1980 and 1997—age-standardized incidence rate (ASIR) in Maoris was higher (1.49 in men and 1.59 in women) than in New Zealanders (0.41 in men and 0.74 in women) (Koea et al. 2002). A retrospective cohort study utilizing an online database in Waitemata District Health Board in New Zealand (2002–2003) found that the age-standardized incidence rate (ASIR) of GBC was 0.6 per 100,000 per year. ASIR in Maoris was higher (males 0.96 vs. 0.21, females 1.37 vs. 0.76) as compared to the overall ASIR (Lilic et al. 2015). In Israel, women born in Europe have higher incidence of GBC than those born in Asia or Africa (Hart et al. 1971).

3.2 GBC in Various Countries

3.2.1 GBC in Chile

Central and South America (CSA), specifically Chile, has one of the highest incidence rates of GBC in the world. Data from 48 population-based cancer registries in 13 countries in CSA revealed that Chile had the highest incidence and mortality rates from GBC in CSA (17.1 and 12.9 in women and 7.3 and 6.0 in men) (Izarzugaza et al. 2016). Age-adjusted rate of incidence (ARI) was 9.7 new cases for every 100,000 inhabitants each year in Chile and 8.1 in Bolivia; age-adjusted rate of mortality (ARM) was 7.8 in Chile and 7.5 in Bolivia (Villanueva 2016). Biliary tract cancer BTC (incidence 17.2) is the third commonest (following breast 43.2 and skin 19.2) cancer in women in Chile (Villanueva 2016). Even within Chile, there are geographical variations; GBC is more common in the South—the highest rates (incidence 28.5) were reported in women in Los Lagos and Los Rios (Southern Chile) (Villanueva 2016). Chilean Mapuche Indian women have one of the highest incidence rates of GBC in the Andean populations in South America. In Chile, GBC is the leading cause of cancer death, exceeding even breast and cervix, among women. WHO Cancer Mortality Database (2009–2013) from 50 countries showed 21 deaths per 100,000 in women and 9 deaths per 100,000 in men in Chile to be due to GBC. In 2000, GBC was the third most common (following stomach and lungs) cause of cancer death in men; in 2013, it became the sixth (following stomach, lung, colo-rectal, prostate, and breast). In women, GBC was the second most common (following stomach) cause of cancer death in 2000; in 2013, it became the fourth (following stomach, lungs, and breast) (Torre et al. 2018). Because of the very high incidence rates of GBC in females in Bolivia (21.0), Chile (11.7), and Peru (6.0) (Miranda-Filho et al. 2020). GBC has become an important public health problem in Chile (Salazar et al. 2019).

3.2.2 GBC in the United States

GBC is uncommon in the United States; 11,420 new cases of and 3710 deaths due to BTC (including GBC and cholangiocarcinoma) were reported in the United States in 2016 cf. 1.3 million new cases of and 700,000 deaths due to colorectal cancer (CRC) in 2012 (American Cancer Society website). GBC is the fifth most common (following colon, pancreas, stomach, and esophagus) GI tract cancer in the United States. Estimated incidence of GBC is about 2 per 100,000 population per year. In the National Cancer Database (NCDB), which captures approximately 75% of all newly diagnosed cancer cases, 15,131 new cases of GBC were registered in the United States during 1989–1996 (Fong et al. 2006).

3.2.3 GBC in India

India with a population of about 1.2 billion has about 1.5 million new cancer cases every year. Five most common cancers in India are breast, cervix, oral cavity, lung, and colorectal. GBC accounts for about 26,000 new cases (with 25,000 deaths) of cancer in India every year (Cancer incidence and mortality worldwide). It is estimated that India contributes to more than 10% of the global GBC burden (Dutta et al. 2019). GBC is an "Indian Disease"—common in south Asian Indians and Native American Indians (Kapoor and McMichael 2003).

GBC was earlier (Bartlett 2000), and is still in many texts and publications, reported to be rare in India. This was based on data from Mumbai (earlier called Bombay) in West India—the only data available earlier. There are, however, wide geographical variations in the incidence rates of GBC within India itself. Data from 23 population-based cancer registries (PBCR) of the Indian Council of Medical Research (ICMR), which cover about 7% (20% of urban but only 1% of rural population) of 1.2 billion population of India, has shown that there is great geographical variation in the incidence rates of GBC even within India, incidence rates in Delhi in northern India being almost ten times higher than those in Chennai (earlier called Madras) in southern India. In northern India, GBC is the fourth most common (after breast, cervix, and ovary) cancer and the commonest GI cancer in women. GBC is the commonest cause of surgical obstructive jaundice in north India (Sikora et al. 1994). GBC accounted for 6% of all cancer cases in Delhi in 2012 (Malhotra et al. 2017). In an interesting case–control study of 1170 GBC cases and 2525 controls, cases more often reported current residence in the high incidence Northern (56%) and Northeast (34%) regions—residence in low incidence South

India (0.3%) was reported by the least number of cases. The odds ratio (OR) of developing GBC was 4.82 (3.87–5.99) in those reporting birth in a high-risk region versus those born in a low-risk region. This risk was more in women (6.04, 4.52–8.07) than in men (3.17; 2.23–4.50). This risk increased with the increasing duration of residence in a high-risk region. Those who were born in a high-risk region continued to remain susceptible to develop GBC even after migration from the high-risk region to a low-risk region (OR 1.36, 1.02–1.82) (Mhatre et al. 2016).

There is a huge divide between north and south India as far as the incidence rates of GBC are concerned (Behari and Kapoor 2010). Ganges (called Ganga in Hindi) is one of the major rivers in north India originating in the Himalayas and draining in the Bay of Bengal. GBC has been described in some reports as a cancer of the Gangetic belt or the Indo-Gangetic basin, i.e., states of Uttarakhand, Uttar Pradesh (Fig. 3.7), Bihar (Fig. 3.8), and Bengal (Gupta et al. 2016; Madhawi et al. 2018) but even other countries in south Asia, e.g., Pakistan, Nepal (Fig. 3.9), and Bangladesh and many other states of India, e.g., Jammu & Kashmir, Himachal Pradesh, Chandigarh, Punjab, Haryana, Rajasthan, Delhi, and the northeastern states, all areas outside the Gangetic belt or the Indo-Gangetic basin, have also reported high incidence rates of GBC.

In Pakistani women, GBC was the fourth most common GI cancer (Atique et al. 2008); in another report, it was the second commonest GI cancer in Pakistani women (Alvi et al. 2011). The incidence rate of GBC in women in South Karachi Pakistan is as high as 13.8. In Nepal, GBC is the sixth commonest overall and the second most common GI cancer (Tamrakar et al. 2016). In Bangladesh, GBC was the second most common (following stomach) primary source of liver metastases (Rahman et al. 2013). GBC is, therefore, common in the entire north Indian subcontinent.

The Author (VKK), for these reasons, does not believe in the Gangetic belt or the Indo-Gangetic basin theory of high incidence of GBC in north India.

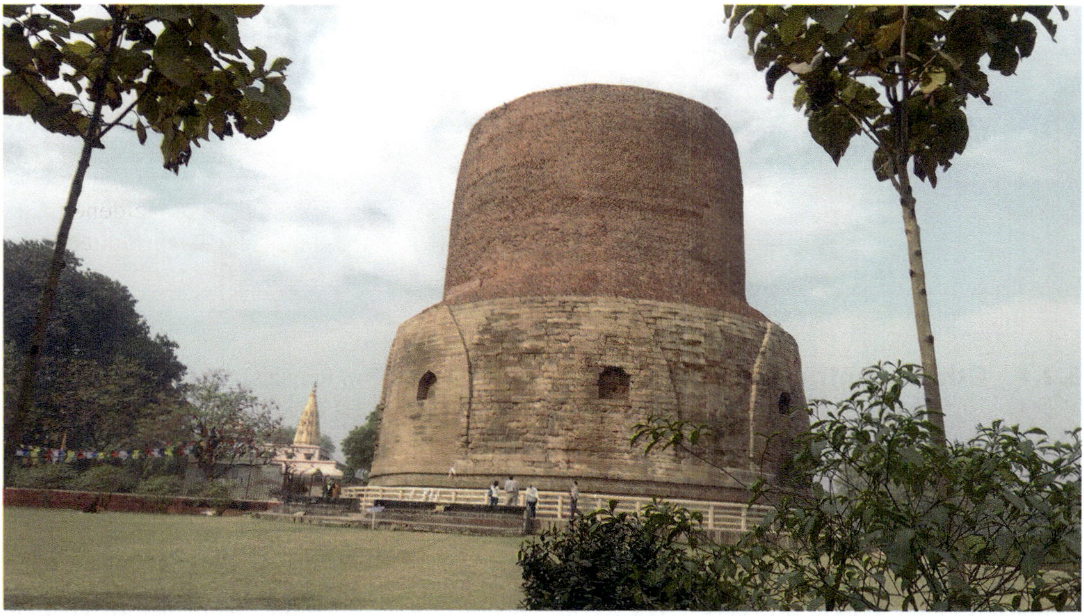

Fig. 3.7 Dhamekh Stupa at Sarnath Varanasi in Uttar Pradesh in north India—gall bladder cancer is very common in north and east India

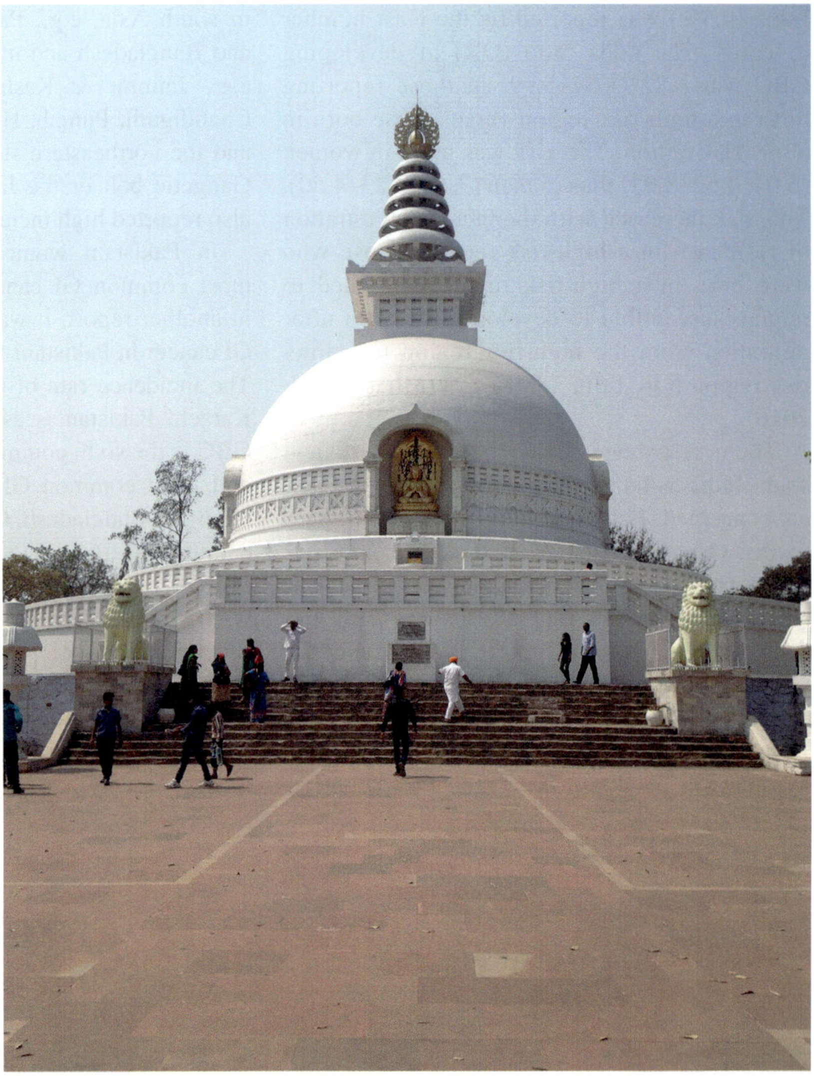

Fig. 3.8 Buddha Stupa at Rajgir Bihar in north India—gall bladder cancer is very common in north and east India

3.2.4 Other Countries

The incidence rates of GBC were 6.3 in 2006 and 5.2 per 1,000,000 in 2015 in South Korea (Kim et al. 2019). GBC was one of the cancers with expected years of life lost >10 years in both men and women in Taiwan (Wu et al. 2018). The National Central Cancer Registry (NCCR) in China collects data from 339 cancer registries covering a population of 288 million. Crude incidence rate of GBC in 2014 was 3.82 (3.59 in males and 4.05 in females); ASIR was 2.37. GBC accounted for 1.4% of all new cancer cases in China (Tuo et al. 2018).

Migrant studies provide good evidence to elucidate genetic and environmental factors in the etiopathogenesis of a cancer. GBC is common even in Indians settled abroad, e.g., Fiji, Kuwait, and Singapore. Incidence of GBC in Indian women in Fiji was 4.3 versus 0.5 in Fijians. Similarly, incidence of GBC in non-Kuwaitis (most of whom are Indians) in Kuwait

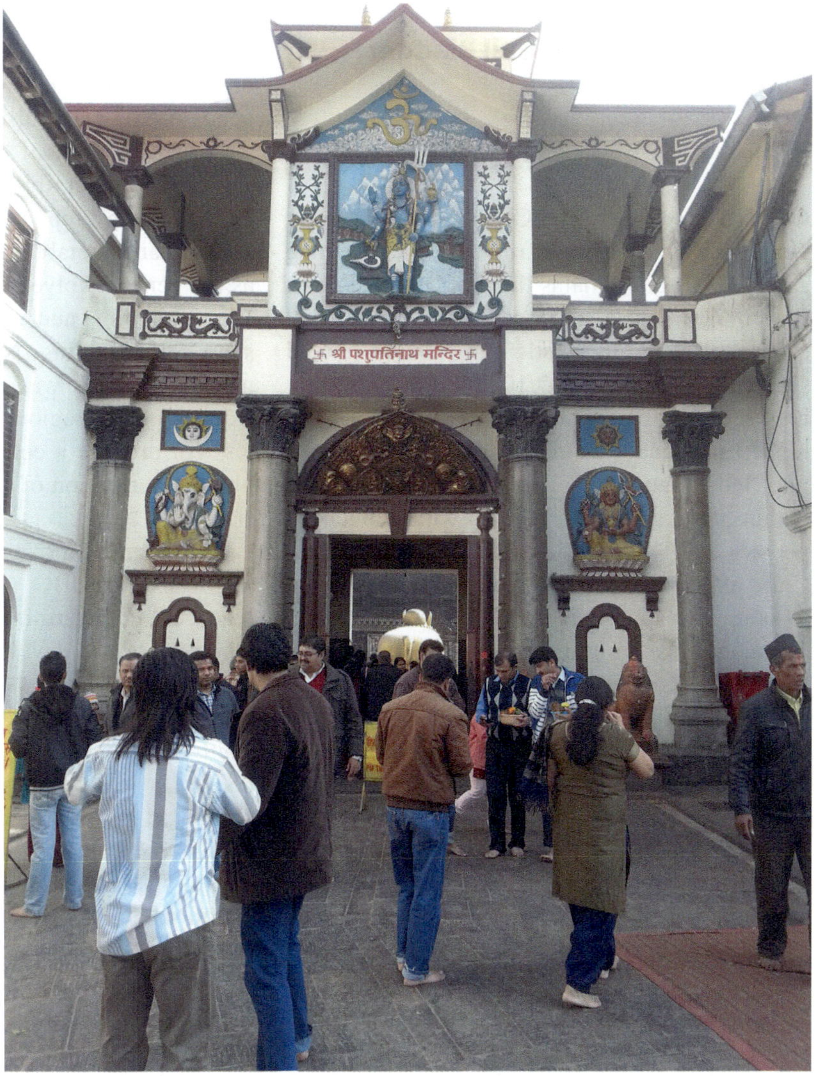

Fig. 3.9 Pashupatinath Temple in Kathmandu Nepal—gall bladder cancer is very common in countries of the Indian subcontinent, e.g., Nepal, India, Pakistan, and Bangladesh

was 3.4 versus 1.8 in Kuwaitis. In Singapore, Indian women had the highest (2.0) incidence rates as compared to Chinese (0.9) and Malay (0.7) women (Parkin 1986). In the Swedish family cancer database, among the first-generation immigrants, women from India and Chile had an increased risk of GBC (Hemminki and Li 2003). Indians in United Kingdom had higher (males 3.4, 2.4–4.7, females 6.6, 5.1–8.5) risk of mortality from GBC versus native UK-born population (Swerdlow et al. 1995). All cancer standardized mortality ratio (SMR) for GBC in South Asian women in the United Kingdom was 3.3 for Indians, 4.3 for Pakistanis, and 8.3 for Bangladeshis (Mangtani et al. 2010). Age-standardized rate per 100,000 person-years of GBC in south Asian women in England was 2.0 (Indian 1.5, Pakistani 3.0, and Bangladeshi 2.9) vs. Whites 0.9 (Ali et al. 2013). In the New South Wales (NSW) Central Cancer Registry in Australia (1972–1990) overall ASIR of GBC was lower but Asian (Indian and Sri Lankan) immigrants, especially women had a higher (2.9 vs. 0.5) incidence rate of GBC (Grulich et al. 1995). Incidence rates were 5.9 (much higher than those in native white people) in Korean men in Los Angeles USA (Eslick 2010).

India, unfortunately, qualifies to be called the 'GBC capital' of the world.

Invited Commentary on Epidemiology of Gall Bladder Cancer

Jonathan Koea

Gallbladder cancer (GBC) is a rare cancer worldwide (global standardized incidence rate 2.3/100,000) but remains the world's most common biliary cancer and one of the most lethal cancers affecting the world's population (global standardized death rate 1.7/100,000). Significantly it is a cancer of the developing world and the highest incidences are recorded in Korea, China, Lao, India, and Chile. There is further variation within these, and other, regions with indigenous peoples and Hispanics in the United States and Chile affected disproportionately in comparison to other ethnicities. In India, GBC is far more common in the north than the south of the country and in all regions women are more likely to develop the disease than males. Importantly, territories with the highest incidence of GBC have the highest mortality rates (Mahdavifar et al. 2018).

The observed geographical and ethnic variations remain largely unexplained. However, the presence of untreated, symptomatic cholelithiasis for at least two decades, recurrent or chronic gallbladder infections with *Salmonella* and other bacteria (*Helicobacter pylori*), porcelain gallbladder and gallbladder polyps are regarded as strong risk factors for the development of cancer. Similarly, the presence of an anomalous pancreaticobiliary duct junction, estrogen exposure, carcinogen exposure (heavy metals, radiation, vinyl chloride), pregnancy, adenomyomatosis, polyposis coli, Mirizzi syndrome, tobacco usage, and obesity are regarded as weak or moderate risk factors. Diets with emphasis on fruits and green vegetables appear to have a protective effect (Mahdavifar et al. 2018; Sharma et al. 2017).

Numerous contemporary investigations have attempted to define the genetic profile of GBC. A large multinational investigation showed that no single gene was mutated in all GBCs but mutations in BAP1, ARID1A, and PBRM1 were most common. Other investigators have demonstrated mutations in the TP53 and c-erb-B2 genes in late-stage disease (Jiao et al. 2013). A worldwide review of potential candidate genes for GBC susceptibility showed mutations in DNA pathway repair genes, hormonal, inflammatory, and metabolic pathway genes, as well as for genes involved in the apoptosis pathway, Wnt signaling, nuclear receptor synthesis, and stem cell signaling. No single gene or combination of genes was representative of tumors from any given region, making it unlikely genetics will provide a cohesive explanation for the global distribution of GBC (Sharma et al. 2017; Jiao et al. 2013).

However, while a genetic determinant for the cause of GBC may be currently out of reach, social determinants are not. GBC is most common in the developing world. Low socioeconomic status and untreated gallstones are independent risk factors for early onset and death from GBC. Low socioeconomic status results in low health literacy and reduces the ability to access medical and surgical care. Employment options are also limited, often to hazardous occupations, tobacco use is high, and healthy dietary options are not readily available (Dutta et al. 2005). Consequently, GBC could be regarded as a "bell weather" condition for any territory, its incidence and mortality reflecting the socioeconomic status and healthcare available to the affected communities. The presence of global outposts of high GBC incidence and mortality should be a stimulus for a concerted effort to assist these affected communities to raise their standard of living, ensure that healthcare services are available to provide prompt and effective care for gallstone-related conditions as well as gallbladder polyps and porcelain gallbladder, ensure that workplaces and home environments are safe and that exposure to carcinogens is eliminated. The worldwide incidence and mortality from GBC would then almost certainly decline.

References

Chapter References

ACS. www.cancer.org.

Alberts SR, Kelly JJ, Ashokkumar R, Lanier AP. Occurrence of pancreatic, biliary tract, and gallbladder cancers in Alaska Native people, 1973–2007. Int J Circumpolar Health. 2012;71:17521. https://doi.org/10.3402/IJCH.v71i0.17521.

Ali R, Barnes I, Cairns BJ, Finlayson AE, Bhala N, Mallath M, Beral V. Incidence of gastrointestinal cancers by ethnic group in England, 2001–2007. Gut. 2013;62(12):1692–703. https://doi.org/10.1136/gutjnl-2012-303000. Epub 2012 Oct 23.

Alvi AR, Siddiqui NA, Zafar H. Risk factors of gallbladder cancer in Karachi-a case-control study. World J Surg Oncol. 2011;9(9):164. https://doi.org/10.1186/1477-7819-9-164.

Are et al. Cancer incidence in five continents. 2017. http://ci5.iarc.fr/.

Are C, Ahmad H, Ravipati A, Croo D, Clarey D, Smith L, Price RR, Butte JM, Gupta S, Chaturvedi A, Chowdhury S. Global epidemiological trends and variations in the burden of gallbladder cancer. J Surg Oncol. 2017;115(5):580–90. https://doi.org/10.1002/jso.24546. Epub 2017 Jan 30

Atique M, Leghari MJ, Amin MS, Parveen S, Mushahid N, Ullah Khan MA. Cancer data analysis in the pathology department, combined military hospital, Multan, Pakistan 2002–2007. Asian Pac J Cancer Prev. 2008;9(4):679–81.

Bartlett DL. Gallbladder cancer. Semin Surg Oncol. 2000;19(2):145–55. Review

Behari A, Kapoor VK. Does gallbladder cancer divide India? Indian J Gastroenterol. 2010;29(1):3–7. https://doi.org/10.1007/s12664-010-0008-1.

Cancer incidence and mortality worldwide Arroyo 1. globocan.iarc.fr.

Cancer incidence in five continents. http://ci5.iarc.fr/.

Carey MC, Paigen B. Epidemiology of the American Indians' burden and its likely genetic origins. Hepatology. 2002;36(4 Pt 1):781–91. https://doi.org/10.1053/jhep.2002.36545.

Dutta U, Bush N, Kalsi D, Popli P, Kapoor VK. Epidemiology of gallbladder cancer in India. Chin Clin Oncol. 2019;8(4):33. https://doi.org/10.21037/cco.2019.08.03.

Eslick GD. Epidemiology of gallbladder cancer. Gastroenterol Clin N Am. 2010;39(2):307–30. https://doi.org/10.1016/j.gtc.2010.02.011.

Fong Y, Wagman L, Gonen M, Crawford J, Reed W, Swanson R, Pan C, Ritchey J, Stewart A, Choti M. Evidence-based gallbladder cancer staging: changing cancer staging by analysis of data from the National Cancer Database. Ann Surg. 2006;243(6):767–71; discussion 771–4.

Grulich AE, McCredie M, Coates M. Cancer incidence in Asian migrants to New South Wales, Australia. Br J Cancer. 1995;71(2):400–8.

Gupta S, Kori C, Kumar V, Misra S, Akhtar N. Epidemiological study of gallbladder cancer patients from north Indian Gangetic planes—a high-volume centre's experience. J Gastrointest Cancer. 2016;47(1):27–35. https://doi.org/10.1007/s12029-015-9781-5.

Hart J, Modan B, Shani M. Cholelithiasis in the aetiology of gallbladder neoplasms. Lancet. 1971;1(7710):1151–3.

Hemminki K, Li X. Familial liver and gall bladder cancer: a nationwide epidemiological study from Sweden. Gut. 2003;52(4):592–6.

Henley SJ, Weir HK, Jim MA, Watson M, Richardson LC. Gallbladder cancer incidence and mortality, United States 1999–2011. Cancer Epidemiol Biomark Prev. 2015;24(9):1319–26. https://doi.org/10.1158/1055-9965.EPI-15-0199. Epub 2015 Jun 12

Hundal R, Shaffer EA. Gallbladder cancer: epidemiology and outcome. Clin Epidemiol. 2014;6:99–109.

Incidence in five continents Arroyo 7. iarc.fr/en/publications/pdfs-online/epi/sp160/Cancer.

Izarzugaza MI, Fernández L, Forman D, Sierra MS. Burden of gallbladder cancer in Central and South America. Cancer Epidemiol. 2016;44(Suppl 1):S82–9. https://doi.org/10.1016/j.canep.2016.07.021.

Jaruvongvanich V, Yang JD, Peeraphatdit T, Roberts LR. The incidence rates and survival of gallbladder cancer in the USA. Eur J Cancer Prev. 2019;28(1):1–9. https://doi.org/10.1097/CEJ.0000000000000402.

Kapoor VK, McMichael AJ. Gallbladder cancer: an 'Indian' disease. Natl Med J India. 2003;16(4):209–13.

Kim BW, Oh CM, Choi HY, Park JW, Cho H, Ki M. Incidence and overall survival of biliary tract cancers in South Korea from 2006 to 2015: using the National Health Information Database. Gut Liver. 2019;13(1):104–13. https://doi.org/10.5009/gnl18105.

Koea J, Phillips A, Lawes C, Rodgers M, Windsor J, McCall J. Gall bladder cancer, extrahepatic bile duct cancer and ampullary carcinoma in New Zealand: demographics, pathology and survival. ANZ J Surg. 2002;72(12):857–61.

Lemrow SM, Perdue DG, Stewart SL, Richardson LC, Jim MA, French HT, et al. Gallbladder cancer incidence among American Indians and Alaska natives, US, 1999–2004. Cancer. 2008;113(5 Suppl):1266–73. https://doi.org/10.1002/cncr.23737.

Lilic N, Addison B, Hammodat H. Gallbladder carcinoma: a New Zealand centre's 10-year experience with presentation, ethnic diversity and survival rate. ANZ J Surg. 2015;85(4):260–3. https://doi.org/10.1111/ans.12503. Epub 2014 Jan 20.

Lorenzo Bermejo J, Boekstegers F, González Silos R, Marcelain K, Baez Benavides P, Barahona Ponce C, Müller B, Ferreccio C, Koshiol J, Fischer C, Peil B, Sinsheimer J, Fuentes Guajardo M, Barajas O, Gonzalez-Jose R, Bedoya G, Cátira Bortolini M, Canizales-Quinteros S, Gallo C, Ruiz Linares A, Rothhammer F. Subtypes of Native American ancestry and leading causes of death: Mapuche ancestry-specific associations with gallbladder cancer risk in Chile. PLoS Genet. 2017;13(5):e1006756. https://doi.org/10.1371/journal.pgen.1006756. eCollection 2017 May.

Madhawi R, Pandey A, Raj S, Mandal M, Devi S, Sinha PK, Singh RK. Geographical pattern of carcinoma gallbladder in Bihar and its association with river Ganges and arsenic levels: retrospective individual consecutive patient data from Regional Cancer Centre. South Asian J Cancer. 2018;7(3):167–70. https://doi.org/10.4103/sajc.sajc_37_18.

Malhotra RK, Manoharan N, Shukla NK, Rath GK. Gallbladder cancer incidence in Delhi urban: a 25-year trend analysis. Indian J Cancer. 2017;54(4):673–7. https://doi.org/10.4103/ijc.IJC_393_17.

Mangtani P, Maringe C, Rachet B, Coleman MP, dos Santos Silva I. Cancer mortality in ethnic South Asian migrants in England and Wales (1993–2003): patterns in the overall population and in first and subsequent generations. Br J Cancer. 2010;102(9):1438–43. https://doi.org/10.1038/sj.bjc.6605645.

Mazereeuw MV, Withrow DR, Diane Nishri E, Tjepkema M, Marrett LD. Cancer incidence among First Nations adults in Canada: follow-up of the 1991 Census Mortality Cohort (1992–2009). Can J Public Health. 2018;109(5–6):700–9. https://doi.org/10.17269/s41997-018-0091-0. Epub 2018 Jun 28

Mhatre SS, Nagrani RT, Budukh A, Chiplunkar S, Badwe R, Patil P, et al. Place of birth and risk of gallbladder cancer in India. Indian J Cancer. 2016;53(2):304–8.

Miranda-Filho A, Piñeros M, Ferreccio C, et al. Gallbladder and extrahepatic bile duct cancers in the Americas: incidence and mortality patterns and trends. Int J Cancer. 2020;147(4):978–89. https://doi.org/10.1002/ijc.32863.

Morris DL, Buechley RW, Key CR, Morgan MV. Gallbladder disease and gallbladder cancer among American Indians in tricultural New Mexico. Cancer. 1978;42(5):2472–7.

Nemunaitis JM, Brown-Glabeman U, Soares H, Belmonte J, Liem B, Nir I, Phuoc V, Gullapalli RR. Gallbladder cancer: review of a rare orphan gastrointestinal cancer with a focus on populations of New Mexico. BMC Cancer. 2018;18(1):665. https://doi.org/10.1186/s12885-018-4575-3. Review

Nielsen NH, Storm HH, Gaudette LA, Lanier AP. Cancer in Circumpolar Inuit 1969–1988. A summary. Acta Oncol. 1996;35(5):621–8.

Nir I, Wiggins CL, Morris K, Rajput A. Diversification and trends in biliary tree cancer among the three major ethnic groups in the state of New Mexico. Am J Surg. 2012;203(3):361–5. https://doi.org/10.1016/j.amjsurg.2011.12.002.

Parkin DM. Cancer occurrence in developing countries. IARC Scientific Publications No. 75. Lyon: IARC; 1986.

PBCR. https://icmr.nic.in/sites/default/files/reports/Preliminary_Pages_web.pdf.

Rahman MA, Barua R, Azad AK, Ahmed DS, Raihan MA. Demographic and clinical evaluation of secondaries to liver. Mymensingh Med J. 2013;22(1):131–5.

Randi G, Franceschi S, La Vecchia C. Gallbladder cancer worldwide: geographical distribution and risk factors. Int J Cancer. 2006;118(7):1591–602. Review

Salazar M, Ituarte C, Abriata MG, Santoro F, Arroyo G. Gallbladder cancer in South America: epidemiology and prevention. Chin Clin Oncol. 2019;8(4):32. https://doi.org/10.21037/cco.2019.07.12. Epub 2019 Aug 12.

Shaffer EA. Gallbladder cancer: the basics. Gastroenterol Hepatol (NY). 2008;4(10):737–41.

Sikora SS, Kapoor R, Pradeep R, Kapoor VK, Saxena R, Kaushik SP. Palliative surgical treatment of malignant obstructive jaundice. Eur J Surg Oncol. 1994;20(5):580–4.

Swerdlow AJ, Marmot MG, Grulich AE, Head J. Cancer mortality in Indian and British ethnic immigrants from the Indian subcontinent to England and Wales. Br J Cancer. 1995;72(5):1312–9.

Tamrakar D, Paudel I, Adhikary S, Rauniyar B, Pokharel P. Risk factors for gallbladder cancer in Nepal a case control study. Asian Pac J Cancer Prev. 2016;17(7):3447–53.

Torre LA, Siegel RL, Islami F, Bray F, Jemal A. Worldwide burden of and trends in mortality from gallbladder and other biliary tract cancers. Clin Gastroenterol Hepatol. 2018;16(3):427–37. https://doi.org/10.1016/j.cgh.2017.08.017. Epub 2017 Aug 18.

Tuo JY, Zhang M, Zheng RS, Zhang SW, Li GC, Yang NN, Chen WQ. [Report of incidence and mortality of gallbladder cancer in China, 2014]. Zhonghua Zhong Liu Za Zhi. 2018;40(12):894–899. doi: https://doi.org/10.3760/cma.j.issn.0253-3766.2018.12.004. Chinese.

Villanueva L. Cancer of the gallbladder-Chilean statistics. Ecancermedicalscience. 2016;10:704. https://doi.org/10.3332/ecancer.2016.704. eCollection 2016. Review

Wi Y, Woo H, Won YJ, Jang JY, Shin A. Trends in gallbladder cancer incidence and survival in Korea. Cancer Res Treat. 2018;50(4):1444–51. https://doi.org/10.4143/crt.2017.279. Epub 2018 Jan 24.

Wiggins CL, Becker TM, Key CR, Samet JM. Cancer mortality among New Mexico's Hispanics, American Indians, and non-Hispanic Whites, 1958–1987. J Natl Cancer Inst. 1993;85(20):1670–8.

Wu TY, Chung CH, Lin CN, Hwang JS, Wang JD. Lifetime risks, loss of life expectancy, and health care expenditures for 19 types of cancer in Taiwan. Clin Epidemiol. 2018;10:581–91. https://doi.org/10.2147/CLEP.S155601. eCollection 2018.

Zatonskí W, La Vecchia C, Levi F, Negri E, Lucchini F. Descriptive epidemiology of gall-bladder cancer in Europe. J Cancer Res Clin Oncol. 1993;119(3):165–71.

References for Commentary Notes

Dutta U, Nagi B, Garg PK, Sinha SK, Singh K, Tandon RK. Patients with gallstones develop cancer at an earlier age. Eur J Cancer Prev. 2005;14(4):381–5.

Jiao Y, Pawlik T, Anders RA, Selaru FM, Streppel MM, Lucas DJ, et al. Exome sequencing identifies frequent inactivating mutations in BAP1, ARID1A and PBRM1 in intrahepatic cholangiocarcinomas. Nat Genet. 2013;45:1470–5. https://doi.org/10.1038/ng.2813.

Mahdavifar N, Mohammadian M, Salehiniya H. Gallbladder cancer in the world: epidemiology, incidence, mortality and risk factors. World Cancer Res J. 2018;5(3):e1124–31.

Sharma A, Sharma KL, Gupta A, Yadav A, Kumar A. Gallbladder cancer epidemiology, pathogenesis and molecular genetics: recent update. World J Gastroenterol. 2017;23(22):3978–98. https://doi.org/10.3748/wjg.v23.i22.3978. Review

4 Etiology and Pathogenesis of Gall Bladder Cancer

Vinay K. Kapoor

4.1 Etiology

Etiology of gall bladder cancer (GBC) is not well understood. This is partly because it is an uncommon cancer (overall global incidence being about 2–3 per 100,000 per year) but mainly because it is uncommon in the Western developed world. Very little evidence is available regarding the etiology of GBC and that too is in the form of small size and poor quality cohort studies and case–control studies, and even these studies lack well-matched controls.

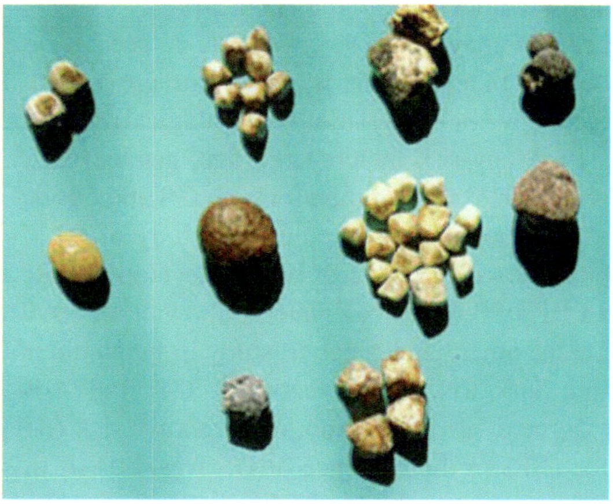

Fig. 4.1 Gallstones are the most important risk factor for gall bladder cancer

4.1.1 Gall Stones

Gallstones (GS) (Fig. 4.1) are the strongest risk factor for the causation of GBC—there is a strong association between the presence of GS and GBC. There are striking similarities between and parallels in the epidemiology of gall stone disease (GSD) and GBC. Incidence rates of GBC parallel the prevalence rates of GS all over the world—areas and populations with high prevalence rates of GS reporting higher incidence rates of GBC, e.g., Native Americans having high prevalence of GS reporting very high incidence rates of GBC, and areas and populations with low prevalence rates of GS reporting lower incidence rates of GBC, e.g., Norway having low prevalence of GSD reporting very low incidence rate (0.2–0.4 per 100,000 per year) of GBC. In Chile, which has one of the highest incidence rates of GBC in the world—40–50% of adult females and 20–30% of adult males in Chile have GS and these prevalence rates are even higher in Mapuche Indians in whom GBC is even more common. GBC is very common in the Native American Indians—a survey of 3296 American Indians

Please also see an Invited Commentary on Etiology and Pathogenesis of Gall Bladder Cancer by Jean Michel Butte (pp **–**)

V. K. Kapoor (✉)
Department of Surgical Gastroenterology, Sanjay Gandhi Post-Graduate Institute of Medical Sciences (SGPGIMS), Lucknow, Uttar Pradesh, India
e-mail: vkkapoor.india@gmail.com

V. K. Kapoor (ed.), *A Pictorial Treatise on Gall Bladder Cancer*,
https://doi.org/10.1007/978-981-15-5289-2_4

revealed that 64% of women and 30% men had either symptoms of GS or a history of cholecystectomy (Everhart et al. 2002).

The prevalence of GS shows large variations within India. The prevalence of GS in women in north India is very high. Symptomatic GSD was much more common in north (quinquennial 1960–1964 incidence being 91.6 per 100,000 per year), northeast (24.4) and east (17.3) than in west (9.5), south (5.4), and central (4.1) India (Malhotra 1968); these rates parallel the incidence rates of GBC in various parts of India as the incidence rates are about ten times higher in north than in south India.

This may, however, be just a coincidence because of a common risk factor or there may be a facultative or even causative (etiological) relationship. Many risk factors, e.g., age, gender, parity, obesity, etc. are common for both GS and GBC.

In a population-based cohort study of 60,176 patients with GS (42 of whom developed GBC) an RR of 3.6 was calculated (Chow et al. 1999). On the other hand, a cohort study in Japan did not find any association between GS and GBC (Yagyu et al. 2004). Summary relative risk (RR) for GBC in the presence of GS was 4.9—it was 2.2 in cohort studies and 7.1 in case–control studies (Randi et al. 2006). As many as 80 of 368 cases of GBC reported from China had GS—the odds ratio (OR) for developing GBC in patients with GS versus those without GS was as high as 24 (Hsing et al. 2007a). Risk of GBC due to GS varies between different races/ethnic groups—Native Americans with GS have 21 times higher risk of developing GBC than those without GS (Lowenfels et al. 1985).

On the other hand, while about 10–15% of the adult population has GS, only a very small proportion (0.3–3.0%) of patients with GS will go on to develop GBC over 20 years (Randi et al. 2006). Also, GBC is uncommon in many areas and populations where GS are common and even in high GBC incidence areas, a significant number of patients with GBC do not have associated GS. GS are present in majority of patients with GBC, but this association varies from region to region—95% of patients with GBC reported from Chile (Roa et al. 1999), 60–70% of patients with GBC reported from India, 55% of GBCs reported from China (Yang et al. 2014), and 50–60% of patients with GBC reported from Japan and Korea have GS, i.e., a significant number of patients with GBC do not have GS. The relationship between GS and GBC remains a mystery. It is presumed that other risk factors act together to increase the risk of GBC in the presence of GS which acts as a promoter in the pathogenesis of GBC.

Size of the stones is also important—there is about ten times higher risk of developing GBC with large (>3 cm) (Fig. 4.2) versus small (<1 cm) GS (Diehl 1983; Lowenfels et al. 1989). Another study, however, did not find any correlation between GS size and the risk of GBC (Moerman et al. 1993). GB packed with stones, i.e., high GS/GB volume ratio also carries higher risk of having GBC (Vitetta et al. 2000). GS weight was more (4.9 g vs. 2.8 g) in GBC than in chronic cholecystitis (CC) in a study from China (Hsing et al. 2007a). In another study, GS weight (9.6 g vs. 6.0 g), number (21 vs. 14), and volume (11.7 ml vs. 6.5 ml) were higher in GBC than in CC. GS volumes of 6, 8, and 10 mL were associated with 5, 7, and 11 times the relative risk (RR) of GBC (Roa et al. 2006b).

Age of GS (which is not the same as the duration of symptoms of GS) and which, in any case, is difficult to know may also be a risk factor. In a case–control study of 228 persons from Chile, 15% of GBC cases had a longer history of GSD

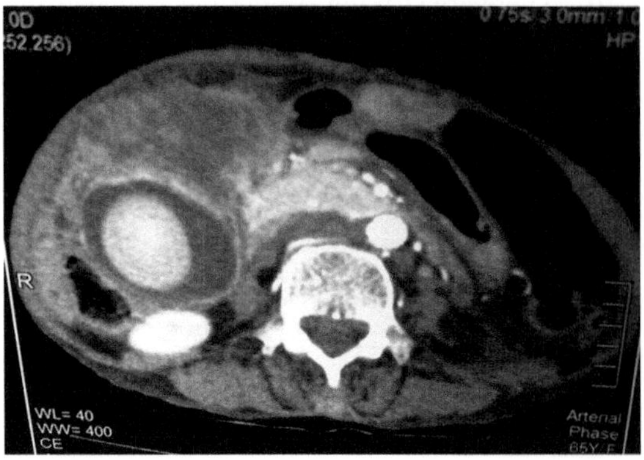

Fig. 4.2 There is some very soft evidence that large (>3 cm) gallstones may be associated with a higher risk of gall bladder cancer

compared to only 4% in controls (OR 11, 1.4–85.2) (Serra et al. 2002). GS are not only more common but form at a much younger age in north Indians, especially women; in a population-based ultrasonography (US) study in Kashmir in north India, the prevalence of GS in women was 9.6% but it was as high as 29% in the age group 51–60 years; even in young women in the age group 21–30 years, it was 5% (Khuroo et al. 1989). The longer duration of exposure of the GB to GS may be one of the factors responsible for very high incidence of GBC in north Indian women. Higher incidence rates of GBC have been reported in low socioeconomic and education groups; this may be because of delay in cholecystectomy for GS thus resulting in longer exposure of the GB to GS (Serra et al. 2002).

GS are common in the West but GBC is uncommon. The type of GS viz. pure cholesterol or cholesterol solitaire (cholesterol contributing to >90% of the dry weight of the stone), cholesterol predominant (cholesterol contributing to 50–90% of the dry weight of the stone), mixed (cholesterol contributing to <50% of the dry weight of the stone), or pigment (calcium bilirubinate; cholesterol contributing to <5% of the dry weight of the stone) stone, is also important. More than 80% of GS in north India, where incidence rates of GBC are very high, are cholesterol predominant stones (Choudhuri et al. 1995), whereas majority (>60%) of GS in south India, where incidence rates of GBC are low, are pigment stones (Fig. 4.3) and only 5% of GS are cholesterol stones (Jayanthi et al. 1998). In China also, patients with GBC were found to have cholesterol stones more frequently than pigment stones (Hsing et al. 2007a). Using NMR spectroscopy, we found some differences in the chemical composition of GS in patients with GBC versus those without GBC (Srivastava et al. 2008; Jayalakshmi et al. 2009).

Clinical picture related to GS is also important. As many as one-third of incidental GBCs, diagnosed for the first time on histopathological examination of a grossly normal GB removed for GSD, were detected in patients who presented with acute cholecystitis (Fig. 4.4); a clinical diagnosis of empyema (Fig. 4.5) is a significant risk factor for the diagnosis of incidental GBC (Lohsiriwat et al. 2009). Mirizzi syndrome, a large GS in the GB neck causing extrinsic compression of the common bile duct (CBD) or a fistula between the GB and the CBD (Fig. 4.6), carries a higher risk of GBC—unsuspected GBC was found more frequently (5/18, 28%) in patients with Mirizzi syndrome than in those

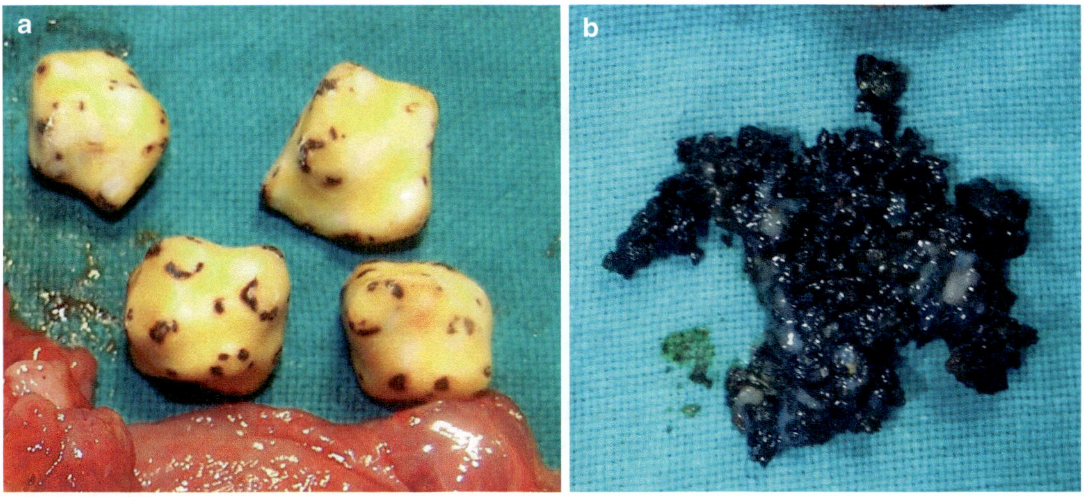

Fig. 4.3 The type of gallstones, whether cholesterol solitaire; mixed stones; and black pigment stones, is also important from the point of view of etiopathogenesis of gallbladder cancer; majority of stones in north India where GBC is very common are cholesterol predominant mixed stones (**a**), whereas majority of stones in south India where GBC is not common are pigment stones (**b**)

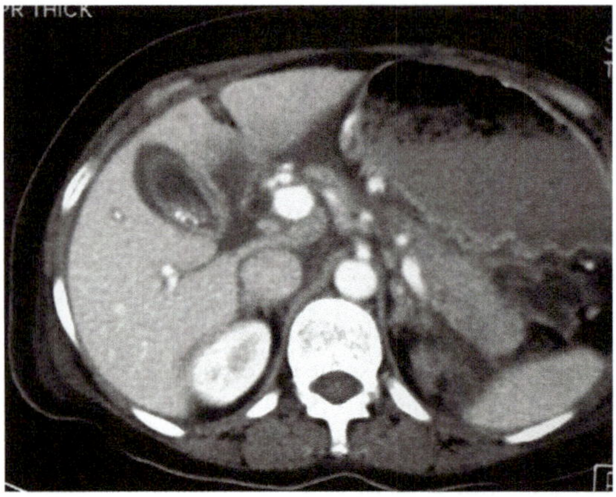

Fig. 4.4 CT showing pericholecystic fluid suggestive of acute cholecystitis—incidental gallbladder cancer is more likely to be found in patients presenting clinically with acute cholecystitis

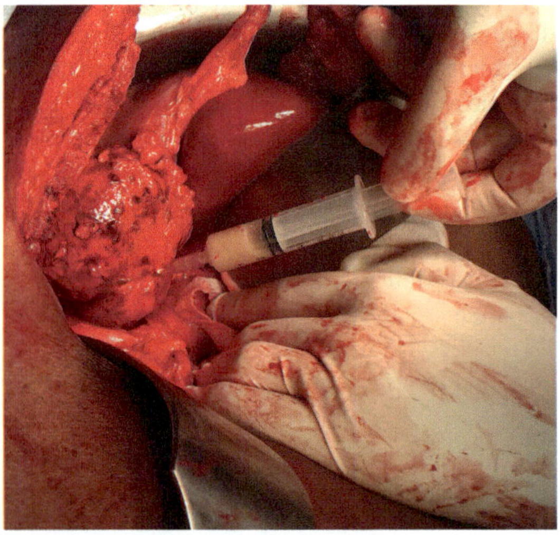

Fig. 4.5 Tense distended gallbladder which on aspiration revealed pus—empyema; a clinical diagnosis of empyema is a significant risk factor for the histopathological diagnosis to turn out to be (incidental) GBC

with GS only (36/175, 2%) (Redaelli et al. 1997). Eight (5%) out of 169 patients with Mirizzi syndrome reported by us had GBC (Kumar et al. 2016b). Xantho-granulomatous cholecystitis (XGC) (Fig. 4.7) is a variant of long-standing CC caused by GS with destructive inflammation. It is seen as diffuse thick-walled GB (TWGB), with submucosal hypoechoic/hypoattenuated nodules

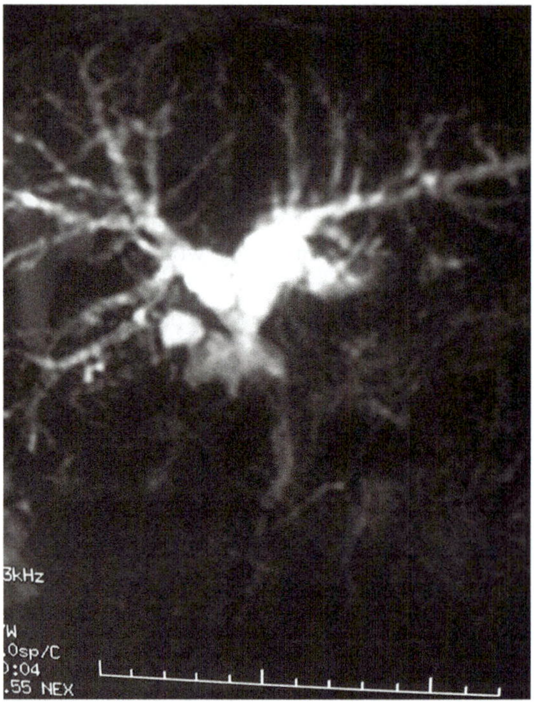

Fig. 4.6 MRC showing a large gallbladder neck stone eroding through a cholecysto-choledochal fistula into the common bile duct—Mirizzi's syndrome; unsuspected gallbladder cancer is more likely to be found at operation in patients presenting with Mirizzi's syndrome

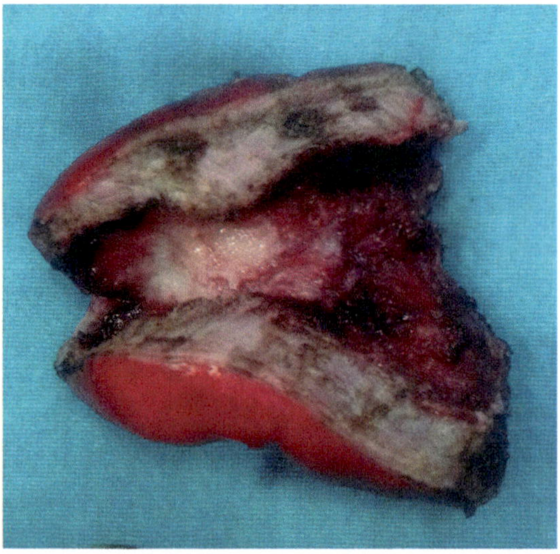

Fig. 4.7 Diffuse thickening of the gallbladder wall—xantho-granulomatous cholecystitis (XGC); XGC carries a higher risk of gallbladder cancer and the two may coexist

in the thick GB wall, GB mass with infiltration of adjacent organs and lymphadenopathy and mimics GBC on imaging and even at operation—XGC also carries a higher risk of GBC and the two (XGC and GBC) may coexist (Rao et al. 2005). Porcelain GB (Fig. 4.8) is intramural calcification of the GB wall—it indicates end-stage GB disease and is a manifestation of long-standing chronic inflammation of the GB wall with GS being present in 95% of cases. GB wall becomes bluish in hue and brittle in consistency. There is conflicting evidence about cancer risk in porcelain GB—earlier porcelain GB was thought to carry a high risk of GBC but the current evidence is in favor of the fact that the risk is low. None of the 13 porcelain GBs found in 1200 cholecystectomies had GBC (Khan et al. 2011). In a systemic review of 60,665 cholecystectomies, 0.2% had porcelain GB and only 15% of those with porcelain GB had GBC (Brown and Geller 2011). Selective focal punctate stippled mucosal versus diffuse dense transmural calcification is more frequently associated with GBC (Stephen and Berger 2001). In a review of the topic, Machado (2016) recommended selective preventive cholecystectomy for porcelain GB and warned that the nonoperative approach may require prolonged (even life-long) follow-up. Cholecysto-enteric (-duodenal or -colonic) fistula (Fig. 4.9) also increases the risk of GBC in a GB with GS. In an interesting analysis, GB length >9.5 cm in women older than 55 years was associated with a five times higher risk of GBC (Roa et al. 2014). All these clinical presentations are, in fact, manifestations of long-standing GSD and probably increase the risk of GBC as a result of the increased duration of exposure of the GB to GS.

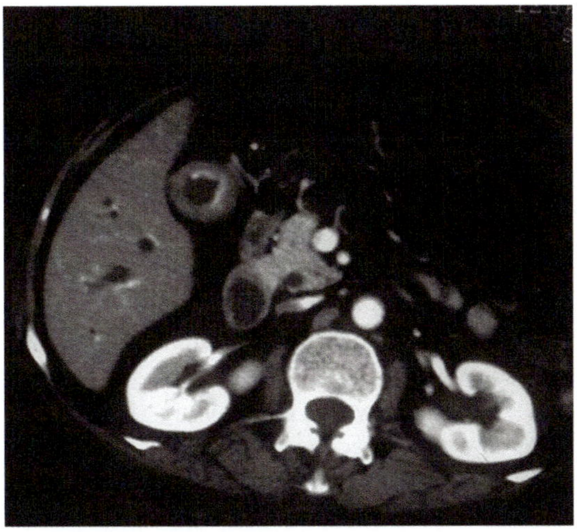

Fig. 4.8 CT showing porcelain gallbladder; focal punctate calcification in the gallbladder mucosa has a higher risk of gallbladder cancer

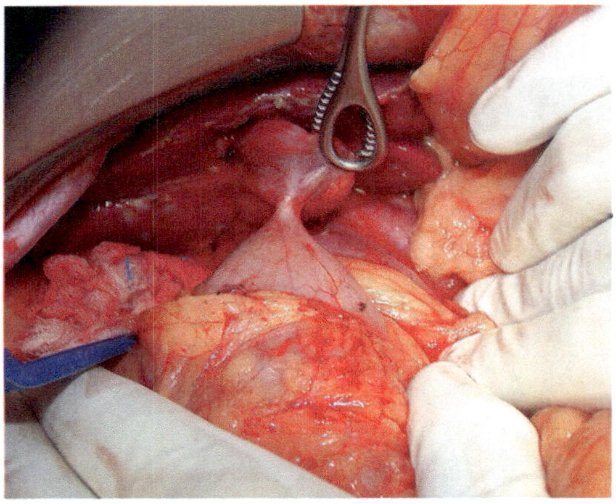

Fig. 4.9 Cholecysto-duodenal fistula increases the risk of gallbladder cancer

4.1.2 Age

GBC is a disease of the elderly with the incidence increasing with age in both sexes but cases are reported even in young patients (Fig. 4.10). GBC occurs at a younger age in the high-risk groups, e.g., American Indians and Hispanics than in the low-risk groups, e.g., in Whites and Blacks, in the same population (United States). Patients with GS develop GBC at a younger (6 years) age than those without GS (Dutta et al. 2005). GBC was found in 3.4% of autopsies conducted on patients with GS over 60 years of age (Mlinarić-Vrbica and Vrbica 2009).

4.1.3 Gender

GBC is one of the few non-genital/non-gender bigender cancers (thyroid being another) which is more common in women than in men. There

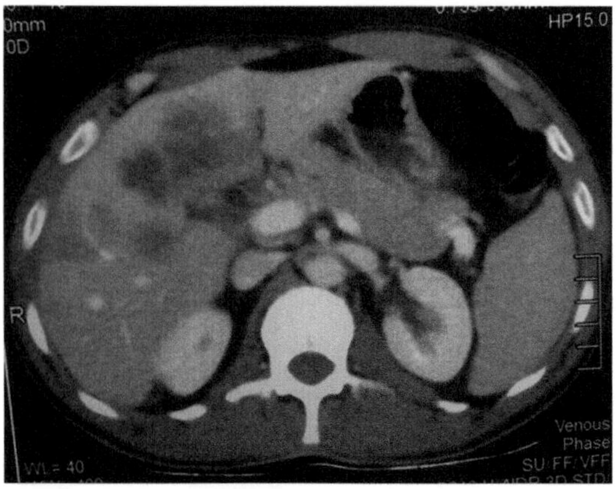

Fig. 4.10 Gallbladder cancer is a disease of elderly but can occur in young patients also; gallbladder cancer with metastasis in a 28-year-old male

is a strong female preponderance with a female to male ratio of 2–3:1 in most areas; but it is as high as 5:1 (age-standardized rate ASR F:M 9.5:1.6) in some high incidence areas, e.g., Chile (Roa et al. 2014). On the other hand, the gender distribution is almost equal in Korea (Central Cancer Registry F 3.9, M 4.4) (Wi et al. 2018), Japan (ASR F:M 7.8:5.5 in Nagasaki and 5.9:4.4 in Osaka), and China. ASR for GBC was lower for females than for males in Korea and Japan (Hori and Saito 2018). A population-based case–control study of 269 GBC, 647 GSD, and 586 healthy controls revealed that older age at menarche, younger age at first pregnancy or childbirth, a higher number of pregnancies or parity, and late age at last birth increase the risk of GBC in women with GS (Andreotti et al. 2010). Irregular and longer menstrual cycles increased the risk of GBC (Makiuchi et al. 2017). All these observations suggest the role of hormonal factors, e.g., estrogen receptors (Saranga Bharathi et al. 2015) and progesterone receptors (Baskaran 2005) in the etiopathogenesis of GBC. Eleven (23%) of 47 patients expressed estrogen/progesterone receptors on IHC; receptor expression correlated with early stages of disease (Saranga Bharathi et al. 2015). On the other hand, no relation has been found with the use of oral contraceptive pills (OCP) or hormone replacement therapy (HRT) with risk of GBC.

GBC in South Asia and South America (both having high prevalence rates of GS) has high F:M ratio and is frequently associated with GS. On the other hand, GBC in East Asia, i.e., Japan, Korea, and China (having low prevalence rates of GS) has near equal F:M ratio and is less frequently associated with GS. This may indicate that GBC in East Asia may be a different disease than the one seen in South Asia or South America.

4.1.4 Family History

Summary relative risk (RR) for GBC with a family history of GS was 3.2 while summary RR with a family history of GBC was 4.8 (Randi et al. 2006). A higher risk of GBC with a family history of GS has been reported from China also (Hsing et al. 2007b). Familial clustering of GBC has been reported (Jackson et al. 2007). Twenty-five out of 229 GBC patients operated at Nagoya between 1977 and 2004 had a second cancer (Nishio et al. 2007). Results from the Biliary Tract Cancers pooling project of the National Cancer Institute (NCI) in USA, however, did not find any relationship between family history of cancer and risk of GBC (Van Dyke et al. 2018).

4.1.5 Lifestyle

Lifestyle factors, e.g., smoking (Aune et al. 2016) have been found to be associated with increased risk of GBC. Higher levels of nicotine were found in GBC tissue in 20 patients (Basu et al. 2012). In a systematic review and meta-analysis including 4676 GBC cases in 11 case control studies and 9 cohort studies, the pooled relative risk (RR) for smoking was 1.33 (1.17–1.51); the risk increased linearly with smoking intensity and duration—it was 1.60 for 30 cigarettes/day and 1.25 for 30 years of smoking (Lugo et al. 2020). Poor socioeconomic and education status (Serra et al. 2002), and poor sanitation, have been shown to be associated with increased risk of GBC. A higher rate of mortality from GBC has been seen in women with the lowest levels of education (Herrera Riquelme et al. 2015).

4.1.6 Diet

High calorie and high carbohydrate diet, higher consumption of red meat, and the use of mustard oil (Tamrakar et al. 2016) are associated with increased risk of GBC. A case–control study of 1170 GBCs and 2525 controls in India revealed that high consumption of mustard oil was associated with GBC risk (Mhatre et al. 2020). Dixit et al. (2013) found higher levels of sanguinarine and diethylnitrosomine, adulterants in mustard oil, in blood and tissue samples in 20 patients with GBC as compared to 20 patients with cholelithiasis. High intake of fiber in the form of green leafy vegetables and fruits and of vitamins (C and E) are protective. Contamination with mutagen aflatoxins (Foerster et al. 2016; Koshiol et al. 2017) in grain-based agriculture and ochratoxins (Ikoma et al. 2015) in red chilli pepper in Chile, Peru, and Bolivia have been incriminated in the etiopathogenesis of GBC. In India, however, we did not find an association between mycotoxin concentration in red chilli pepper and the incidence of GBC (Ikoma et al. 2016).

4.1.7 Obesity

Obesity increases the risk of many cancers including GBC (Avgerinos et al. 2019; Wade et al. 2019). Obesity increases the risk of formation of GS and increases estrogen secretion; fat cells secrete a large amount of inflammatory mediators—all carcinogenic factors. In a case–control study of 4287 cases and 8574 controls, obesity and metabolic syndrome were found to be associated with increased risk of hepatobiliary cancers (Menon and Mathew 2019). A meta-analysis of three case–control studies and eight cohort studies including 3288 GBC cases found a potential relationship between excess body weight (EBW) and risk of GBC—obese women were at a higher (1.35) risk to develop GBC (Larsson and Wolk 2007). The risk of GBC associated with overweight/obesity is more in women 1.59 (1.02–2.47) than in men 1.09 (0.99–1.21). Each 5 kg/m^2 increase in BMI was linearly associated with increased risk of GBC (1.3, 1.1–1.5) (Bhaskaran et al. 2014). Nationwide medical checkup sample cohort data (2002–2015) of 496,390 individuals in South Korea showed disability-adjusted life year (DALY) value attributable to obesity to be 226 per 100,000 in men and 167 per 100,000 in women (Lee et al. 2018). A recent meta-analysis of 14 studies found higher risk (RR 1.78) of GBC in obese (BMI >30) women (Liu et al. 2016).

4.1.8 Diabetes

Type II diabetes is associated with an increased risk of death from any cancer. An increased risk of GBC was observed in 2,186,196 individuals followed from 2002 to 2012 in Israel (Dankner et al. 2016). Asia cohort consortium of 19 prospective population-based cohorts of more than 700,000 persons with diabetes found the hazard ratio (HR) of death from GBC to be 1.33 (Chen et al. 2017).

4.1.9 Anatomical Anomalies

Anomalous pancreaticobiliary ductal union (APBDU) (also called anomalous pancreaticobiliary ductal maljunction APBDJ or pancreaticobiliary maljunction PBM) is a rare anatomic congenital variation in which there is abnormal union of the common bile duct (CBD) and the pancreatic duct outside the duodenal wall with a long (>8 or 10 mm) common channel of the CBD and the pancreatic duct (Fig. 4.11). There is no sphincter in the part of the common channel outside the duodenal wall leading to persistent reflux of the pancreatic juice into the biliary system (including the GB) causing high amylase levels in bile, activation of proteolytic enzymes in the biliary tree, altered composition of bile, damage to the biliary epithelium and inflammation-associated genetic alterations, e.g., k-ras mutation, leading to hyperplasia–metaplasia–dysplasia. APBDU is rare in the West but is common in Japan and Korea. APBDJ has not been reported in patients with GBC in Chile where p53 mutations are seen early in the pathogenesis. PBM with a median

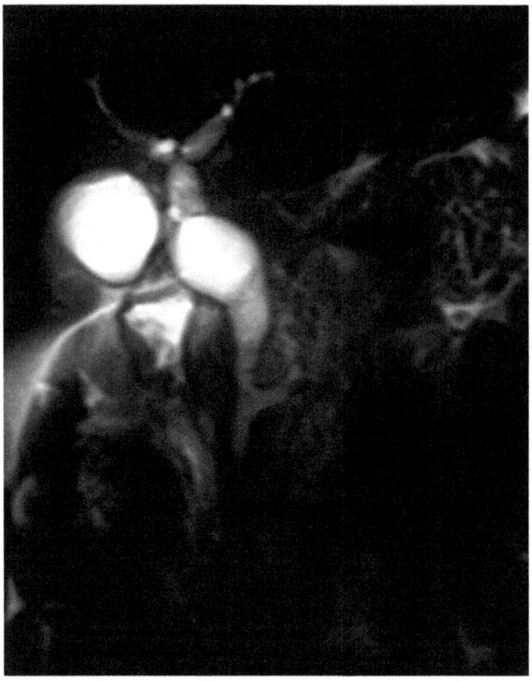

Fig. 4.11 Anomalous pancreaticobiliary ductal union with a long common channel of the common bile duct and the pancreatic duct is associated with a higher risk of gallbladder cancer (note the associated cystic dilatation of the extrahepatic bile duct)

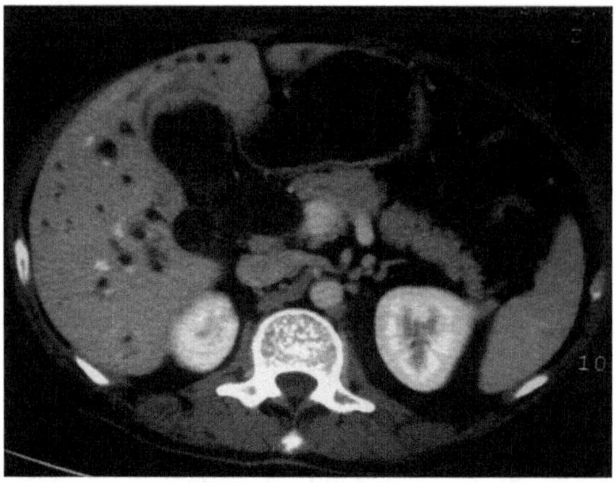

Fig. 4.12 Gallbladder cancer with choledochal cyst; there is disproportionate dilatation of the extrahepatic bile duct as compared to the intrahepatic duct

length of 20 mm (10–23 mm) was identified in 4 (5.5%) out of 73 patients with biliary malignancies in Finland in whom MRC was available (Hyvärinen et al. 2019). APBDJ was thought to be responsible for the causation of GBC in 116 patients in a cohort of 113,394 Japanese people (Yagyu et al. 2004). When looked for (by ERCP, MRCP, or EUS), PBM can be found in 10–20% of patients with GBC. APBDJ was seen in 69 (17%) of 401 patients with GBC who were operated at the Seoul National University Hospital (SNUH) South Korea between 2000 and 2014 (Chang et al. 2016). GBC is the commonest cancer in patients with APBDU, it occurs at a younger age, there is no female gender bias, it is usually not associated with GS and it is associated with papillary tumors which are less invasive and less aggressive; K ras mutations are more common. In a large series of 168 adult patients with PBM in Japan, 87 had associated biliary cancers (including 79 GBC) (Yoshimoto et al. 2019). APBDJ is often associated with a cystic dilatation of the CBD, i.e., choledochal cyst, treatment of which in the form of excision necessitates a cholecystectomy. A choledochal cyst (Fig. 4.12) itself is associated with a higher risk of BTC including GBC. Choledochal cyst was found in 18 (4.5%) of 401 patients with GBC (Chang et al. 2016). Annual follow-up with CA 19-9 is suggested if the patient with choledochal cyst is not operated (Madadi-Sanjani et al. 2019). Preventive cholecystectomy is recommended in patients with APBDJ but without congenital dilatation of the CBD as these patients have a very high risk of GBC.

4.1.10 Biliary Diseases

Adenomyomatosis (Fig. 4.13), a degenerative hyperplasia of the GB mucosal epithelium, especially when it is focal, carries a higher risk of GBC. A single large (>10 mm) sessile polyp in an old (>60 years) person living in a high GBC incidence area may carry a high risk of GBC (see Chap. 5). Primary sclerosing cholangitis (PSC) (Fig. 4.14), a cholestatic liver disease associated with progressive fibro-inflammatory destruction of the bile ducts, carries an increased risk of GBC (and cholangiocarcinoma) (Fung et al. 2019). Annual (or semiannual) surveillance with ultrasonography (US) is recommended to detect a mass lesion in GB—preventive cholecystectomy

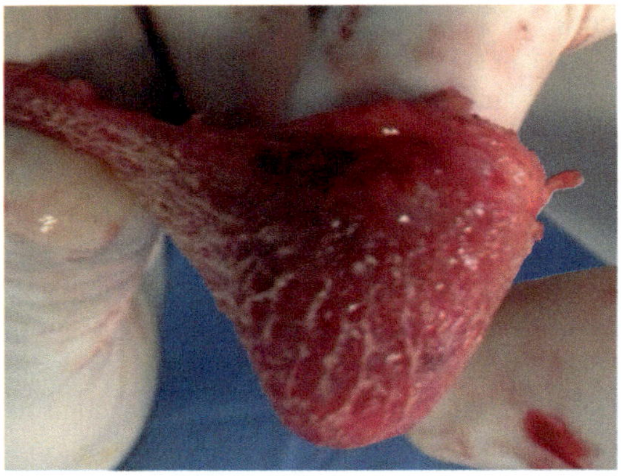

Fig. 4.13 Focal thickening of the gallbladder wall—adenomyomatosis; it may be associated with an increased risk of gallbladder cancer

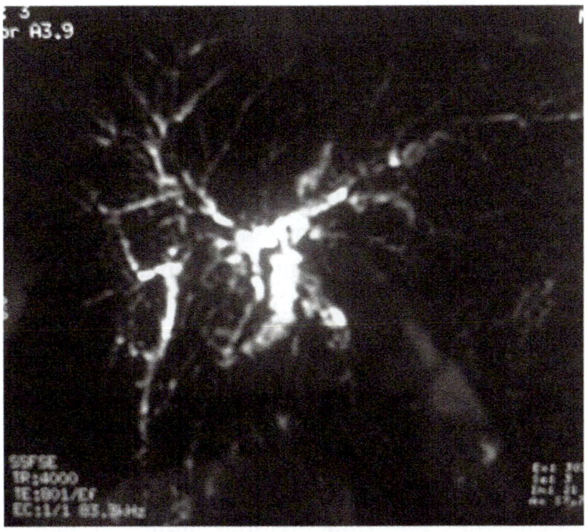

Fig. 4.14 MRC showing diffuse irregularity of the biliary tree with multiple strictures—primary sclerosing cholangitis (PSC) which is associated with an increased risk of biliary tract cancers including gallbladder cancer

should be performed if a mass is seen on US (EASL 2009; Chapman et al. 2010).

4.1.11 Infections

Infection of the bile because of the presence of GS causes degradation of primary bile acids resulting in higher concentrations of secondary bile acids viz. lithocholic and deoxycholic acid, in bile causing chronic irritation and inflammation—leading to mucosal changes of hyperplasia, metaplasia, and dysplasia.

Salmonella typhi bacteria colonize the GB even after the acute infection (enteric fever) has been cured and result in an asymptomatic carrier state. *S. typhi* produces a biofilm which is a key factor in the persistence of chronic infection in the GB. *S. typhi* (and *paratyphi*) carrier state is associated with an increased (six- to eightfold) risk of developing and dying from hepatobiliary cancers (Nagaraja and Eslick 2014). Salmonella carrier state provides inflammatory stimulus in a genetic model of GB carcinogenesis (akin to *Helicobacter pylori* in stomach). Scanu et al. (2015) demonstrated that Salmonella infection promotes carcinogenesis by activation of MAPK and AKT pathways. *S. typhi* produces a toxin which has a carcinogenic potential by inducing DNA damage and causing cell cycle alterations (Di Domenico et al. 2017). In a meta-analysis of >1000 GBC cases, Koshiol et al. (2016) found a summary relative risk (RR) of 4.6 for anti-Vi antibodies. *S. typhi* was found in 11/26 and non-typhoidal salmonella species in 12/26 GBCs (Iyer et al. 2016). Salmonella carrier state is diagnosed by the presence (culture or PCR) of bacteria in bile or Vi antigens in serum.

Helicobacter (Fig. 4.15) is an epsilon proteobacterium which has been categorized as a group I carcinogen by the International Agency for Research on Cancer (IARC) (Segura-López et al.

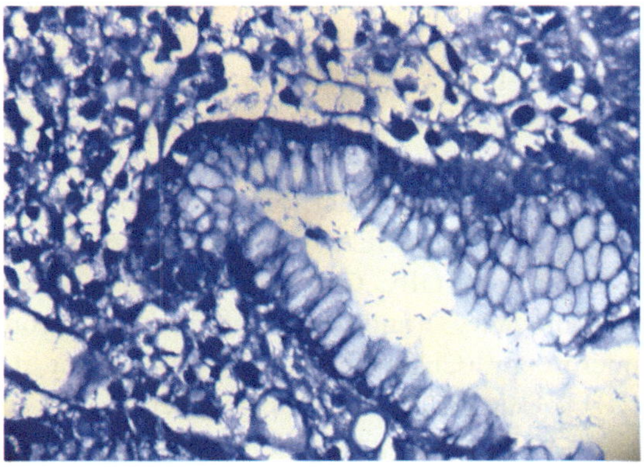

Fig. 4.15 *Helicobacter pylori* (seen here in gastric lumen) infection is associated with an increased risk of gall bladder cancer. (Image courtesy Dr. Pallavi Prasad Pathology SGPGIMS Lucknow)

2015). Fox et al. (1998) identified Helicobacter species in 13/23 bile samples and 9/23 GB tissue samples in Chilean patients with chronic cholecystitis. Seropositivity to *H. pylori* was found to be associated with an increased risk of biliary tract cancers (BTCs) (including GBC) in the Finnish Alpha Tocopherol Beta Carotene Cancer Prevention (ATBC) study including 64 BTCs and 224 age matched controls (Murphy et al. 2014). Hassan et al. (2015) showed the role of *H. pylori* infection in precancerous changes of mucosal hyperplasia and metaplasia. There are inconsistent reports of association of Helicobacter infection with GBC (Mishra 2010); we did not find *H. pylori* (using plasma antibody titers) as an important risk factor for GBC in India (Tsuchiya et al. 2018). *H. pylori* infection can be diagnosed by detecting DNA using PCR analysis using Helicobacter specific 16s ribosomal primers, bacterial culture, histological examination, serological test, and rapid urease test. *H. bilis* (Pandey et al. 2010) and *H. hepaticus* (Segura-López et al. 2015) have also been incriminated in the etiopathogenesis of GBC.

4.1.12 Heavy Metals

Heavy metals, e.g., cadmium, chromium, copper, lead, and nickel in drinking water have been incriminated in the etiopathogenesis of GBC; antioxidants, e.g., selenium and zinc, on the other hand, are protective. Shukla et al. (1998), for the first time, found higher concentrations of heavy metals, i.e., cadmium, chromium, and lead in the bile of 38 GBC patients versus 58 patients with GS. Higher levels of heavy metals, e.g., arsenic, chromium, lead, and zinc were found in Indian GBC tissue samples compared with Japanese GBC tissue samples using spectrophotometry and transmission electron microscopy (Chhabra et al. 2012). Basu et al. (2013) found higher levels of copper and lower levels of selenium and zinc in serum, bile, and tissue from 30 patients with GBC as compared to 30 sex-matched patients with GS. Recently, an association was found between the concentration of arsenic in groundwater and incidence rates of GBC in 52 countries worldwide (Ganesan et al. 2019). Elevated levels of arsenic were found in unregulated water sources in Navajo Nations, where incidence rates of GBC are high (Hoover et al. 2017). In Bihar state in northern India, high arsenic soil content had higher (1.45) odds ratio (OR) for GBC (Madhawi et al. 2018). Lee et al. (2019) created a metallome panel of 18 metals which were studied in serum samples of patients with GBC (n = 259), GS (n = 701), and population-based controls (n = 851) using inductively coupling plasma mass spectroscopy (ICPMS). Boron, lithium, molybdenum, and arsenic levels were associated with GBC versus GS.

4.1.13 Pesticides

Shukla et al. (2001) found higher levels of organochlorine pesticides, e.g., benzene hexachloride (BHC), dichloro-diphenyl-trichloroethane (DDT) in bile in 60 patients with GBC versus 30 with GS. In an ecological study analyzing water and urine samples in areas along the Yangtze river in China, Cui et al. (2017) found a higher standardized rate ratio (SRR) of 3.46 for GBC with high exposure to pentacholorophenol (PCP), used for killing snails, the intermediate host of schistosome.

Other risk factors for GBC are environmental carcinogens, e.g., dimethyl nitrosamine, 3-methyl cholanthrene; exposure to rubber textile, shoe, oil, paper, fiber, and chemicals industry; medications such as estrogens, isoniazid (INH), methyldopa, and blood groups A and AB (Pandey et al. 1995).

Both genetic and environmental etiological risk factors play a role in the pathogenesis of GBC; Japanese immigrants to the United States have lower incidence rates of GBC than those living in Japan but the rates are still higher than in the United States natives.

The index of suspicion for GBC should be higher in a patient with GS who has one or more of the above risk factors. Annual surveillance with ultrasonography (US) is recommended in some high-risk group, e.g., PSC, but unfortunately US does not pick up early GBC.

4.2 Etiopathogenesis of Gallbladder Cancer

GBC, like many other cancers, is a multifactorial disease caused by a complex interplay of various risk factors, both genetic and environmental.

Two main etiopathological pathways have been proposed for GBC (Castillo et al. 2010)

1. Chronic inflammation (cholecystitis)—recurrent infection and irritation (inflammation) of the GB mucosa due to presence of GS in the GB lumen results in release of inflammatory mediators which cause recurrent cycles of epithelial damage and repair/regeneration and adaptive changes, e.g., hyperplasia, metaplasia (which can be either gastric (i.e. pseudopyloric) or intestinal)—leading to dysplasia (low or high grade) (Fig. 4.16) which then progresses to carcinoma-in-situ (CIS) and invasive carcinoma; this progression takes about 15 years; the mean age was 46.3 years for patients with dysplasia, 57.5 years for early carcinoma, 59.0 years for advanced carcinoma, and 61.1 years for metastatic cancer (Roa et al. 1996). Deletion of the TP53 locus was seen in 58%, 85%, and 91% of dysplasia, carcinoma-in-situ, and invasive carcinoma, respectively (Wistuba et al. 1995). Loss of heterozygosity (LoH) at 8 loci of eight tumor suppressor genes (TSGs) was seen in 2–48% of preneoplastic lesions, e.g., metaplasia and dysplasia, in 350 patients with GS and chronic cholecystitis, suggesting a possible causal association of GS with GBC (Jain et al. 2014). Reactive atypia and metaplasia are seen in the GB mucosa in about 1–5% of patients with chronic cholecystitis due to GS. Dysplasia is defined as nuclear enlargement and irregularity, increased nucleus-to-cytoplasm (NC) ratio, hyperchromasia, prominent nucleoli, and atypia, i.e., loss of polarity. Biliary intraepithelial neoplasia (BilIN) is a new alternative term proposed for dysplasia. Dysplasia can be—1 (low grade), 2 (intermediate grade), or 3 (high grade) dysplasia (i.e. CIS). Metaplasia, dysplasia, and CIS are seen very frequently in the mucosa surrounding the cancer in GBC. The close topographic relation between the intraepithelial lesions and infiltrating cancer suggests an etiopathological relation. Metaplasia, dysplasia, and CIS were present adjacent to cancer in 66%, 81%, and 69%, respectively; the average age of dysplasia (52 years), early carcinoma (57 years), and advanced carcinoma (63 years) also suggested progression of these lesions (Roa et al. 2006a). In a histopathological analysis of 350 GBs from patients with GS, hyperplasia (32%), metaplasia (48%), dysplasia (16%), and CIS (0.6%) were seen very frequently (Jain et al. 2014). Total sampling of 140 consecutive cholecystectomy specimens from Chilean women revealed 3 (2%) incidental invasive (T2) GBC with high-grade dysplasia (HGD); 14 (10%) other cases had low-grade dysplasia (LGD), 5 of which could have been missed on routine longitudinal diagnostic sectioning of the GB (Koshiol et al. 2018).

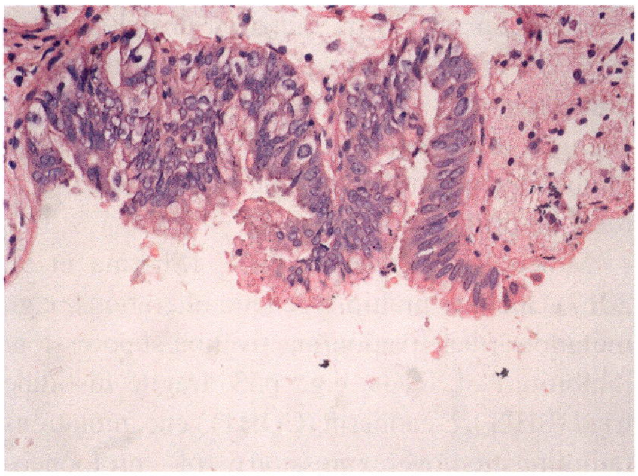

Fig. 4.16 Inflammation-induced hyperplasia, metaplasia, and dysplasia play an important role in the etiopathogenesis of GBC

2. Unlike in colon cancer, adenoma (a benign glandular neoplasm) (Fig. 4.17)—carcinoma sequence is not common in GBC; very few GBCs arise in a preexisting adenoma. Remnants of an adenoma were seen in only 6 (2.8%) out of 210 cases (Roa et al. 2006b). There is some evidence for the association of a GB adenoma with Peutz Jeghers and Gardner syndromes.

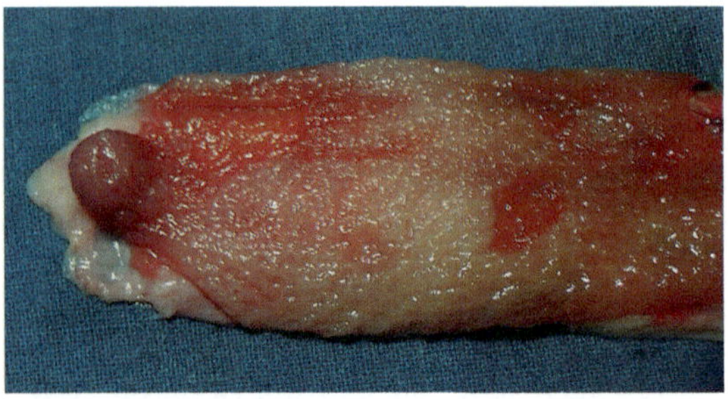

Fig. 4.17 Adenomatous polyp; adenoma—carcinoma sequence does not play a major role in the etiopathogenesis of gallbladder cancer; inflammation is more important

There are virtually no animal models for GBC—Suzuki and Takahashi (1983) induced GBC in hamsters by inserting methylcholanthrene beeswax pellets in GB lumen.

4.3 Molecular Biology of Gallbladder Cancer

From the basic research point of view, GBC is an "orphan" cancer—rarity in the Western world, low resectability rate resulting in scarcity of tumor tissue, very few available cell lines and no reliable animal model. Very little translational research has been done in GBC so that there is a poor understanding of the genetic and molecular aspects of GBC. No specific oncogenes or tumor suppressor genes (TSG) have been found for GBC; not many GBC specific signaling pathways are known.

GBC, however, offers a unique opportunity for research in terms of a wide variety of tissue samples available viz. GB tumor tissue, normal (noncancerous) tissue in the GB around the tumor, normal (noncancerous) liver tissue from the same patient, inflammatory (CC and XGC) tissues in patients with GS, preneoplastic lesions, e.g., hyperplasia, metaplasia, and dysplasia around CC and GBC, normal (noncancerous, non-inflammatory) GB removed during operations for the diseases of liver (e.g. right hepatectomy), CBD (e.g. choledochal cyst excision), and pancreas (e.g. pancreatoduodenectomy).

The genetic landscape of GBC and the molecular changes in GBC can be studied by various

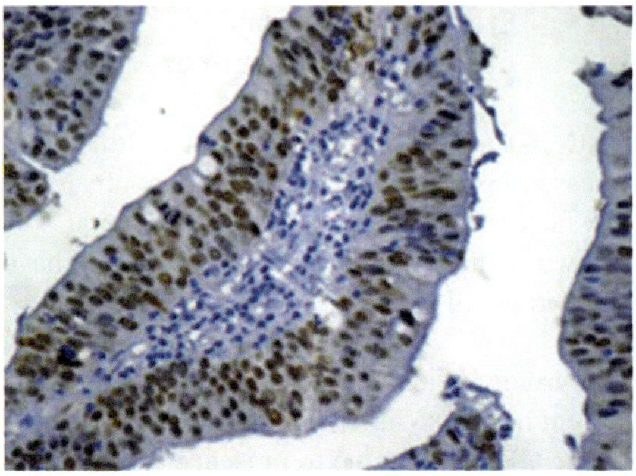

Fig. 4.18 Immunohistochemistry (IHC) is an important technique to study protein expression

techniques, e.g., protein expression by immunohistochemistry (IHC) (Fig. 4.18), aneuploidy by flow cytometry, fluorescent in situ hybridization (FISH), real time polymerase chain reaction (RT PCR) (Fig. 4.19), genome-wide association studies (GWAS), and high throughput methods, e.g., targeted gene sequencing, whole-exome sequencing (WES), transcriptome sequencing, next-generation sequencing (NGS), etc. (Mehrotra et al. 2018).

GS-related chronic inflammation causes sustained release of excessive reactive oxygen and nitrogen, and inflammatory mediators, e.g., cytokines, chemokines, and prostaglandins. They cause DNA damage which promotes mutational defects, e.g., activation of oncogenes and suppression of TSGs. Inflammation causes oxidative stress and increased cell turnover resulting in deactivation of p53 by mutation or deletion (Li et al. 2014; Espinoza et al. 2016). Environmental mutagens, e.g., aflatoxins can also cause these changes. Inflammation, combined with genetic predisposition and environmental exposure, may result in progression to cancer.

Molecular changes in GBC (Sharma et al. 2017) include multiple genetic alterations, e.g., mutations (deactivation/inactivation/suppression/inhibition) of TSGs, e.g., p53, fragile histidine triad (FHIT), e-cadherin (CDH1) gene, mutations (amplification/overexpression) of protooncogenes, e.g., K-ras, cErb B2, HER2/neu, DNA repair genes, adhesion molecules, e.g., beta-catenin (CTNNBI), genomic instability in the form of polymorphisms (Fig. 4.20) in genes

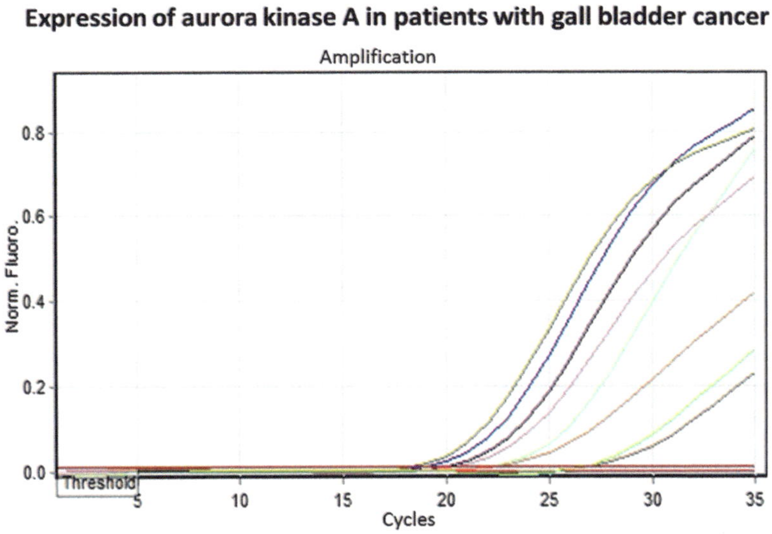

No.	Colour	Name	Ct
1		NC	NEG (NTC)
2		1.1 B-Actin	22.48
3		1.2 B-Actin	22.45
4		2.1 GBC	19.17
5		2.2 GBC	18.48
6		3.1 GBC	19.97
7		3.2 GBC	20.66
8		4.1 CC	26.96
9		4.2 CC	26.87

Fig. 4.19 Real time polymerase chain reaction (RT PCR) curve for mRNA expression of aurora kinase A in biopsy samples of two patients with gall bladder cancer (GBC) and one with chronic cholecystitis (CC). Samples were run in duplicate and B-actin was used as housekeeping gene. Cycle threshold (Ct) is inversely proportional to the relative expression level of the gene of interest

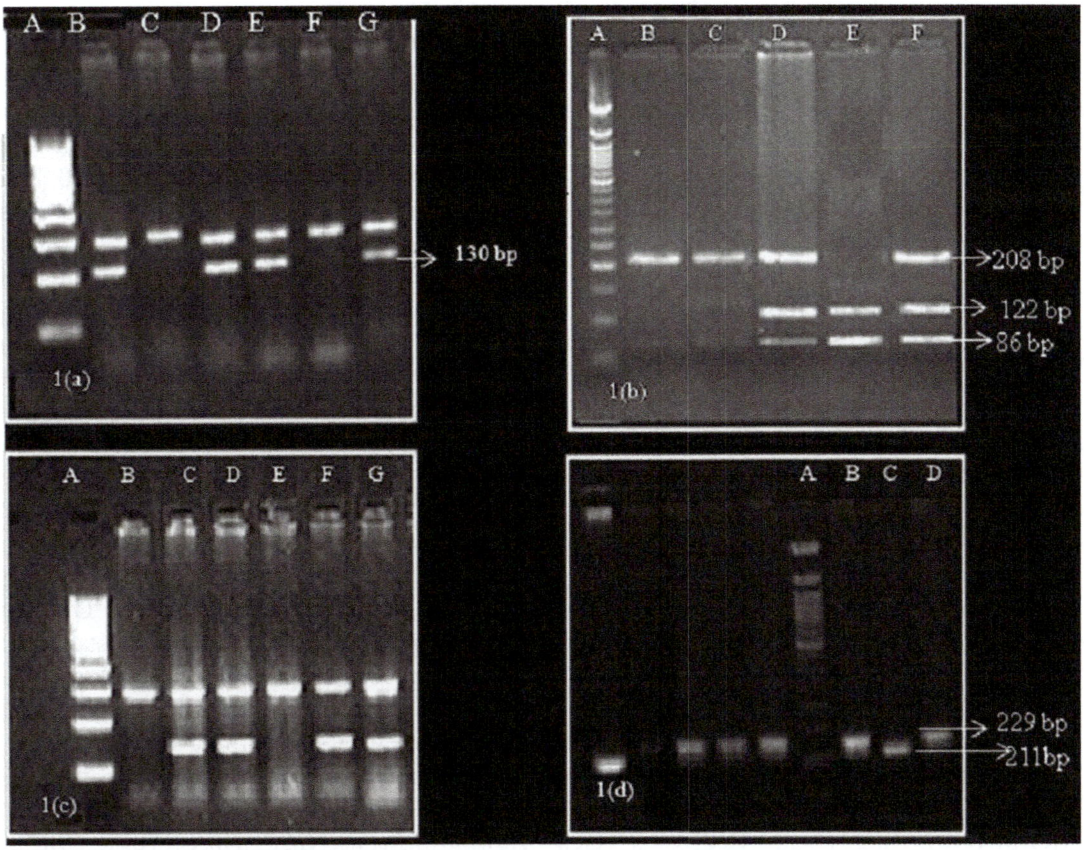

Fig. 4.20 Vascular endothelial growth factor (VEGF) polymorphism (Lane-A shows 50bp DNA ladder against the single nucleotide polymorphisms SNPs)

(Baez et al. 2010), loss of heterozygosity (LoH), and microsatellite instability (MSI) indicating mismatch repair deficiency, and epigenetic changes, e.g., hypermethylation of gene promoter regions (Sharma et al. 2016).

Li et al. (2014) identified about 1500 somatic changes at the genome level using whole-exome sequencing (WES) and targeted gene sequencing—the commonest genes involved were TP 53, KRAS, and Erb B. Using next generation sequencing (NGS), Zuo et al. (2016) found that TP53 and PIK3CA were the most common mutations. In the Indian population, we found PIK3CA and KRAS as the commonest mutations (Kumari et al. 2014). In whole exome sequencing (WES) analysis of 157 GBC patients, Li et al. (2019) identified mutations in TP53 (27%), KMT2C (11%), SMAD4 (11%), PER3 (8%), ERBB3 (8%), ERBB2 (7%), ARID2 (7%), and ARID1A (7%). The most common genetic alterations in another study were TP53, KRAS, and cyclin-dependent kinase (CDKN) 2A (Hirata et al. 2019). Small noncoding (snc) RNAs, e.g., micro RNA (miRNA) (Chandra et al. 2016) and long noncoding RNAs which can act as oncogenes or TSGs (Tekcham and Tiwari 2016; Chen et al. 2018) have also been implicated in the pathogenesis of GBC.

A recent review (Tulsyan et al. 2020) has summarized the studies on the transcriptomic profile of GBC with emphasis on studies pertaining to coding (mRNA) and noncoding (micro and long noncoding) RNA along with aberrant promoter methylation studies, ranging from a single gene to global gene to high throughput RNA sequencing approaches, published between 2000 to May, 2019.

4.4 Therapeutic Options

Actionable mutations of molecules such as EGFR, VEGF, VEGFR, mTOR, HER2, PDL-1, PD-1, MET, PI3K, cadherin, MEK1, MEK2 which can be targets for potential therapy are being studied in GBC (Mishra et al. 2019). Various cell signaling pathways, e.g., Erb B, AKT/MAPK/ERK, Notch, Hedgehog, etc., which can play an important role in carcinogenesis, are also being studied. Small molecules and antibodies against components of various signaling pathways are being increasingly used in various cancers, e.g., breast, colorectal, etc. and may play a role in GBC also in future.

Celecoxib—a selective inhibitor of cyclooxygenase (COX) was found to have an inhibitory effect on the proliferation of GBC cells (Deng 2017); this may have a therapeutic implication as cox-2 overexpression was seen by us in 57/64 GBCs (Ghosh et al. 2000). EGFR overexpression was seen on immunohistochemistry in 44/50 patients with GBC (weak in 10, moderate in 26, and strong in 8) (Kumar et al. 2016a). HER2-positive GBC can be treated with trastuzumab. MSI as a sign of mismatch repair deficiency is a predictor of response to anti-PD-1 therapy (Le et al. 2015). Li et al. (2019) demonstrated the therapeutic activity of PD-L1 monoclonal antibodies (sapitinib and atezolizumab) in GBC cells.

Differences have been found in genetic changes in GBC samples from different geographical areas. K-ras mutations are more common in APBDJ-related GBC seen in Japan and in papillary GBC; p53 mutations, on the other hand, are more common in GS and chronic inflammation-related GBC seen in Chile. k-ras codon 12 mutation was seen in as many as 16/39 GBCs in India (Kazmi et al. 2013) but in only 2/21 GBCs in Chile (Wistuba et al. 1995) and in 2/29 GBCs in the United States (Pai et al. 2011). Targeted sequencing of known cancer-associated genes in GBC tumors from Japan ($n = 11$), Chile ($n = 21$), and the United States ($n = 49$) revealed different mutation patterns, thus suggesting different etiopathogenesis in different populations (Narayan et al. 2019).

The Author (VKK) is of the opinion that GBC with and without GS are two different diseases; also, GBC in East Asia, i.e., Japan, Korea, and China is biologically different from GBC in South Asia, i.e., India, Nepal, Pakistan, and Bangladesh, which in itself is different from GBC in central and south America (CSA), i.e., Chile and Bolivia.

Do GS cause GBC? Do some types of GS cause GBC? Do GS cause GBC in some people? How do GS cause GBC? Do GS cause GBC in the presence of some other carcinogens? We don't know!

Invited Commentary on Etiology and Pathogenesis of Gallbladder Cancer

Jean Michel Butte

Gallbladder cancer (GBC) is an aggressive malignancy and most patients are diagnosed with advanced disease. Thus, recognizing factors associated with its origin is not only important to identify a population of patients who have a higher risk of developing this disease but also to implement national programs against these factors to decrease the progression to cancer and improve survival.

Despite the fact that GBC is a rare disease, it has a higher incidence in some areas of the world such as India, Japan, and Chile, where most of the risk factors are shared. However, local and environmental factors may produce a different disease in nonrelated areas of the world.

In this chapter, Dr. Kapoor has analyzed in detail the etiology and pathogenesis of GBC. The presence of gallstones (GS) and resultant chronic inflammation seems to be a strong risk factor for developing GBC. However, it has always been debated if there are other factors playing a major role in conjunction with GS, considering that most patients with GS do not develop this malignancy around the world. As the Author (VKK) has mentioned, GBC seems to be more commonly found in areas where GS are more frequent, when the GS have a larger size and when the symptoms are longer. This is highly associated with the socioeconomic status of the patient and there is a real option of getting an elective cholecystectomy to cut this line of cancer development. Other clinical presentations analyzed in this chapter i.e. acute cholecystitis, gallbladder empyema, Mirizzi syndrome, obstruction of the gallbladder neck, xantho-granulomatous cholecystitis (XGC), porcelain gallbladder, and cholecysto-enteric fistula confirm that chronic inflammation is a known pathway with a higher chance of developing GBC.

There are other risk factors reported in this chapter that have been associated with GBC viz. personal (age, gender, and family history), biliary (anatomical biliary anomalies and diseases and chronic infection), environmental (lifestyle, diet, heavy metals, and pesticides), and comorbid situations (obesity and diabetes). GBC may present at any age and gender, but in the majority of areas it is more frequent in females. Patients diagnosed at a younger age seems to have longer periods of symptomatic GS to explain the development of cancer, but it is not clear why in some areas there is a female preponderance but in others it is not. However, it looks like that there is a synergism among long periods of chronic inflammation secondary to GS, female gender, and hormonal status. On the other hand, family history, lifestyle, diet, obesity and diabetes are found in similar population and most of the time associated with low economic status. Thus, people with less access to fruits and vegetables (protective factors) usually have a diet based in high calorie and carbohydrate, with a higher propensity of developing GS, obesity, and diabetes, and then altering their hormonal status. This lifestyle is usually common in some communities and families, explaining a common pathway in some areas of the world, as the Author (VKK) says.

An interesting theory about developing GBC around the world has been linked to gallbladder's chronic infection. As the Author (VKK) mentioned, after having an acute Salmonella infection, this bacteria may colonize the gallbladder and produce chronic inflammation as it has been shown in genetic models. This also has been associated with Helicobacter infection, increasing the relative risk of developing GBC. This theory also has been considered in Chile where an important epidemic of Salmonella infection occurred in the 1970s and could be related to current cases of GBC, but it is difficult to prove this with certainty. The presence of heavy metals and pesticides has been found in patients with GBC, but it seems that these factors need further investigation to prove real association with the development of GBC.

Two main pathways have been described by the Author (VKK); the first is related to chronic inflammation and the second to the development of an adenoma. The first mechanism is significantly more common and has been vastly referred and mainly associated with GS, while the second is less common and associated with the presence of polyps.

In summary, this chapter describes in detail different risk factors and pathogenesis related to GBC. Similarly, it suggests that GBC may arise from a specific pathway in different areas of the world. This is important to define clinical methods to diagnose this disease in precancerous or early stages with the aim of improving survival and having a better chance of cure.

References

Andreotti G, Hou L, Gao YT, Brinton LA, Rashid A, Chen J, Shen MC, Wang BS, Han TQ, Zhang BH, Sakoda LC, Fraumeni JF Jr, Hsing AW. Reproductive factors and risks of biliary tract cancers and stones: a population-based study in Shanghai, China. Br J Cancer. 2010;102(7):1185–9. https://doi.org/10.1038/sj.bjc.6605597. Epub 2010 Mar 9.

Aune D, Vatten LJ, Boffetta P. Tobacco smoking and the risk of gallbladder disease. Eur J Epidemiol. 2016;31(7):643–53. https://doi.org/10.1007/s10654-016-0124-z. Epub 2016 Feb 22. Review.

Avgerinos KI, Spyrou N, Mantzoros CS, Dalamaga M. Obesity and cancer risk: emerging biological mechanisms and perspectives. Metabolism. 2019;92:121–35. https://doi.org/10.1016/j.metabol.2018.11.001. Epub 2018 Nov 13. Review

Báez S, Tsuchiya Y, Calvo A, Pruyas M, Nakamura K, Kiyohara C, Oyama M, Yamamoto M. Genetic variants involved in gallstone formation and capsaicin metabolism, and the risk of gallbladder cancer in Chilean women. World J Gastroenterol. 2010;16(3):372–8.

Baskaran V, Vij U, Sahni P, Tandon RK, Nundy S. Do the progesterone receptors have a role to play in gallbladder cancer? Int J Gastrointest Cancer. 2005;35(1):61–8. https://doi.org/10.1385/IJGC:35:1:061. PMID: 15722575.

Basu S, Priya R, Singh TB, Srivastava P, Mishra PK, Shukla VK. Role of nicotine in gallbladder carcinoma: a preliminary report. J Dig Dis. 2012 Oct;13(10):536–40. https://doi.org/10.1111/j.1751-2980.2012.00623.x.

Basu S, Singh MK, Singh TB, Bhartiya SK, Singh SP, Shukla VK. Heavy and trace metals in carcinoma of the gallbladder. World J Surg. 2013;37(11):2641–6. https://doi.org/10.1007/s00268-013-2164-9.

Bhaskaran K, Douglas I, Forbes H, dos-Santos-Silva I, Leon DA, Smeeth L. Body-mass index and risk of 22 specific cancers: a population-based cohort study of 5·24 million UK adults. Lancet. 2014;384(9945):755–65. https://doi.org/10.1016/S0140-6736(14)60892-8. Epub 2014 Aug 13.

Brown KM, Geller DA. Porcelain gallbladder and risk of gallbladder cancer. Arch Surg. 2011;146(10):1148.

Castillo J, García P, Roa JC. [Genetic alterations in preneoplastic and neoplastic injuries of the gallbladder]. Rev Med Chil. 2010;138(5):595–604. Epub 2010 Jul 12. Review. Spanish.

Chandra V, Kim JJ, Mittal B, Rai R. MicroRNA aberrations: an emerging field for gallbladder cancer management. World J Gastroenterol. 2016;22(5):1787–99. https://doi.org/10.3748/wjg.v22.i5.1787. Review.

Chang J, Jang JY, Kang MJ, Jung W, Shin YC, Kim SW. Clinicopathologic differences in patients with gallbladder cancer according to the presence of anomalous biliopancreatic junction. World J Surg. 2016;40(5):1211–7. https://doi.org/10.1007/s00268-015-3359-z.

Chapman R, Fevery J, Kalloo A, Nagorney DM, Boberg KM, Shneider B, Gores GJ, American Association for the Study of Liver Diseases. Diagnosis and management of primary sclerosing cholangitis. Hepatology. 2010;51(2):660–78. https://doi.org/10.1002/hep.23294.

Chen Y, Wu F, Saito E, Lin Y, Song M, Luu HN, Gupta PC, Sawada N, Tamakoshi A, Shu XO, Koh WP, Xiang YB, Tomata Y, Sugiyama K, Park SK, Matsuo K, Nagata C, Sugawara Y, Qiao YL, You SL, Wang R, Shin MH, Pan WH, Pednekar MS, Tsugane S, Cai H, Yuan JM, Gao YT, Tsuji I, Kanemura S, Ito H, Wada K, Ahn YO, Yoo KY, Ahsan H, Chia KS, Boffetta P, Zheng W, Inoue M, Kang D, Potter JD. Association between type 2 diabetes and risk of cancer mortality: a pooled analysis of over 771,000 individuals in the Asia Cohort Consortium. Diabetologia. 2017;60(6):1022–32. https://doi.org/10.1007/s00125-017-4229-z. Epub 2017 Mar 7.

Chen B, Li Y, He Y, Xue C, Xu F. The emerging roles of long non-coding RNA in gallbladder cancer tumorigenesis. Cancer Biomark. 2018;22(3):359–66. https://doi.org/10.3233/CBM-170979. Review.

Chhabra D, Oda K, Jagannath P, Utsunomiya H, Takekoshi S, Nimura Y. Chronic heavy metal exposure and gallbladder Cancer risk in India, a comparative study with Japan. Asian Pac J Cancer Prev. 2012;13(1):187–90. https://doi.org/10.7314/APJCP.2012.13.1.187.

Choudhuri G, Agarwal DK, Negi TS. Polarizing microscopy of partially dissolved gallstone powder: a simple technique for studying gallstone composition. J Gastroenterol Hepatol. 1995;10(3):241–5.

Chow WH, Johansen C, Gridley G, Mellemkjaer L, Olsen JH, Fraumeni JF Jr. Gallstones, cholecystectomy and risk of cancers of the liver, biliary tract and pancreas. Br J Cancer. 1999;79(3–4):640–4.

Cui Y, Liang L, Zhong Q, He Q, Shan X, Chen K, Huang F. The association of cancer risks with pentachlorophenol exposure: focusing on community population in the areas along certain section of Yangtze River in China. Environ Pollut. 2017;224:729–38. https://doi.org/10.1016/j.envpol.2016.12.011. Epub 2017 Jan 13.

Dankner R, Boffetta P, Balicer RD, Boker LK, Sadeh M, Berlin A, Olmer L, Goldfracht M, Freedman LS. Time-dependent risk of cancer after a diabetes diagnosis in a cohort of 2.3 million adults. Am J Epidemiol. 2016;183(12):1098–106. https://doi.org/10.1093/aje/kwv290. Epub 2016 Jun 2.

Deng M, Qin Y, Chen X, Li D, Wang Q, Zheng H, Gu L, Deng C, Xue Y, Zhu D, Wang Q, Wang J. Combination of celecoxib and PD184161 exerts synergistic inhibitory effects on gallbladder cancer cell proliferation. Oncol Lett. 2017;13(5):3850–58. https://doi.org/10.3892/ol.2017.5914. Epub 2017 Mar 27. PMID: 28521485; PMCID: PMC5431146.

Di Domenico EG, Cavallo I, Pontone M, Toma L, Ensoli F. Biofilm producing Salmonella Typhi: chronic colonization and development of gallbladder cancer. Int J Mol Sci. 2017;18(9):E1887. https://doi.org/10.3390/ijms18091887. Review.

Diehl AK. Gallstone size and the risk of gallbladder cancer. JAMA. 1983;250(17):2323–6.

Dixit R, Srivastava P, Basu S, Srivastava P, Mishra PK, Shukla VK. Association of mustard oil as cooking media with carcinoma of the gallbladder. J Gastrointest Cancer. 2013;44(2):177–81. https://doi.org/10.1007/s12029-012-9458-2.

Dutta U, Nagi B, Garg PK, Sinha SK, Singh K, Tandon RK. Patients with gallstones develop gallbladder cancer at an earlier age. Eur J Cancer Prev. 2005;14(4):381–5.

Espinoza JA, Bizama C, Garcia P, Ferreccio P, Javle M, Miguel JF, et al. The inflammatory inception of gallbladder cancer. Biochim Biophys Acta. 2016;1865(2):245–54.

European Association for the Study of the Liver. EASL Clinical Practice Guidelines: management of cholestatic liver diseases. J Hepatol. 2009;51(2):237–67. https://doi.org/10.1016/j.jhep.2009.04.009. Epub 2009 Jun 6.

Everhart JE, Yeh F, Lee ET, Hill MC, Fabsitz R, Howard BV, Welty TK. Prevalence of gallbladder disease in American Indian populations: findings from the Strong Heart Study. Hepatology. 2002;35(6):1507–12.

Foerster C, Koshiol J, Guerrero A, Kogan M, Ferrecio C. The case for aflatoxins in the causal chain of gallbladder cancer. Med Hypotheses. 2016;86:47–52. https://doi.org/10.1016/j.mehy.2015.11.026.

Fox JG, Dewhirst FE, Shen Z, Feng Y, Taylor NS, Paster BJ, Ericson RL, Lau CN, Correa P, Araya JC, Roa I. Hepatic Helicobacter species identified in bile and gallbladder tissue from Chileans with chronic cholecystitis. Gastroenterology. 1998;114(4):755–63.

Fung BM, Lindor KD, Tabibian JH. Cancer risk in primary sclerosing cholangitis: epidemiology, prevention, and surveillance strategies. World J Gastroenterol. 2019;25(6):659–71. https://doi.org/10.3748/wjg.v25.i6.659. Review.

Ganesan N, Bambino K, Boffetta P, Labgaa I. Exploring the potential carcinogenic role of arsenic in gallbladder cancer. Eur J Cancer Prev. 2019; https://doi.org/10.1097/CEJ.0000000000000521.

Ghosh M, Kawamoto T, Koike N, Fukao K, Yoshida S, Kashiwagi H, Kapoor VK, Agarwal S, Krishnani N, Uchida K, Miwa M, Todoroki T. Cyclooxygenase expression in the gallbladder. Int J Mol Med. 2000;6(5):527–32.

Hassan EH, Gerges SS, El-Atrebi KA, El-Bassyouni HT. The role of H. pylori infection in gall bladder cancer: clinicopathological study. Tumour Biol. 2015;36(9):7093–8. https://doi.org/10.1007/s13277-015-3444-9. Epub 2015 Apr 16.

Herrera Riquelme CA, et al. Trends in mortality from cancer in Chile according to differences in educational level, 2000–2010. Rev Panam Salud Publica. 2015;37(1):44–51.

Hirata K, Kuwatani M, Suda G, Ishikawa M, Sugiura R, Kato S, Kawakubo K, Sakamoto N. A novel approach for the genetic analysis of biliary tract cancer specimens obtained through endoscopic ultrasound-guided fine needle aspiration using targeted amplicon sequencing. Clin Transl Gastroenterol. 2019;10(3):e00022. https://doi.org/10.14309/ctg.0000000000000022.

Hoover J, Gonzales M, Shuey C, Barney Y, Lewis J. Elevated arsenic and uranium concentrations in unregulated water sources on the Navajo nation, USA. Expo Health. 2017;9(2):113–24. https://doi.org/10.1007/s12403-016-0226-6.

Hori M, Saito E. Gallbladder cancer incidence rates in the world from the cancer incidence in five continents XI. Jpn J Clin Oncol. 2018;48(9):866–7. https://doi.org/10.1093/jjco/hyy119.

Hsing AW, Gao YT, Han TQ, Rashid A, Sakoda LC, Wang BS, Shen MC, Zhang BH, Niwa S, Chen J, Fraumeni JF Jr. Gallstones and the risk of biliary tract cancer: a population-based study in China. Br J Cancer. 2007a;97(11):1577–82. Epub 2007 Nov 13

Hsing AW, Bai Y, Andreotti G, Rashid A, Deng J, Chen J, et al. Family history of gallstones and the risk of biliary tract cancer and gallstones: a population-based study in Shanghai, China. Int J Cancer. 2007b;121(4):832–8.

Hyvärinen I, Hukkinen M, Kivisaari R, Parviainen H, Nordin A, Pakarinen MP. Increased prevalence of pancreaticobiliary maljunction in biliary malignancies. Scand J Surg. 2019;11:1457496918822617. https://doi.org/10.1177/1457496918822617.

Ikoma T, Tsuchiya Y, Asai T, Okano K, Ito N, Endoh K, Yamamoto M, Nakamura K. Ochratoxin A contamination of red chili peppers from Chile, Bolivia and Peru, countries with a high incidence of gallbladder cancer. Asian Pac J Cancer Prev. 2015;16(14):5987–91.

Ikoma T, Kapoor VK, Behari A, Mishra K, Tsuchiya Y, Asai T, Endoh K, Okano K, Nakamura K. Lack of an apparent association between mycotoxin concentrations in red chili peppers and incidence of gallbladder cancer in India: an ecological study. Asian Pac J Cancer Prev. 2016;17(7):3499–503.

Iyer P, Barreto SG, Sahoo B, Chandrani P, Ramadwar MR, Shrikhande SV, Dutt A. Non-typhoidal Salmonella

DNA traces in gallbladder cancer. Infect Agent Cancer. 2016;11:12. https://doi.org/10.1186/s13027-016-0057-x. eCollection 2016.

Jackson HH, Glasgow RE, Mulvihill SJ, Cannon-Albright LA. Familial risk in gallbladder cancer. J Am Coll Surg. 2007;205:S38–S138.

Jain K, Mahapatra T, Das P, Misra MC, Gupta SD, Ghosh M, et al. Sequential occurrence of preneoplastic lesions and accumulation of loss of heterozygosity in patients with gallbladder stones suggest causal association with gallbladder cancer. Ann Surg. 2014;260(6):1073–80. https://doi.org/10.1097/SLA.0000000000000495.

Jayalakshmi K, Sonkar K, Behari A, Kapoor VK, Sinha N. Solid state (13)C NMR analysis of human gallstones from cancer and benign gall bladder diseases. Solid State Nucl Magn Reson. 2009;36(1):60–5. https://doi.org/10.1016/j.ssnmr.2009.06.001. Epub 2009 Jun 16.

Jayanthi V, Palanivelu C, Prasanthi R, Mathew S, Srinivasan V. Composition of gallstones in Coimbatore District of Tamil Nadu state. Indian J Gastroenterol. 1998;17(4):134–5.

Kazmi HR, Chandra A, Nigam J, Noushif M, Parmar D, Gupta V. Prognostic significance of K-ras codon 12 mutation in patients with resected gallbladder cancer. Dig Surg. 2013;30(3):233–9. https://doi.org/10.1159/000353133. Epub 2013 Jul 6. PMID: 23838952.

Khan ZS, Livingston EH, Huerta S. Reassessing the need for prophylactic surgery in patients with porcelain gallbladder: case series and systematic review of the literature. Arch Surg. 2011;146(10):1143–7. https://doi.org/10.1001/archsurg.2011.257. Review.

Khuroo MS, Mahajan R, Zargar SA, Javid G, Sapru S. Prevalence of biliary tract disease in India: a sonographic study in adult population in Kashmir. Gut. 1989;30(2):201–5.

Koshiol J, Wozniak A, Cook P, Adaniel C, Acevedo J, Azócar L, Hsing AW, Roa JC, Pasetti MF, Miquel JF, Levine MM, Ferreccio C, Gallbladder Cancer Chile Working Group. Salmonella enterica serovar Typhi and gallbladder cancer: a case-control study and meta-analysis. Cancer Med. 2016;5(11):3310–235. https://doi.org/10.1002/cam4.915. Epub 2016 Oct 11. Review.

Koshiol J, Gao YT, Dean M, Egner P, Nepal C, Jones K, Wang B, Rashid A, Luo W, Van Dyke AL, Ferreccio C, Malasky M, Shen MC, Zhu B, Andersen JB, Hildesheim A, Hsing AW, Groopman J. Association of aflatoxin and gallbladder cancer. Gastroenterology. 2017;153(2):488–494.e1. https://doi.org/10.1053/j.gastro.2017.04.005. Epub 2017 Apr 17.

Koshiol J, Bellolio E, Vivallo C, Cook P, Roa JC, McGee EE, Losada H, Van Dyke AL, Van De Wyngard V, Prado R, Villaseca M, Riquelme P, Acevedo J, Olivo V, Pettit K, Hildesheim A, Medina K, Memis B, Adsay V, Ferreccio C, Araya JC. Distribution of dysplasia and cancer in the gallbladder: an analysis from a high cancer-risk population. Hum Pathol. 2018;82:87–94. https://doi.org/10.1016/j.humpath.2018.07.015. Epub 2018 Jul 21.

Kumar N, Khan MA, Kumar N, Rigvardhan, Ranjan R, Hazra N. Epidermal growth factor receptor expression in carcinoma gallbladder: a prospective study in Indian scenario. J Cancer Res Ther. 2016a;12(2):959–62. https://doi.org/10.4103/0973-1482.179063.

Kumar A, Senthil G, Prakash A, Behari A, Singh RK, Kapoor VK, Saxena R. Mirizzi's syndrome: lessons learnt from 169 patients at a single center. Korean J Hepatobiliary Pancreat Surg. 2016b;20(1):17–22. https://doi.org/10.14701/kjhbps.2016.20.1.17. Epub 2016 Feb 19.

Kumari N, Corless CL, Warrick A, Beadling C, Nelson D, Neff T, Krishnani N, Kapoor VK. Mutation profiling in gallbladder cancer in Indian population. Indian J Pathol Microbiol. 2014;57(1):9–12. https://doi.org/10.4103/0377-4929.130849.

Larsson SC, Wolk A. Obesity and the risk of gallbladder cancer: a meta-analysis. Br J Cancer. 2007;96(9):1457–61. Epub 2007 Mar 20.

Le DT, Uram JN, Wang H, Bartlett BR, Kemberling H, Eyring AD, Skora AD, Luber BS, Azad NS, Laheru D, Biedrzycki B, Donehower RC, Zaheer A, Fisher GA, Crocenzi TS, Lee JJ, Duffy SM, Goldberg RM, de la Chapelle A, Koshiji M, Bhaijee F, Huebner T, Hruban RH, Wood LD, Cuka N, Pardoll DM, Papadopoulos N, Kinzler KW, Zhou S, Cornish TC, Taube JM, Anders RA, Eshleman JR, Vogelstein B, Diaz LA Jr. PD-1 blockade in tumors with mismatch-repair deficiency. N Engl J Med. 2015;372(26):2509–20. https://doi.org/10.1056/NEJMoa1500596. Epub 2015 May 30.

Lee JE, Nam CM, Lee SG, Park S, Kim TH, Park EC. The health burden of cancer attributable to obesity in Korea: a population-based cohort study. Cancer Res Treat. 2018; https://doi.org/10.4143/crt.2018.301.

Lee MH, Gao YT, Huang YH, McGee EE, Lam T, Wang B, Shen MC, Rashid A, Pfeiffer RM, Hsing AW, Koshiol J. A metallomic approach to assess associations of serum metal levels with gallstones and gallbladder cancer. Hepatology. 2019;71:917. https://doi.org/10.1002/hep.30861.

Li M, Zhang Z, Li X, Tan Z, Liu C, Shen B, et al. Whole-exome and targeted gene sequencing of gallbladder carcinoma identifies recurrent mutations in the ErbB pathway. Nat Genet. 2014;46(8):872–6. https://doi.org/10.1038/ng.3030.

Li M, Liu F, Zhang F, Zhou W, Jiang X, Yang Y, Qu K, Wang Y, Ma Q, Wang T, Bai L, Wang Z, Song X, Zhu Y, Yuan R, Gao Y, Liu Y, Jin Y, Li H, Xiang S, Ye Y, Zhang Y, Jiang L, Hu Y, Hao Y, Lu W, Chen S, Gu J, Zhou J, Gong W, Zhang Y, Wang X, Liu X, Liu C, Liu H, Liu Y, Liu Y. Genomic *ERBB2*/*ERBB3* mutations promote PD-L1-mediated immune escape in gallbladder cancer: a whole-exome sequencing analysis. Gut. 2019;68(6):1024–33. https://doi.org/10.1136/gutjnl-2018-316039. Epub 2018 Jun 28

Liu H, Ziang Y, Ai M, Wang J, Jin B, Wo M, et al. Body mass index can increase the risk of gallbladder cancer: a meta-analysis of 14 cohort studies. Med Sci Monit Basic Res. 2016;22:146–55. https://doi.org/10.12659/MSMBR.901651.

Lohsiriwat V, Vongjirad A, Lohsiriwat D. Value of routine histopathologic examination of three common surgical specimens: appendix, gallbladder, and hemorrhoid. World J Surg. 2009;33(10):2189–93. https://doi.org/10.1007/s00268-009-0164-6.

Lowenfels AB, Lindström CG, Conway MJ, Hastings PR. Gallstones and risk of gallbladder cancer. J Natl Cancer Inst. 1985;75(1):77–80.

Lowenfels AB, Walker AM, Althaus DP, Townsend G, Domellöf L. Gallstone growth, size, and risk of gallbladder cancer: an interracial study. Int J Epidemiol. 1989;18(1):50–4.

Lugo A, Peveri G, Gallus S. Should we consider gallbladder cancer a new smoking-related cancer? A comprehensive meta-analysis focused on dose-response relationships. Int J Cancer. 2020;146(12):3304–11. https://doi.org/10.1002/ijc.32681.

Machado NO. Porcelain gallbladder: decoding the malignant truth. Sultan Qaboos Univ Med J. 2016;16(4):e416–21. https://doi.org/10.18295/squmj.2016.16.04.003. Epub 2016 Nov 30. Review.

Madadi-Sanjani O, Wirth TC, Kuebler JF, Petersen C, Ure BM. Choledochal cyst and malignancy: a plea for lifelong follow-up. Eur J Pediatr Surg. 2019;29(2):143–9. https://doi.org/10.1055/s-0037-1615275. Epub 2017 Dec 19. Review.

Madhawi R, Pandey A, Raj S, Mandal M, Devi S, Sinha PK, Singh RK. Geographical pattern of carcinoma gallbladder in Bihar and its association with river Ganges and arsenic levels: retrospective individual consecutive patient data from Regional Cancer Centre. South Asian J Cancer. 2018;7(3):167–70. https://doi.org/10.4103/sajc.sajc_37_18.

Makiuchi T, Sobue T, Kitamura T, Sawada N, Iwasaki M, Sasazuki S, Yamaji T, Shimazu T, Tsugane S. Reproductive factors and gallbladder/bile duct cancer: a population-based cohort study in Japan. Eur J Cancer Prev. 2017;26(4):292–300. https://doi.org/10.1097/CEJ.0000000000000260.

Malhotra SL. Epidemiological study of cholelithiasis among railroad workers in India with special reference to causation. Gut. 1968;9(3):290–5.

Mehrotra R, Tulsyan S, Hussain S, Mittal B, Singh Saluja S, Singh S, Tanwar P, Khan A, Javle M, Hassan MM, Pant S, De Aretxabala X, Sirohi B, Rajaraman P, Kaur T, Rath GK. Genetic landscape of gallbladder cancer: global overview. Mutat Res. 2018;778:61–71. https://doi.org/10.1016/j.mrrev.2018.08.003. Epub 2018 Aug 23. Review.

Menon S, Mathew R. Association between metabolic syndrome and hepatobiliary cancers: a case-control study. Indian J Gastroenterol. 2019;38(1):61–8. https://doi.org/10.1007/s12664-018-0925-y. Epub 2019 Jan 10.

Mhatre S, Rajaraman P, Chatterjee N, et al. Mustard oil consumption, cooking method, diet and gallbladder cancer risk in high- and low-risk regions of India. Int J Cancer. 2020;147(6):1621–8. https://doi.org/10.1002/ijc.32952.

Mishra RR, Tewari M, Shukla HS. Helicobacter species and pathogenesis of gallbladder cancer. Hepatobiliary Pancreat Dis Int. 2010;9(2):129–34. PMID: 20382581.

Mishra SK, Kumari N, Krishnani N. Molecular pathogenesis of gallbladder cancer: an update. Mutat Res. 2019;816–818:111674. https://doi.org/10.1016/j.mrfmmm.2019.111674.

Mlinarić-Vrbica S, Vrbica Z. Correlation between cholelithiasis and gallbladder carcinoma in surgical and autopsy specimens. Coll Antropol. 2009;33(2):533–7.

Moerman CJ, Lagerwaard FJ, Bueno de Mesquita HB, van Dalen A, van Leeuwen MS, Schrover PA. Gallstone size and the risk of gallbladder cancer. Scand J Gastroenterol. 1993;28(6):482–6.

Murphy G, Michel A, Taylor PR, Albanes D, Weinstein SJ, Virtamo J, Parisi D, Snyder K, Butt J, McGlynn KA, Koshiol J, Pawlita M, Lai GY, Abnet CC, Dawsey SM, Freedman ND. Association of seropositivity to Helicobacter species and biliary tract cancer in the ATBC study. Hepatology. 2014;60(6):1963–71. https://doi.org/10.1002/hep.27193. Epub 2014 Jul 30

Nagaraja V, Eslick GD. Systematic review with meta-analysis: the relationship between chronic Salmonella typhi carrier status and gall-bladder cancer. Aliment Pharmacol Ther. 2014;39(8):745–50. https://doi.org/10.1111/apt.12655. Epub 2014 Feb 20. Review.

Narayan RR, Creasy JM, Goldman DA, Gönen M, Kandoth C, Kundra R, Solit DB, Askan G, Klimstra DS, Basturk O, Allen PJ, Balachandran VP, D'Angelica MI, DeMatteo RP, Drebin JA, Kingham TP, Simpson AL, Abou-Alfa GK, Harding JJ, O'Reilly EM, Butte JM, Matsuyama R, Endo I, Jarnagin WR. Regional differences in gallbladder cancer pathogenesis: insights from a multi-institutional comparison of tumor mutations. Cancer. 2019;125(4):575–85. https://doi.org/10.1002/cncr.31850. Epub 2018 Nov 14.

Nishio H, Nagino M, Ebata T, Yokoyama Y, Igami T, Nimura Y. Aggressive surgery for stage IV gallbladder carcinoma; what are the contraindications? J Hepatobiliary Pancreat Surg. 2007;14(4):351–7. Epub 2007 Jul 30

Pai RK, Mojtahed K, Pai RK. Mutations in the RAS/RAF/MAP kinase pathway commonly occur in gallbladder adenomas but are uncommon in gallbladder adenocarcinomas. Appl Immunohistochem Mol Morphol. 2011;19(2):133–40. https://doi.org/10.1097/PAI.0b013e3181f09179.

Pandey M, Gautam A, Shukla VK. ABO and Rh blood groups in patients with cholelithiasis and carcinoma of the gall bladder. BMJ. 1995;310(6995):1639.

Pandey M, Mishra RR, Dixit R, et al. Helicobacter bilis in human gallbladder cancer: results of a case-control study and a meta-analysis. Asian Pac J Cancer Prev. 2010;11(2):343–7.

Randi G, Franceschi S, La Vecchia C. Gallbladder cancer worldwide: geographical distribution and risk factors. Int J Cancer. 2006;118(7):1591–602. Review.

Rao RV, Kumar A, Sikora SS, Saxena R, Kapoor VK. Xanthogranulomatous cholecystitis: differentiation from associated gall bladder carcinoma. Trop Gastroenterol. 2005;26(1):31–3.

Redaelli CA, Büchler MW, Schilling MK, Krähenbühl L, Ruchti C, Blumgart LH, Baer HU. High coincidence of Mirizzi syndrome and gallbladder carcinoma. Surgery. 1997;121(1):58–63.

Roa I, Araya JC, Villaseca M, De Aretxabala X, Riedemann P, Endoh K, Roa J. Preneoplastic lesions and gallbladder cancer: an estimate of the period required for progression. Gastroenterology. 1996;111(1):232–6.

Roa I, Araya JC, Villaseca M, Roa J, de Aretxabala X, Ibacache G. Gallbladder cancer in a high risk area: morphological features and spread patterns. Hepatogastroenterology. 1999;46(27):1540–6.

Roa I, de Aretxabala X, Araya JC, Roa J. Preneoplastic lesions in gallbladder cancer. J Surg Oncol. 2006a; 93(8):615–23. Review.

Roa I, Ibacache G, Roa J, Araya J, de Aretxabala X, Muñoz S. Gallstones and gallbladder cancer-volume and weight of gallstones are associated with gallbladder cancer: a case-control study. J Surg Oncol. 2006b;93(8):624–8.

Roa I, Ibacache G, Muñoz S, de Aretxabala X. Gallbladder cancer in Chile: pathologic characteristics of survival and prognostic factors: analysis of 1,366 cases. Am J Clin Pathol. 2014;141(5):675–82. https://doi.org/10.1309/AJCPQT3ELN2BBCKA.

Saranga Bharathi R, Singh R, Gupta R, Verma GR, Kalra N, Kiran K, Joshi K. Female sex hormone receptors in gallbladder cancer. J Gastrointest Cancer. 2015;46(2):143–8. https://doi.org/10.1007/s12029-015-9698-z.

Scanu T, Spaapen RM, Bakker JM, Pratap CB, Wu LE, Hofland I, Broeks A, Shukla VK, Kumar M, Janssen H, Song JY, Neefjes-Borst EA, te Riele H, Holden DW, Nath G, Neefjes J. Salmonella manipulation of host signaling pathways provokes cellular transformation associated with gallbladder carcinoma. Cell Host Microbe. 2015;17(6):763–74. https://doi.org/10.1016/j.chom.2015.05.002. Epub 2015 May 28.

Serra I, Yamamoto M, Calvo A, Cavada G, Báez S, Endoh K, Watanabe H, Tajima K. Association of chili pepper consumption, low socioeconomic status and longstanding gallstones with gallbladder cancer in a Chilean population. Int J Cancer. 2002;102(4):407–11. Erratum in: Int J Cancer. 2003;104(6):798.

Segura-López FK, Güitrón-Cantú A, Torres J. Association between Helicobacter spp. infections and hepatobiliary malignancies: a review. World J Gastroenterol. 2015;21(5):1414–23. https://doi.org/10.3748/wjg.v21.i5.1414. Review.

Sharma P, Bhunia S, Poojary SS, Tekcham DS, Barbhuiya MA, Gupta S, Shrivastav BR, Tiwari PK. Global methylation profiling to identify epigenetic signature of gallbladder cancer and gallstone disease. Tumour Biol. 2016;37(11):14687–99. Epub 2016 Sep 14

Sharma A, Sharma KL, Gupta A, Yadav A, Kumar A. Gallbladder cancer epidemiology, pathogenesis and molecular genetics: recent update. World J Gastroenterol. 2017;23(22):3978–98. https://doi.org/10.3748/wjg.v23.i22.3978. Review.

Shukla VK, Prakash A, Tripathi BD, Reddy DC, Singh S. Biliary heavy metal concentrations in carcinoma of the gall bladder: case-control study. BMJ. 1998;317(7168):1288–9.

Shukla VK, Rastogi AN, Adukia TK, Raizada RB, Reddy DC, Singh S. Organochlorine pesticides in carcinoma of the gallbladder: a case-control study. Eur J Cancer Prev. 2001;10(2):153–6.

Srivastava M, Sharma A, Kapoor VK, Nagana Gowda GA. Stones from cancerous and benign gallbladders are different: a proton nuclear magnetic resonance spectroscopy study. Hepatol Res. 2008;38(10):997–1005. https://doi.org/10.1111/j.1872-034X.2008.00356.x. Epub 2008 May 27.

Stephen AE, Berger DL. Carcinoma in the porcelain gallbladder: a relationship revisited. Surgery. 2001;129(6):699–703.

Suzuki A, Takahashi T. Histogenesis of the gallbladder carcinoma induced by methylcholanthrene beeswax pellets in hamsters. Jpn J Surg. 1983;13(1):55–9.

Tamrakar D, Paudel I, Adhikary S, Rauniyar B, Pokharel P. Risk factors for gallbladder cancer in Nepal a case control study. Asian Pac J Cancer Prev. 2016;17(7):3447–53.

Tekcham DS, Tiwari PK. Non-coding RNAs as emerging molecular targets of gallbladder cancer. Gene. 2016;588(1):79–85. https://doi.org/10.1016/j.gene.2016.04.047. Epub 2016 Apr 27. Review

Tsuchiya Y, Mishra K, Kapoor VK, Vishwakarma R, Behari A, Ikoma T, Asai T, Endoh K, Nakamura K. Plasma Helicobacter pylori antibody titers and Helicobacter pylori infection positivity rates in patients with gallbladder cancer or cholelithiasis: a hospital-based case-control study. Asian Pac J Cancer Prev. 2018;19(7):1911–5.

Tulsyan S, Hussain S, Mittal B, Saluja SS, Tanwar P, Rath GK, Goodman M, Kaur T, Mehrotra R. A systematic review with in silico analysis on transcriptomic profile of gallbladder carcinoma. Semin Oncol. 2020:S0093-7754(20)30100–7. https://doi.org/10.1053/j.seminoncol.2020.02.012. Epub ahead of print. PMID: 33162112.

Van Dyke AL, Langhamer MS, Zhu B, Pfeiffer RM, Albanes D, Andreotti G, Beane Freeman LE, Chan AT, Freedman ND, Gapstur SM, Giles GG, Grodstein F, Liao LM, Luo J, Milne RL, Monroe KR, Neuhouser ML, Poynter JN, Purdue MP, Robien K, Schairer C, Sinha R, Weinstein S, Zhang X, Petrick JL, McGlynn KA, Campbell PT, Koshiol J. Family history of cancer and risk of biliary tract cancers: results from the biliary tract cancers pooling project. Cancer Epidemiol Biomarkers Prev. 2018;27(3):348–51. https://doi.org/10.1158/1055-9965.EPI-17-1003. Epub 2018 Jan 16.

Vitetta L, Sali A, Little P, Mrazek L. Gallstones and gall bladder carcinoma. Aust N Z J Surg. 2000;70(9):667–73. Review.

Wade KH, Carslake D, Tynelius P, Davey Smith G, Martin RM. Variation of all-cause and cause-specific mortality with body mass index in one million Swedish parent-son pairs: an instrumental variable analysis. PLoS Med. 2019;16(8):e1002868. https://doi.org/10.1371/journal.pmed.1002868. eCollection 2019 Aug.

Wi Y, Woo H, Won YJ, Jang JY, Shin A. Trends in gallbladder cancer incidence and survival in Korea. Cancer Res Treat. 2018;50(4):1444–51. https://doi.org/10.4143/crt.2017.279. Epub 2018 Jan 24.

Wistuba II, Sugio K, Hung J, Kishimoto Y, Virmani AK, Roa I, Albores-Saavedra J, Gazdar AF. Allele-specific mutations involved in the pathogenesis of endemic gallbladder carcinoma in Chile. Cancer Res. 1995;55(12):2511–5.

Yagyu K, Lin Y, Obata Y, Kikuchi S, Ishibashi T, Kurosawa M, Inaba Y, Tamakoshi A, JACC Study Group. Bowel movement frequency, medical history and the risk of gallbladder cancer death: a cohort study in Japan. Cancer Sci. 2004;95(8):674–8.

Yang XW, Yuan JM, Chen JY, Yang J, Gao QG, Yan XZ, Zhang BH, Feng S, Wu MC. The prognostic importance of jaundice in surgical resection with curative intent for gallbladder cancer. BMC Cancer. 2014;14:652. https://doi.org/10.1186/1471-2407-14-652.

Yoshimoto K, Kamisawa T, Kikuyama M, Kuruma S, Chiba K, Igarashi Y. Classification of pancreaticobiliary maljunction and its clinical features in adults. J Hepatobiliary Pancreat Sci. 2019;26:541. https://doi.org/10.1002/jhbp.691.

Zuo M, Rashid A, Wang Y, Jain A, Li D, Behari A, Kapoor VK, Koay EJ, Chang P, Vauthey JN, Li Y, Espinoza JA, Roa JC, Javle M. RNA sequencing-based analysis of gallbladder cancer reveals the importance of the liver X receptor and lipid metabolism in gallbladder cancer. Oncotarget. 2016;7(23):35302–12. https://doi.org/10.18632/oncotarget.9181.

Surgical Pathology of Gall bladder Cancer

5

Vinay K. Kapoor

Biliary tract cancer (BTC) is a heterogeneous group of cancers including histologically similar intrahepatic or cholangiocellular carcinoma (IHC or CCC), extrahepatic perihilar and distal (periampullary or perivaterian) cholangiocarcinoma (CC), and gallbladder cancer (GBC).

5.1 Gross Morphology

Most GBCs occur in the fundus (about 60%) (Fig. 5.1a, b) and/or the body (about 30%) (Fig. 5.2) of the gallbladder (GB); GBC neck (Fig. 5.3) is an uncommon site (10%) for GBC. A GBC in the GB body can cause an hourglass deformity of the GB. GBC neck causes cystic duct obstruction resulting in a mucocele. Cystic duct carcinoma is defined as a GBC either confined (limited) to the cystic duct or the center of which is located in the cystic duct. Yokoyama et al. (2008) classified cystic duct carcinomas based on the geometric center of the tumor into hepatic hilum (HH) and cystic confluence (CC) types; overall median survival was less (11.9 vs. 45.8 months) in HH than in the CC type.

The tumor in GBC is grayish white in color; mucinous tumors may have a gelatinous surface. Gross pathological types include diffuse infiltrative (resulting in a thick-walled GB TWGB), nodular infiltrative (invading through the GB wall into the adjacent organs), ulceroproliferative, and papillary (intraluminal polypoidal) (Fig. 5.4); combined forms may be seen. Wakai (2012) classified GBCs as superficial (elevated, flat, or depressed) and protruding (pedunculated or sessile) types. Papillary (polypoidal cauliflower) tumors result from malignant degeneration of papillary adenoma; they are exfoliative in nature and can have intramural (intraductal) discontiguous embolic spread giving rise to multiple lesions in the GB and/or the CBD. They are less commonly associated with GS; are more common with APBDJ and have associated k-ras mutation. They do not usually infiltrate the adjacent organs and have better prognosis. Most GBCs in India are infiltrating type while in Japan, papillary tumors are more common. This may be one of the reasons for better outcome of GBC in Japan.

Please also see an Invited Commentary on Surgical Pathology of Gall Bladder Cancer by Juan Carlos Roa (pp **_**)

V. K. Kapoor (✉)
Department of Surgical Gastroenterology, Sanjay Gandhi Post-Graduate Institute of Medical Sciences (SGPGIMS), Lucknow, Uttar Pradesh, India
e-mail: vkkapoor.india@gmail.com

V. K. Kapoor (ed.), *A Pictorial Treatise on Gall Bladder Cancer*,
https://doi.org/10.1007/978-981-15-5289-2_5

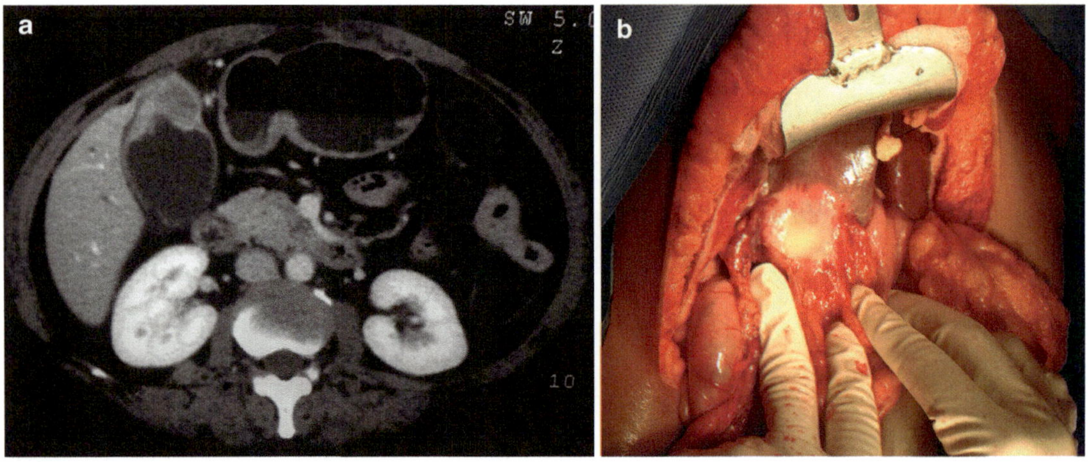

Fig. 5.1 Gallbladder cancer at fundus (**a**) on CT (**b**) at operation

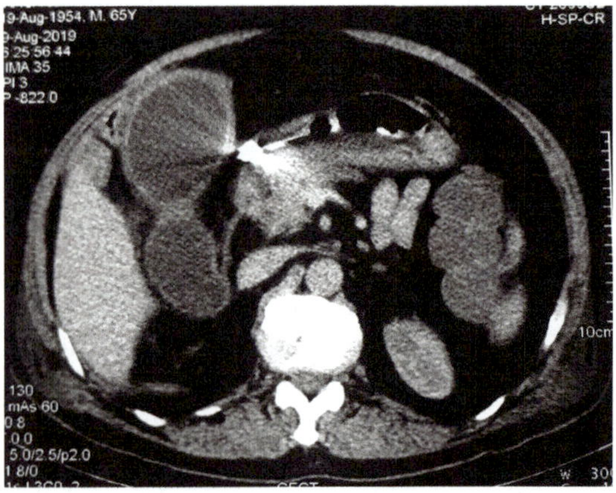

Fig. 5.2 Gallbladder cancer at body producing an hourglass gallbladder

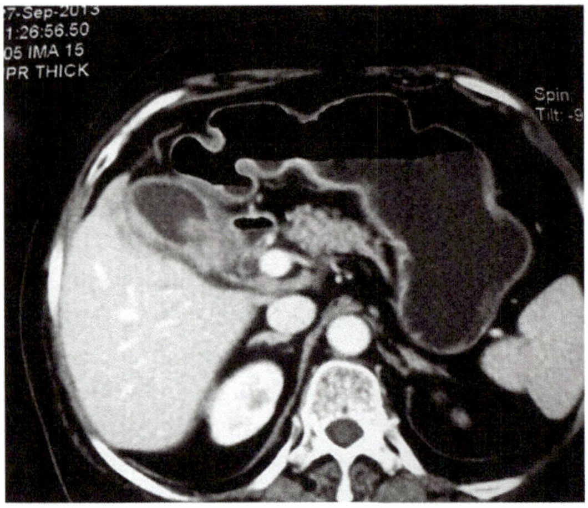

Fig. 5.3 Gallbladder cancer at neck

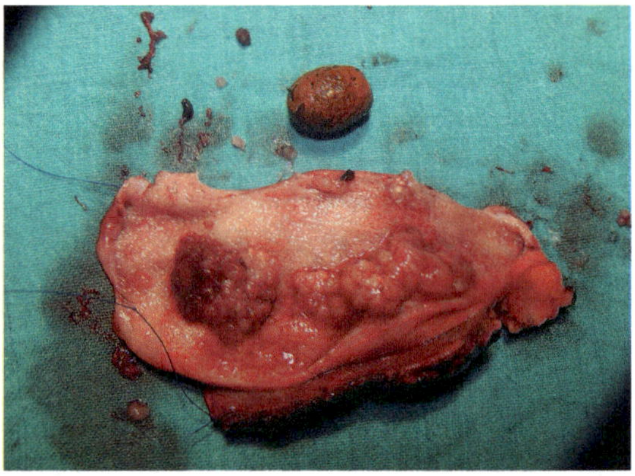

Fig. 5.4 Polypoidal gallbladder cancer; note the multicentricity of the tumor

5.2 Microscopic Pathology

Most GBCs are epithelial in origin. Histologically, adenocarcinoma (Fig. 5.5) is the commonest (90%) type—it could be biliary, gastric, or intestinal type and clear cell, mucinous, or signet ring cell; adenosquamous (Fig. 5.6)/squamous carcinomas are uncommon. Rarely, non-epithelial mesenchymal tumors, e.g., lymphoma, sarcoma, neuroendocrine tumor (NET), and melanoma may be seen in the GB. Benign tumors of GB may be epithelial (adenoma) or mesenchymal (e.g., hemangioma, lipoma, fibroma, etc.). Chronic

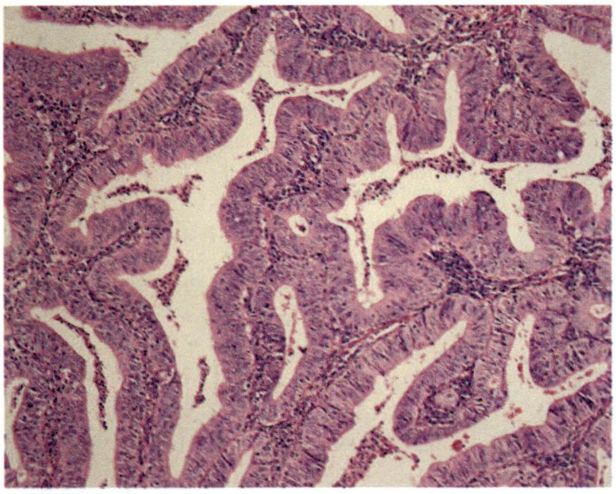

Fig. 5.5 Histologically, most gallbladder cancers are adenocarcinoma

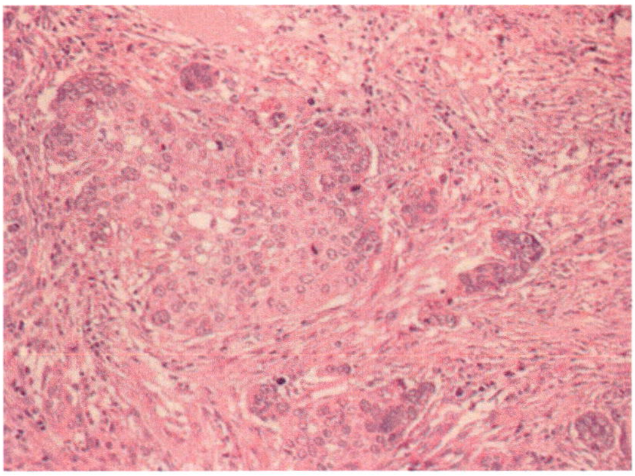

Fig. 5.6 Adenosquamous carcinoma may also be uncommonly seen in the gallbladder

inflammation (cholecystitis) caused by the presence of GS in the GB can cause hyperplasia and metaplasia (gastric or intestinal type) which is very frequently seen in patients with GS and CC. Metaplasia–dysplasia–carcinoma sequence has been proposed as a mechanism of carcinogenesis in GBC. Dysplasia is characterized by nuclear enlargement (increased nucleus:cytoplasm (N:C) ratio), irregularity, hyperchromasia, prominent nucleoli, and loss of polarity. Severe dysplasia and carcinoma-in-situ are found very frequently in the mucosa surrounding the GBC. Biliary intraepithelial neoplasia (BilIN) arising from or extending into the Rokitansky Aschoff (RA) sinuses may look like an invasive carcinoma.

5.2.1 Local Spread

Locally advanced GBC is one which has gone beyond the GB wall into the adjacent organs/structures and/or has spread to the regional lymph nodes. Organs/structures commonly involved in GBC are liver (Fig. 5.7), hepatoduodenal ligament (Fig. 5.8) containing the common bile duct (CBD), proper hepatic artery (PHA) and main portal vein (MPV), duodenum (Fig. 5.9), pancreas (Fig. 5.10), colon (Fig. 5.11), omentum, and parietes. GBC involving liver, CBD, colon, and omentum is resectable. GBC involving the biliary ductal confluence and/or the right portal pedicle can be resected with extended right hepatectomy (ERH) and GBC involving duo-

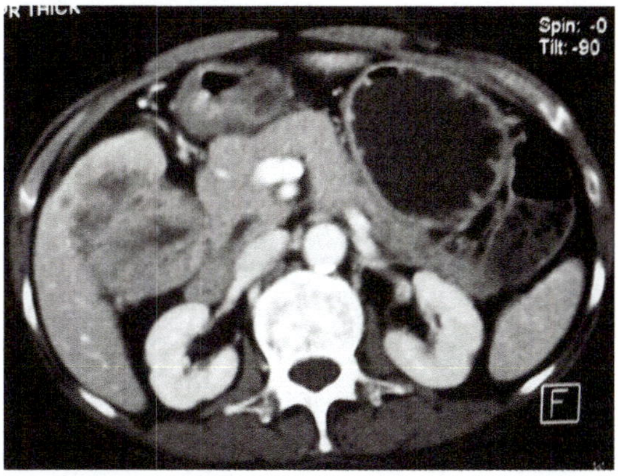

Fig. 5.7 Gallbladder cancer infiltrating liver; liver infiltration requires liver resection in the form of segments IVB + V resection or extended right hepatectomy

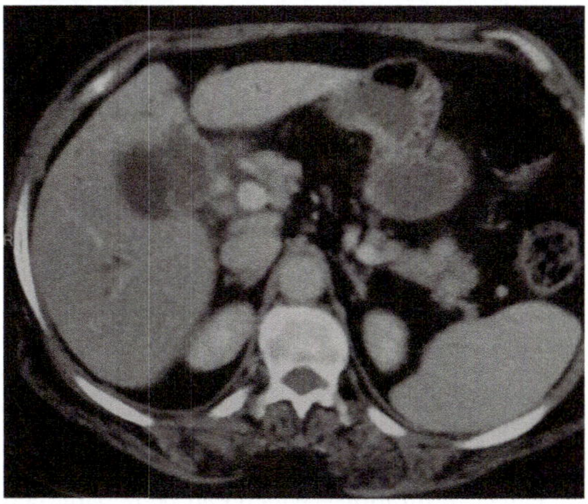

Fig. 5.8 Gallbladder cancer infiltrating the hepatoduodenal ligament; this is unresectable disease

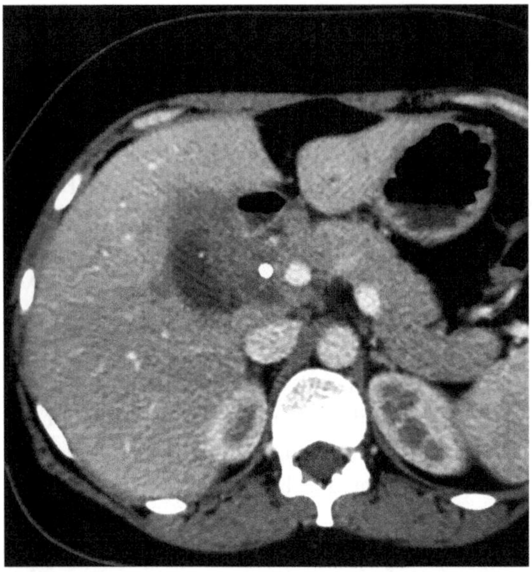

Fig. 5.9 Gallbladder cancer infiltrating the duodenum; duodenal infiltration requires pancreatoduodenectomy or segmental/sleeve resection of the duodenum

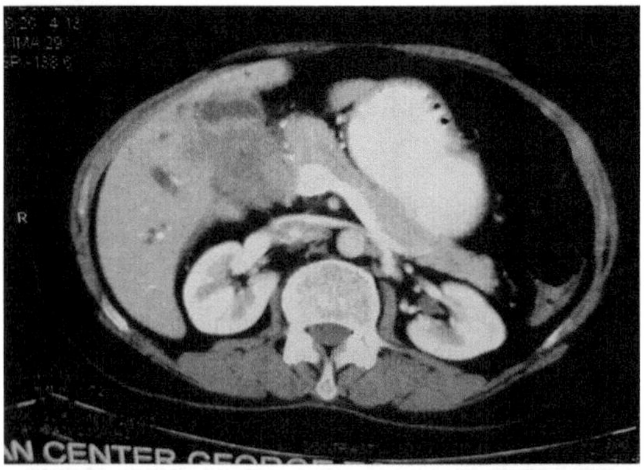

Fig. 5.10 Gallbladder cancer infiltrating the pancreas; pancreatic infiltration requires pancreatoduodenectomy

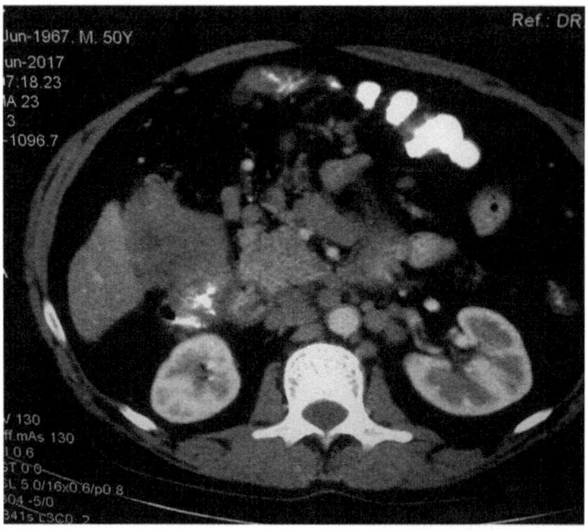

Fig. 5.11 Gallbladder cancer infiltrating the colon; colonic infiltration is not a contraindication for resection and can be managed with segmental colonic resection

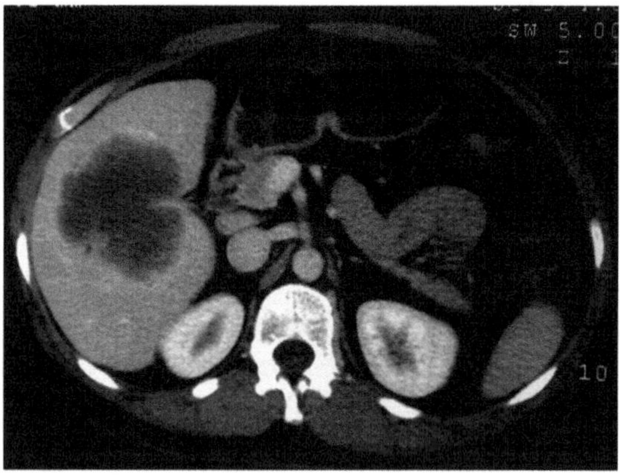

Fig. 5.12 Gallbladder cancer hepatic bed type; this can be managed with liver resection in the form of segments IVB + V resection or extended right hepatectomy

denum/pancreas can be resected if additional pancreatoduodenectomy is performed. GBC involving the proper hepatic artery (PHA) and/or the main portal vein (MPV), though technically resectable (with vascular resection and reconstruction, as in cholangiocarcinoma), is considered unresectable because of poor outcome.

Liver can be involved in GBC by

1. Direct infiltration—which can be hepatic bed type (Fig. 5.12) (an expansive mass) or hepatic hilum type (Fig. 5.13) (infiltrating into the loose connective tissue with lymphovascular invasion (LVI) and perineural invasion (PNI)).
2. Liver metastases due to spread via the cholecysto-hepatic veins.
3. Portal tract invasion including intrahepatic stromal invasion, intrahepatic lymphatic invasion, and intrahepatic venous invasion (Wakai et al. 2010).

Miyazaki et al. (1996) classified involvement of adjacent organs in GBC as follows

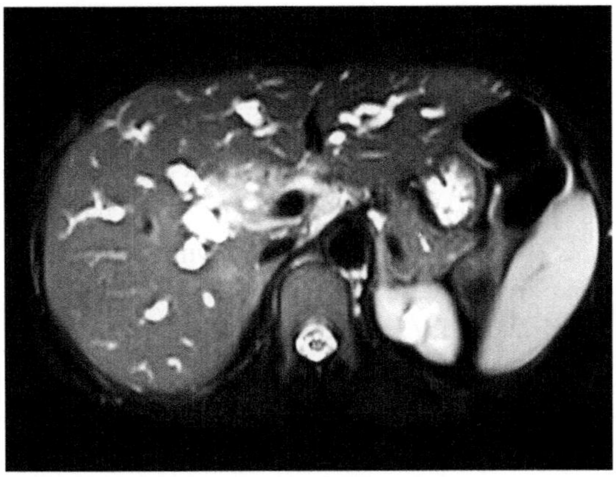

Fig. 5.13 Gallbladder cancer hepatic hilum type; this will require a major liver resection, e.g., extended right hepatectomy along with common bile duct excision

- Type I: a: hepatic involvement
  - b: hepatic involvement + gastrointestinal (gastroduodenal, colonic) involvement
- II: a: bile duct involvement
  - b: bile duct involvement + gastrointestinal (gastroduodenal, colonic) involvement
- III: a: both hepatic and bile duct involvement
  - b: both hepatic and bile duct involvement + gastrointestinal (gastroduodenal, colonic) involvement
- IV: gastrointestinal (gastroduodenal, colonic) involvement alone (without hepatic or bile duct involvement)

Involvement of the hepatoduodenal ligament (proper hepatic artery and main portal vein) and pancreas was, however, not mentioned in this classification.

GBC neck tumor may infiltrate the hepatoduodenal ligament—CBD, proper hepatic artery and main portal vein, and the loose areolar connective tissue in the hepatoduodenal ligament. Kaneoka et al. (2003) defined HDL invasion as a combination of two components—lymph node involvement (LNI) and bile duct invasion (BDI). Shimizu et al. (2004) defined four types of invasion of the HDL:

- I direct extramural spread—this type has the poorest survival in all types
- II continuous intramural spread
- III distant spread from a papillary tumor
- IV spread from metastatic LNs

Hepatoduodenal ligament involvement maybe small in the form of microscopic spread into the loose connective areolar tissues, lymphatic permeation, lymphovascular invasion (LVI), and perineural invasion (PNI) without gross/obvious infiltration of the structures in the hepatoduodenal ligament viz. CBD, proper hepatic artery, and main portal vein which are apparently free (uninvolved)—R0 resection status is difficult to achieve in such cases. Moreover, such involvement of the hepatoduodenal ligament is more frequently associated with paraaortic lymph node (PALN) involvement, which again indicates unresectable disease because of poor prognosis. Perineural invasion (PNI) is a predictor of poor prognosis. It was seen in 48/68 (71%) patients who underwent attempted curative resection—5-year survival was 7% versus 72% in patients with and without perineural invasion (PNI) (Yamaguchi et al. 2002).

Kondo et al. (2002) classified GBC on the basis of the types of tumor spread

1. Hepatic (liver) bed type—a large mass in the GB fundus/body with expansive extension into the liver parenchyma in the GB bed away from the hepatic hilum (porta hepatis)—R0 resection can be achieved with wedge resection or segment IVB + V resection; large amount of infiltration of the liver parenchyma may necessitate a major resection, e.g., extended right hepatectomy (ERH).
2. Hepatic (liver) hilum type—GB neck tumor (not necessarily large) with infiltration into the liver hilum—involvement of the biliary ductal confluence (requires bile duct resection) and/or the proper hepatic artery (PHA) and/or the main portal vein (MPV) (which makes it unresectable) or the right portal pedicle (which requires major hepatectomy) even though the primary tumor may be small.
3. Hepatic bed + hilum type.
4. Lymph node (LN) type (primary tumor being confined to the GB)—extended cholecystectomy (including lymphadenectomy) is adequate.

5. Cystic duct type—small cystic duct tumor infiltrating the CBD (but no liver infiltration)—patient presents with jaundice—can be managed with CBD excision along with extended cholecystectomy.
6. Localized type—localized to the GB—can be treated with extended cholecystectomy.

Kurahara et al. (2018) classified GBC into proximal type, i.e., involving GB neck or cystic duct and distal type, i.e., located in GB body and fundus. Patients with proximal type tumor had >3 metastatic LNs and higher rate of perineural invasion (PNI). Five-year survival was much lower (33% vs. 74%) in proximal type than in distal type.

5.2.2 Lymph Nodal Spread

GBC is characterized by early lymphatic spread which increases with increasing T stage (<5% in T1a, up to 10% in T1b, 40–60% in T2, and about 80% in T3–T4). Japanese surgeons classify regional LNs into

1. First echelon—cystic (12c) (Fig. 5.14), pericholedochal (12b)
2. Second echelon—hepatic artery (12a), periportal (12p), hilar (12h), posterosuperior pancreaticoduodenal (13a) (Fig. 5.15a, b)

Aortocaval (Fig. 5.16a, b), celiac, and superior mesenteric LNs are considered as distant LNs. Lymphatic spread from GBC may, however, not follow a predictable pattern. Cystic LN is not a sentinel LN for GBC—i.e. the disease may spread to other regional LNs without first involving the cystic LN. Hepatoduodenal ligament lymph nodes can compress the CBD and get adhered to the vessels (PHA and MPV) in the hepatoduodenal ligament. LN metastasis is usually diagnosed on cytological examination (image-guided fine needle aspiration

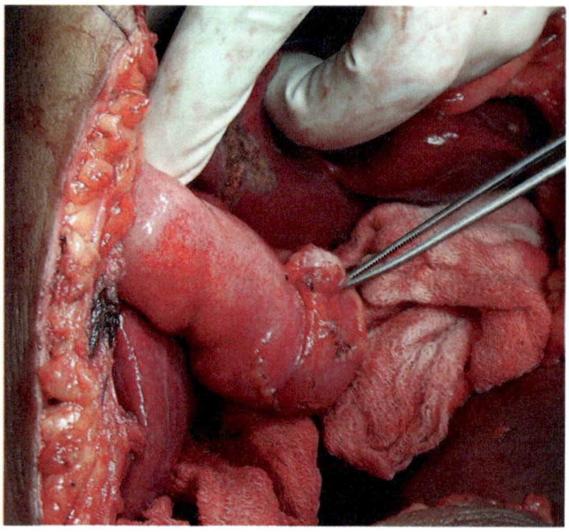

Fig. 5.14 Cystic lymph node is frequently involved in gallbladder cancer but is not a sentinel lymph node

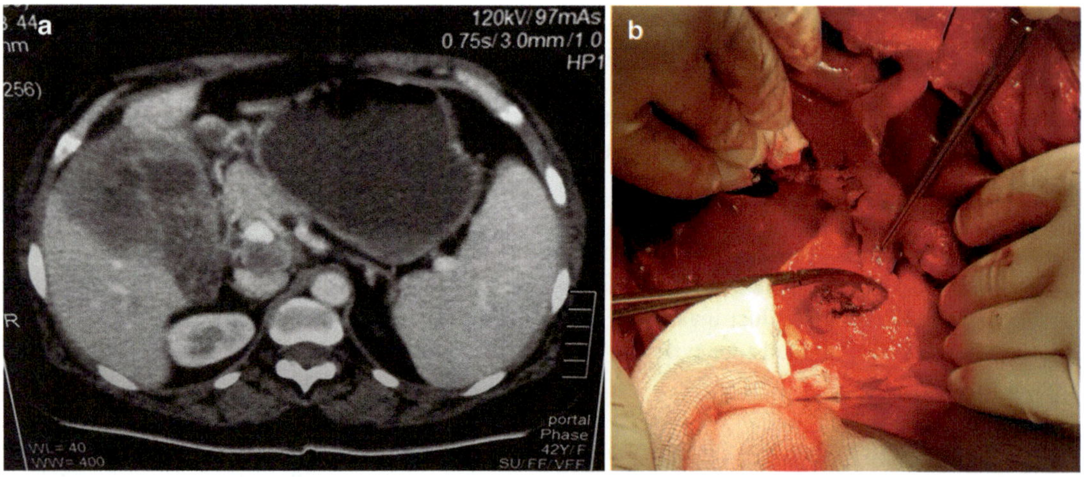

Fig. 5.15 Retroportal lymph node (**a**) on CT (**b**) at operation

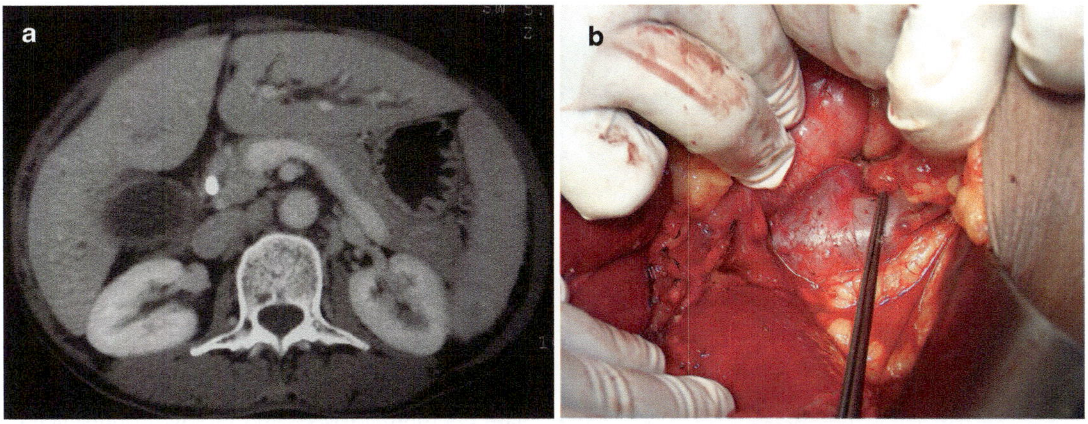

Fig. 5.16 Aortocaval lymph node (**a**) on CT (**b**) at operation

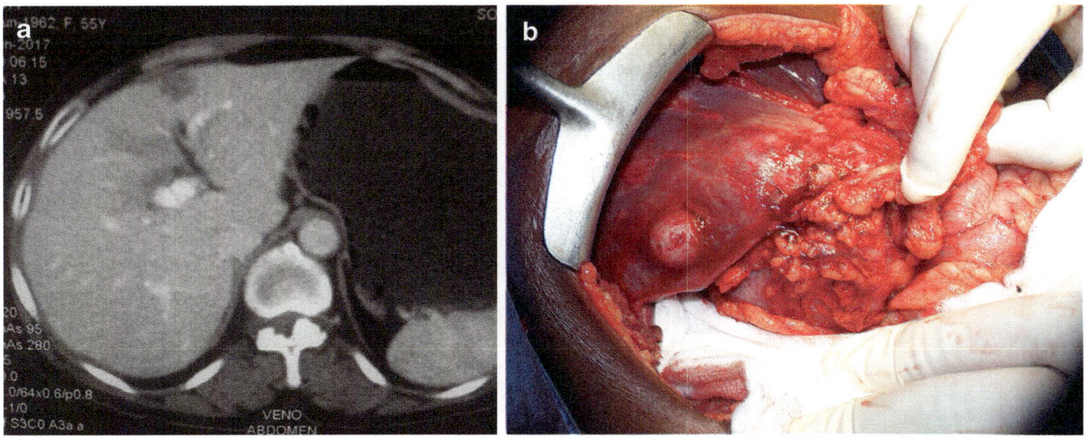

Fig. 5.17 Liver metastasis (**a**) on CT (**b**) at operation

cytology (FNAC)) or histopathological examination of removed LNs. Monoclonal antibody (MCA) against cytokeratins 8 and 18 can be demonstrated in the LNs. Immunohistochemically (IHC) detected metastasis was seen in 23/67 (34%) patients with pT2–4 in whom 1476 nodes were examined—5-year survival was worse (17% vs. 53%) in 23 patients with versus 44 without IHC detected metastasis in the LN (Sasaki et al. 2006). Metastases can occur to LNs at unusual sites, e.g., left supraclavicular, axillary, and inguinal LNs.

5.2.3 Distant Spread

Hematogenous spread results in distant metastases. Blood-borne metastases occur to liver (Fig. 5.17a, b), lungs (Fig. 5.18), bones, and brain; subcutaneous metastases and metastasis to the umbilicus producing a palpable hard umbilical nodule (Fig. 5.19) are rarely seen. GBC with tumor thrombus in the portal vein has been reported (Zhang et al. 2018).

GBC has propensity for transperitoneal spread resulting in peritoneal (Fig. 5.20), omental (Fig. 5.21a, b), diaphragmatic, pelvic (Fig. 5.22), and ovarian deposits, diffuse peritoneal dissemination (carcinomatosis), needle tract implantation following percutaneous interventions, e.g., FNAC, percutaneous transhepatic biliary drainage (PTBD): and port site metastases (PSM) (Fig. 5.23) following laparoscopic cholecystectomy.

GB may be involved in Hodgkin's lymphoma, and myeloma. Metastases can occur to the GB from a primary tumor in the GI tract, renal cell carcinoma (RCC), melanoma, and bronchogenic carcinoma.

5.3 Prognosis

Histological features, e.g., poor differentiation (Fig. 5.24a, b), lymphovascular invasion (LVI) (Fig. 5.25), and perineural invasion (PNI) (Fig. 5.26) in the primary tumor and pericapsular invasion (PCI) in the LNs indicate aggressive biology and poor outcome; threshold for adjuvant chemotherapy should be low in presence of any of these features.

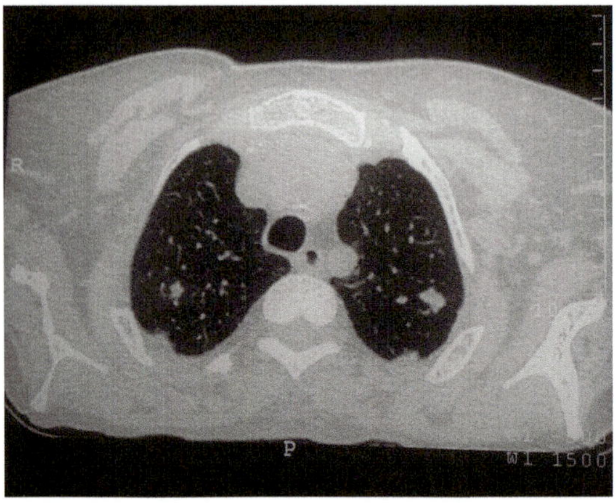

Fig. 5.18 Bilateral lung nodules on CT chest

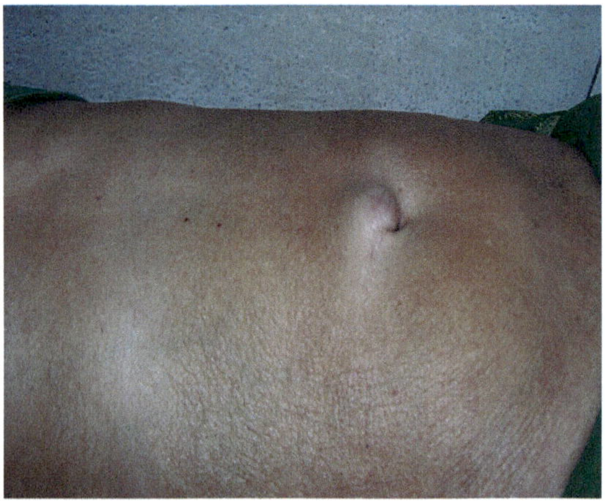

Fig. 5.19 Umbilical metastatic nodule

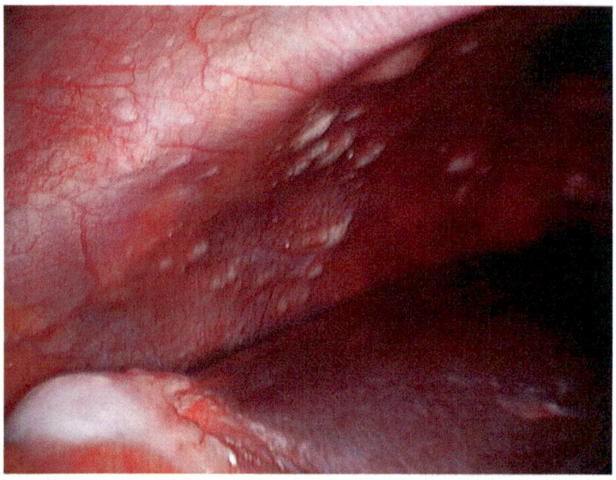

Fig. 5.20 Peritoneal metastatic nodules seen on staging laparoscopy

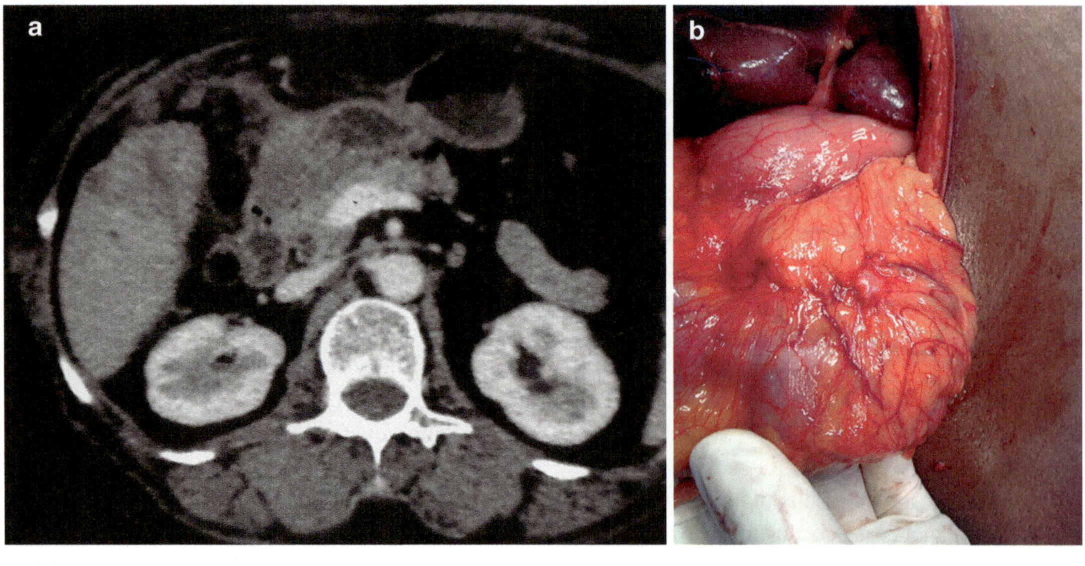

Fig. 5.21 Omental metastatic nodule (**a**) on CT (**b**) at operation

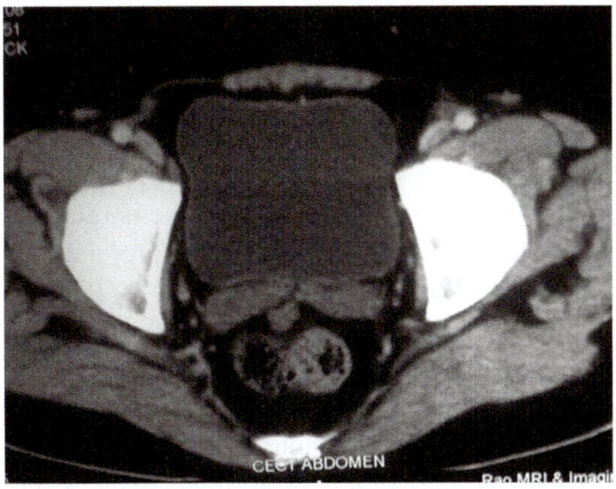

Fig. 5.22 Pelvic metastatic deposit

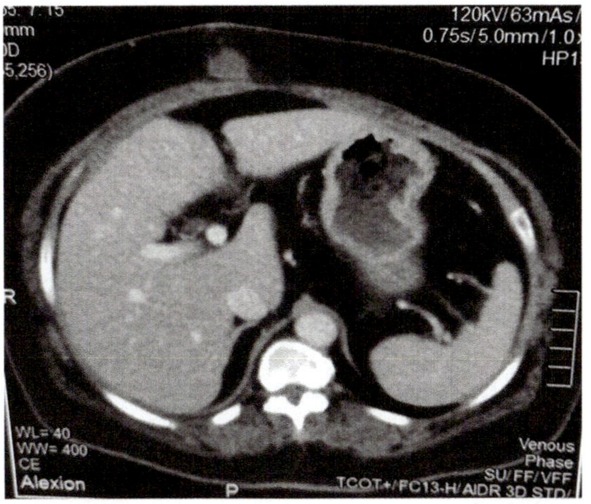

Fig. 5.23 Port site metastasis after laparoscopic cholecystectomy

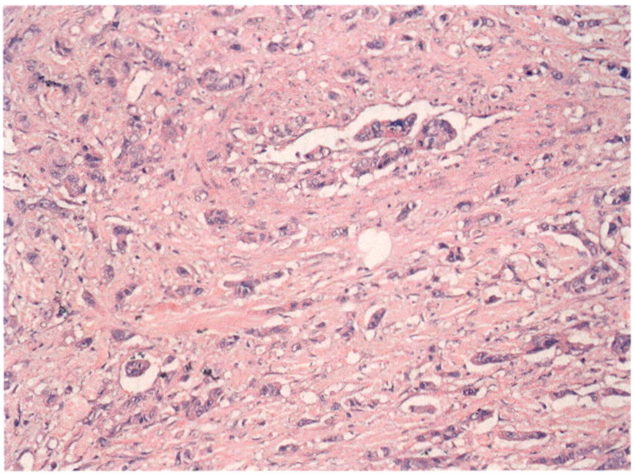

Fig. 5.25 Lymph-vascular invasion (LVI) in the primary tumor indicates poor prognosis

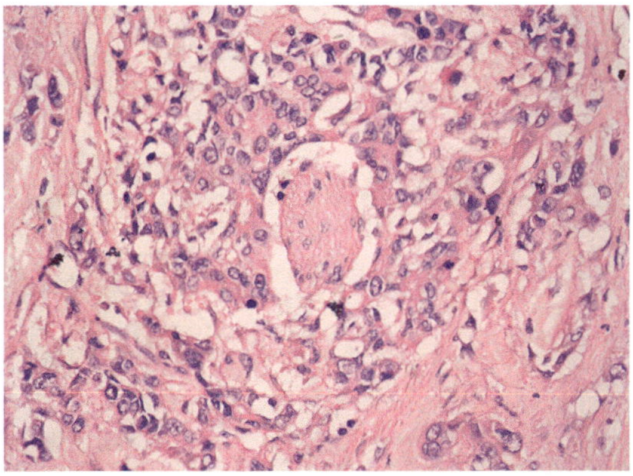

Fig. 5.26 Perineural invasion (PNI) in the primary tumor indicates poor prognosis

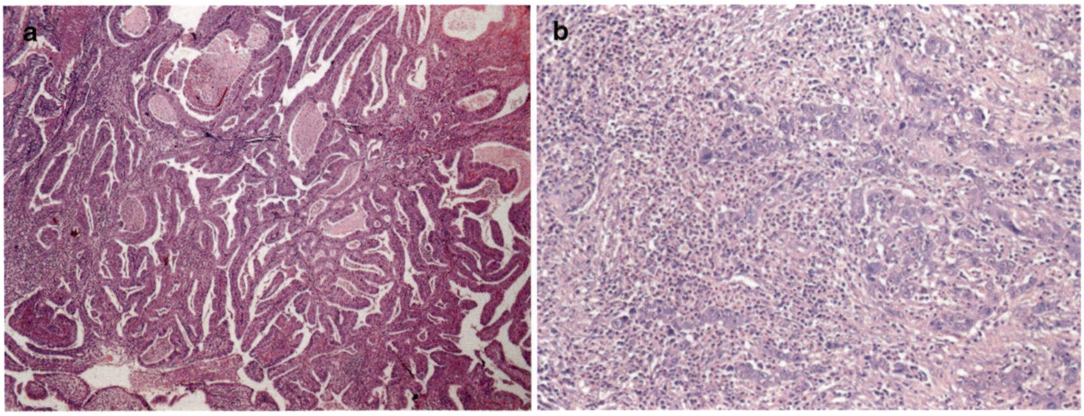

Fig. 5.24 (**a**) Well-differentiated tumors have a better prognosis than (**b**) poorly differentiated tumors

5.4 Benign Conditions

5.4.1 Xantho-Granulomatous Cholecystitis (XGC)

Xantho-granulomatous cholecystitis (XGC) is an uncommon variant of CC. It is a destructive inflammatory process caused by extravasation of bile from the GB lumen into the GB wall through a mucosal ulcer (tear). XGC is seen as diffuse (cf. focal in GBC) GB wall thickness of >3 mm on US (thick-walled GB TWGB). A TWGB on US merits further evaluation with CT and/or MRI. CT shows diffuse GB wall thickening, continuous mucosal enhancement, luminal surface enhancement (LSE) with focal breach in mucosa, submucosal hypodense nodules (Fig. 5.27) or bands in the GB wall, even mass formation with infiltration of adjacent structures, e.g., liver, CBD, duodenum, colon, etc., and lymph node enlargement. MRI also shows diffusely TWGB (Fig. 5.28). It is, however, difficult to differentiate XGC from malignant (GBC) TWGB even after imaging (US, CT, MRI, and PET). At operation, dense adhesions may be seen between GB and omentum, duodenum, and colon. GB wall is diffusely thickened, sometimes even more than 1 cm (Fig. 5.29). A mass may be present which may be infiltrating adjacent organs and may even have lymphadenopathy XGC is invariably associated with GS; CBD stones or Mirizzi's syndrome are frequently present. Grayish or brownish-yellow nodules/streaks are present in the diffusely thick GB wall (Fig. 5.30).

XGC mimics GBC clinically, on imaging and even, at operation and may undergo EC with a suspicion of GBC: most reports of EC done for a preoperative or intraoperative presumed diagnosis of GBC include a significant proportion of patients who are finally found to have XGC on histopathological examination (Rammohan et al. 2014). There

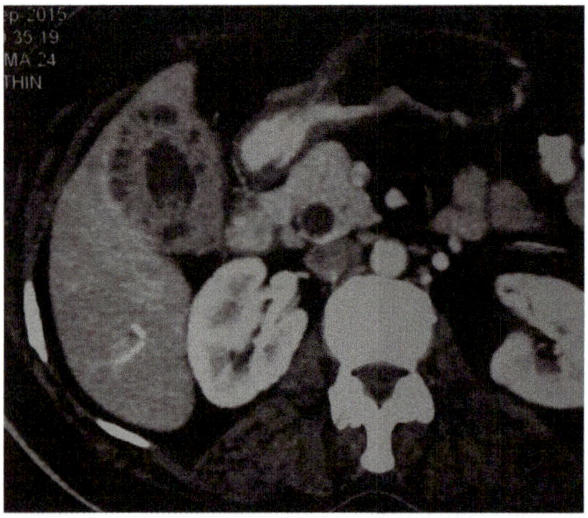

Fig. 5.27 CT shows diffuse thick-walled gallbladder (TWGB) with hypodense nodules in the gallbladder wall—xantho-granulomatous cholecystitis (XGC)

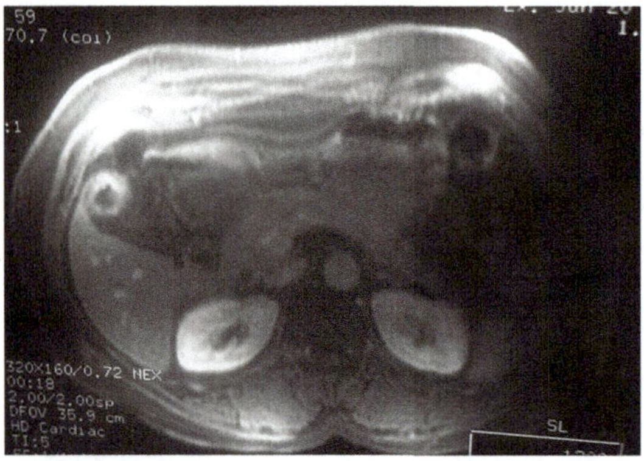

Fig. 5.28 MRI shows diffuse thick walled gallbladder (TWGB)—xantho-granulomatous cholecystitis (XGC)

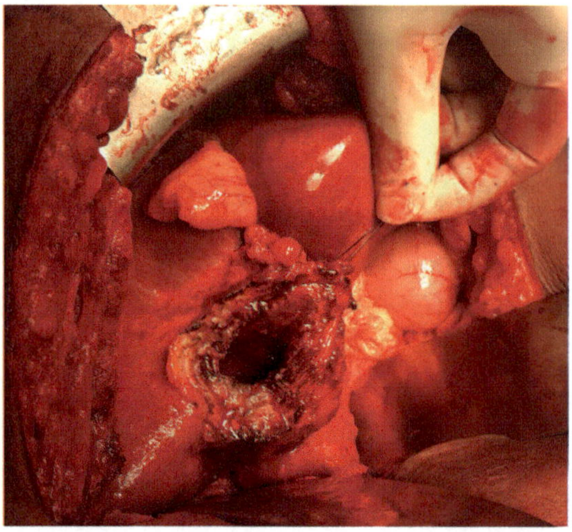

Fig. 5.29 GB wall is diffusely thickened (GB has been opened at the fundus to remove the stones and examine the GB mucosa from inside as the Calot's triangle was obliterated)

are even reports of major resections in patients with XGC with a preoperative diagnosis of GBC.

Histopathology (Fig. 5.31) shows foam (xanthoma) cells—lipid and bile laden macrophages (histiocytes), acute and chronic inflammatory cells, microabscesses in the GB wall, severe fibrosis, and even atypia. XGC may coexist in as many as 10% of cases of GBC; at the same time, a small focus of malignancy in a GB with XGC may be missed by the pathologist resulting in recurrence of cancer at a later date during the follow-up (missed GBC).

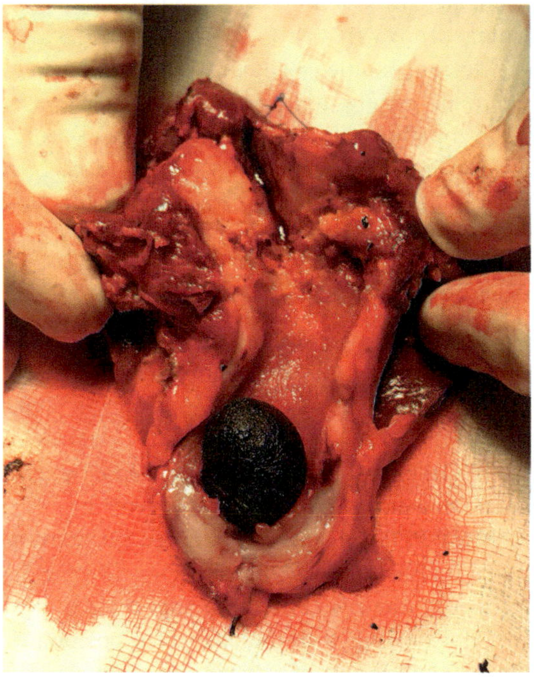

Fig. 5.30 Diffusely thick-walled GB (TWGB) with yellowish nodules in GB wall—xantho-granulomatous cholecystitis (XGC)

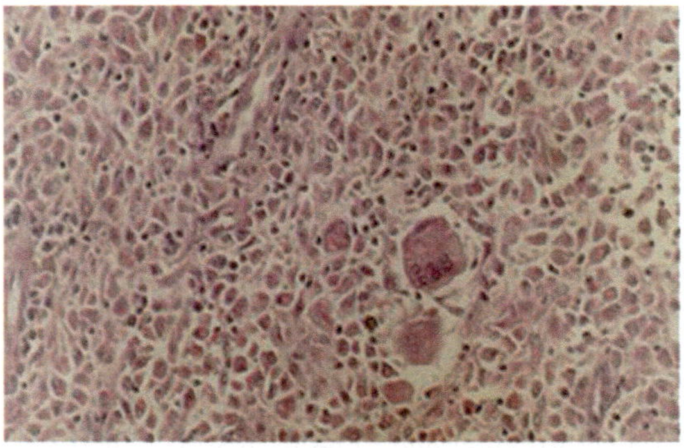

Fig. 5.31 Microphotograph shows foamy macrophages—xantho-granulomatous cholecystitis (XGC)

5.4.2 GB Polyp

Polypoidal lesions of the GB (PLG or PLGB) are mucosal outgrowths or elevations presenting as protuberant lesions of the GB wall into its lumen. They may be pedunculated (polyp) or sessile (nodule), and may have a smooth, granular, or cauliflower surface.

More and more PLGBs are being detected as an incidental finding on ultrasonography (US) following easy and universal availability and application of abdominal US in the evaluation of any and every abdominal symptoms whether related to the GI/HPB, urinary, or genital system. A wide range of prevalence, i.e., 0.3–12% has been reported in various series.

PLGB can be

1. Neoplastic
   (a) Epithelial
   Benign, i.e., adenoma (Fig. 5.32)—the most common neoplastic PLGB but still only 5% of all PLGBs; usually (90%) single, may be sessile or pedunculated
   Malignant, i.e., adenocarcinoma
   (b) Mesenchymal (fibroma, lipoma, leiomyoma)—rare
2. Non-neoplastic (pseudopolyp)
   (a) Cholesterol polyp—the commonest (60%) PLGB. Cholesterol polyps are usually small and multiple (Fig. 5.33); they

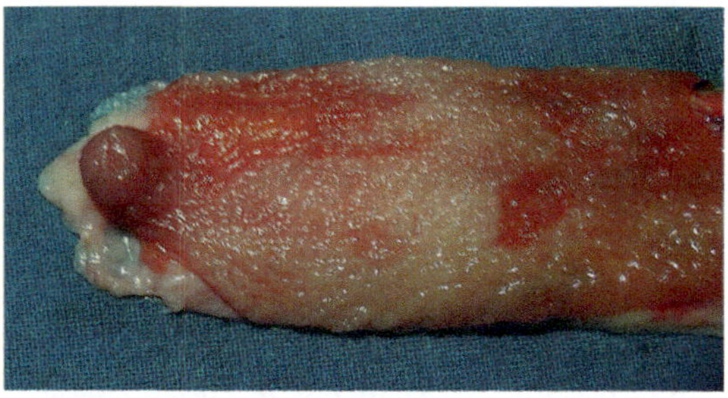

Fig. 5.32 Adenomatous polyp

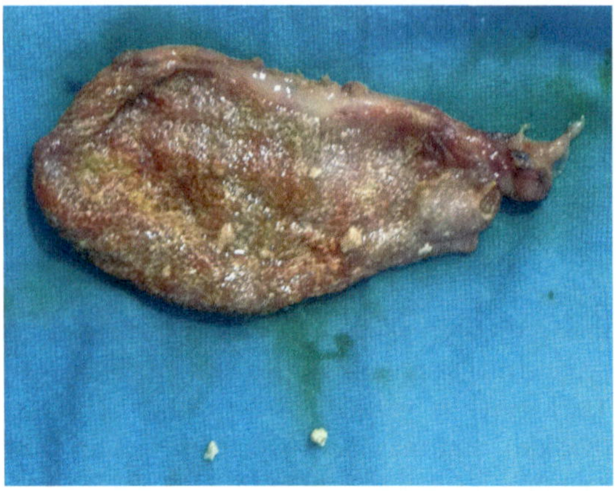

Fig. 5.33 Multiple cholesterol polyps

are echogenic on US but without posterior acoustic shadowing (cf. GS)
(b) Adenomyomatosis (25%) has a characteristic comet tail appearance
(c) Inflammatory (10%)

Large majority of PLGBs detected on US turn out to be pseudopolyps; only about 5% are true polyps, i.e., adenoma or adenocarcinoma. Histopathologically, they may be tubular, papillary, or tubulo-papillary.

Adenoma may be associated with Peutz Jeghers (PJS) and Gardner syndromes. Only neoplastic polyp, i.e., adenoma, has malignant potential. Unlike in colorectum, adenoma-carcinoma sequence is a less common mechanism of carcinogenesis in GBC; inflammation—dysplasia—carcinoma being more common.

Most PLGBs are asymptomatic; even if any symptoms, e.g., dyspepsia, are present they are usually not due to the polyp meaning thereby that the cause of symptoms, e.g., gastroduodenal or pancreatic disease has to be investigated and that they are very likely to persist after cholecystectomy; counseling of the patient before cholecystectomy is, therefore, very important. PLGBs may, though uncommonly, cause biliary colic or acute cholecystitis (due to cystic duct obstruction) or rarely acute cholangitis (a fragment of the polyp breaking off and "embolizing" in the CBD). PLGBs are not usually associated with GS; when a PLGB is associated with GS, it is usually impossible to say whether the symptoms are caused by

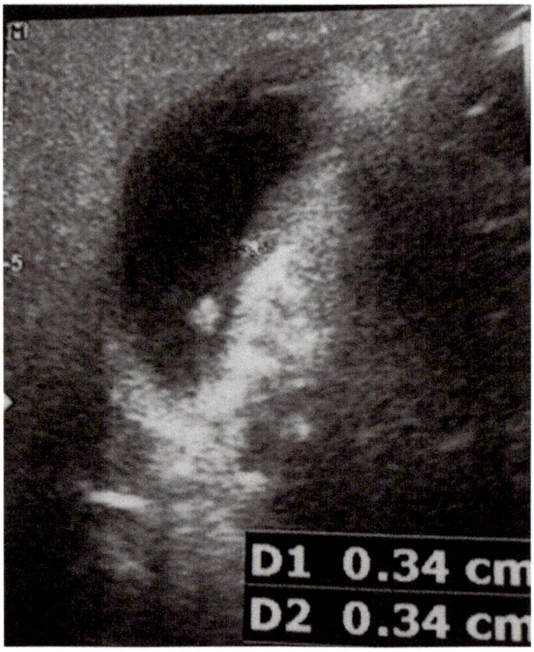

Fig. 5.34 US shows a small gallbladder polyp—at operation, it turned out to be a stone adherent to the gallbladder mucosa

the PLGB or the stone but it is immaterial because the treatment is same, i.e., cholecystectomy.

Most PLGBs can be diagnosed on conventional transabdominal US using a low (2–5 MHz) frequency transducer. A polyp appears as a fixed (i.e. not moving with the change in position of the patient) lesion cf. stones which move (i.e. change their position) and do not have posterior acoustic shadowing (cf. stones, which have); an impacted GS may, however, not move on US and look like a polyp (Fig. 5.34). Hypoechoic foci are seen in neoplastic polyps. Once diagnosed on US, the PLGBs are better evaluated by a high-resolution US (HRUS) using a 5–7 MHz transducer. HRUS had 90% sensitivity and 63% accuracy which was better than even EUS (86% and 56%) and CT (72% and 44%) to diagnose malignancy in 144 patients with PLGB >1 cm (Jang et al. 2009). Contrast-enhanced US (CEUS) using perflubutane or galactose palmitic acid shows heterogeneous contrast enhancement and dilated, irregular and tortuous vessels in neoplastic polyps (Miwa et al. 2019). Quantitative CEUS has been shown to differentiate between neoplas-

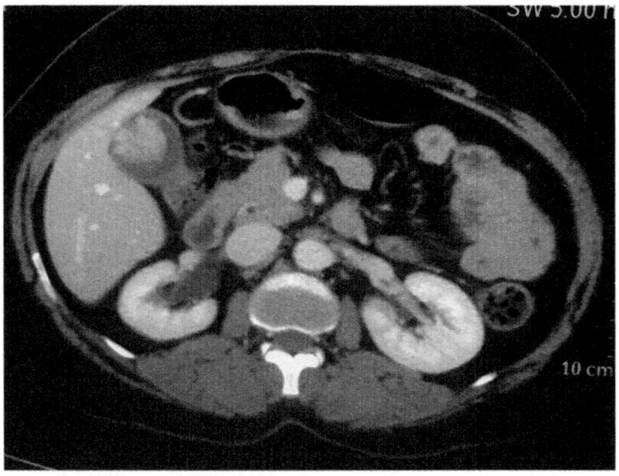

Fig. 5.35 CT shows a large gallbladder polyp—it turned out to be gallbladder cancer

tic (*n* = 17) and nonneoplastic polyps (*n* = 12) with high sensitivity and specificity (Bae et al. 2019). Real-time color Doppler US shows strong blood flow in neoplastic polyps. Endoscopic US (EUS) using high (5–12 MHz) frequency transducer is semi-invasive with risks of bleeding and perforation. Contrast-enhanced EUS has also been used. CT (Fig. 5.35) and MRI are more for staging of GBC than for evaluation of PLGB. A sludge ball may look like a polyp on US, CT, or MRI. Diffusion-weighted MRI shows lower apparent diffusion coefficient (ADC) rates in malignant polyps. On dual time point, i.e., early (62 min) and delayed (146 min) imaging postinjection PET/CT, SUV max of polyp/SUV mean of liver >1.14 suggests malignancy (Nishiyama et al. 2006). Tumor markers, e.g., CEA and CA 19.9 are not of much value to detect malignancy in a PLGB. Intravenous (IV) cholecystography and percutaneous transhepatic cholecystoscopy have been described but are rarely used as they are invasive.

The key issue in the management of a PLGB is whether it has a malignant potential or is already malignant. Management of a PLGB depends on several factors—i. patient related, e.g., age, ethnicity, symptoms, fitness for surgery, fear of risk of cancer; i.e. GB–related, e.g., associated GS, GB wall thickness; i.e. polyp–related, e.g., size, number, stalk, and iv. social factors. Increasing age (50 or 60+), single or few (<3) in number, large (>10 mm) size, enlarging (on serial US every 3–6 months), sessile, associated GS, and polyp in primary sclerosing cholangitis (PSC) are risk factors for malignancy in a PLGB. Comorbidities and fitness for surgery, biliary symptoms, and patient attitude, i.e., fear of or anxiety about risk of malignancy, eager or unwilling for surgery, willing for regular, long-term follow-up, or unlikely to come back for follow-up, are also considered while deciding for or against the operation. The most important factor, which dictates the management of a PLGB, i.e., whether cholecystectomy or only follow-up, is its size. The European Association for Endoscopic Surgery (EAES) and European Society of Gastrointestinal Endoscopy (ESGE) guidelines (Wiles et al. 2017) state that a large (>18 mm) polyp should be treated as GBC. On the other hand, a small (<4 mm) polyp has virtually no risk of malignancy. These are, however, arbitrary cutoffs with very soft data to support them. In an analysis of 256 benign and 35 malignant PLGBs—age >60 year (OR 8.2), single sessile polyp (OR 7.7), and size >10 mm (OR 8.9) were found to be risk factors for malignancy (Kwon et al. 2009). European Society of Gastrointestinal and Abdominal Radiology (ESGAR) guidelines use 10 mm (>6 mm for sessile polyp; 6–9 mm Indian ethnicity) as cutoff, but in a systematic review, (Bhatt et al. 2016), a significant number of malignant polyps were less than 10 mm in size but the probability of malignancy was virtually 0 when it was <4.5 mm. As many as one-third (32%) of 524 PLGBs <1 cm in size were neoplastic (123 premalignant and 61 malignant) and 27% of PLGBs >1 cm in size were nonneoplastic (Wennmacker et al. 2019). Some reports (Zielinski et al. 2009) suggest a cutoff of 6 mm; this will pick up 90% of neoplastic polyps but cholecystectomy rate for nonneoplastic polyps will increase to 50%. Several other risk factors are also taken into account along with size. Age >50 years—probability of malignancy is 20% even if the polyp is <10 mm. Solitary sessile polyp has a high probability of malignancy and should be operated. Indian ethnicity was a risk factor for malignancy in PLGB (Wiles et al. 2017). Prevalence of cancer in PLGB was much higher (5.5% vs. 0.1%) in patients with Indian ethnic background as compared to Caucasians (Aldouri et al. 2009). Polyp in PSC should be operated irrespective of size; 71 (16%) of 453 patients with PSC had GBP—cholecystectomy was performed in 17—3 were found to have GBC (van Erp et al. 2020).

Natural history of GBPs is not very well known—27 patients who were found to have PLGB in 2002 were followed up in 2013—polyps disappeared in 13/27 and persisted in 14/27. The number increased in 6, decreased in 6, and remained the same in 2. Size increased in 5, decreased in 7, and remained the same in 2 (Heitz 2019).

PLGBs are important because GBC has an extremely poor prognosis. One has to aim to strike a balance between missing (i.e. not operating upon) a malignant or premalignant polyp on one hand and doing an unnecessary operation for a pseudopolyp on the other. Single large sessile polyp or a polyp in an elderly patient, or a patient of East Asian or South Asian ethnicity, a polyp with focal GB wall thickening, or with intralesional blood flow or in a patient with PSC may be operated irrespective of its size (Sun 2019). While every cholecystectomy should be safe, every attempt must be made to ensure that cholecystectomy for an asymptomatic polyp is safe. Surveillance of a polyp which is not operated upon involves two US scans at 6-month intervals—a 2-mm increase in size indicates surgery. If there is no increase in size, yearly US scans should be done for 5 years.

5.4.3 Adenomyomatosis

Adenomyomatous hyperplasia is an acquired degenerative disease characterized by proliferation of mucosal epithelium, which invaginates and extends into the thickened muscularis propria causing intramural diverticula. US shows multiple anechoic areas in the GB wall—the pearl necklace or comet tail appearance; but only 71 (47%) out of 150 GBs with comet tail artifacts found on US turned out to be adenomyomatosis the remaining were CC (n = 74) cholesterosis (n = 3), and XGC (n = 2) (Oh 2019). CT shows the rosary sign showing mucosal epithelium with intramural diverticula (Pang 2018). Adenomyomatosis can be focal (localized) or diffuse; focal adenomyomatosis carries a higher risk of GBC.

5.4.4 Porcelain GB

Porcelain (calcified) GB (Fig. 5.36a, b) is the effect of long-standing inflammation—end-stage GB disease. Focal stippled mucosal calcification carries a higher risk of GBC.

5.4.5 ICPN

Intra-cholecystic papillary-tubular neoplasm (ICPN) homologous to intraductal papillary mucinous neoplasm (IPMN) of pancreas and bili-

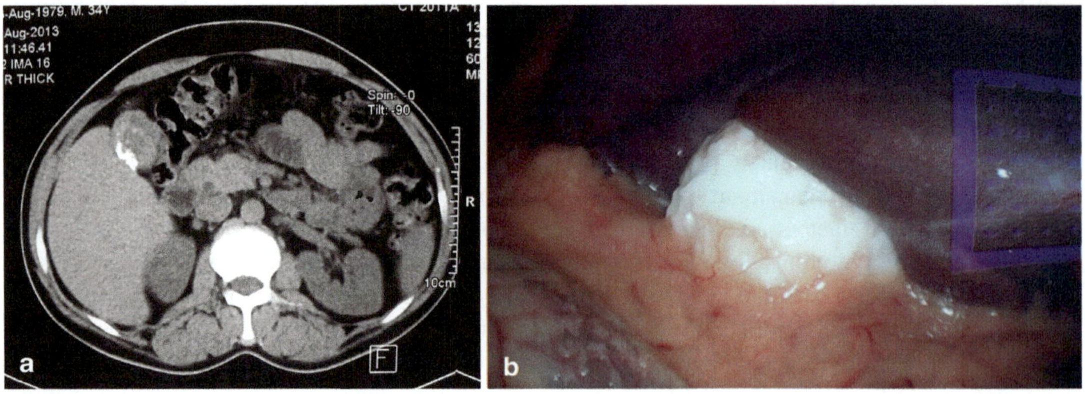

Fig. 5.36 Porcelain (calcified) gallbladder (**a**) on CT (**b**) at operation

ary intraductal papillary neoplasm of the bile duct is a mass forming neoplastic lesion of the GB. Biliary phenotype and papillary configuration are associated with invasive adenocarcinoma component (Kiruthiga et al. 2019)—it may look like adenomyomatosis on imaging but needs radical resection. Diligent long-term follow-up is required as ICPN may be associated with other biliary malignancies.

Several benign conditions of the GB viz. xantho-granulomatous cholecystitis (XGC), GB polyp, and adenomyomatosis can mimic GBC.

Invited Commentary on Surgical Pathology of Gallbladder Cancer

Juan Carlos Roa

Some anatomical and histological aspects of the gallbladder are important to understanding the surgical pathology and prognostic value of morphological aspects of gallbladder cancer (GBC). The absence of muscularis mucosae tunic as well as the characteristic presence of its discontinuous muscle layer offer less resistance to tumor infiltration. The presence of diverticular structures of mucosa that can reach even the subserosal layer (Rokitansky–Aschoff sinuses (RAS)) also promotes easy spread of the disease. This is similar to what is seen in diverticulosis of the colon, caused by increased intra-vesicular pressure. In a normal gallbladder, there are no glandular structures but rather a coating of glandular epithelium of the mucosa that is gradually replaced by pseudopyloric and/or intestinal metaplasia in the histogenic sequence of GBC produced by inflammation related to GB stone disease (Espinoza et al. 2016). For the diagnosis of pre-neoplastic lesions, it is extremely difficult to have uniformity about infiltration among pathologists from the East and West (Vieth et al. 2014; Adsay et al. 2016).

Unlike other organs, the histological analysis of GB lesions has methodological limitations because the pathologist examines only a small fraction of the total surface of the lesion; therefore, he must trust empirically that what is observed in these sections corresponds to the real condition of the entire surgical specimen, unaware of what happens spatially in front of and behind the histological section analyzed. This aspect is particularly important when the mucosal lesions extend to the Rokitansky–Aschoff sinuses, there is no obvious infiltration of the muscle layer but the tumor behaves in terms of survival similar to subserosal tumors (pT2). For this reason, the extension of early GBC (pT1a) to RAS should potentially be considered for a wedge liver resection and selective lymphadenectomy (Roa et al. 2013).

The position of the GB under the liver and its partial peritoneal lining incorporate variables that should be considered when processing and reporting on surgical pathology. This has been published to be useful specifically in the subserosal tumor group (pT2). In the liver-side lesion (without positive surgical margin), patients have a lower survival and have benefited by a second surgery with liver resection and selective lymphadenectomy (Shindoh et al. 2015).

There is a no standard protocol for processing the cholecystectomy specimen for screening, which can make it possible to identify most pre-neoplastic and neoplastic lesions with the fewest number of histological sections needed to avoid overburdening the pathology laboratory (Aloia et al. 2015; Koshiol et al. 2018). This deficiency also extends to the nomenclature used to diagnose flat and polypoid pre-neoplastic lesions although this was addressed in the last classification of tumors by introducing concepts and definitions such as ICNNs and pyloric gland adenoma (Roa et al. 2019). Additionally, the absence of a protocolized full mapping in the event of early lesions (pT1a, T1b) or subserosal cases (pT2) (Memis et al. 2016), which would ensure detection of the maximum infiltration of the vesicular wall, prevents the reproducibility of studies conducted on different populations, affecting not only the consolidation of knowledge about surgical pathology of GBC but also the comparison of different groups of patients who undergo surgical treatment and/or adjuvant therapies (Akkas et al. 2015).

Most lesions are caused de novo associated with lithiasis-related inflammation in the metaplasia-dysplasia-carcinoma sequence (usually extensive flat lesions) and not the less frequent histogenic adenoma-carcinoma sequence apparently more related to non-lithiasic inflammatory conditions (e.g., biliary pancreatic abnormal junction) (Roa et al. 1996; Roa and Arias 2011). They make understandable a high frequency of incidental GBC (one-third of advanced carcinomas and two-thirds of early carcinomas), the granular macroscopic or micropapillary pattern of which is often undetectable in the absence of careful, standardized gross processing in the pathological anatomy laboratory (Goldin and Roa 2009).

Due to the endoscopic inaccessibility of the GB and the fact that once it is removed it becomes impossible to follow its evolution, the accumulated knowledge regarding the histogenic/carcinogenic pathways of GB has basically been gained through extrapolation and recapitulation of information from other neoplasms of the digestive tract such as colo-rectal cancer, gastric and intestinal carcinoma, and adenocarcinoma developing in Barrett's esophagus or inflammatory bowel disease carcinoma. This makes it absolutely necessary to develop a good animal model associated with lithiasis inflammation as a tool to further discover and plan new prevention and treatment strategies.

Finally, it is important to emphasize that the modern molecular genetic analysis of these tumors will certainly be important for prognostic stratification, therapy selection, and predictive purposes. Beyond that, however, is the correct and complete handling and sampling of the cholecystectomy (neoplastic and non-neoplastic) surgical specimen as well as the anatomopathological report of pre-neoplastic and neoplastic lesions, which includes on the one hand a standardized nomenclature and on the other the morphological aspect that has been shown to have prognostic value and ensures maximum wall depth infiltration for a correct categorization of the pT. To date, these are the main prognostic elements that help determine the management of patients with GBC (Roa et al. 2014).

References

Chapter References

Aldouri AQ, Malik HZ, Waytt J, Khan S, Ranganathan K, Kummaraganti S, Hamilton W, Dexter S, Menon K, Lodge JP, Prasad KR, Toogood GJ. The risk of gallbladder cancer from polyps in a large multiethnic series. Eur J Surg Oncol. 2009;35(1):48–51. https://doi.org/10.1016/j.ejso.2008.01.036. Epub 2008 Mar 12

Bae JS, Kim SH, Kang HJ, Kim H, Ryu JK, Jang JY, Lee SH, Paik WH, Kwon W, Lee JY, Han JK. Quantitative contrast-enhanced US helps differentiating neoplastic vs non-neoplastic gallbladder polyps. Eur Radiol. 2019;29(7):3772–81. https://doi.org/10.1007/s00330-019-06123-w. Epub 2019 Apr 8

Bhatt NR, Gillis A, Smoothey CO, Awan FN, Ridgway PF. Evidence based management of polyps of the gall bladder: a systematic review of the risk factors of malignancy. Surgeon. 2016;14(5):278–86. https://doi.org/10.1016/j.surge.2015.12.001. Epub 2016 Jan 26. Review

Heitz L, Kratzer W, Gräter T, Schmidberger J; EMIL study group. Gallbladder polyps - a follow-up study after 11 years. BMC Gastroenterol. 2019;19(1):42. https://doi.org/10.1186/s12876-019-0959-3. PMID: 30885181; PMCID: PMC6423886.

Jang JY, Kim SW, Lee SE, Hwang DW, Kim EJ, Lee JY, Kim SJ, Ryu JK, Kim YT. Differential diagnostic and staging accuracies of high resolution ultrasonography, endoscopic ultrasonography, and multidetector computed tomography for gallbladder polypoid lesions and gallbladder cancer. Ann Surg. 2009;250(6):943–9. https://doi.org/10.1097/SLA.0b013e3181b5d5fc.

Kaneoka Y, Yamaguchi A, Isogai M, Harada T, Suzuki M. Hepatoduodenal ligament invasion by gallbladder carcinoma: histologic patterns and surgical recommendation. World J Surg. 2003;27(3):260–5. https://doi.org/10.1007/s00268-002-6702-0.

Kiruthiga KG, Kodiatte TA, Burad D, Kurian R, Raju RS, Rymbai ML, Jagannathan AM, Vyas FL. Intracholecystic papillary-tubular neoplasms of the gallbladder - a clinicopathological study of 36 cases. Ann Diagn Pathol. 2019;40:88–93. https://doi.org/10.1016/j.anndiagpath.2019.04.014.

Kondo S, Nimura Y, Kamiya J, Nagino M, Kanai M, Uesaka K, Hayakawa N. Mode of tumor spread and surgical strategy in gallbladder carcinoma. Langenbecks Arch Surg. 2002;387(5–6):222–8. Epub 2002 Oct 2

Kurahara H, Maemura K, Mataki Y, Sakoda M, Iino S, Kawasaki Y, Mori S, Arigami T, Kijima Y, Shinchi H, Natsugoe S. Indication of extrahepatic bile duct resection for gallbladder cancer. Langenbecks Arch Surg. 2018;403(1):45–51. https://doi.org/10.1007/s00423-017-1620-7. Epub 2017 Sep 5

Kwon W, Jang JY, Lee SE, Hwang DW, Kim SW. Clinicopathologic features of polypoid lesions of the gallbladder and risk factors of gallbladder cancer.

J Korean Med Sci. 2009;24(3):481–7. https://doi.org/10.3346/jkms.2009.24.3.481. Epub 2009 Jun 12
Miwa H, Numata K, Sugimori K, Sanga K, Hirotani A, Tezuka S, Goda Y, Irie K, Ishii T, Kaneko T, Tanaka K, Maeda S. Differential diagnosis of gallbladder polypoid lesions using contrast-enhanced ultrasound. Abdom Radiol (NY). 2019;44(4):1367–78. https://doi.org/10.1007/s00261-018-1833-4.
Miyazaki M, Itoh H, Ambiru S, Shimizu H, Togawa A, Gohchi E, Nakajima N, Suwa T. Radical surgery for advanced gallbladder carcinoma. Br J Surg. 1996;83(4):478–81.
Nishiyama Y, Yamamoto Y, Fukunaga K, Kimura N, Miki A, Sasakawa Y, Wakabayashi H, Satoh K, Ohkawa M. Dual-time-point 18F-FDG PET for the evaluation of gallbladder carcinoma. J Nucl Med. 2006;47(4):633–8. Erratum in: J Nucl Med. 2006;47(8):1266.
Oh SH, Han HY, Kim HJ. Comet tail artifact on ultrasonography: is it a reliable finding of benign gallbladder diseases? Ultrasonography. 2019;38(3):221–30. https://doi.org/10.14366/usg.18029. Epub 2018 Oct 3. PMID: 30481951; PMCID: PMC6595125.
Pang L, Zhang Y, Wang Y, Kong J. Pathogenesis of gallbladder adenomyomatosis and its relationship with early-stage gallbladder carcinoma: an overview. Braz J Med Biol Res. 2018;51(6):e7411. https://doi.org/10.1590/1414-431x20187411. Epub 2018 May 21. PMID: 29791592; PMCID: PMC6002143.
Rammohan A, Cherukuri SD, Sathyanesan J, Palaniappan R, Govindan M. Xanthogranulomatous cholecystitis masquerading as gallbladder cancer: can it be diagnosed preoperatively? Gastroenterol Res Pract. 2014;2014: 253645. https://doi.org/10.1155/2014/253645. Epub 2014 Oct 27.
Sasaki E, Nagino M, Ebata T, Oda K, Arai T, Nishio H, Nimura Y. Immunohistochemically demonstrated lymph node micrometastasis and prognosis in patients with gallbladder carcinoma. Ann Surg. 2006;244(1): 99–105.
Shimizu Y, Ohtsuka M, Ito H, Kimura F, Shimizu H, Togawa A, Yoshidome H, et al. Should the extrahepatic bile duct be resected for locally advanced gallbladder cancer? Surgery. 2004;136(5):1012–1017; . discussion 1018. https://doi.org/10.1016/j.surg.2004.04.032.
Sun Y, Yang Z, Lan X, Tan H. Neoplastic polyps in gallbladder: a retrospective study to determine risk factors and treatment strategy for gallbladder polyps. Hepatobiliary Surg Nutr. 2019;8(3):219–27. https://doi.org/10.21037/hbsn.2018.12.15. PMID: 31245402; PMCID: PMC6561872.
van Erp LW, Cunningham M, Narasimman M, Ale Ali H, Jhaveri K, Drenth JPH, Janssen HLA, Levy C, Hirschfield GM, Hansen BE, Gulamhusein AF. Risk of gallbladder cancer in patients with primary sclerosing cholangitis and radiographically detected gallbladder polyps. Liver Int. 2020;40(2):382–92. https://doi.org/10.1111/liv.14326. Epub 2019 Dec 20
Wakai T, Shirai Y, Sakata J, Nagahashi M, Ajioka Y, Hatakeyama K. Mode of hepatic spread from gallbladder carcinoma: an immunohistochemical analysis of 42 hepatectomized specimens. Am J Surg Pathol. 2010;34(1):65–74. https://doi.org/10.1097/PAS.0b013e3181c467d4.
Wakai T, Ajioka Y, Nagino N, Yamaguchi N, Shirai Y, Hatakeyama K. Morphological features of early gallbladder carcinoma. Hepatogastroenterology. 2012;59(116):1013–7. https://doi.org/10.5754/hge11923. PMID: 22366390.
Wennmacker SZ, van Dijk AH, Raessens JHJ, van Laarhoven CJHM, Drenth JPH, de Reuver PR, Nagtegaal ID. Polyp size of 1 cm is insufficient to discriminate neoplastic and non-neoplastic gallbladder polyps. Surg Endosc. 2019;33(5):1564–71. https://doi.org/10.1007/s00464-018-6444-1. Epub 2018 Sep 10.
Wiles R, Thoeni RF, Barbu ST, Vashist YK, Rafaelsen SR, Dewhurst C, Arvanitakis M, Lahaye M, Soltes M, Perinel J, Roberts SA. Management and follow-up of gallbladder polyps: joint guidelines between the European Society of Gastrointestinal and Abdominal Radiology (ESGAR), European Association for Endoscopic Surgery and other Interventional Techniques (EAES), International Society of Digestive Surgery - European Federation (EFISDS) and European Society of Gastrointestinal Endoscopy (ESGE). Eur Radiol. 2017;27(9):3856–66. https://doi.org/10.1007/s00330-017-4742-y. Epub 2017 Feb 9
Yamaguchi R, Nagino M, Oda K, Kamiya J, Uesaka K, Nimura Y. Perineural invasion has a negative impact on survival of patients with gallbladder carcinoma. Br J Surg. 2002;89(9):1130–6.
Yokoyama Y, Nishio H, Ebata T, Abe T, Igami T, Oda K, Nimura Y, Nagino M. New classification of cystic duct carcinoma. World J Surg. 2008;32(4):621–6. https://doi.org/10.1007/s00268-007-9324-8.
Zhang XZ, Tu JJ, Chen W, Ma T, Bai XL, Liang TB. Gallbladder cancer with tumor thrombus in the portal vein: a case report. Medicine (Baltimore). 2018;97(16):e0271. https://doi.org/10.1097/MD.0000000000010271.
Zielinski MD, Atwell TD, Davis PW, Kendrick ML, Que FG. Comparison of surgically resected polypoid lesions of the gallbladder to their pre-operative ultrasound characteristics. J Gastrointest Surg. 2009;13(1):19–25. https://doi.org/10.1007/s11605-008-0725-2. Epub 2008 Oct 30

References for Commentary Notes

Adsay V, et al. Epithelial atypia in the gallbladder: diagnosis and classification in an international consensus study. Pancreas and biliary tree. Mod Pathol. 2016;29:438–51. https://doi.org/10.1038/modpathol.2016.19.
Akkas G, et al. Pathologic diagnosis as the reason for wide discrepancies in the literature regarding the incidence and behavior of T1 gallbladder cancer (GBC): an analysis of 473 GBC and comparison with literature.

Pancreas and biliary tree. Mod Pathol. 2015;28:438–52. https://doi.org/10.1038/modpathol.2015.25.

Aloia TA, Járufe N, Javle M, Maithel SK, Roa JC, Adsay V, Coimbra FJ, Jarnagin WR. Gallbladder cancer: expert consensus statement. HPB (Oxford). 2015;17(8):681–90. https://doi.org/10.1111/hpb.12444.

Espinoza JA, Bizama C, Garcia P, Ferreccio P, Javle M, Miguel JF, et al. The inflammatory inception of gallbladder cancer. Biochim Biophys Acta. 2016;1865(2):245–54. https://doi.org/10.1016/j.bbcan.2016.03.004. Epub 2016 Mar 12. Review.

Goldin RD, Roa JC. Gallbladder cancer: a morphological and molecular update. Histopathology. 2009;55(2):218–29. https://doi.org/10.1111/j.1365-2559.2008.03192.x. Epub 2009 Mar 12. Review.

Koshiol J, Bellolio E, Vivallo C, Cook P, Roa JC, McGee EE, Losada H, Van Dyke AL, Van De Wyngard V, Prado R, Villaseca M, Riquelme P, Acevedo J, Olivo V, Pettit K, Hildesheim A, Medina K, Memis B, Adsay V, Ferreccio C, Araya JC. Distribution of dysplasia and cancer in the gallbladder: an analysis from a high cancer-risk population. Hum Pathol. 2018;82:87–94. https://doi.org/10.1016/j.humpath.2018.07.015. Epub 2018 Jul 21.

Memis B, et al. Prognosis of T2 gallbladder carcinomas: an analysis of 326 cases highlights a prognosis better than the current impression in the West, but incomparably worse than what is reported in Asia. Pancreas and biliary tree. Mod Pathol. 2016;29:438–51. https://doi.org/10.1038/modpathol.2016.19.

Roa JC, Arias JAC. Molecular genetic alterations in preneoplastic and neoplastic lesions of the gallbladder. In: Field cancerization: basic science and clinical applications. New York: Nova Science Publishers, Inc.; 2011. p. 241–76.

Roa I, Araya JC, Villaseca M, De Aretxabala X, Riedemann P, Endoh K, Roa J. Preneoplastic lesions and gallbladder cancer: an estimate of the period required for progression. Gastroenterology. 1996;111(1):232–6.

Roa JC, Tapia O, Manterola C, Villaseca M, Guzman P, Araya JC, Bagci P, Saka B, Adsay V. Early gallbladder carcinoma has a favorable outcome but Rokitansky–Aschoff sinus involvement is an adverse prognostic factor. Virchows Arch. 2013;463(5):651–61. Epub 2013 Sep 11. Erratum in: Virchows Arch. 2013;463(6):851.

Roa I, Ibacache G, Muñoz S, de Aretxabala X. Gallbladder cancer in Chile: pathologic characteristics of survival and prognostic factors: analysis of 1,366 cases. Am J Clin Pathol. 2014;141(5):675–82. https://doi.org/10.1309/AJCPQT3ELN2BBCKA.

Roa J, Adsay NV, et al. Carcinoma of the gallbladder. In: WHO Classification of Tumours Editorial Board, editor. Digestive system tumours, vol. 1. Lyon: IARC; 2019. p. 283–8.

Shindoh J, de Aretxabala X, Aloia TA, Roa JC, Roa I, Zimmitti G, Javle M, Conrad C, Maru DM, Aoki T, et al. Tumor location is a strong predictor of tumor progression and survival in T2 gallbladder cancer: an international multicenter study. Ann Surg. 2015;261(4):733–9. https://doi.org/10.1097/SLA.0000000000000728.

Vieth M, Riddell RH, Montgomery EA. High-grade dysplasia versus carcinoma: east is east and west is west, but does it need to be that way? Am J Surg Pathol. 2014;38(11):1453–6. https://doi.org/10.1097/PAS.0000000000000288.

6 Clinical Presentation of Gall Bladder Cancer

Vinay K. Kapoor

The National Comprehensive Cancer Network (NCCN 2015) has described four modes of presentation of gall bladder cancer (GBC)

1. Incidental finding at surgery
2. Incidental finding at histopathology
3. Mass on imaging
4. Jaundice

The Author (VKK), however, disagrees with this terminology as GBC detected at surgery is not "incidental".

6.1 Presentations

The Author (Kapoor et al. 1996) had earlier suggested a nomenclature based on the time in clinical presentation at which a diagnosis (or suspicion) of GBC is made.

1. Obvious—(also called overt GBC in some reports) clinically evident, viz. dull continuous non-colicky pain in the right upper abdomen, jaundice, gastric outlet obstruction (GOO), anorexia and weight loss, and palpable GB mass (cf. distended GB of mucocele due to gall stone disease GSD).
2. Suspected—clinical picture (symptoms and signs) is suggestive of benign GSD, i.e., biliary colic, a distended GB (mucocele) may be palpable but a suspicion of GBC is raised on imaging (US/CT) which shows GB wall thickening, mass, or polyp.
3. Unsuspected—preoperative (clinical as well as imaging) diagnosis is benign, i.e., GSD and there is no suspicion of malignancy on imaging but at operation (laparoscopy or laparotomy), the GB is found to be thick walled and/or there is difficulty in dissection of the GB from its bed in the liver or there is a suspicious finding, viz. wall thickening, nodule, polyp, or ulcer (which should then be subjected to frozen section histopathological examination) on gross examination of the GB specimen (Fig. 6.1).
4. Incidental—preoperative and even intraoperative diagnosis is benign, i.e., GSD and there is no suspicion of malignancy even on gross examination of the GB specimen; GBC is found for the first time on histopathological examination of the GB specimen. This, according to the Author (VKK), is true incidental GBC.
5. Missed—either the GB was not sent for histopathological examination (because it looked grossly normal) or an early GBC was missed

Please also see Invited Commentaries on Clinical Presentation of Gall Bladder Cancer by Yuman Fong (pp **–**), Pradeep Ghimire (pp **–**) and Prabin Bikram Thapa (pp **–**)

V. K. Kapoor (✉)
Department of Surgical Gastroenterology, Sanjay Gandhi Post-Graduate Institute of Medical Sciences (SGPGIMS), Lucknow, Uttar Pradesh, India
e-mail: vkkapoor.india@gmail.com

V. K. Kapoor (ed.), *A Pictorial Treatise on Gall Bladder Cancer*,
https://doi.org/10.1007/978-981-15-5289-2_6

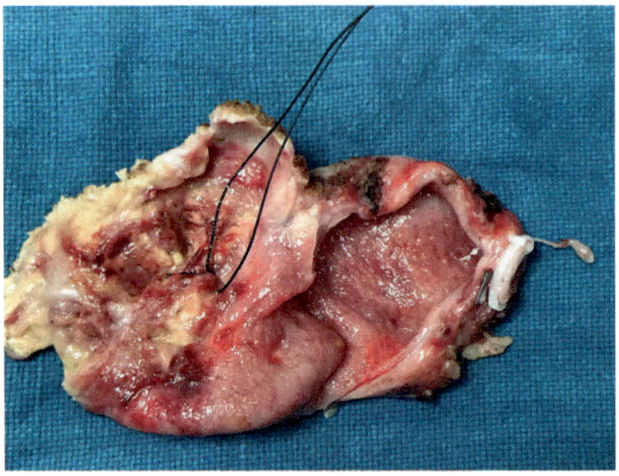

Fig. 6.1 During cholecystectomy for presumed gall stone disease if the specimen reveals a wall thickening, nodule, polyp, or ulcer, it should be called unsuspected (NOT incidental) gall bladder cancer

even by the pathologist on routine histopathological examination of the GB.

Relative proportion of these presentations varies depending on the incidence rates of GBC in the geographical area/ethnic group, the level of index of suspicion of GBC and prevalence and timing of cholecystectomy for GSD. In high GBC incidence areas with a high index of suspicion of GBC and/or low prevalence rates and delayed timing of cholecystectomy for GSD, e.g., India and Japan, obvious/suspected GBC is more common and incidental GBC is less common. At the Tokyo Women's Medical University Japan, only 26 (7%) out of 389 GBCs who underwent surgery between 1969 and 2012 were incidental (Higuchi et al. 2014). On the other hand, 37% of 669 GBC cases in Chile were incidental (Roa et al. 1999). In low GBC incidence areas with a low index of suspicion of GBC and high prevalence rates and early timing of cholecystectomy for GBC, e.g., the USA, obvious/suspected GBC is less common and incidental GBC is more common. Less than one-third of GBCs in the USA are diagnosed preoperatively; majority are diagnosed either at operation or on histopathology. In the USA, 47% of 435 GBCs were incidental (Duffy et al. 2008). In the 10-institution Extrahepatic Biliary Malignancy Consortium in the USA, out of 445 patients with GBC who underwent resection, 266 (60%) were incidental GBC (Ethun et al. 2017). Butte et al. (2011) compared patients with GBC treated in the USA ($n = 130$), Chile ($n = 85$), and Japan ($n = 46$); only 15% of GBCs treated in Japan were incidental (cf. 60% in the USA).

6.2 Symptoms

GBC, in its early stages (i.e., when it is confined to the GB wall), can remain silent (asymptomatic) for a long time. Even when symptomatic, it has no pathognomonic clinical features to enable early diagnosis as symptoms of early GBC are either vague or nonspecific, e.g., dyspepsia or indigestion, or mimic those of GSD, i.e., biliary colic and chronic cholecystitis. Even ultrasonography (US) does not pick up early GBC; these patients undergo cholecystectomy with a preoperative diagnosis of GSD and GBC is suspected either at operation or in the GB specimen on gross examination (unsuspected GBC) or is serendipitously detected after histopathological examination of the grossly normal GB (incidental GBC).

Symptomatic GBC presents with a wide range of symptoms including local, metastatic, and cancer related. Commonest symptom of obvious GBC is pain but patients with GBC may have pain (biliary colic) due to associated GS also; there may be a change in the character of pain from long standing intermittent biliary colic to recent dull continuous diffuse pain (because of local infiltration) in the right upper quadrant or epigastrium of the abdomen. Pain was present in 89% of 385 patients reported by Mishra et al. (2017). Jaundice is seen in about one-fourth to one-third of patients with clinically obvious GBC. Jaundice was seen in 110/424, 26% (Regimbeau et al. 2011), 82/240, 34% (Hawkins et al. 2004), 152/385, 39% (Mishra et al. 2017), and 65/179, 40% (Ethun et al. 2017) patients with GBC. GBC is the commonest cause of malignant jaundice in north India (Sikora et al. 1994). These patients present with yellow eyes (and skin), high colored urine (Fig. 6.2), clay colored stools, and may have associated pruritus.

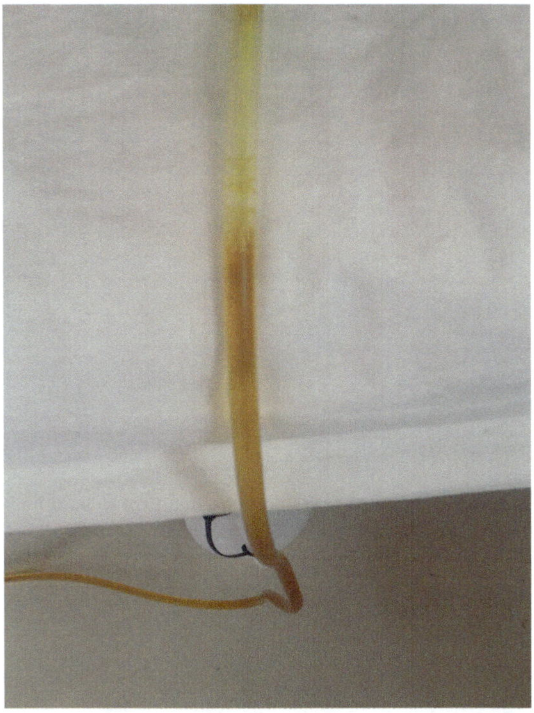

Fig. 6.2 Gall bladder cancer patients with biliary obstruction have jaundice and pass high colored urine

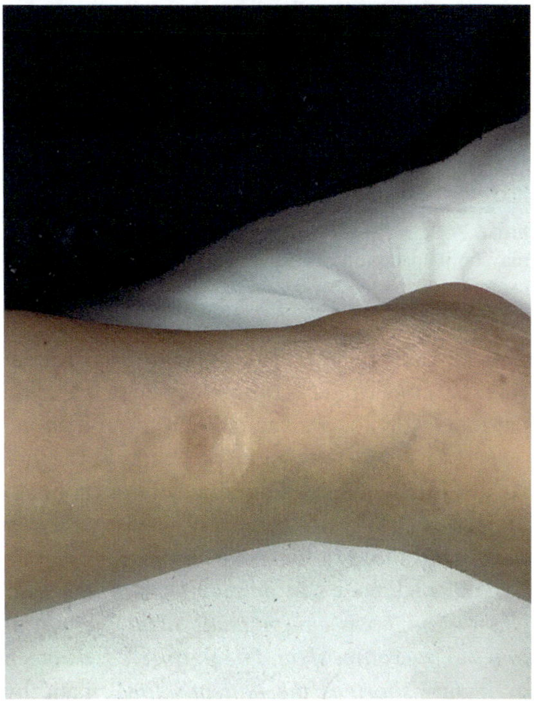

Fig. 6.3 Patients with advanced/metastatic gall bladder cancer may be malnourished and have bilateral pitting pedal edema

Cholangitis, i.e., high-grade fever with chills and rigors, though not as common in complete malignant biliary obstruction of GBC as in incomplete biliary obstruction due to benign causes, e.g., CBD stones, may supervene in patients with GBC and jaundice. Jaundice is caused by direct infiltration of the CBD by GBC neck or by compression of the common bile duct (CBD) by enlarged metastatic lymph nodes (LNs) in the hepatoduodenal ligament (HDL). Jaundice in GBC is usually associated with pain but may rarely present as painless progressive jaundice and thus mimic periampullary carcinoma and cholangiocarcinoma. Anorexia and weight loss, and generalized weakness, malaise, and lethargy are frequently present in patients with GBC and usually indicate advanced disease. Loss of appetite (60%) and loss of weight (63%) were very common in 385 patients with GBC seen at a tertiary level hospital in north India from 2003 to 2014 (Mishra et al. 2017). Symptomatic (obvious) GBC is usually in advanced stage as the symptoms are a result of infiltration of adjacent organs.

Metastatic symptoms include

1. Liver—no specific symptoms other than anorexia and weight loss; rarely, a large metastasis near the hepatic hilum can cause biliary obstruction and jaundice (it must, however, be noted that the common mechanism of causation of jaundice in GBC is infiltration of the common bile duct by a GBC neck)
2. Lungs—persistent cough, chest pain, shortness of breath, hemoptysis
3. Bones—bone pain, fracture (spontaneous or after trivial trauma)
4. Brain—persistent headache and vomiting, convulsions.

6.3 Signs

Patients with advanced GBC may be malnourished with loss of body fat and pedal edema (Fig. 6.3); they may even be cachectic. Jaundice (icterus) may be present (Fig. 6.4) and pruritic scratch marks (Fig. 6.5) are frequently present in patients with jaundice. A firm to hard non-tender

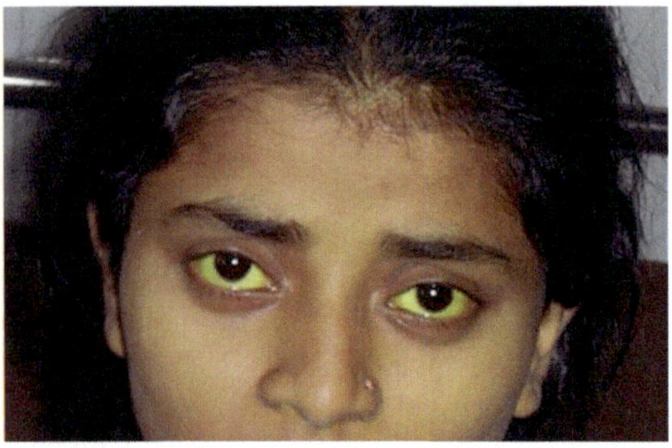

Fig. 6.4 Jaundice (icterus) is present in as many as one-fourth to one-third of patients with clinically obvious gall bladder cancer

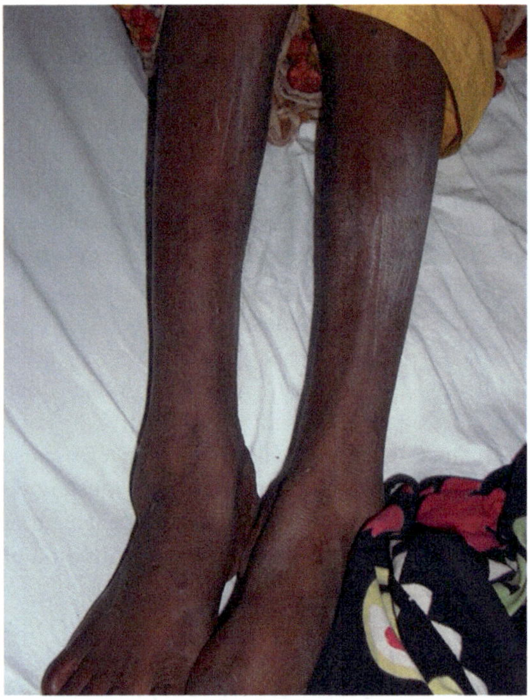

Fig. 6.5 Patients with obstructive jaundice also have pruritus—scratch marks can be seen on examination

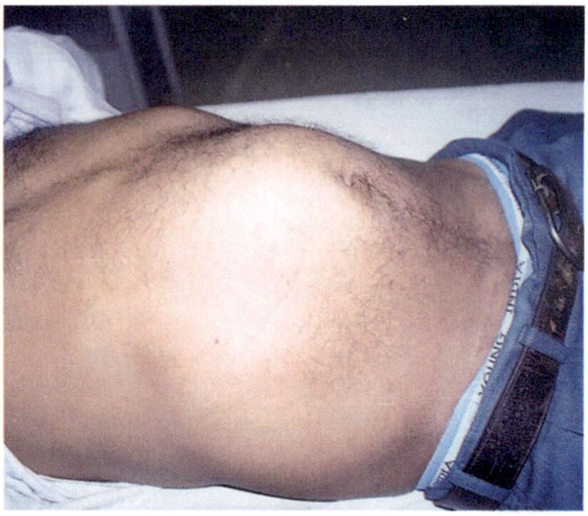

Fig. 6.6 Advanced GBC presents as a firm to hard non-tender palpable GB lump

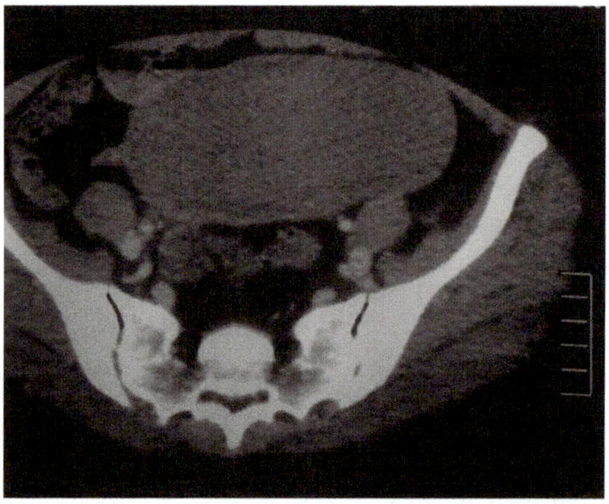

Fig. 6.7 A large ovarian deposit from gall bladder cancer may be palpable on per vaginal (PV) or per rectal (PR) examination

GB lump (Fig. 6.6) (cf. distended GB of mucocele) is palpable in a large number of cases. Hepatomegaly, which may be hard nodular (metastases) or firm diffuse (cholestasis due to biliary obstruction), may be present. Ascites which may be metastatic (peritoneal dissemination) or nutritional (when it is associated with pedal edema) should be looked for. Pelvic (recto-vesical and recto-uterine pouch) or ovarian (Fig. 6.7) metastatic deposits may be palpable on per rectal (PR) or per vaginal (PV) examination.

Most patients in whom a preoperative diagnosis of GBC is made either clinically or on imaging (US, CT, or MRI) have advanced, i.e., either locally advanced or metastatic disease.

The statement "*In malignancy of the GB, when a diagnosis can be made without exploration, no operation should be performed, as much as it only shortens the patient's life.*" made by Alfred Blalock a century ago in 1924 is not far from truth even today.

6.4 Unusual Clinical Presentations

Like any other disease, GBC has several unusual and atypical clinical presentations, which make the diagnosis difficult (Haribhakti et al. 1997). They should be kept in mind to have a suspicion of GBC, especially in high GBC incidence areas/populations. Locally advanced GBC can infiltrate (the first part of) the duodenum or (the antro-pyloric region of) the stomach and cause mechanical gastric outlet obstruction (GOO) (Fig. 6.8) causing early satiety, post-prandial fullness, nausea, and frank (non-bilious) vomiting. GOO was present in 8% of 385 patients with GBC reported by Mishra et al. (2017). Some patients may have symptoms suggestive of GOO but without mechanical gastro-duodenal obstruction—this is malignant gastroparesis (similar to the one seen in locally advanced pancreatic cancer). We showed delayed gastric emptying on radioisotope scintigraphy in a significant proportion of patients with GBC (Singh et al. 1998). While mechanical GOO will respond to gastro-jejunostomy (GJ) or antro-duodenal stenting, malignant gastroparesis may not. GBC may result in intestinal obstruction—colonic (due to direct infiltration of the hepatic flexure or proximal transverse colon) and small bowel (due to a large peritoneal deposit). GBC may also cause gastro-intestinal (GI) bleed due to direct infiltration of the duodenum/stomach (upper GI bleed) or colon (lower GI bleed). A tumor in the GB neck or the cystic duct may result in a mucocele (distended palpable GB) (Fig. 6.9) thus mimicking GSD. This is an exception to the usual clinical scenario where a distended palpable GB in malignant obstructive jaundice suggests a lower biliary obstruction due to a pancreatic head or periampullary cancer. Patients with GBC may present with acute cholecystitis and empyema due to obstruction of the cystic duct. In fact, the incidence of incidental GBC is higher in patients with acute cholecystitis than in those with chronic cholecystitis. Clinical diagnosis of empyema in an elderly (>60 years) patient should raise the suspicion of GBC (Lohsiriwat et al. 2009). Perforated GBC presenting as a sinus/fistula has been reported. A large GB mass can undergo central necrosis and look like a liver abscess on imaging (Fig. 6.10); fever of tumor necrosis may also be present further confusing the clinical diagnosis. Unusual sites of metastases, e.g., umbilical nodule (Fig. 6.11), left supra-clavicular (Fig. 6.12), axillary (Fig. 6.13), or inguinal LN and scalp nodule

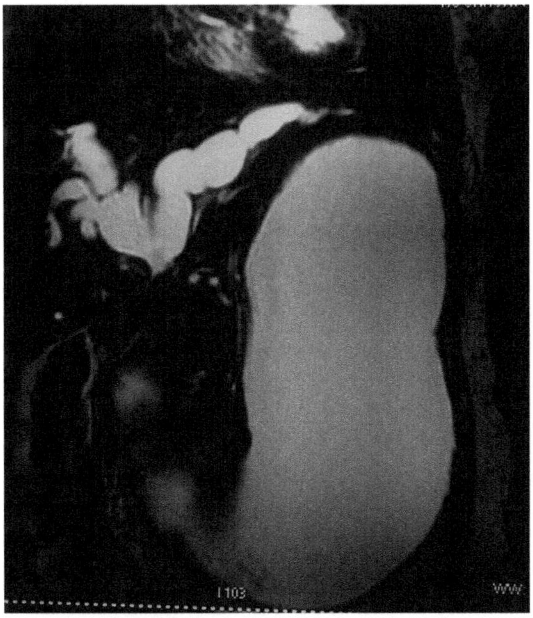

Fig. 6.8 Patients with advanced gall bladder cancer can have gastric outlet obstruction due to infiltration of the first part of the duodenum

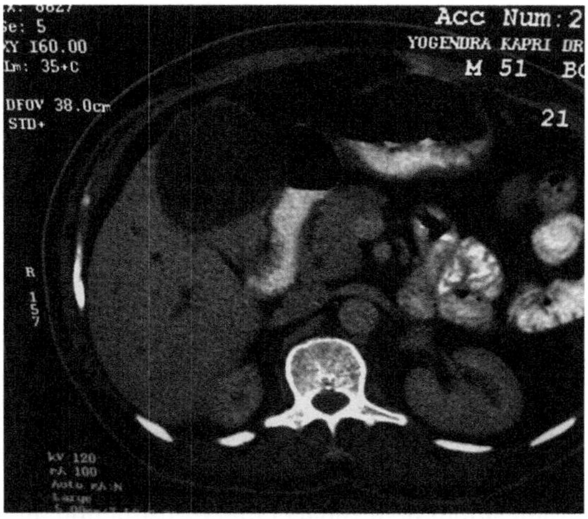

Fig. 6.9 Patients with GBC at neck can have a firm distended GB—mucocele

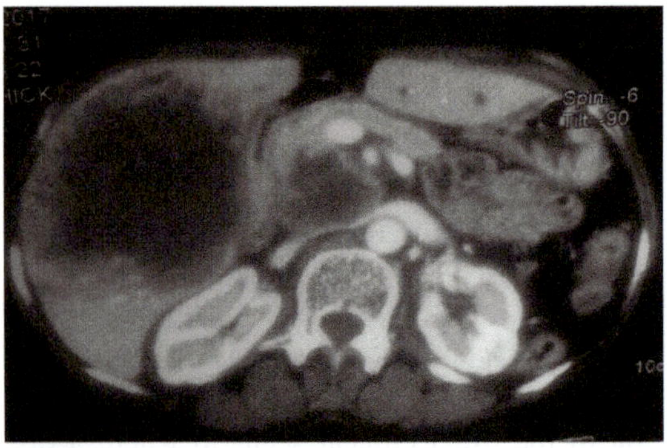

Fig. 6.10 A large gall bladder cancer can undergo central necrosis and look like a liver abscess; fever of tumor necrosis may also be present

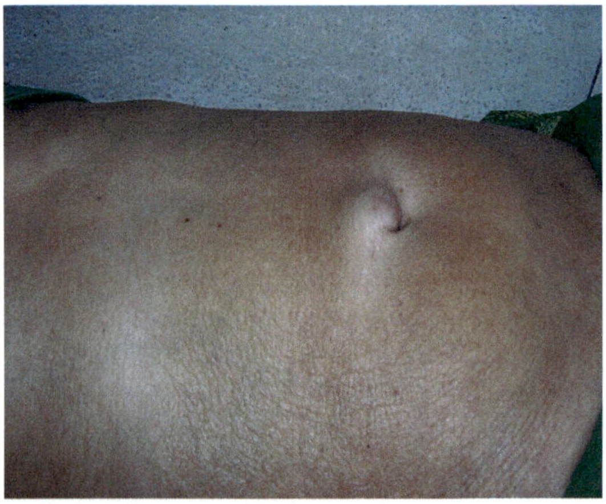

Fig. 6.11 An unusual but easily detectable site of metastasis from gall bladder cancer is the umbilicus (hard palpable nodule)

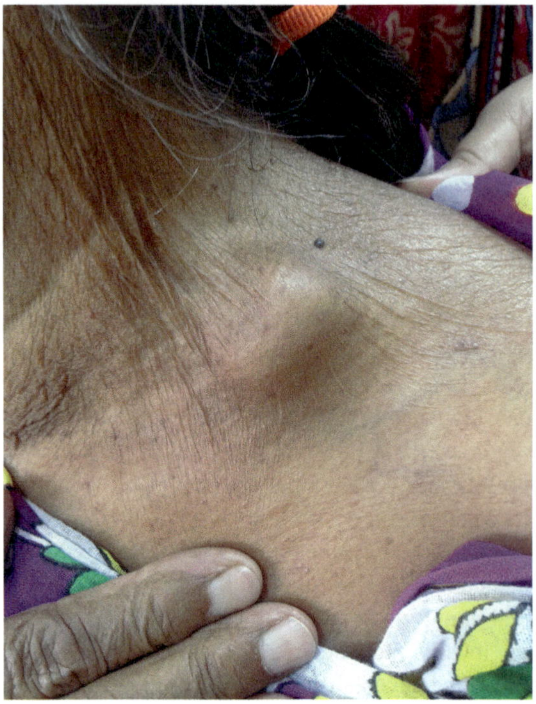

Fig. 6.12 Gall bladder cancer may spread to the left supraclavicular lymph nodes which are easily palpable and can be subjected to fine needle aspiration cytology (FNAC)

have been reported. Patients with incidental GBC may present with scar (following open cholecystectomy) or port-site (following laparoscopic cholecystectomy) metastasis, especially if long time has elapsed since the index cholecystectomy. Post-cholecystectomy jaundice is usually benign, either due to retained CBD stones or because of a bile duct injury and benign biliary stricture; it may rarely be malignant due to recurrence of a missed GBC (Fig. 6.14). An uneventful postoperative course, i.e., no bile leak after cholecystectomy, GB not sent for histopathological examination, high (hilar) biliary obstruction and the presence of a mass on imaging should suggest the possibility that the post-cholecystectomy jaundice is not benign but malignant (Sharma et al. 2008). Recurrent/missed GBC may present as scar site (after open cholecystectomy)/port-site (after laparoscopic cholecystectomy) metastases in the form of hard non-tender nodules.

6.5 Differential Diagnosis

Differential diagnosis of GBC may include

1. Gall stone disease as symptoms of early GBC may be same as that of GSD.
2. GB perforation (on the hepatic side) due to complications of GS may look like a GBC on imaging (US, CT, or MRI) (Fig. 6.15). At the same time, patients with a clinical diagnosis of acute cholecystitis or empyema are more likely to turn out to have an incidental GBC.
3. Clinical picture of GBC patients with jaundice may resemble that of patients with CBD stones and Mirizzi syndrome (Fig. 6.16)—

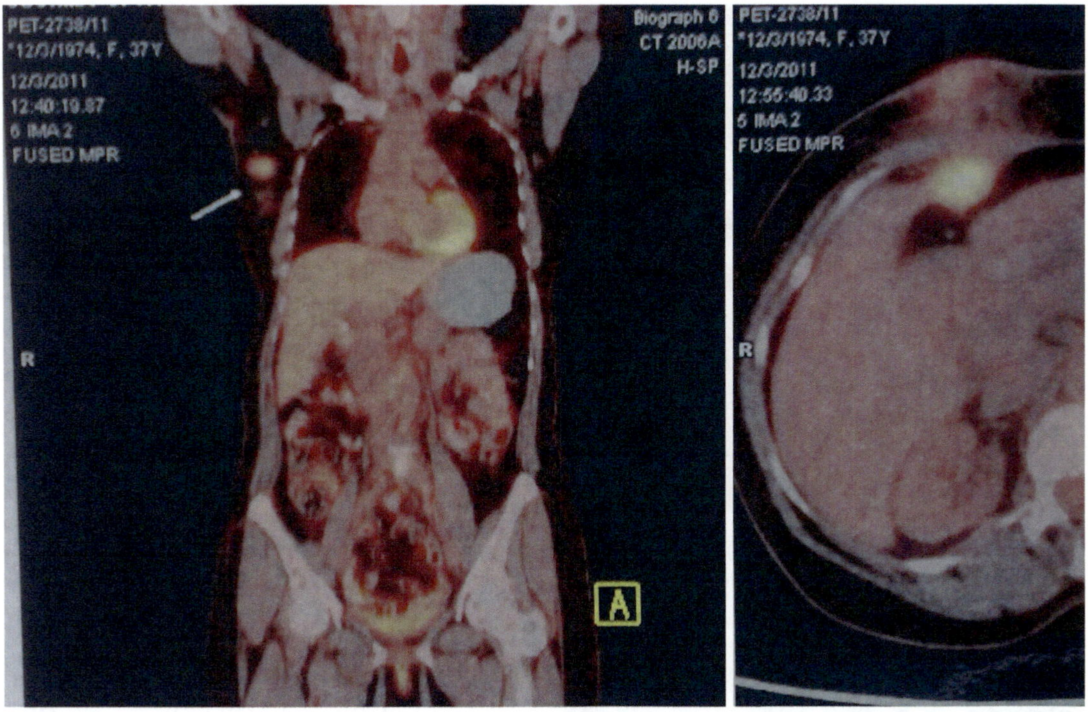

Fig. 6.13 PET scan shows FDG avid lesions in the right axilla and the GB. (Image courtesy Dr. Amit Javed GB Pant Hospital New Delhi)

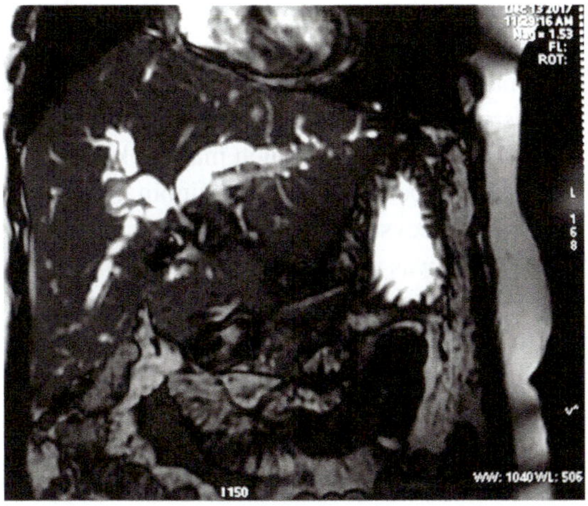

Fig. 6.14 Post-cholecystectomy jaundice may be due to recurrence of a gall bladder cancer which was missed at cholecystectomy because the gall bladder was not sent for histopathological examination

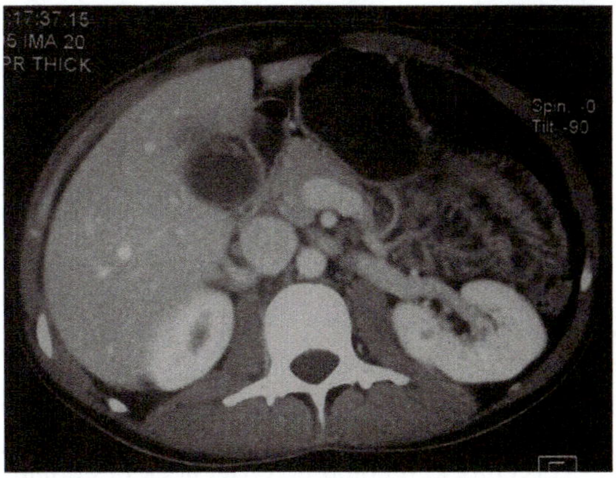

Fig. 6.15 Gall bladder perforation into the liver parenchyma and the resulting abscess may look like a gall bladder cancer infiltrating the liver on imaging

there is a higher chance of finding incidental GBC in these scenarios. Jaundice due to associated CBD stones in a patient with GBC is a favorable scenario where the CBD stones can be cleared endoscopically and then the GBC can be treated on its own merits.

4. In a patient presenting with obstructive jaundice, which on clinical grounds appears to be malignant, if the US shows a high (Fig. 6.17) or mid (Fig. 6.18) CBD (cf. low

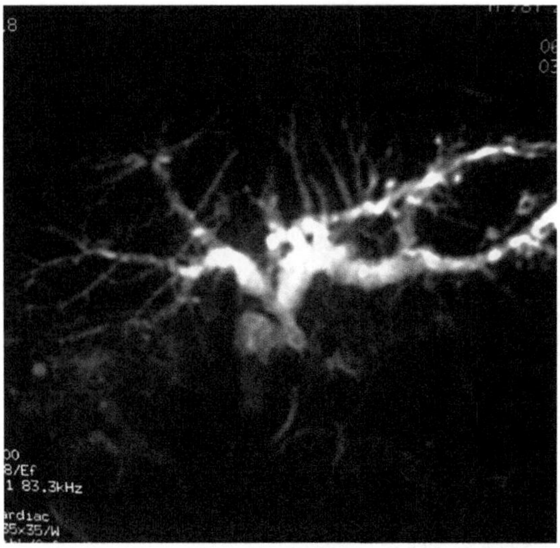

Fig. 6.16 Mirizzi syndrome may look like gall bladder cancer with common bile duct infiltration

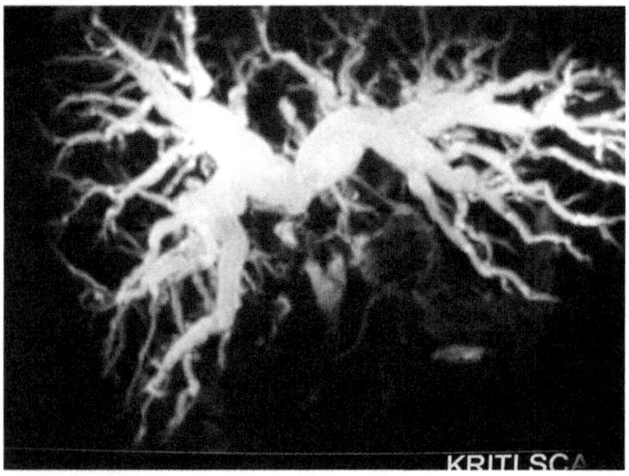

Fig. 6.17 Gall bladder cancer can infiltrate into the common hepatic duct (CHD) or the biliary ductal confluence and look like a hilar (high) cholangiocarcinoma

block in pancreatic and periampullary cancers) block, it could be GBC neck or cholangiocarcinoma (hilar and mid CBD) and differentiation between them is not easy (Kapoor 2015). The presence of pain (either biliary colic due to associated GS or dull diffuse continuous ache of liver infiltration) suggests GBC as cholangiocarcinoma is usually painless, but cholangiocarcinoma may also be associated with GS which cause pain and and a small GBC neck may be painless. The presence of a mass on imaging (US, CT, MRI) is more in favor of a GBC than cholangiocarcinoma. On cholangiogram, selective involvement of the right anterior sectoral pedicle (which lies in the GB bed) suggests GBC whereas involvement of the left hepatic duct (and segment IV duct) indicates hilar cholangiocarcinoma. Similarly, involvement of the left hepatic artery and/or the left portal vein suggests cholangiocarcinoma. Uncommonly, a patient with GBC may have lower CBD obstruction due to enlarged periduodenal/peripancreatic LNs which may look like pancreatic or periampullary carcinoma.

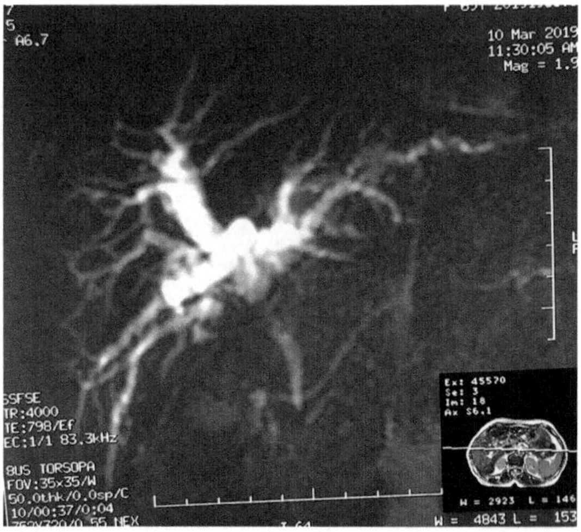

Fig. 6.18 Gall bladder cancer can infiltrate the common bile duct (CBD) and look like a mid CBD cholangiocarcinoma

5. Post-cholecystectomy jaundice, especially if the GB was not sent for histopathological examination, may be because of a missed (rather than CBD stones or biliary stricture which are more common).
6. GBC presenting as thick-walled GB (TWGB) on imaging (US or CT) (Fig. 6.19) or at operation may finally (fortunately) turn out to be benign, e.g., chronic cholecystitis (CC) or xantho-granulomatous cholecystitis (XGC) on histopathological examination—most reports of extended cholecystectomy with a presumed diagnosis of GBC include a significant proportion of patients in whom the final histology is benign, i.e., CC or XGC.
7. A GB fossa mass on imaging which looks like GBC may be a hepatocellular carcinoma

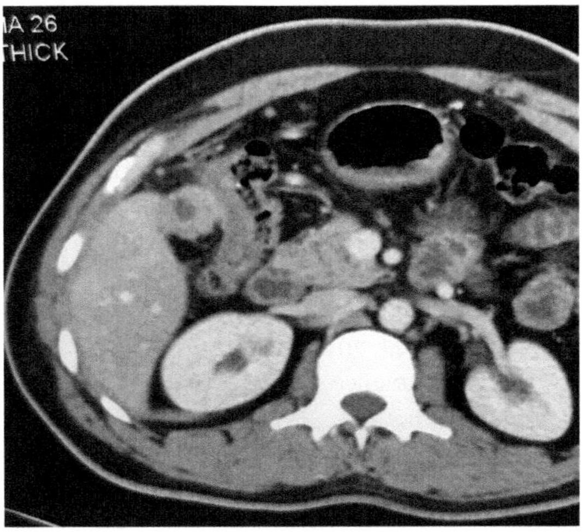

Fig. 6.19 A thick-walled gall bladder (TWGB) on US or CT is usually benign but may turn out to be gall bladder cancer

(HCC) or a metastasis (from another primary).

8. Rare entities, e.g., hepatobiliary tuberculosis (Haque et al. 2019), IgG4-related sclerosing cholecystitis (Ichinokawa et al. 2019; Jearth et al. 2020).

A high index of suspicion is required, especially in geographical areas and ethnic groups with high incidence rates of GBC, for the clinical diagnosis of GBC. In geographical areas and ethnic groups with low incidence rates of GBC, it should be considered as a possible differential diagnosis when dealing with above-mentioned conditions/situations.

Early GBC is difficult to diagnose; clinically obvious GBC is usually advanced and is difficult to treat.

Invited Commentary on Clinical Presentation of Gall Bladder Cancer

Yuman Fong

In this chapter on clinical presentation of gallbladder cancer (GBC), Professor Kapoor summarizes the recommendations of the National Comprehensive Cancer Network (NCCN) for classifying GBC into (1) incidental finding at surgery, (2) incidental finding at histopathology, (3) mass on imaging, and (4) jaundice. Professor Kapoor then recommends an alternative classification system as (1) obvious clinical symptoms and signs, (2) suspected, (3) unsuspected, (4) incidental, and (5) missed GBC.

A much simpler way of classifying GBC is as to when the mass is noted. Gallbladder cancers are masses that can be recognized as cancer prior to surgery (radiologic diagnosis), at the time of surgery (surgical diagnosis), or after surgery (pathologic diagnosis).

Pathologically diagnosed: For those patients with pathologically diagnosed GBC, it is very important to ask the pathologist to report (1) whether the gross specimen was intact or ruptured, i.e., bile spill occurred during cholecystectomy, (2) whether the tumor was on the liver side or the peritoneal side of the specimen, (3) the deep margin status, (4) the cystic duct margin status, and (5) the cancer status of the Calot's (cystic) lymph node, if available. The data is very clear that patients with intact specimens, negative margins, and carcinoma in situ or T1a GBC do not need additional surgery. All other patients including those with T1b GBC deserve further radiologic staging. If resectable localized disease is found, additional resection is warranted.

Surgically diagnosed: The cases of GBC diagnosed in the operating room can either be (1) disseminated disease, (2) advanced localized disease (liver invasion or nodal dissemination of cancer), or (3) gallbladder-confined disease resectable by cholecystectomy.

For disseminated disease, biopsy of peritoneal or non-contiguous liver tumor proves unresectable disease, and obtaining sufficient sample for molecular analysis (BRAF mutational status, microsatellite instability MSI, and mutational burden) helps drive trials and the treatment of disseminated disease.

For disease found at surgery that has advanced local extension to liver or lymph nodes, most surgeons will biopsy the liver tumor (through normal liver parenchyma in order to minimize spillage of tumor) or sample a lymph node and stop. Most will return later after obtaining full informed consent for more extensive resection, and possibly after neoadjuvant chemotherapy.

For those found to have gallbladder-confined disease which is highly suspected to be gallbladder cancer (intraoperative sonographically confirmed mass or clear mass on the external portion of the gallbladder), operative conduct should be modified. (1) Consideration should be given to avoiding of grabbing the gallbladder to avoid spillage of gallbladder contents. (2) The cystic plate (serosa of the gallbladder) on the liver side of the gallbladder should be removed. Taking off the cystic plate gets rid of all the lymphatics in the gallbladder and avoids the plane of T1 and T2 gallbladder cancers. (3) Immediate documentation of the cystic duct margin status reduces the need for a second operative procedure (to excise the CBD). (4) Cystic duct node or suspicious nodes should be sent for frozen section evaluation. These steps provide a strong possibility for immediate resection of early gallbladder cancer and minimize the need for second operations.

Radiologically diagnosed: Radiologically diagnosed GBC comes in four forms: (1) advanced disseminated disease, (2) advanced local disease including jaundiced patients, (3) resectable obvious masses, and (4) small masses including gallbladder polyps.

The first two radiologic presentations constitute non-surgical disease. In particular, the reason that the NCCN segregates out jaundice as a symptom in that most patients with GBC as the cause of their jaundice are incurable (Hawkins et al. 2004). When patients are found to have advanced disease, biopsy of a deposit to prove stage IV disease allows for appropriate systemic cancer therapy or palliative therapies.

Obvious resectable masses demand further imaging for cancer staging. FDG-PET is recommended for these patients to document local and regional disease to define the extent of surgical resection or to document distant disease to rule out resection (Ramos-Font et al. 2014). Patients with stage III GBC should have resections at high volume centers for HPB surgery.

For those with small luminal masses including polyps, one should follow the surgical process as outlined above for intraoperatively discovered small masses to avoid cancer spillage, and to ensure the highest cure rate in as few operative procedures as possible.

Discovering GBC and performing the right operation for potential cure requires vigilance when examining preoperative scans. The rate of diagnosing GBC is related to the vigilance, with as high a rate as >90% preoperative diagnosis in Japan (Higuchi et al. 2014), versus >60% in Chile (Roa et al. 1999), and only approximately 40% in the USA (Ethun et al. 2017; Butte et al. 2011).

Invited Commentary on Clinical Presentation of Gall Bladder Cancer

Pradeep Ghimire

Gallbladder carcinoma (GBC) is known to show an unusual geographic distribution worldwide, with quite a substantial geographic variation noted. In Asia, the northern Indian population and southern Pakistani population from Karachi appear to be the highest of affected, showing a rate of 21.5 and 13.8 per 100,000 population, respectively.

With the pre-operative diagnosis occurring in less than 20% of afflicted patients; in spite of the recent advancement and the availability of various diagnostic approaches and modalities, the preoperative diagnosis of GBC is still regarded as an exception, rather than the diagnosis being a rule. Most of the cases of GBC are diagnosed during or after surgery performed for stones or benign biliary diseases. Lack of timely diagnosis and subsequent poor prognosis at the time of discovery can be considered a major problem in the treatment of GBC, with poor outcomes encountered.

GBC is more commonly encountered in the females; however, the mortality rate appears to be higher in the males. The etiology of GBC has been attributed to the presence of cholelithiasis, various genetic and environmental causes, infection of the gallbladder, porcelain gallbladder, Mirizzi syndrome, gallbladder polyps, choledochal cyst, and biliary reflux. A positive family history of gallbladder calculi, chemical exposure (including wood dust and coal dust), tobacco consumption, longer interval between meals, higher concentration of secondary bile acids, and excessive intake of fried food are also associated risk factors. Interestingly, patients residing in the Gangetic belt have also shown an increased risk in the development of GBC, probably due to exposure to high cadmium, chromium, and lead particles. Consumption of fruits on a regular basis has been associated with protective effect against GBC.

GBC is widely considered as the fifth most common cancer of the digestive tract and the most common malignancy of the biliary tract. Among the fatal carcinomas afflicting the Nepalese population, GBC is regarded as a relatively common entity. According to the American Institute for Cancer Research, of the top 20 countries with the highest rates of GBC in 2018, Nepal had the sixth highest rate of 6.7 per 100,000 population for both the sexes, the fifth highest rate of 6.0 per 100,000 population for males and the third highest rate of 7.3 per 100,000 population for females. In a study conducted by our team at Fishtail Hospital and Research Center, Pokhara, Nepal, the incidence of GBC in cases of routine cholecystectomy among 783 patients operated over 11 years was found to be 1.28% (Ghimire et al. 2011). As also recommended in the study, it is a standard practice to perform routine histopathological examinations for all cholecystectomy specimens. Various studies, including the working report of the Royal College of Pathologists have recommended for this routine standard practice, as it helps in detection of a large number of cases of occult (incidental) GBC. Also, given that primary GBCs are known for their late presentation and hence poor survival rates; occult GBC diagnosed incidentally on histopathological examination of post-cholecystectomy specimen are usually detected at earlier stages and thus have better prognosis.

Invited Commentary on Clinical Presentation of Gall Bladder Cancer

Prabin Bikram Thapa

Gallbladder cancer (GBC) is notorious for being asymptomatic in early stages of the disease. While there are many clinical scenarios in which GBC can be detected by the clinician, as enumerated by the Author (VKK), their presentation can be characterized into the following categories:

1. Asymptomatic
2. Symptoms pertaining to gallstone disease
3. Symptoms of locally advanced disease
4. Symptoms of metastatic disease

Up to 90% of cases of GBC are associated with gallstone disease, and in most instances they mimic symptoms of cholelithiasis such as right upper quadrant pain (Grobmyer et al. 2004). However, they are more often than not characterized by constant pain rather than the typical colicky type of pain seen in biliary colic. Elderly patients with above-mentioned features who are from high-incidence areas should be suspected of having GBC, particularly when the symptoms are associated with anorexia, weight loss, and jaundice.

Locally advanced disease may clinically manifest as obstructive jaundice, usually from the direct invasion of the biliary tree. Invasion of the tumor into the gastro-duodenum may also result in gastric outlet obstruction (Sharma et al. 2010).

Palpable gall bladder, hepatomegaly, ascites, weight loss, and anorexia usually are tell-tale signs of advanced disease. Metastatic disease may also manifest as jaundice due to the involvement of the hepatoduodenal ligament or as a peri-umbilical nodule or left supraclavicular lymphadenopathy. Rarely, GBC may present with paraneoplastic syndromes (due to ectopic hormone secretion) such as Cushing syndrome, hypercalcemia, acanthosis nigricans, bullous pemphigoid, dermatomyositis, and the Leser-Trélat sign, i.e., explosive onset of multiple seborrheic keratoses (many pigmented skin lesions) (Uribe-Uribe et al. 2009).

Given the myriad nature of presentations of GBC, a high degree of clinical suspicion is warranted for the timely detection and appropriate treatment of the disease.

References

Chapter References

Butte JM, Matsuo K, Gönen M, D'Angelica MI, Waugh E, Allen PJ, Fong Y, DeMatteo RP, Blumgart L, Endo I, De La Fuente H, Jarnagin WR. Gallbladder cancer: differences in presentation, surgical treatment, and survival in patients treated at centers in three countries. J Am Coll Surg. 2011;212(1):50–61. https://doi.org/10.1016/j.jamcollsurg.2010.09.009. Epub 2010 Nov 12.

Duffy A, Capanu M, Abou-Alfa GK, Huitzil D, Jarnagin W, Fong Y, D'Angelica M, Dematteo RP, Blumgart LH, O'Reilly EM. Gallbladder cancer (GBC): 10-year experience at Memorial Sloan-Kettering Cancer Centre (MSKCC). J Surg Oncol. 2008;98(7):485–9.

Ethun CG, Le N, Lopez-Aguiar AG, Pawlik TM, Poultsides G, Tran T, Idrees K, Isom CA, Fields RC, Krasnick BA, Weber SM, Salem A, Martin RCG, Scoggins CR, Shen P, Mogal HD, Schmidt C, Beal E, Hatzaras I, Shenoy R, Russell MC, Maithel SK. Pathologic and prognostic implications of incidental versus nonincidental gallbladder cancer: a 10-institution study from the United States Extrahepatic Biliary Malignancy Consortium. Am Surg. 2017;83(7):679–86.

Haque MMU, Whadva RK, Luck NH, Mubarak M. Primary hepaticobiliary tuberculosis mimicking gall bladder carcinoma with liver invasion: a case report. Pan Afr Med J. 2019;32:68. https://doi.org/10.11604/pamj.2019.32.68.10519. eCollection 2019.

Haribhakti SP, Awasthi S, Pradeep R, Kapoor VK, Kaushik SP. Carcinoma gallbladder: atypical presentations and unusual associations. Trop Gastroenterol. 1997;18(1):32–4.

Hawkins WG, DeMatteo RP, Jarnagin WR, Ben-Porat L, Blumgart LH, Fong Y. Jaundice predicts advanced disease and early mortality in patients with gallbladder cancer. Ann Surg Oncol. 2004;11(3):310–5.

Higuchi R, Ota T, Araida T, Kajiyama H, Yazawa T, Furukawa T, Yoshikawa T, Takasaki K, Yamamoto M. Surgical approaches to advanced gallbladder cancer: a 40-year single-institution study of prognostic factors and resectability. Ann Surg Oncol. 2014;21(13):4308–16. https://doi.org/10.1245/s10434-014-3885-1. Epub 2014 Jul 15.

Ichinokawa M, Matsumoto J, Kuraya T, Kuwabara S, Wada H, Kato K, Ikeda A, Murakawa K, Ono K. A rare case of localized IgG4-related sclerosing cholecystitis mimicking gallbladder cancer. J Rural Med. 2019;14(1):138–42. https://doi.org/10.2185/jrm.2998. Epub 2019 May 30.

Jearth V, Patil P, Patkar S, et al. Immunoglobulin G4-related cholecystitis mimicking a locally advanced gallbladder cancer-a case report and review of literature. Clin J Gastroenterol. 2020; https://doi.org/10.1007/s12328-020-01168-7.

Kapoor VK. Gallbladder neck cancer and perihilar cholangiocarcinoma - siblings, cousins or look alike? Korean J Hepatobiliary Pancreat Surg. 2015;19(2):86–8. https://doi.org/10.14701/kjhbps.2015.19.2.86. Epub 2015 May 31.

Kapoor VK, Pradeep R, Haribhakti SP, Sikora SS, Kaushik SP. Early carcinoma of the gallbladder: an elusive disease. J Surg Oncol. 1996;62(4):284–7.

Lohsiriwat V, Vongjirad A, Lohsiriwat D. Value of routine histopathologic examination of three common surgical specimens: appendix, gallbladder, and hemorrhoid. World J Surg. 2009;33(10):2189–93. https://doi.org/10.1007/s00268-009-0164-6.

Mishra PK, Saluja SS, Prithiviraj N, Varshney V, Goel N, Patil N. Predictors of curative resection and long term survival of gallbladder cancer—a retrospective analysis. Am J Surg. 2017;214(2):278–86. https://doi.org/10.1016/j.amjsurg.2017.02.006. Epub 2017 Feb 9.

NCCN Clinical Practice Guidelines in Oncology (NCCN Guidelines™) Hepatobiliary Cancers. Version 2.2015. 2015. Available from: www.NCCN.org.

Regimbeau JM, Fuks D, Bachellier P, Le Treut YP, Pruvot FR, Navarro F, Chiche L, Farges O. Prognostic value of jaundice in patients with gallbladder cancer by the AFC-GBC-2009 study group. Eur J Surg Oncol. 2011;37(6):505–12. https://doi.org/10.1016/j.ejso.2011.03.135. Epub 2011 Apr 21.

Roa I, Araya JC, Villaseca M, Roa J, de Aretxabala X, Ibacache G. Gallbladder cancer in a high risk area: morphological features and spread patterns. Hepatogastroenterology. 1999;46(27):1540–6.

Sharma A, Behari A, Sikora SS, Kumar A, Saxena R, Kapoor VK. Post-cholecystectomy biliary strictures: not always benign. J Gastroenterol Hepatol. 2008;23(7 Pt 2):e63–6. Epub 2007 Jul 20.

Sikora SS, Kapoor R, Pradeep R, Kapoor VK, Saxena R, Kaushik SP. Palliative surgical treatment of malignant obstructive jaundice. Eur J Surg Oncol. 1994;20(5):580–4.

Singh B, Kapoor VK, Sikora SS, Kalawat TC, Das BK, Kaushik SP. Malignant gastroparesis and outlet obstruction in carcinoma gall bladder. Trop Gastroenterol. 1998;19(1):37–9.

References for Commentary Notes by Yuman Fong

Ramos-Font C, Gomez-Rio M, Rodriguez-Fernandez A, Jimenez-Heffernan A, Sanchez Sanchez R, Llamas-Elvira JM. Ability of FDG-PET/CT in the detection of gallbladder cancer. J Surg Oncol. 2014;109(3):218–24.

Reference for Commentary Notes by Pradeep Ghimire

Ghimire P, Yogi N, Shrestha BB. Incidence of incidental carcinoma gall bladder in cases of routine cholecystectomy. Kathmandu Univ Med J. 2011;9(34):3–6.

References for Commentary Notes by Prabin Bikram Thapa

Grobmyer SR, Lieberman MD, Daly JM. Gallbladder cancer in the twentieth century: single institution's experience. World J Surg. 2004;28(1):47–9.

Sharma D, Jakhetia A, Agarwal L, Baruah D, Rohtagi A, Kumar A. Carcinoma gall bladder with Bouveret's syndrome: a rare cause of gastric outlet obstruction. Indian J Surg. 2010;72(4):350–1.

Uribe-Uribe NO, Jimenez-Garduño AM, Henson DE, Albores-Saavedra J. Paraneoplastic sensory neuropathy associated with small cell carcinoma of the gallbladder. Ann Diagn Pathol. 2009;13(2):124–6. https://doi.org/10.1016/j.anndiagpath.2007.08.003.

7 Investigations for Diagnosis of Gall Bladder Cancer

Vinay K. Kapoor

Investigations in a patient with clinical diagnosis or suspicion of gall bladder cancer (GBC) are aimed at

1. Confirmation of the diagnosis
2. Staging of the disease, with the aim to assess operability/resectability—T1–T3 disease is potentially resectable, T4 disease is usually unresectable, and M1 disease is inoperable
3. To differentiate GBC from benign diseases (chronic cholecystitis CC and xanthogranulomatous cholecystitis XGC) in a thick-walled GB (TWGB)
4. To find out/rule out any residual disease or dissemination in a patient with incidental GBC before reoperation
5. To detect recurrence during follow-up
6. Overall evaluation of the patient for management, i.e., general investigations, e.g., hemogram, blood sugar, liver function tests, renal function tests, coagulation profile, chest X-ray, EKG.

Please also see an Invited Commentary on Investigations for Diagnosis of Gall Bladder Cancer by Thomas A. Aloia (pp **–**)

V. K. Kapoor (✉)
Department of Surgical Gastroenterology, Sanjay Gandhi Post-Graduate Institute of Medical Sciences (SGPGIMS), Lucknow, Uttar Pradesh, India
e-mail: vkkapoor.india@gmail.com

7.1 Blood Tests

Routine blood tests, including liver function tests (LFT), do not have a role in the diagnosis of GBC. There are, however, some reports which suggest that elevated alkaline phosphatase (ALP) and/or gamma glutamyl transpeptidase (GGTP) in the absence of jaundice, i.e., normal serum bilirubin, may raise a suspicion of GBC in a patient with gall stone disease (GSD).

7.2 Ultrasonography (US)

Transabdominal US is an easily and universally available, non-invasive, no-radiation, inexpensive, quick, and easy to perform and repeat first investigation in a patient with symptoms to suggest biliary disease—whether benign or malignant. The following findings on US suggest malignancy

1. Mass replacing the GB (Fig. 7.1)
2. Irregular non-uniform asymmetric focal thickening (>3 mm) (Fig. 7.2) of the GB wall (cf. smooth uniform symmetric generalized thickening of the GB wall which suggests benign disease, i.e., CC or XGC)
3. Intraluminal polypoidal heterogeneous, predominantly hypoechoic but may be isoechoic, mass (Fig. 7.3) with no posterior acoustic shadowing which does not move with change in the patient's position (cf. stones which have

V. K. Kapoor (ed.), *A Pictorial Treatise on Gall Bladder Cancer*,
https://doi.org/10.1007/978-981-15-5289-2_7

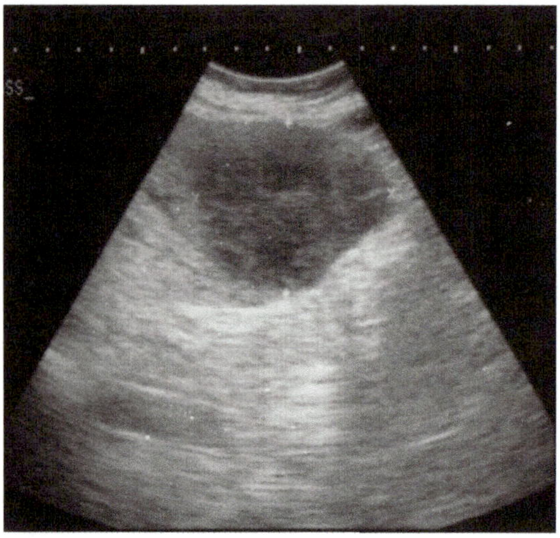

Fig. 7.1 US shows a mass replacing the gall bladder

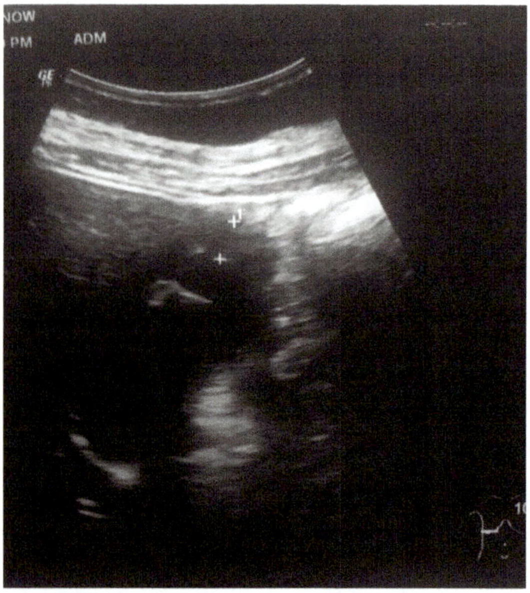

Fig. 7.2 US shows focal thickening of the gall bladder wall—this is highly suspicious of gall bladder cancer and should be further investigated with CT

posterior acoustic shadowing and move with change in the patient's position)

4. Echogenic mucosa, discontinuity of the mucosa and submucosal echolucency

Pearl necklace appearance and posterior comet tail artifact (Fig. 7.4) on US suggest adenomyomatosis.

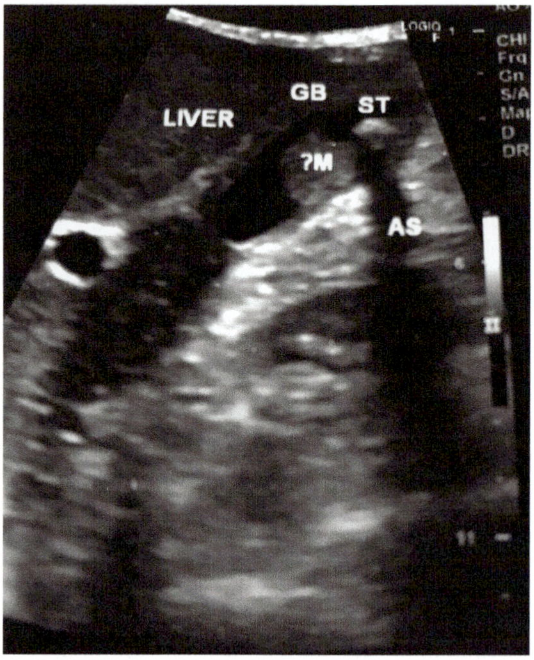

Fig. 7.3 US shows an intraluminal polypoidal lesion—this can be further evaluated with CT, high-resolution US (HRUS), or endoscopic US (EUS)

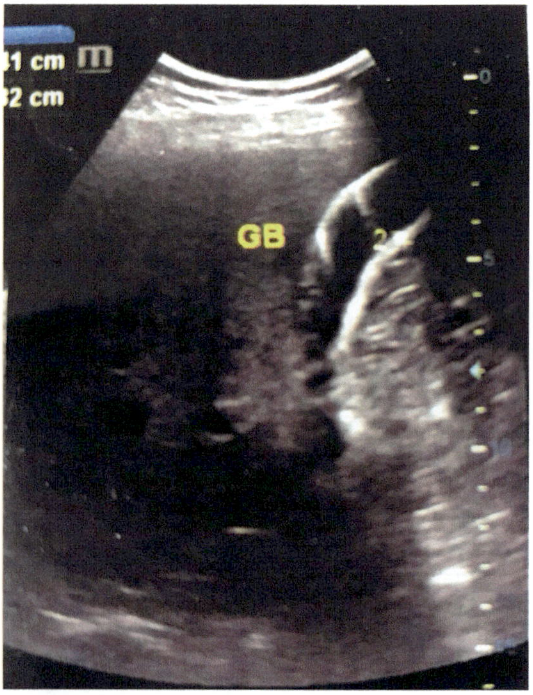

Fig. 7.4 US shows the comet tail appearance suggestive of adenomyomatosis

US can evaluate liver infiltration (loss of interface between the GB and liver); it can detect liver metastases (Fig. 7.5) and cholangiolytic abscesses which are seen as space-occupying lesions (SOL), enlarged lymph nodes (LNs) (Fig. 7.6), large omental/peritoneal deposits (Fig. 7.7) and ascites. If US shows metastases (which are then proved on fine needle aspiration cytology FNAC), further imaging, viz. CT or MRI will not be indicated. Intrahepatic biliary radicle dilatation (IHBRD) (Fig. 7.8) suggests biliary obstruction; the level of biliary obstruction (high, mid, or low) can be easily discerned on US. GBC can cause biliary obstruction at all levels—intrahepatic (segment V duct or right anterior sectoral pedicle) due to infiltration of the GB bed, high (due to hilar, i.e., biliary ductal confluence involvement), mid (due to direct infiltration of a GBC neck into the common bile duct CBD), or low (caused by enlarged metastatic peri-duodenal or peri-pancreatic lymph nodes). In patients with high biliary obstruction, US can also show whether the primary and secondary (right) biliary ductal confluence are patent or involved (blocked).

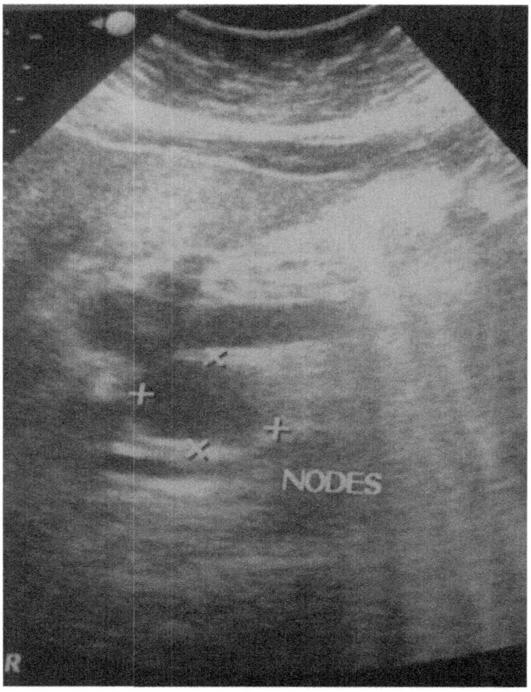

Fig. 7.6 US shows an enlarged lymph node

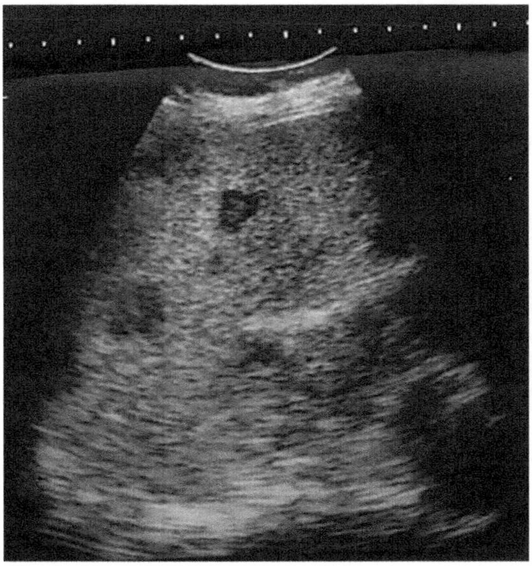

Fig. 7.5 US shows space-occupying lesion (SOL) in liver suggestive of liver metastasis; it could be a cholangiolytic abscess also if the patient has jaundice and cholangitis

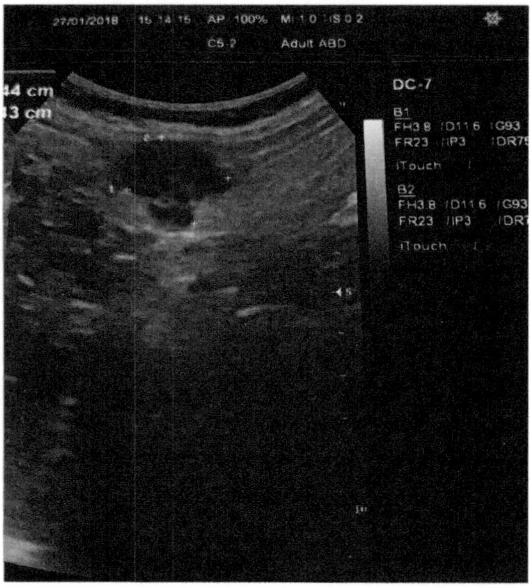

Fig. 7.7 US shows a large omental nodule; small omental (and peritoneal) nodules cannot, however, be picked up on US (or even CT) but will be very easily seen on staging laparoscopy

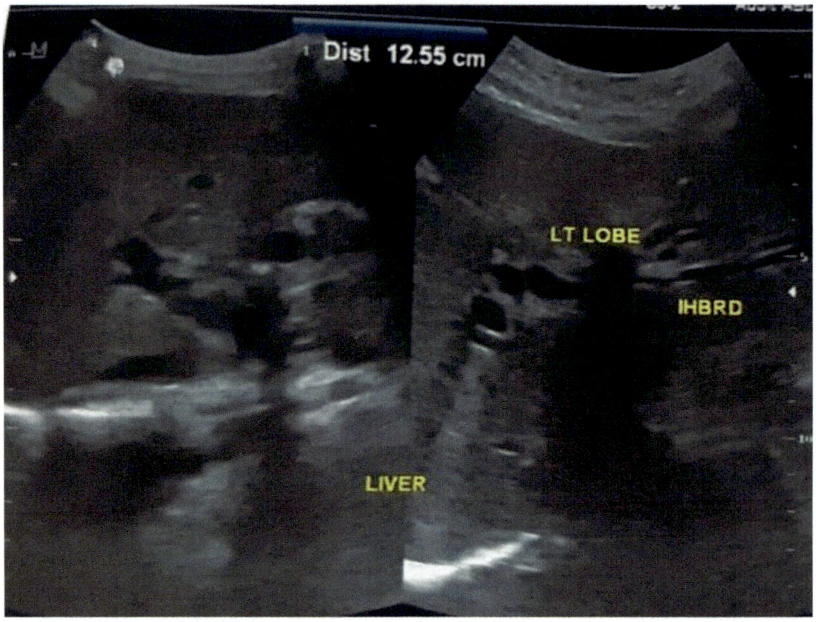

Fig. 7.8 US shows intrahepatic biliary radical dilatation (IHBRD) in a patient with jaundice; US is a good investigation to document the level of biliary obstruction, i.e., intrahepatic, high (hilar), mid, or low

a b

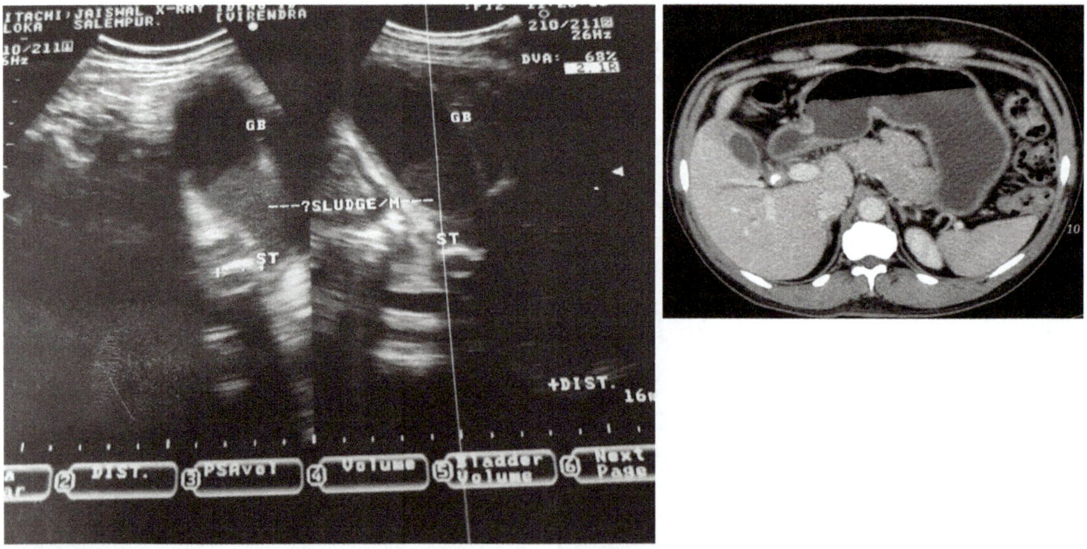

Fig. 7.9 (**a**) US shows gall bladder sludge (no distal acoustic shadowing). (**b**) CT showed that it was not sludge but a gall bladder mass

US, however, has several limitations. It is highly operator dependent. Early GBC is very likely to be missed on US as US, which though sensitive to diagnose advanced GBC, fails to pick up flat and sessile early lesions, especially in the presence of GS. US may not differentiate between GB sludge (Fig. 7.9a, b) and an intraluminal GB mass. It is not good for staging (especially involvement of adjacent hollow visceral organs such as colon or duodenum). The sensitivity of US can be increased to some extent by using high-resolution US (HRUS).

Doppler US can be used for evaluation of vessels, viz. portal vein (PV) and hepatic artery

(HA), in advanced GBC; it can also evaluate the vascularity of a polypoidal lesion. Evaluation of the GB wall arterial blood flow velocity and resistive index by color Doppler-guided spectral analysis can differentiate benign from malignant (Hayakawa et al. 1998). A sludge ball (tumefactive sludge) in the GB may look like an intraluminal mass—color Doppler US shows blood flow within the lesion which suggests GBC. Contrast-enhanced US (CEUS) uses intravenous (IV) signal enhancers, e.g., perflubutane. The micro-bubble contrast agents enhance the contrast between the blood and the surrounding tissues and make it possible to detect blood flow. CEUS can also differentiate a sludge ball from neoplasm; continuous staining of the lesion (eruption sign) suggests GBC. Sludge showed the absence of enhancement in 16/16 cases (vs. 0/23 in neoplasm); washout of the contrast within 60 s was seen in 9/9 cancer vs. 2/14 benign cases (Serra et al. 2018). A meta-analysis and systemic review of 12 studies including 1044 patients revealed that the sensitivity and specificity of CEUS to differentiate between malignant and benign GB lesions was 81% and 87%, respectively (Cheng et al. 2018). CEUS was found to be more accurate (84% vs. 65%) than US to differentiate between benign and malignant GB lesions (Kong et al. 2018).

Endoscopic US (EUS) using 5–12 MHz 360° probe is useful for evaluation of TWGB and GB polyp, diagnosis of early GBC, to evaluate the depth of invasion and to select cases for laparoscopic extended cholecystectomy and for celiac plexus neurolysis (CPN) for palliation of pain in unresectable GBC. A large aorto-caval LN can be picked up on US or CT, but EUS is more sensitive and EUS-guided fine needle aspiration cytology (FNAC) yields better results (Sharma et al. 2018). Contrast-enhanced harmonic EUS can evaluate the microvasculature and real-time perfusion to differentiate between benign and malignant GB mass (Leem et al. 2018).

Real-time elastography with acoustic radiation force impulse (ARFI) using high intensity focused US can also differentiate between benign and malignant GB lesions.

7.3 Computed Tomography (CT)

The Author (VKK) advocates a very low threshold for CT to better evaluate the GB which should be done at the slightest suspicion of GBC on US; CT abdomen and pelvis (and chest) should be obtained. CT shows the following findings:

1. Heterogeneous but primarily hypodense mass replacing the GB (i.e., GB is not seen) (Fig. 7.10) with or without liver infiltration in 40–65% of cases
2. GB wall (mural) focal, asymmetrical, non-uniform, and irregular (vs. diffuse, symmetrical, uniform, and regular in benign disease) thickening (Fig. 7.11) in 20–30% cases
3. Intraluminal polypoidal mass (Fig. 7.12) in 15–25% cases

Good quality IV contrast-enhanced triple-phase multi-slice spiral (helical) CT with three-dimensional volume rendered images helps to interpret the vascular (portal vein, hepatic artery, and hepatic veins) anatomy better. Multi-detector row CT (MDCT) ensures fast scanning and thin sections, and high-resolution axial and coronal views allow multi-planar reconstruction (MPR).

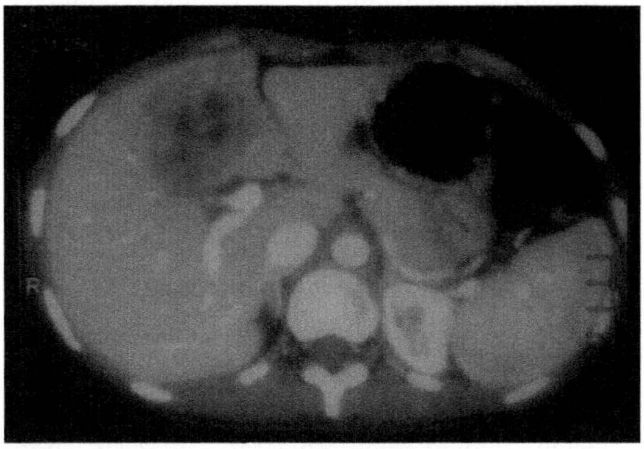

Fig. 7.10 CT shows a mass replacing the gall bladder

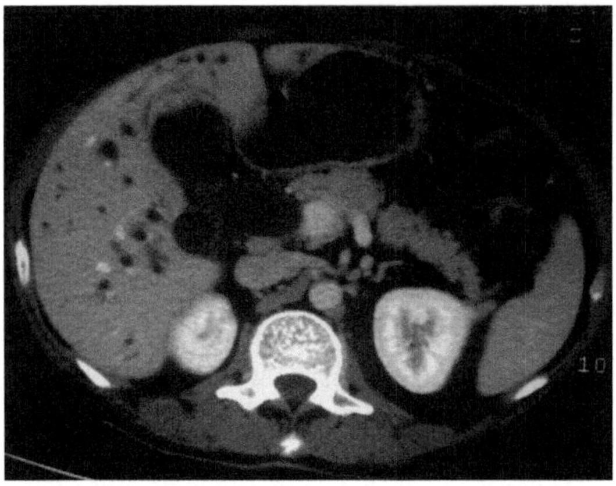

Fig. 7.11 CT shows focal gall bladder wall thickening—this is highly suspicious of gall bladder cancer and should be treated as gall bladder cancer with extended cholecystectomy (note the associated choledochal cyst)

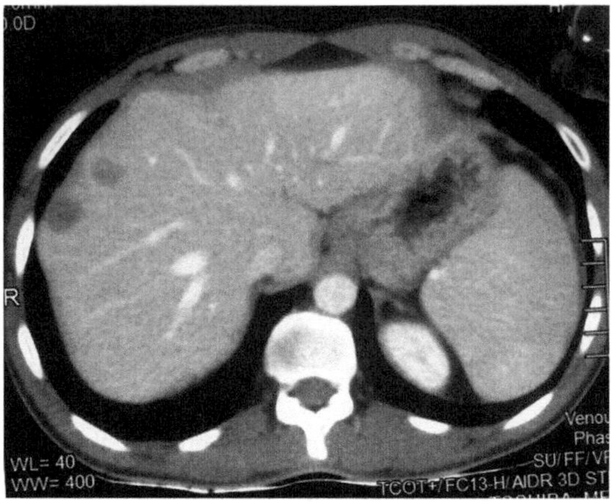

Fig. 7.13 CT shows space-occupying lesion (SOL) in liver suggestive of liver metastasis; it could be a cholangiolytic abscess also if the patient has jaundice and cholangitis

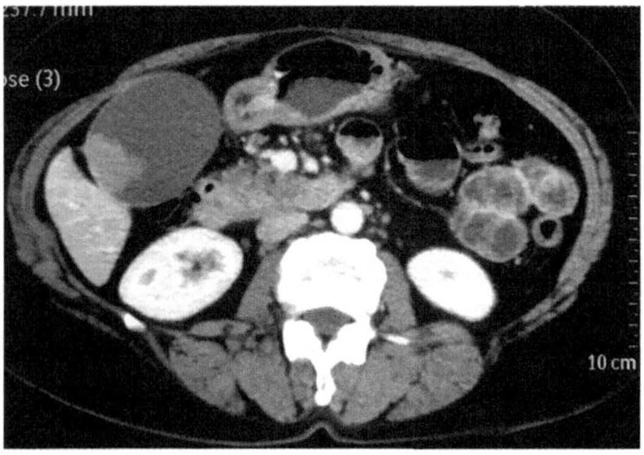

Fig. 7.12 CT shows an intraluminal polypoidal lesion

In chronic cholecystitis, CT shows enhancement of the GB wall in both arterial and venous phases, i.e., isoattenuation in both phases. CT has low sensitivity for detecting early (T1) GBC but shows advanced lesions well. CT detects liver metastases (Fig. 7.13), large omental, peritoneal and pelvic deposits (Fig. 7.14a–c), and can evaluate duodenal (Fig. 7.15) and pancreatic (Fig. 7.16) infiltration and involvement of the hepatoduodenal ligament (Fig. 7.17) and parietes (Fig. 7.18). The presence of a fat plane between the tumor and the adjacent organ/structure/vessel suggests non-involvement (Fig. 7.19) while the absence of a fat plane suggests involvement. Size (>10 mm), shape (round), architecture (heterogeneous), and peripheral (rim or ring like) enhancement suggest metastatic LN involvement (Fig. 7.20). CT has good sensitivity to detect aorto-caval LNs, but enlarged LNs are not necessarily metastatic; on the other hand, metastatic LNs may be normal in size. CT has poor sensitivity to detect peritoneal or omental metastases (unless they are large). CT is poor for evaluation of duodenum (which can be confirmed with UGIE) and colon (which is best evaluated at operation) and the biliary tract (for which MRI and MRC is better). Positive predictive value (PPV) of CT for detecting duodenal involvement was 51%; it increased to 66% with the addition of UGIE (Kalayarasan et al. 2013). Two of three factors, viz. liver invasion, CBD invasion, and hepatic artery invasion on CT predicted positive resection margin in 83% cases (Choi et al. 2019).

CT can also be used to guide FNAC to obtain tissue diagnosis, whenever indicated. CT volumetry (Fig. 7.21) should be done to calculate the remnant liver volume (RLV) if a major hepatic resection, e.g., extended right hepatectomy (ERH) is planned/anticipated; MRI or isotope hepatobiliary scintigraphy can also be used for calculation of the RLV. Some groups perform CT chest (along with abdomen and pelvis) as a routine to pick up pulmonary (Fig. 7.22) and pleural metastases.

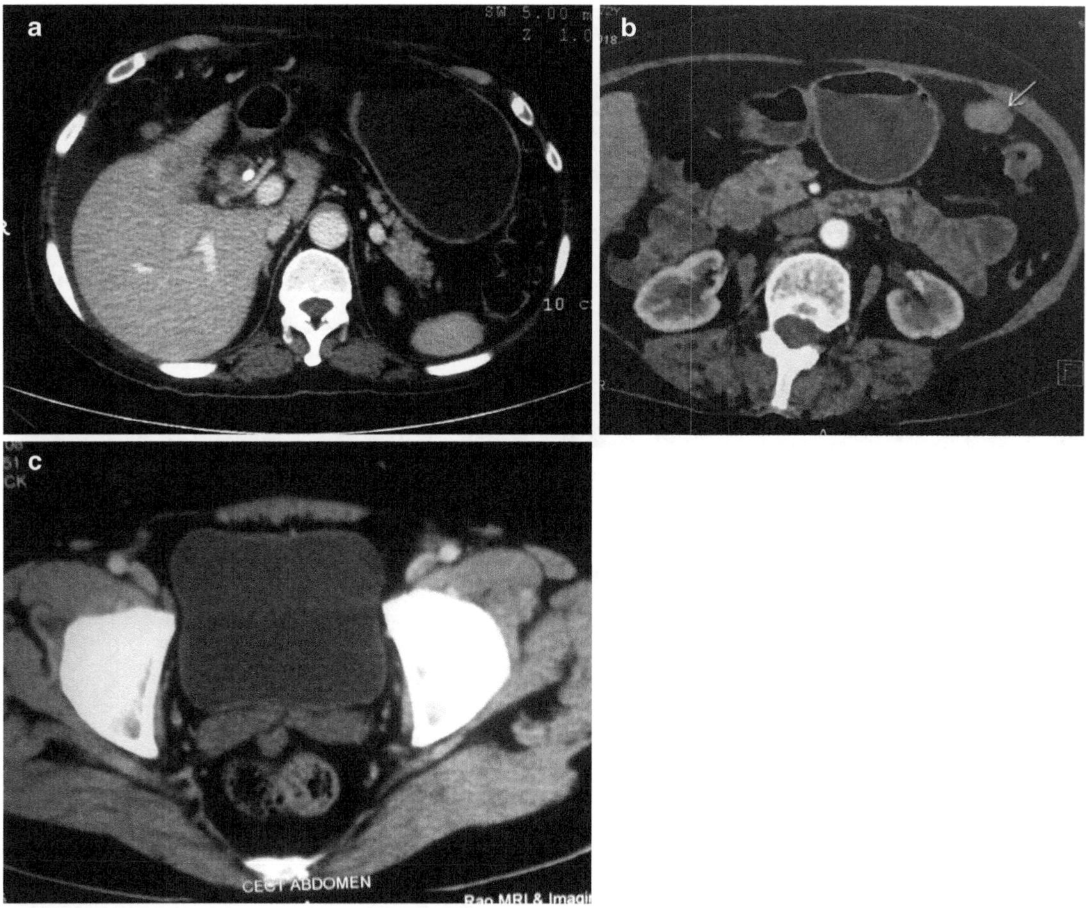

Fig. 7.14 CT shows (**a**) omental (**b**) peritoneal (**c**) pelvic deposit; gall bladder cancer has great propensity for intraperitoneal dissemination

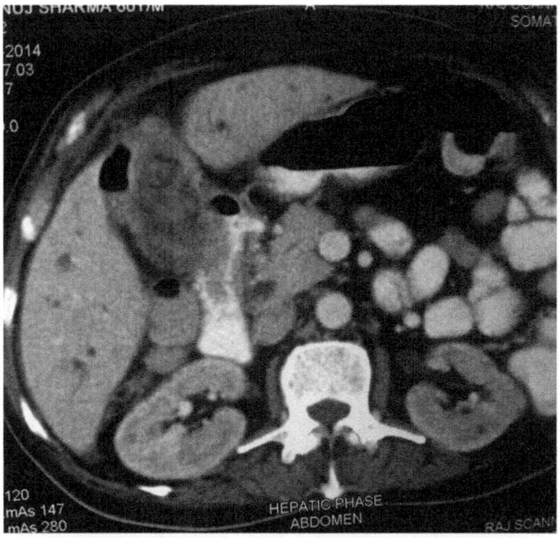

Fig. 7.15 CT shows gall bladder cancer infiltrating duodenum; duodenal infiltration requires pancreato-duodenectomy or segmental/sleeve resection of the duodenum

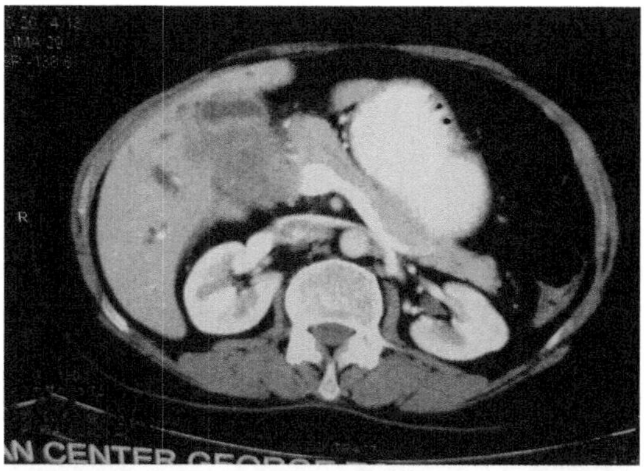

Fig. 7.16 CT shows gall bladder cancer infiltrating pancreas; pancreatic infiltration requires pancreato-duodenectomy

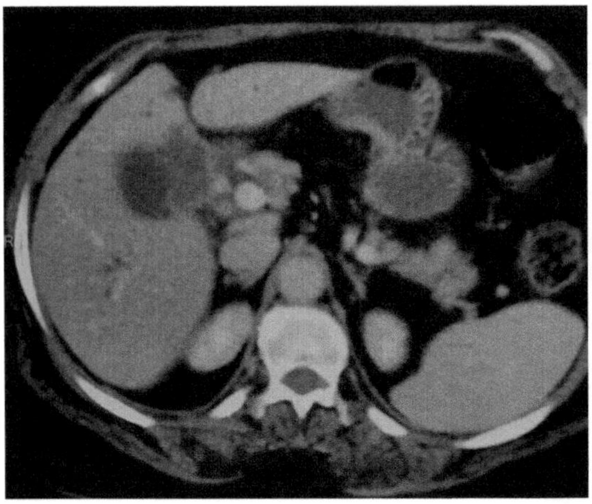

Fig. 7.17 CT shows gall bladder cancer infiltrating the hepatoduodenal ligament; this is unresectable disease

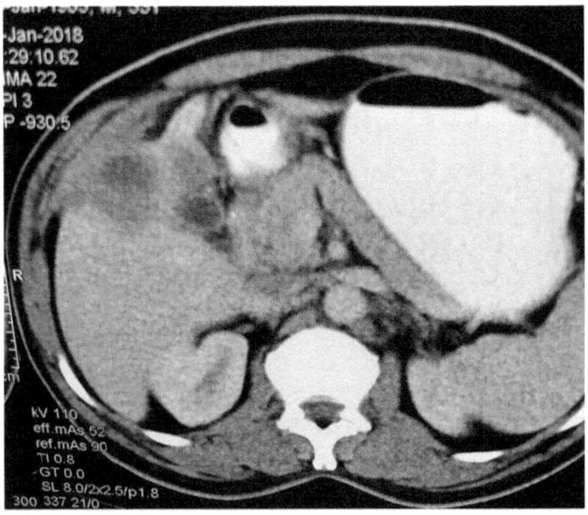

Fig. 7.18 CT shows gall bladder cancer infiltrating the parietes

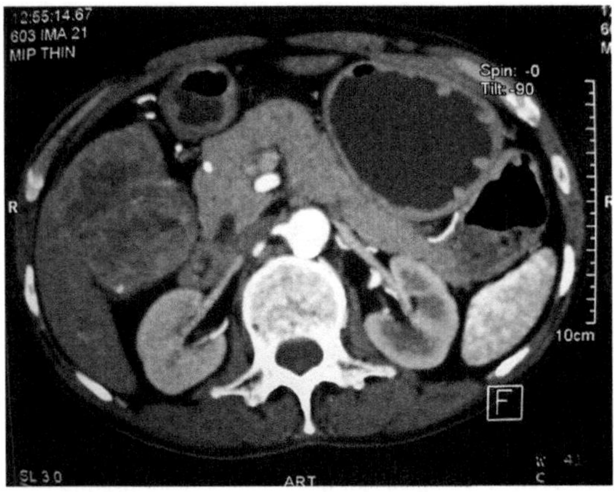

Fig. 7.19 CT shows a clear fat plane between the gall bladder mass and the pancreas indicating that the pancreas is free and is not involved

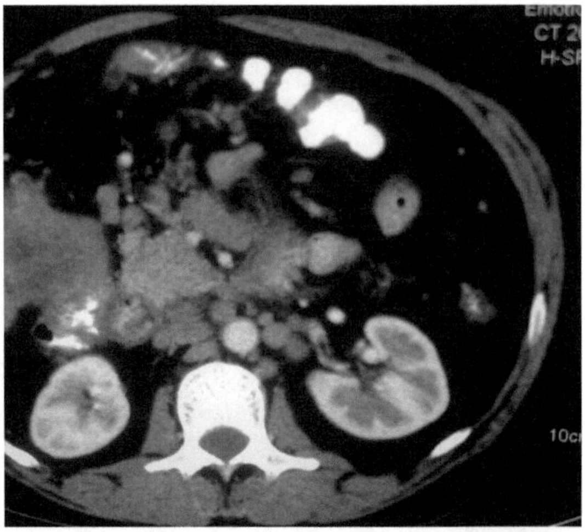

Fig. 7.20 CT shows enlarged retropancreatic lymph node

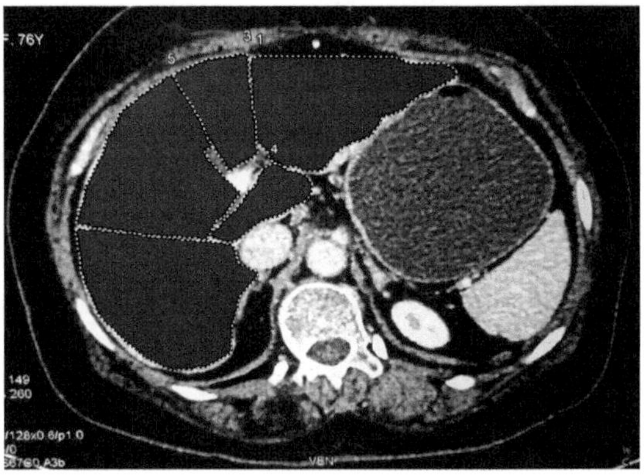

Fig. 7.21 CT volumetry should be done to calculate the remnant liver volume (RLV) if a major liver resection, e.g., extended right hepatectomy (ERH) is planned

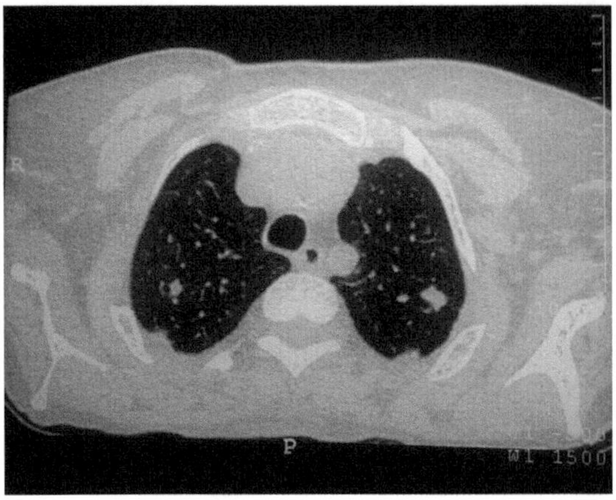

Fig. 7.22 CT chest shows bilateral lung nodules suggestive of pulmonary metastasis; some groups perform CT chest (along with abdomen and pelvis) as routine for evaluation of gall bladder cancer

7.4 Magnetic Resonance Imaging (MRI)

Magnetic resonance imaging (MRI) with magnetic resonance cholangiography (MRC) and magnetic resonance angiography (MRA) is a one-stop single investigational modality to evaluate GBC. MRI shows same finding as CT, viz.

1. Heterogeneous but primarily hypointense mass replacing the GB (i.e., GB is not seen) with or without liver infiltration (Fig. 7.23) or at the hilum (Fig. 7.24)
2. GB wall (mural) focal, asymmetrical, non-uniform and irregular (vs. diffuse, symmetrical, uniform and regular in benign disease) thickening
3. Intraluminal polypoidal mass

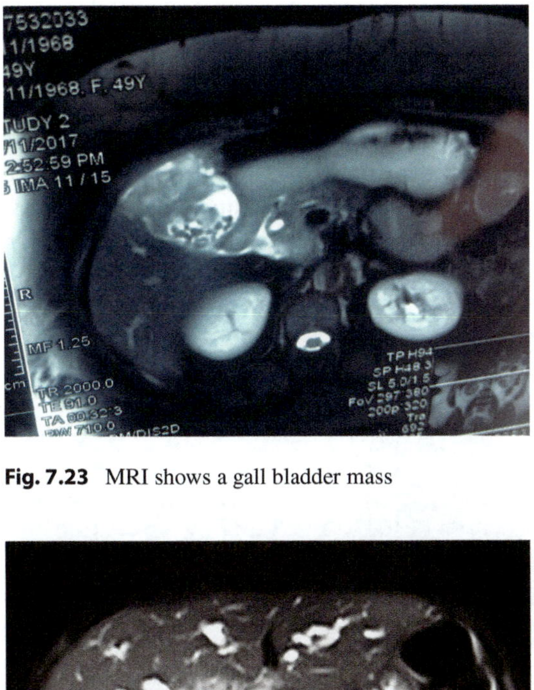

Fig. 7.23 MRI shows a gall bladder mass

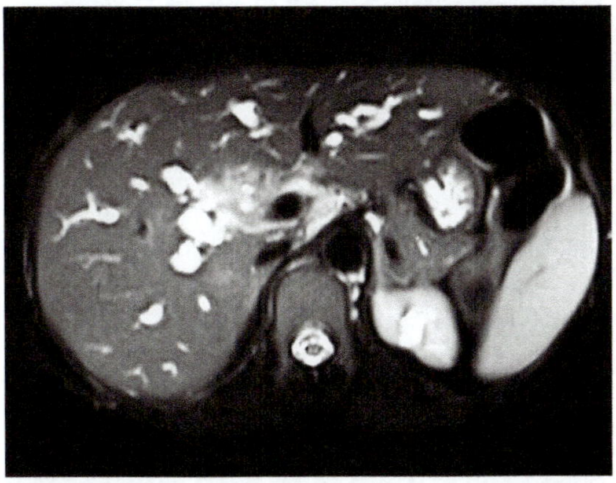

Fig. 7.24 MRI shows a hilar mass—it could be gall bladder cancer at neck or a hilar cholangiocarcinoma which sometimes are difficult to differentiate from each other

GBC is hypointense on T1 and hyperintense on T2 images; contrast enhancement shows early phase enhancement which persists in the delayed phase (cf. early enhancement with subsequent washout in benign masses). MRI is good to detect liver invasion and LN metastases but is poor for detecting duodenum or colon infiltration and peritoneal metastases. Moreover, interpretation of MR images is highly dependent on the skill and expertise of the radiologist. Non-contrast MRI was found to be a useful alternative to gadolinic acid-enhanced MRI to differentiate between 36 GBC and 65 benign causes of focal GB wall thickening (Cha et al. 2019). Diffusion-weighted MRI (DW MRI) has been used to differentiate between GBC and benign disease—apparent diffusion coefficient (ADC) of less than 1.2 and lesion to spinal cord ratio (LSR) of more than 0.5 suggested a diagnosis of GBC with sensitivity of 73%, specificity of 96% and accuracy of 93% (Kitazume et al. 2016). ADC value negatively correlated with tumor stage and differentiation, i.e., lower ADC values in higher stage and poor differentiation; ADC values also predicted survival (Min et al. 2019).

Imaging (CT or MRI) should be performed before any preoperative biliary drainage (PBD) is done because tubes and stents produce artifacts and interfere with radiological resolution.

A systematic review of nine studies including 292 patients and meta-analysis of five studies including 58 patients however, revealed that the value of CT and MRI for evaluation of nodal status was unclear especially for detection of small LN metastases (de Savornin Lohman et al. 2019).

7.5 Tumor Markers

Tumor markers, e.g., carcinoma-embryonic antigen (CEA) and carbohydrate antigen (CA) 19.9 are not specific for GBC and are not recommended for the diagnosis of GBC. Elevated levels of these tumor markers may, however, raise a suspicion of GBC in a patient with TWGB. Elevated CEA level is specific for GBC but sensitivity of CEA to diagnose GBC is low. Sakamoto et al. (2019) developed a scoring system including tumor diameter and serum CEA level to preoperatively predict pT2. CA 19.9 also has low sensitivity for GBC—only 73/217 (34%) patients in a USA consortium report had high (>37 U/mL) CA 19.9 level (Margonis et al. 2016). In an analysis of 292 patients operated between 2000 and 2016 in China, CA 19.9 > 99 U/mL predicted unresectability (Liu et al. 2019a). Zhang et al. (2018) used a normal CA 19.9 level as a selection criteria for laparoscopic management of GBC confined to the GB wall. Baseline CA 19.9 predicts the burden of disease and predicts prognosis; it can also be used to monitor response to neoadjuvant therapy (NAT) (Agrawal et al. 2018). Tumor marker level may also predict survival; in a 10 institutions (USA) experience of 108 GBCs with jaundice, better (40 vs. 12 months) survival was seen in patients with low CA 19.9 (Tran et al. 2017). CA 19.9 > 37 IU/mL predicts poor prognosis (Chang et al. 2016; Liu et al. 2019b). CA 19-9 kinetics during palliative chemotherapy for unresectable GBC is a reliable prognosticator for survival (overall survival OS and disease-free survival DFS) (Lee et al. 2018). Wen et al. (2017) reported that a combination of elevated CEA and CA 19.9 was associated with poor prognosis.

7.6 Positron Emission Tomography (PET)

Imaging, e.g., US, CT, or MRI has low sensitivity in detecting small metastases. 18 Fluorodeoxy-glucose (FDG) positron emission tomography (PET) is a functional nuclear imaging based on selective high utilization of glucose in cancer cells. It can detect radiologically occult abdominal, e.g., lymph nodes (Fig. 7.25) and peritoneum (Fig. 7.26)/extra-abdominal disease not detected on CT/MRI and avoids unnecessary non-therapeutic laparotomy. PET has high sensitivity in GBC due to its aggressive biology and FDG avidity—mean standard uptake value (SUV) was 4.1 in GBC and 1.8 in

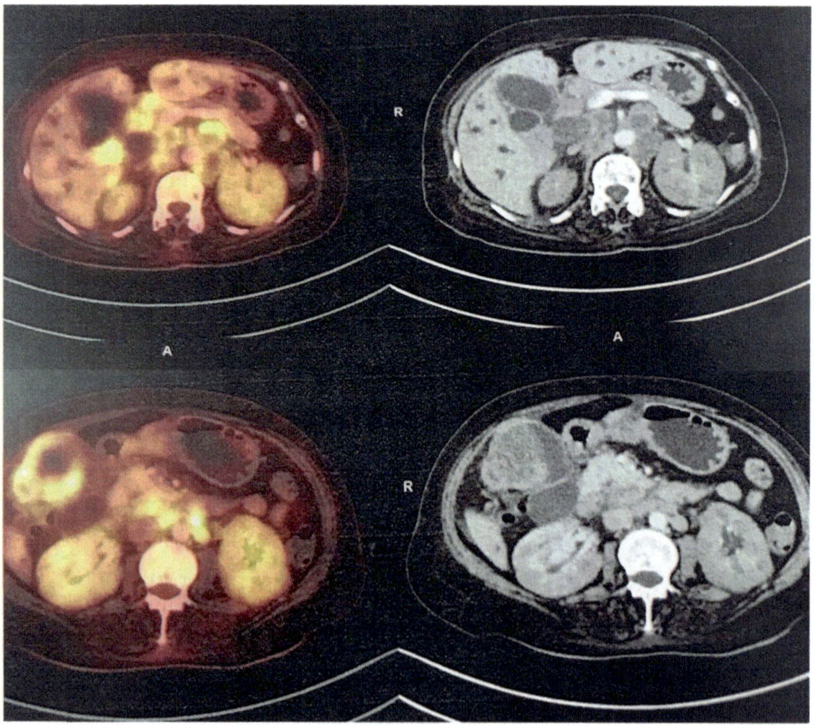

Fig. 7.25 PET shows FDG avid lymph node mass

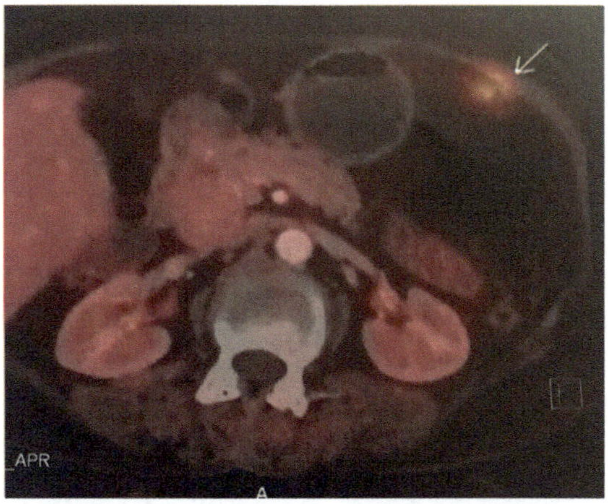

Fig. 7.26 PET shows FDG avid peritoneal nodule

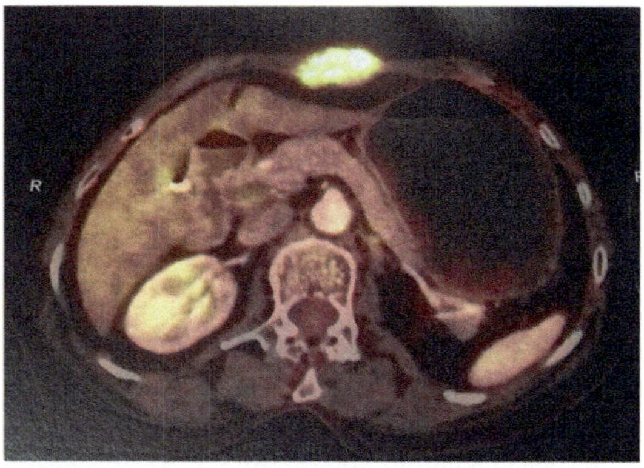

Fig. 7.27 PET shows FDG avid port site metastasis in a patient with incidental gall bladder cancer

benign; it was useful for differentiating GBC from benign, especially XGC, with 80% sensitivity and 82% specificity (Rodríguez-Fernández et al. 2004). SUV max was 7.9 ± 6.3 in GBC; SUVmax cutoff value of 3.62 had 78% sensitivity and 88% specificity for malignancy; PET changed the surgical plans in 22% of 49 (34 malignant and 15 benign) patients (Ramos-Font et al. 2014). PET's larger scan area (cf. US, MR) allows evaluation of multiple organs in one scan with less radiation (cf. CT). Poor resolution and anatomical localization of PET can be covered by combining it with CT. PET-CT is better than MD CT in detecting metastases. Metabolic tumor volume (MTV) and total lesional glycolysis (TLG) (SUV × MTV), as measured on PET-CT, predicted the survival (Chun et al. 2019). PET is useful to detect recurrence (locoregional and distant) in follow-up; in an analysis of 62 patients, sensitivity and specificity were 98% and 90%, respectively (Kumar et al. 2012 AA 53/28).

PET has also been used to detect residual disease including port site metastases (Fig. 7.27) in incidental GBC. PET-CT is recommended in patients with incidental GBC in whom MDCT is normal or shows locally advanced disease (Shukla et al. 2008). The Tata Memorial Hospital (TMH) Mumbai India group suggested that a negative PET may avoid reoperation in T1b incidental GBC (Goel et al. 2016). FDG PET is, however, less useful in incidental GBC than in primary non-incidental GBC; it changed the management in only 13% of 63 patients with incidental GBC vs. 31% of 37 patients with a preoperative diagnosis of GBC (Leung et al. 2014).

PET can be false negative in small (<0.5 cm) size peritoneal disease, in mucinous adenocarcinoma, and in the presence of uncontrolled diabetes with elevated blood glucose. It can be false-positive if it is done too early (within 4 weeks) of surgery (cholecystectomy) in patients with incidental GBC and in inflammatory lesions, e.g., XGC, adenomyomatosis, and in tubercular LNs. PET lesions, therefore, need to be confirmed by tissue diagnosis before curative intent treatment is denied to a patient.

Patkar et al. (2020) found PET to be a valuable tool to rule out metastatic disease in 103 patients with locally advanced GBC. In another recent retrospective but large analysis of 149 patients in whom PET was performed after CECT chest, abdomen, and pelvis showed resectable disease, the management plan changed in as many as 35 (23%) patients; this was more frequent (i.e., 27%) in patients with node-positive disease on CT (Goel et al. 2020). If availability and costs are not a constraint, PET may be done in all patients, especially those going for operation, but the Author (VKK) definitely recommends PET in locally advanced GBC before a major operation, e.g., extended right hepatectomy (ERH) or hepato-pancreato-duodenectomy (HPD) or in patients with incidental GBC who are delayed (say >4 weeks) for reoperation, to rule out any distant disease. PET may also be used to assess the response to NAT.

All imaging investigations including PET, however, have poor sensitivity for detecting small peritoneal and omental deposits thus highlighting the place of staging laparoscopy (*vide infra*) in even PET-negative cases.

7.7 Cholangiography

Non-invasive cholangiography, i.e., MRC should be done in patients with jaundice or suspected biliary obstruction (deranged LFTs, IHBRD on US) to better delineate the level of biliary obstruction—mid-CBD (Fig. 7.28), hilar (Fig. 7.29), or intrahepatic (Fig. 7.30). Invasive cholangiography (endoscopic retrograde cholangiography ERC or percutaneous transhepatic cholangiography PTC, Fig. 7.31) is not indicated as a diagnostic procedure (for which MRC is preferred) and should be done only as a part of a therapeutic intervention for biliary drainage. ERC may be performed if US suggests CBD stones, especially Mirizzi's syndrome, as a cause of jaundice.

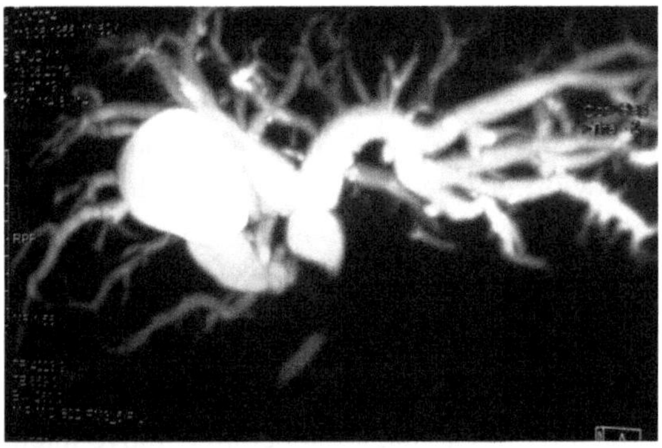

Fig. 7.28 MRC shows mid-biliary obstruction—it could be gall bladder cancer neck involving the common bile duct (CBD) or mid-CBD cholangiocarcinoma

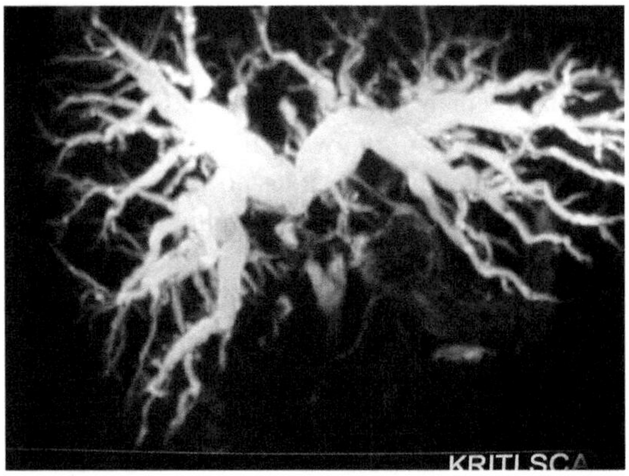

Fig. 7.29 MRC shows high (hilar) biliary obstruction—it could be gall bladder cancer neck involving the hepatic hilum or hilar cholangiocarcinoma

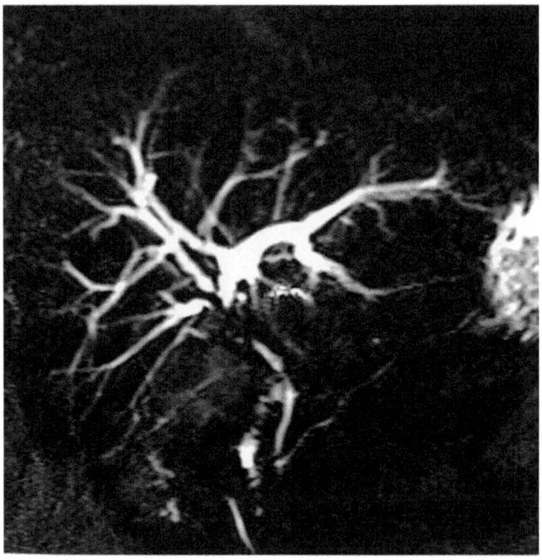

Fig. 7.30 MRC shows intrahepatic biliary obstruction—it could be gall bladder cancer neck involving the intrahepatic bile ducts or hilar cholangiocarcinoma with extension into the right ducts

7.8 Other Investigations

Upper gastro-intestinal endoscopy (UGIE) is indicated in the presence of symptoms of gastric outlet obstruction (GOO) or gastroparesis or in case of suspicion of duodenal involvement on CT. Plasma clearance rate of indo-cyanine green (ICG) can predict surgical outcome after a major liver resection (Yokoyama et al. 2010).

7.9 Tissue Diagnosis (Cytodiagnosis)

Tissue diagnosis is not required if there is a radiological suspicion of malignancy and the

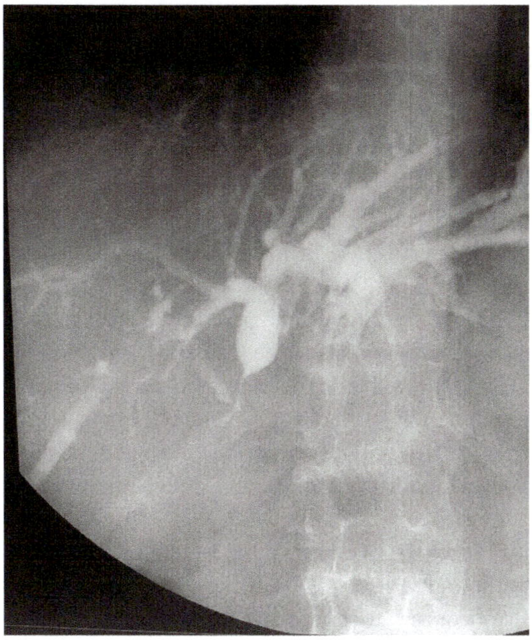

Fig. 7.31 Percutaneous transhepatic cholangiography (PTC) shows mid-biliary obstruction—it could be gall bladder cancer neck involving the common bile duct (CBD) or mid-CBD cholangiocarcinoma; invasive cholangiography, e.g., PTC (or ERC) is, however, not preferred for diagnosis only, it is performed as a part of a therapeutic intervention only

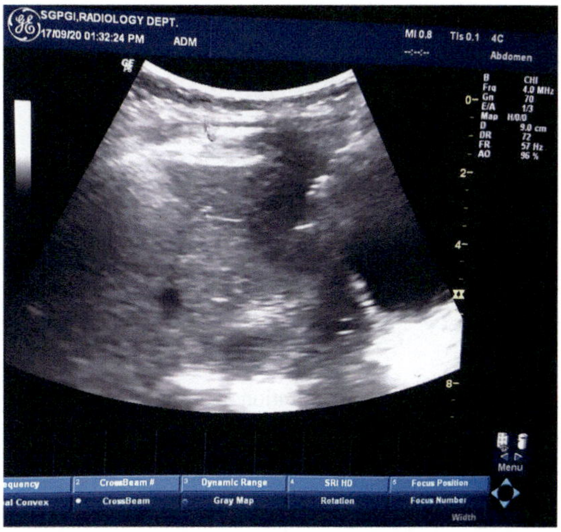

Fig. 7.32 Tissue for confirmation of diagnosis can be obtained by US guided fine needle aspiration cytology (FNAC); tissue diagnosis is not required if the disease is resectable—it should be obtained if the disease is not resectable. (Image courtesy Dr. Rajni Kant Yadav Radiology SGPGIMS Lucknow)

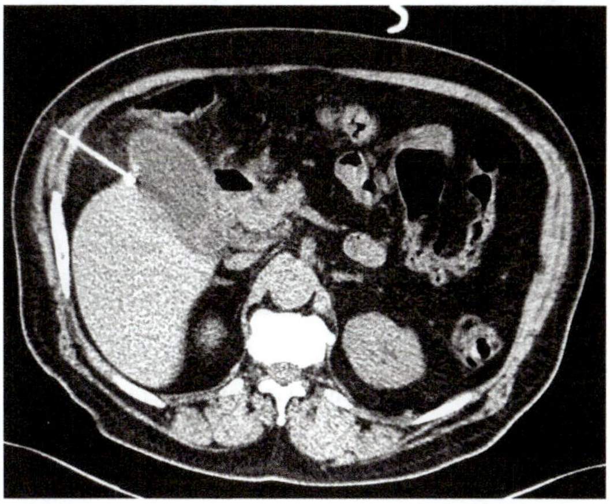

Fig. 7.33 Tissue for confirmation of diagnosis can be obtained by CT-guided fine needle aspiration cytology (FNAC); tissue diagnosis is not required if the disease is resectable—it should be obtained if the disease is not resectable (Image courtesy Dr. Rajni Kant Yadav Radiology SGPGIMS Lucknow)

lesion is resectable. This is because resection will (should) still be performed even if FNAC is negative. FNAC is not preferred in resectable lesions because GBC has high propensity for tumor seeding of the needle track (thus converting eminently curable disease into metastatic); moreover, bleeding and bile leak (from an obstructed biliary system) can occur following FNAC. Preoperative FNAC or intraoperative frozen section is, however, desirable before a major resection, e.g., hepatectomy or pancreato-duodenectomy (as there are anecdotal reports of histology after major resections showing XGC). Tissue diagnosis should also be obtained if the disease is unresectable and non-surgical management is planned (there are anecdotal reports of tuberculosis and lymphoma, which can be managed with medical therapy, mimicking GBC on imaging) or in locoregionally (non-metastatic) advanced disease planned for neo-adjuvant therapy (NAT).

Tissue diagnosis can be obtained using a fine (25–20 G) needle with a stylet or a core (19–14 G) needle—it can be percutaneous direct (if a lump is palpable) or image (US Fig. 7.32 or CT Fig. 7.33) guided. Sensitivity of FNAC (Fig. 7.34) is 80–90%; it can be false negative because of sampling error, i.e., sampling from non-

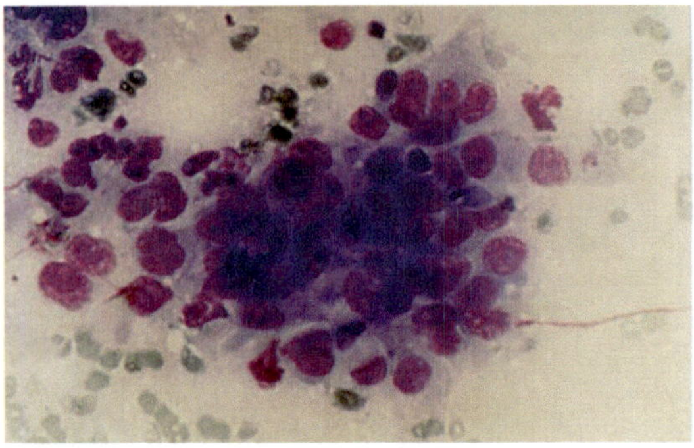

Fig. 7.34 Fine needle aspiration cytology (FNAC) showing malignant cells; FNAC can be obtained from a metastasis (liver or lymph node) or the primary lesion (if the disease is unresectable)

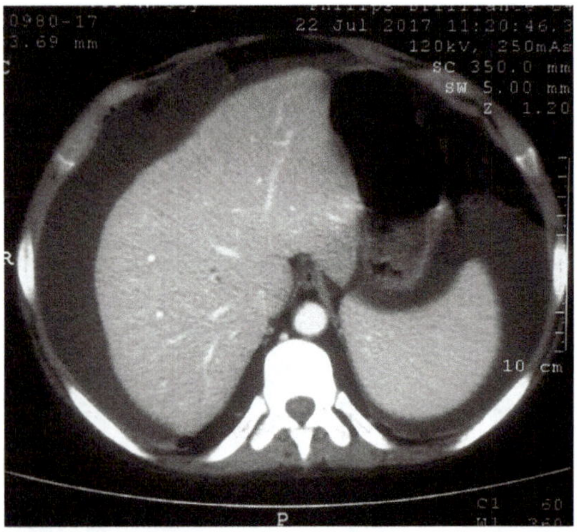

Fig. 7.35 CT shows ascites; ascitic fluid should be aspirated and subjected to fluid cytology if there is no pedal edema and hypoalbuminemia to account for the ascites

representative areas and because of the presence of necrosis or fibrosis in the tumor. MR guidance for FNAC has the advantage of the diagnostic intervention in coronal plane. EUS-guided FNAC of GB mass or regional LNs was performed in 50 (60%) out of 83 suspected GBC patients—sensitivity was 95% (Hijioka et al. 2012). Bile cytology obtained at ERC or PTC can also yield the tissue diagnosis. Endoscopic transpapillary gall bladder drainage (ETGD) and GB bile cytology has been described to differentiate between benign and malignant GB lesions (Itsuki et al. 2018). Liquid biopsy of bile, i.e., analysis of DNA for mutations in oncogenes using next-generation sequencing (NGS) has been shown to be better than bile cytology (Kinugasa et al. 2018). Percutaneous transhepatic cholangioscopic (PTCS) brush biopsy or endoscopic brush biopsy has also been used for diagnosis of GBC invading the CBD. US/EUS/CT-guided FNAC can be performed from an enlarged aorto-caval LN. If US and/or CT show ascites (Fig. 7.35), and more so if there is no pedal edema (to suggest hypoalbuminemia as the cause of ascites), the ascitic fluid should be aspirated for cytological examination to find out if it is malignant. Hirata et al. (2019) recently described even genetic analysis using targeted amplicon sequencing in EUS-FNA specimens.

Intraoperative biopsy and frozen section histopathological examination may be done to confirm cancer, to confirm distant metastases and LNs and the cystic duct margin but it is not good for assessing the depth of invasion.

7.10 Staging Laparoscopy

GBC is an aggressive cancer; in addition to the usual lymphatic and vascular (hematogenous) spread, it has a very high propensity for peritoneal dissemination resulting in small deposits on the surface of liver (Fig. 7.36), parietal and visceral peritoneum (Fig. 7.37), omentum, pelvis, and undersurface of diaphragm. All imaging investigations, i.e., US, CT, MRI, and even PET, have poor sensitivity to detect these small metastases. Staging laparoscopy (SL) very easily detects these small surface peritoneal (parietal and visceral)/omental metastatic deposits which are invariably missed on preoperative imaging, i.e., US/CT/MRI and may not be detectable even on PET-CT (i.e., they are radiographically occult). In addition to the peritoneal nodules, a small parenchymal metastasis on the surface of the liver which was missed on preoperative imaging may also be seen on SL. If a peritoneal or liver lesion is seen on SL, one or two more 5 mm working ports need to be placed and the lesion should be biopsied (Fig. 7.38) and subjected to frozen section histopathological examination to

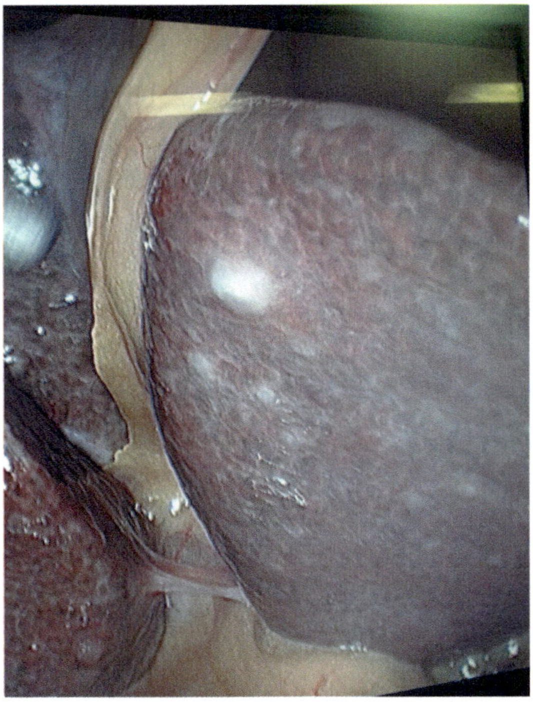

Fig. 7.36 Staging laparoscopy shows small liver surface deposits

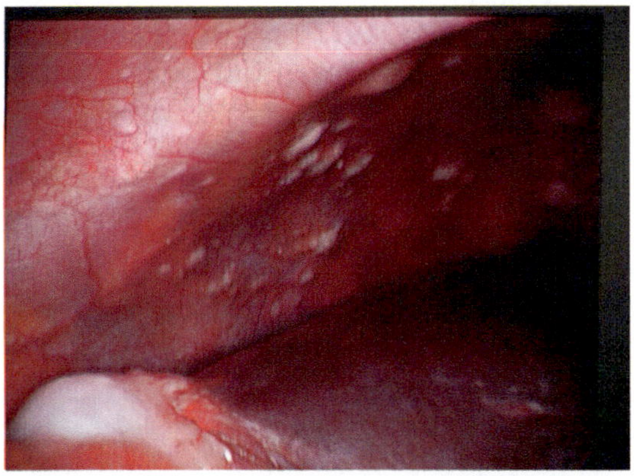

Fig. 7.37 Staging laparoscopy shows small peritoneal deposits

confirm the diagnosis of metastasis. This is important because in areas and populations where tuberculosis is still common, a peritoneal tubercle may look like a peritoneal metastasis. If ascites is found at SL, ascitic fluid cytology should be performed; peritoneal lavage cytology (PLC) may be performed if there is no ascites. The presence of peritoneal dissemination (nodule, positive ascitic fluid cytology, or positive PLC) or liver metastasis on SL is a contraindication for laparotomy—SL, thus, avoids an unnecessary non-therapeutic laparotomy. PET-CT may detect some of these deposits; yield of SL may, therefore, decrease with the routine use of PET-CT in preoperative staging of GBC.

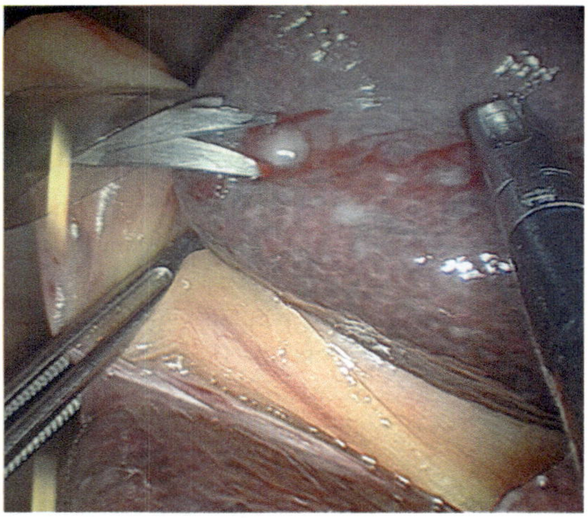

Fig. 7.38 Metastatic deposit seen at staging laparoscopy being biopsied to confirm the metastasis

Many texts (Russolillo et al. 2016) call it "diagnostic" laparoscopy (DL), but the correct term is "staging" laparoscopy because laparoscopy is performed not for the diagnosis of GBC (which is made on imaging, i.e., US, CT, or MRI) but to stage the disease after a diagnosis has been made/is suspected on imaging. Laparoscopy for staging of pancreatic cancer was first reported by Cuschieri et al. (1978). Jarnagin et al. (2000) used it for primary and secondary hepatobiliary cancers. Weber et al. (2002) described it in 100 patients with extrahepatic biliary cancers including 44 patients with potentially resectable GBC out of which 21 patients were found to have unresectable disease. We (Agrawal et al. 2005) reported SL in 91 patients with GBC who were assessed to have resectable disease on CT (PET was not done)—unnecessary laparotomy was avoided in 34 patients with metastases and 6 with extensive unresectable locoregional disease. SL detected disseminated disease in 95 (23%) of 409 potentially resectable GBC patients managed at the GB Pant Hospital, New Delhi, India (2006–2011). The yield was higher (25%, 89/353) in advanced (T3, T4) disease but as many as 11% (6/56) patients with even early (T1, T2) disease had metastases detected on SL. Non-therapeutic laparotomy was avoided in 23% overall and in 56% cases with unresectable disease; overall resectability rate was 58% (Agarwal et al. 2013). In an analysis of 1090 patients with resectable extrahepatic biliary tumors (EHBT) including GBC, the yield of SL was 17% but it increased to a high of 53% in high-risk (increased CA 19.9 and decreased serum albumin) GBC patients (Davidson et al. 2019). The Nagoya University Japan group performs SL before preoperative biliary drainage (PBD)/portal vein embolization (PVE) (Nagino et al. 2006) and then again before surgery. Agarwal et al. (2013) classified lesions indicating unresectability as detectable on SL, viz. peritoneal or liver surface metastases and undetectable on SL, viz. deep intraparenchymal liver metastases, distant (e.g., celiac, superior mesenteric, aorto-caval) LNs, and locally advanced unresectable disease in the form of local adjacent organ infiltration. SL could identify as many as 94% of detectable lesions. The undetectable lesions can, however, be detected if laparoscopic US is used or by doing some laparoscopic dissection after placement of two working ports. Laparoscopic US can increase the yield of SL by detecting intraparenchymal liver metastases, assessing the extent of liver infiltration, and by evaluation of involvement of the hepatoduodenal ligament and involvement of duodenum/pancreas. Laparoscopic US increased the accuracy of detecting these lesions. Laparoscopic celiac, superior mesenteric, and aorto-caval LN biopsy can be performed. Laparoscopic narrow band imaging (NBI) has recently been reported for intraoperative diagnosis and evaluation of the depth of invasion of GBC (Iwashita and Inomata 2019).

The yield of SL in incidental GBC is low because most of these are early lesions; moreover, adhesions of previous surgery may hinder a complete evaluation on SL. The yield of SL in incidental GBC was 4% (2/46) in a series from the Memorial Sloan Kettering Cancer Center (MSKCC) New York, USA (Butte et al. 2011) and 7% (6/83) in another from India (Agarwal et al. 2013). SL is recommended in high-risk patients with incidental GBC, viz. bile spill during the index cholecystectomy, delayed presentation after the index cholecystectomy, advanced T stage and poor differentiation, as the yield of SL was higher in these cases.

In GBC, *always peep (SL) before you enter (laparotomy)* (Kapoor 2017).

7.11 Thick-Walled GB (TWGB)

Normal gall bladder (GB) wall thickness is 3 mm or less; GB wall thickness of 4 mm or more on US is described as TWGB (Fig. 7.39). TWGB is seen in acute cholecystitis, long-standing chronic cholecystitis, xantho-granulomatous cholecystitis (XGC), adenomyomatosis, and gall bladder cancer (GBC). GB wall may be thickened in acute hepatitis, portal hypertension, congestive heart failure (CHF), and chronic renal failure (CRF) also. A TWGB on US merits further evaluation with contrast-enhanced CT (Fig. 7.40) and/or MRI (Fig. 7.41); it can also be evaluated with CEUS, EUS, and real-time elastography.

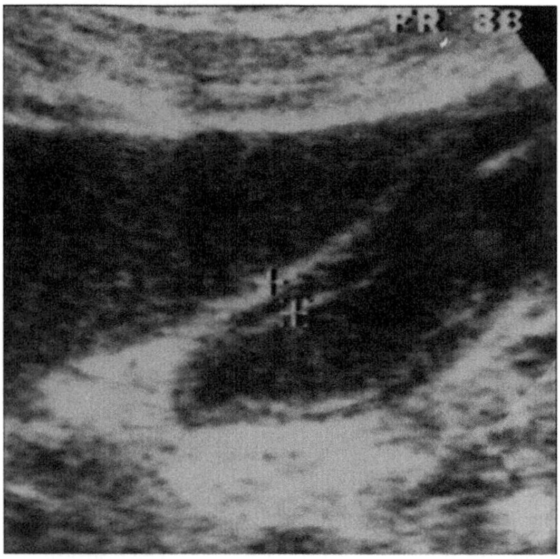

Fig. 7.39 US shows thick (>3 mm)-walled gall bladder (TWGB); this requires further evaluation with CT

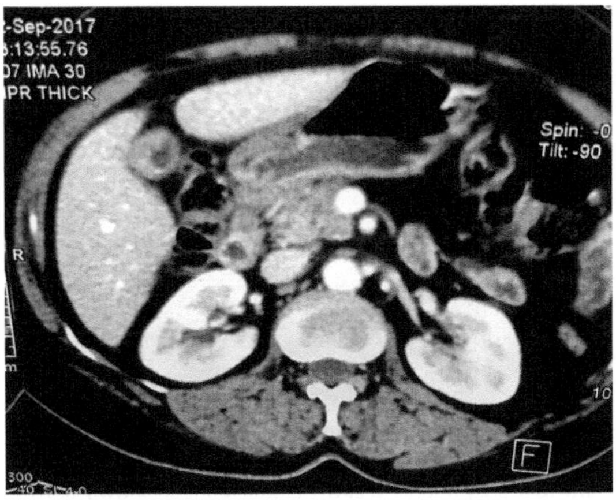

Fig. 7.40 CT shows thick (>3 mm)-walled gall bladder (TWGB)

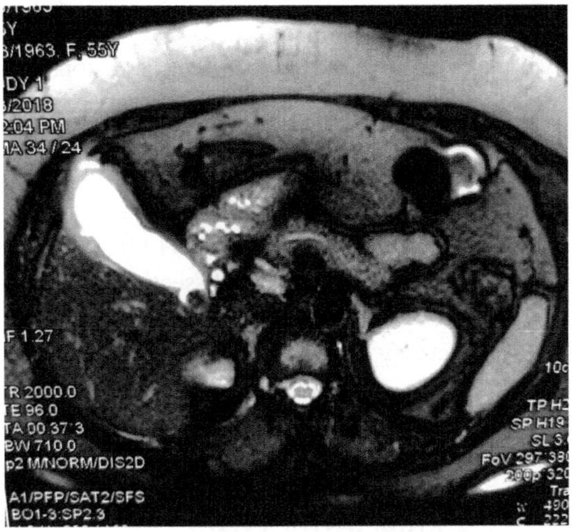

Fig. 7.41 MRI shows thick (>3 mm)-walled gall bladder (TWGB)

TWGB poses a big therapeutic dilemma as it can be benign (CC or XGC) or malignant (GBC). Focal (Fig. 7.42), localized, non-uniform, irregular (Fig. 7.43) thickening of the GB wall should be considered and treated as malignant. Diffuse, generalized, uniform, regular thickening of the GB wall (Fig. 7.44) is usually benign, i.e., chronic cholecystitis or xantho-granulomatous cholecystitis (XGC) but may be malignant. Prospective analysis of 60 consecutive diffuse TWGBs revealed that 30 were due to CC, 28 due to XGC, and 2 turned out to have incidental GBC (Srikanth et al. 2004). PET has been used to differentiate

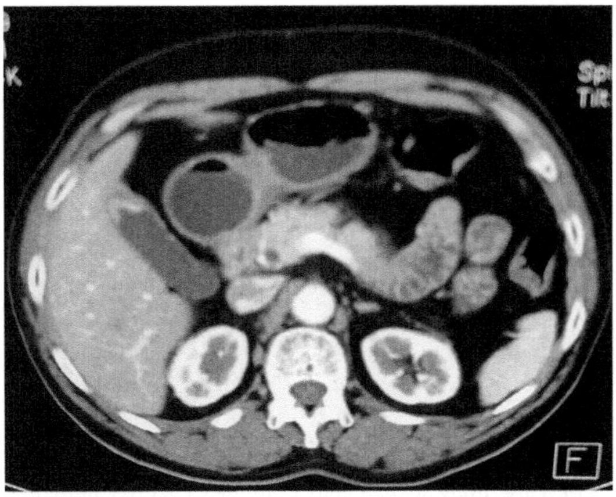

Fig. 7.42 Focal thickening of the gall bladder wall—high suspicion of gall bladder cancer; such cases should be treated as gall bladder cancer with extended cholecystectomy

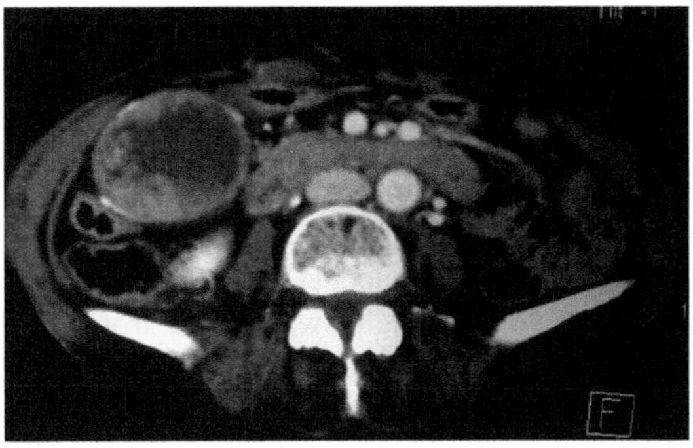

Fig. 7.43 Irregular thickening of the gall bladder wall—high suspicion of gall bladder cancer; such cases should be treated as gall bladder cancer with extended cholecystectomy

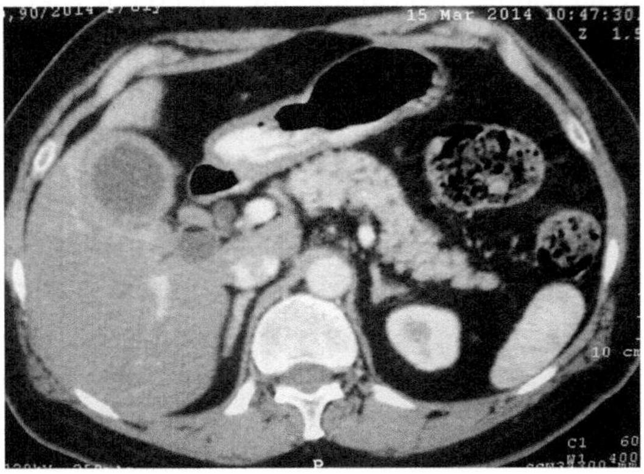

Fig. 7.44 Diffuse thickening of the gall bladder wall—low suspicion of gall bladder cancer; we have described anticipatory extended cholecystectomy (AEC) for such cases

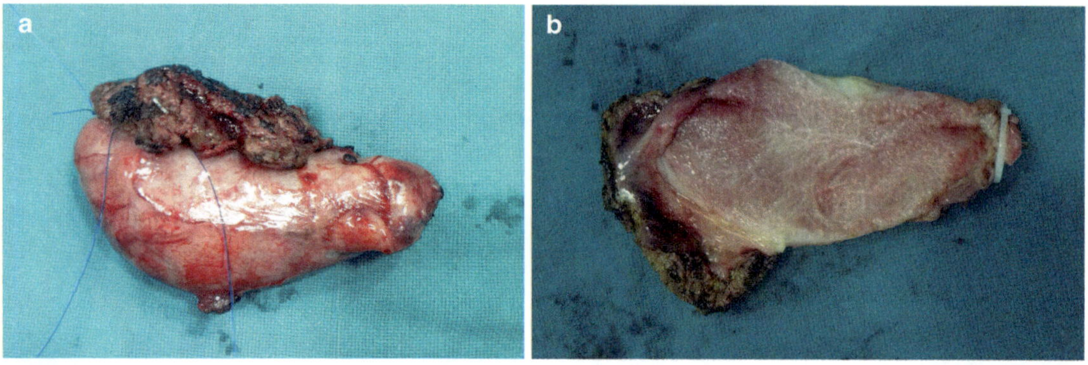

Fig. 7.45 (**a**) Anticipatory extended cholecystectomy (AEC) for thick-walled gall bladder (TWGB) with low suspicion of GBC; the gall bladder is removed with a small wedge of liver and subjected to frozen section histopathological examination. (**b**) AEC specimen in a patient with low suspicion of gall bladder cancer shows normal mucosa—unlikely to be malignant

between benign and malignant TWGB-mean SUV uptake in malignancy was higher (7.46 vs. 4.51) than in benign in an experience of 30 cases of TWGB (GBC n = 12, CC n = 11, XGC n = 4, IgG related n = 2, and GB polyp n = 1). At a median cutoff SUV of 5.95, sensitivity and specificity of PET to detect malignancy were 92% and 79%, respectively (Gupta et al. 2018). A scoring system to differentiate between XGC from GBC has been described (Rajaguru et al. 2018).

All TWGBs (except those seen during acute cholecystitis) should be operated because it is difficult to differentiate benign (CC or XGC) from malignant (GBC) TWGB even after imaging (US, CT, MRI, or PET). While simple cholecystectomy is enough for CC or XGC, extended cholecystectomy will be required for GBC. If TWGB is presumed to be benign and simple cholecystectomy alone is performed, but it turns out to be GBC (on histopathological examination) it will be an inappropriate operation. If TWGB is suspected to be malignant and extended cholecystectomy is performed, but it turns out to be benign (on histopathological examination) it will be on over kill. If there is a high suspicion of GBC on imaging, extended cholecystectomy should be performed—some patients will turn out to have a benign pathology but that is acceptable. Full-thickness cholecystectomy (FTC) including the cystic plate (Shirai et al. 2012) followed by frozen section histopathological examination is an option. In patients with TWGB with a low suspicion of malignancy, we have described anticipatory extended cholecystectomy (AEC) (Fig. 7.45a, b), i.e., removal of the GB with a small wedge of liver in the GB bed in segments IVB and V followed by frozen section histopathological examination of the specimen. Lymphadenectomy is added if the frozen section histopathological examination reveals cancer. Tokumitsu et al. (2020) described laparoscopic whole-layer cholecystectomy (LWLC) (n = 12) and laparoscopic GB bed dissection (LGBD) (n = 3), a procedure similar to anticipatory extended cholecystectomy (AEC) described by the Author (VKK) (2016), suspected malignant lesions.

7.12 Xantho-Granulomatous Cholecystitis (XGC)

XGC is an uncommon variant of CC; it is a diffuse (sometimes focal) destructive inflammatory process which can be infiltrating and even have lymphadenopathy. 22/462 GB operations at Sir Ganga Ram Hospital (SGRH) New Delhi India between 2000 and 2014 were for XGC—only 10/22 XGC could be diagnosed on CT; on the other hand, 5 out of 102 GBCs were diagnosed as XGC on CT (Kishore et al. 2017). In Turkey, 108 (14%) of 7916 cholecystectomy specimens showed XGC (Yucel et al. 2017). In Spain, 25 (11%) of 2206 laparoscopic cholecystectomies performed between 2003 and 2017 had XGC (Domínguez-Comesaña et al. 2019).

Clinical diagnosis of XGC is difficult; symptoms resemble those of GSD, i.e., biliary colic and cholecystitis or those of GBC. In one study, 22 patients with XGC were found to have pain, fever, and leucoytosis more often than 101 patients with GBC. Patients with XGC had a longer history of recurrent episodes of pain for an average of 11.4 months vs. constant pain for 4.7 months in GBC (Kishore et al. 2017).

US shows diffuse, symmetrical, uniform, and regular (cf. focal, asymmetrical, non-uniform, and irregular in GBC) thickening of the GB wall with hypoechoic nodules or bands in the GB wall. XGC is invariably associated with GS; CBD stones or Mirizzi's syndrome are frequently present. CT shows diffuse GB wall thickening, continuous mucosal enhancement, luminal surface enhancement (LSE) with focal breach in mucosa, submucosal hypodense nodules (Fig. 7.46), or bands. GB gets adherent to adjacent duodenum (Fig. 7.47) or colon and a fistula may form between the GB and the viscus resulting in presence of air in the GB (Fig. 7.48). Even mass formation with infiltration of adjacent structures, e.g., liver, CBD, colon, and duodenum and lymph node enlargement (pseudotumor) may be present. MRI again shows diffuse GB wall thickening with intramural nodules (Fig. 7.49). EUS-guided FNAC may be done to rule out malignancy but is helpful only if positive for cancer. The Author (VKK) does not usually obtain preoperative tissue diagnosis and decides the plan of management based on the degree of suspicion of GBC.

XGC mimics GBC clinically, on imaging and even at operation and may undergo extended cholecystectomy with a suspicion of GBC (Fig. 7.50). Most reports of extended cholecystectomy done for a preoperative or intraoperative presumed diagnosis of GBC include a significant proportion of patients who are finally found to have XGC on histopathological examination. Sixteen out of 76 cases who underwent extended cholecystectomy were found to have XGC (Rammohan et al. 2014). In another report, 3 out of 22 XGC patients underwent radical (extended) cholecystectomy (with a presumed diagnosis of GBC) (Kishore et al. 2017). There are even reports of major resections

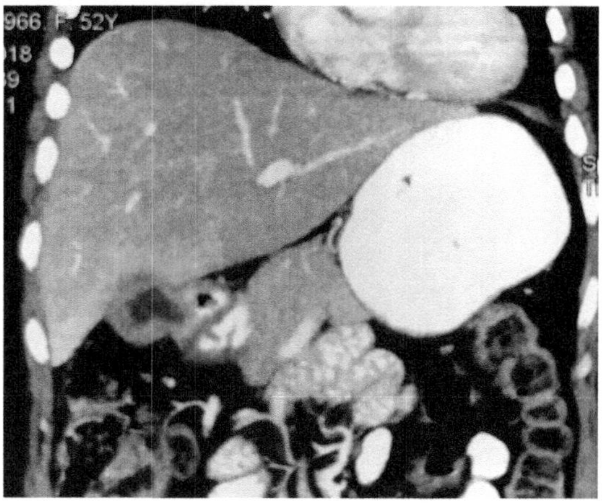

Fig. 7.47 Thick-walled gall bladder (TWGB) adherent to the duodenum

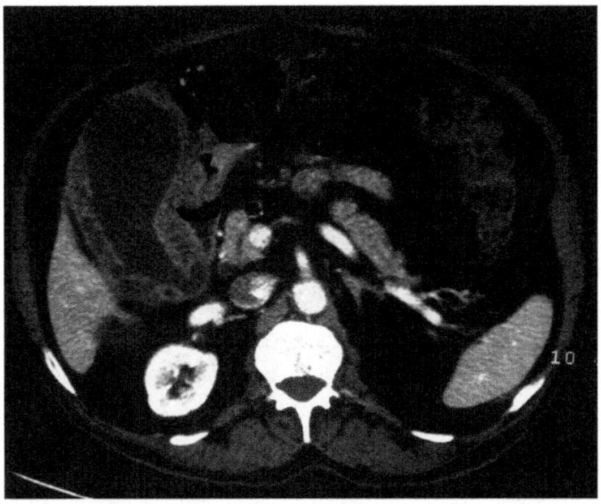

Fig. 7.46 CT shows diffuse thick-walled gall bladder (TWGB) with hypodense intramural nodules—suggestive of xantho-granulomatous cholecystitis (XGC)

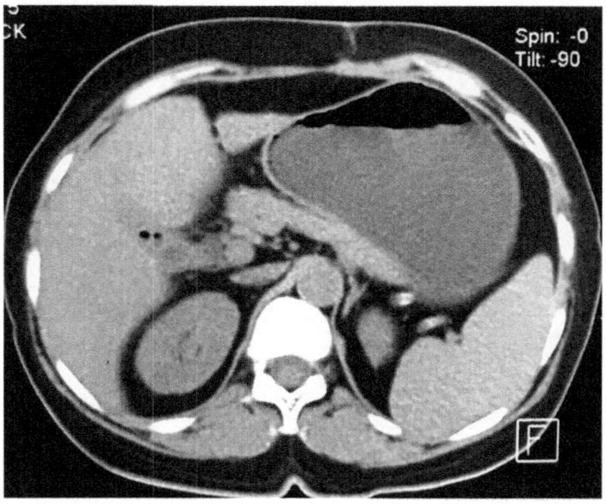

Fig. 7.48 CT shows air in the gall bladder suggesting the presence of an internal, i.e., cholecysto-enteric (duodenal or colonic) fistula

performed in patients with XGC with a preoperative diagnosis of GBC. Khan and Begum (2019) described four cases in whom extended right hepatectomy + right hemicolectomy, segment IVB + V liver resection + segmental colonic resection, radical cholecystectomy + enbloc resection of the bile duct and radical cholecystectomy were performed with a presumed diagnosis of GBC but final histology was XGC. We now end up performing AEC (Fig. 7.51) (*vide supra*) in most patients with XGC as they present with a TWGB, and it is difficult to rule out GBC. XGC and GBC may coexist in as many 10% of cases of GBC; 2/22 patients with XGC had coexistent XGC and GBC (Kishore et al. 2017); at the same time, a small focus of cancer may be missed by the pathologist in the background of XGC and the patient may present after a few months with "missed" recurrent GBC.

At operation, GB wall is thickened (Fig. 7.52) and dense adhesions may be present with duodenum, colon, etc. GB specimen shows grayish or

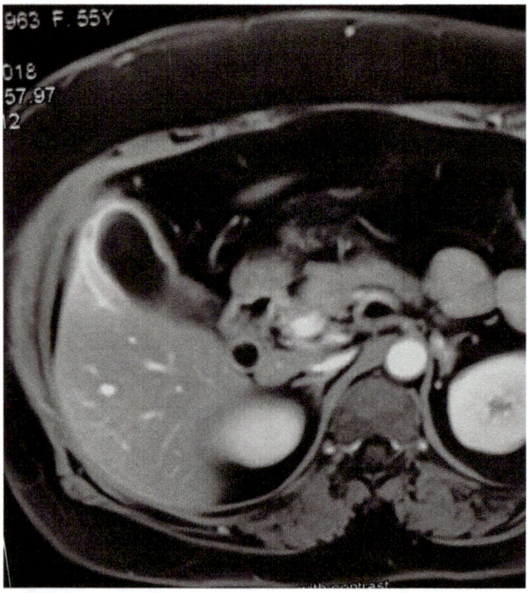

Fig. 7.49 MRI shows diffuse thick-walled gall bladder (TWGB)—suggestive of xantho-granulomatous cholecystitis (XGC)

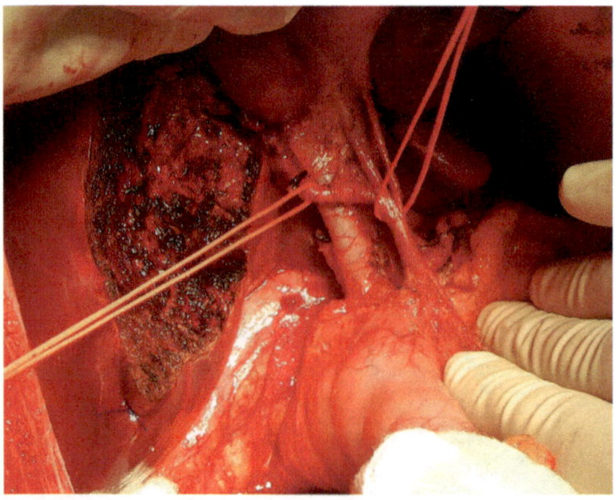

Fig. 7.50 Many patients with xantho-granulomatous cholecystitis (XGC) end up having an extended cholecystectomy with a suspicion of gall bladder cancer

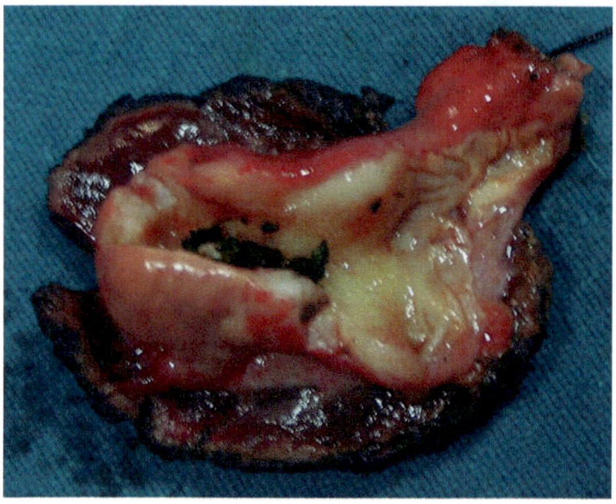

Fig. 7.51 We have described anticipatory extended cholecystectomy (AEC), i.e., removal of the gall bladder with a small wedge of liver followed by frozen section histopathological examination in patients with a low suspicion of gall bladder cancer

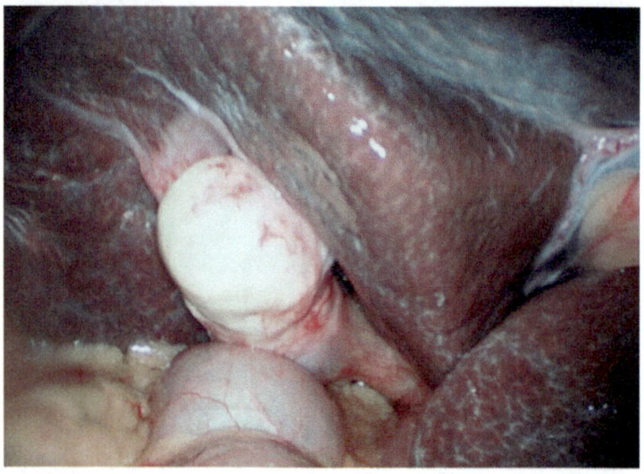

Fig. 7.52 Operative picture shows diffuse thick-walled gall bladder (TWGB)—suggestive of xantho-granulomatous cholecystitis (XGC)

brownish yellow nodules/streaks in the thick GB wall (Fig. 7.53). Etiopathogenesis of XGC is extravasation of bile from the GB lumen into the GB wall through a mucosal ulcer (tear). Histopathology shows acute and chronic inflammatory cells, foam (xanthoma) cells—lipid and bile-laden macrophages (histiocytes), micro-abscesses in the thick GB wall and severe fibrosis (Fig. 7.54); even atypia may be seen. Kishore et al. (2017) described a scoring system including 13 parameters (clinical and imaging) to differentiate XGC from GBC—a score of 12–13 had 81% sensitivity and 95% specificity for XGC, but in spite of recent advances in imaging, no radiological investigation can accurately diagnose XGC; it can be confirmed on histological examination of the GB specimen alone (Pandey et al. 2019).

The aim of investigations in GBC is to find a reason not to operate upon the patient because if such a reason is present and is missed or ignored,

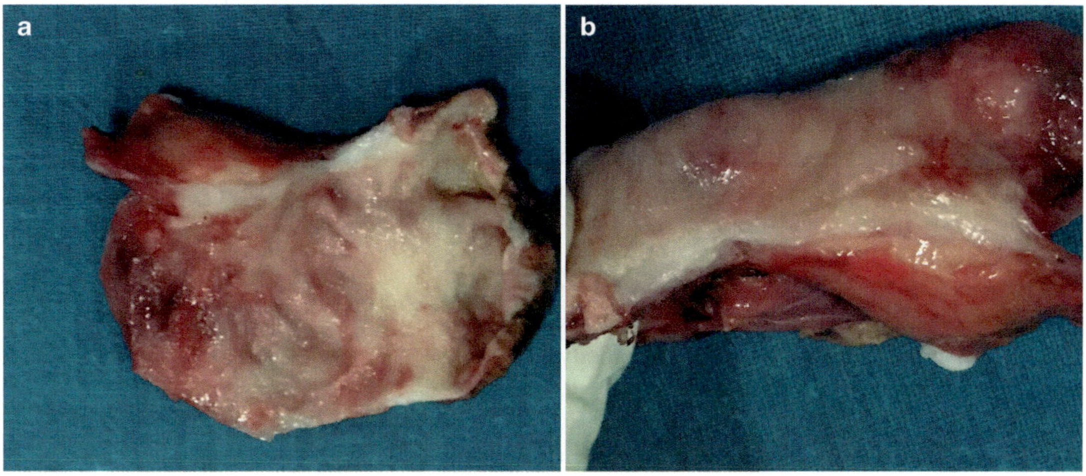

Fig. 7.53 Specimen shows diffuse thick-walled gall bladder (TWGB)—suggestive of xantho-granulomatous cholecystitis (XGC)

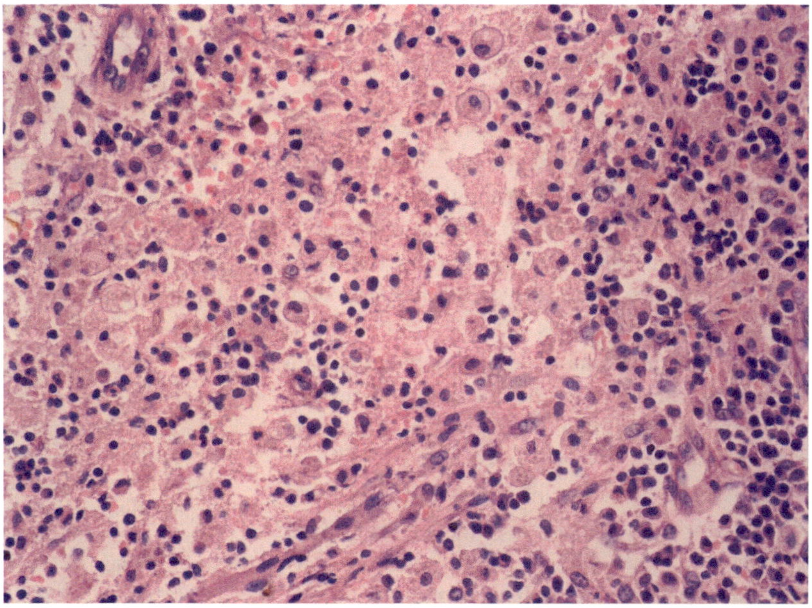

Fig. 7.54 Microphotograph shows foamy macrophages suggestive of xantho-granulomatous cholecystitis (XGC)

the outcome is going to be poor. No patient with GBC should be denied the benefit of staging laparoscopy before laparotomy, even if imaging, i.e., US, CT. MRI and even PET show no metastases and suggest resectable disease.

Invited Commentary on Investigations for Diagnosis of Gall Bladder Cancer

Thomas A. Aloia

In this well-written chapter, Dr. Kapoor, a world-leader and expert in gallbladder cancer (GBC) management, well describes the various modalities for the diagnosis and staging of patients with incidentally discovered GBC, those with suspicious GB masses, and those with biopsy-proven GBC in place.

The review is comprehensive and has much strength. Primarily, the Author (VKK) provides important data on the sensitivity and specificity of each modality based on presentation. As well, the inclusion of data on the indications for biopsy, the benefits of including staging laparoscopy in the workup, and raising awareness of xanthogranulomatous cholecystitis (XGC) masquerading as GBC are outstanding.

There are only a few areas of contention and/or further emphasis that I would submit for reader consideration. These include:

- LFTs may have a role in diagnosis and are requisite to initiate any diagnostic or therapeutic procedures in this setting, and therefore should be included in the workup of these patients.
- Jaundice in GBC is a dire finding that typically indicates both unresectability and very poor overall prognosis.
- MRCP is situationally helpful in patients with jaundice but may not be absolutely necessary when CT imaging provides adequate information.
- It could be further emphasized that in order to maximize diagnostic acumen in jaundiced patients, either CT or MRI should be performed *prior* to endobiliary stenting.
- The value of PET may be somewhat overstated. It is an expensive examination that has high false-negative and false-positive rates, poorly accounts for lymph node involvement and rarely identifies carcinomatosis. We would advocate for its use in rare situations with known GBC and indeterminate masses on cross-sectional imaging that cannot be biopsied. In these circumstances, confirmation of PET avidity may obviate the need for surgical staging.
- In patients with prior laparoscopic cholecystectomy with incidental GBC, careful physical and imaging examination of port sites for signs of local recurrence is recommended.

References

Agarwal AK, Kalayarasan R, Javed A, Gupta N, Nag HH. The role of staging laparoscopy in primary gall bladder cancer—an analysis of 409 patients: a prospective study to evaluate the role of staging laparoscopy in the management of gallbladder cancer. Ann Surg. 2013;258(2):318–23. https://doi.org/10.1097/SLA.0b013e318271497e.

Agrawal S, Sonawane RN, Behari A, Kumar A, Sikora SS, Saxena R, Kapoor VK. Laparoscopic staging in gallbladder cancer. Dig Surg. 2005;22(6):440–5. Epub 2006 Feb 10.

Agrawal S, Lawrence A, Saxena R. Does CA 19-9 have prognostic relevance in gallbladder carcinoma (GBC)? J Gastrointest Cancer. 2018;49(2):144–9. https://doi.org/10.1007/s12029-016-9914-5.

Butte JM, Gönen M, Allen PJ, D'Angelica MI, Kingham TP, Fong Y, Dematteo RP, Blumgart L, Jarnagin WR. The role of laparoscopic staging in patients with incidental gallbladder cancer. HPB (Oxford). 2011;13(7):463–72. https://doi.org/10.1111/j.1477-2574.2011.00325.x. Epub 2011 Jun 7.

Cha SY, Kim YK, Min JH, Lee J, Cha DI, Lee SJ. Usefulness of noncontrast MRI in differentiation between gallbladder carcinoma and benign conditions manifesting as focal mild wall thickening. Clin Imaging. 2019;54:63–70. https://doi.org/10.1016/j.clinimag.2018.12.001. Epub 2018 Dec 4.

Chang J, Jang JY, Lee KB, Kang MJ, Jung W, Shin YC, Kim SW. Improvement of clinical outcomes in the patients with gallbladder cancer: lessons from periodic comparison in a tertiary referral center. J Hepatobiliary Pancreat Sci. 2016;23(4):234–41. https://doi.org/10.1002/jhbp.330. Epub 2016 Mar 1.

Cheng Y, Wang M, Ma B, Ma X. Potential role of contrast-enhanced ultrasound for the differentiation of malignant and benign gallbladder lesions in East Asia: a meta-analysis and systematic review. Medicine (Baltimore). 2018;97(33):e11808. https://doi.org/10.1097/MD.0000000000011808. Review.

Choi SY, Kim JH, Park HJ, Han JK. Preoperative CT findings for prediction of resectability in patients with gallbladder cancer. Eur Radiol. 2019; https://doi.org/10.1007/s00330-019-06323-4.

Chun YJ, Jeung HC, Park HS, Park JS, Rha SY, Choi HJ, Lee JH, Jeon TJ. Significance of metabolic tumor volume and total lesion glycolysis measured using ^{18}F-FDG PET/CT in locally advanced and metastatic gallbladder carcinoma. Yonsei Med J. 2019;60(7):604–10. https://doi.org/10.3349/ymj.2019.60.7.604.

Cuschieri A, Hall AW, Clark J. Value of laparoscopy in the diagnosis and management of pancreatic carcinoma. Gut. 1978;19(7):672–7.

Davidson JT IV, Jin LX, Krasnick B, Ethun CG, Pawlik TM, Poultsides GA, Idrees K, Weber SM, Martin RCG, Shen P, Hatzaras I, Maithel SK, Fields RC, The U.S. Extrahepatic Biliary Malignancy Consortium. Staging laparoscopy among three subtypes of extra-hepatic biliary malignancy: a 15-year experience from 10 institutions. J Surg Oncol. 2019;119(3):288–94. https://doi.org/10.1002/jso.25323. Epub 2018 Dec 26.

de Savornin Lohman EAJ, de Bitter TJJ, van Laarhoven CJHM, Hermans JJ, de Haas RJ, de Reuver PR. The diagnostic accuracy of CT and MRI for the detection of lymph node metastases in gallbladder cancer: a systematic review and meta-analysis. Eur J Radiol. 2019;110:156–62. https://doi.org/10.1016/j.ejrad.2018.11.034. Epub 2018 Nov 28.

Domínguez-Comesaña E, Tojo-Artos I, Domínguez-Fernández R, Tojo-Ramallo S, Rial-Durán A, Estévez-Fernández SM. Clinical outcomes of elective laparoscopic cholecystectomy: retrospective comparative study between patients with and without xanthogranulomatous cholecystitis. Surg Laparosc Endosc Percutan Tech. 2019;29(3):212–5. https://doi.org/10.1097/SLE.0000000000000608.

Goel M, Tamhankar A, Rangarajan V, Patkar S, Ramadwar M, Shrikhande SV. Role of PET CT scan in redefining treatment of incidental gall bladder carcinoma. J Surg Oncol. 2016;113(6):652–8. https://doi.org/10.1002/jso.24198. Epub 2016 Feb 5.

Goel S, Aggarwal A, Iqbal A, Gupta M, Rao A, Singh S. 18-FDG PET-CT should be included in preoperative staging of gall bladder cancer. Eur J Surg Oncol. 2020;46(9):1711–6. https://doi.org/10.1016/j.ejso.2020.04.015.

Gupta V, Vishnu KS, Yadav TD, Sakaray YR, Irrinki S, Mittal BR, Kalra N, Vaiphei K. Radio-pathological correlation of 18F-FDG PET in characterizing gallbladder wall thickening. J Gastrointest Cancer. 2018; https://doi.org/10.1007/s12029-018-0176-2.

Hayakawa S, Goto H, Hirooka Y, Itoh A, Taki T, Watanabe Y, Hayakawa T, Naitoh Y. Colour Doppler-guided spectral analysis of gall-bladder wall flow. J Gastroenterol Hepatol. 1998;13(2):181–5.

Hijioka S, Hara K, Mizuno N, Imaoka H, Ogura T, Haba S, Mekky MA, Bhatia V, Hosoda W, Yatabe Y, Shimizu Y, Niwa Y, Tajika M, Kondo S, Tanaka T, Tamada K, Yamao K. Diagnostic yield of endoscopic retrograde cholangiography and of EUS-guided fine needle aspiration sampling in gallbladder carcinomas. J Hepatobiliary Pancreat Sci. 2012;19(6):650–5. https://doi.org/10.1007/s00534-011-0482-6.

Hirata K, Kuwatani M, Suda G, Ishikawa M, Sugiura R, Kato S, Kawakubo K, Sakamoto N. A novel approach for the genetic analysis of biliary tract cancer specimens obtained through endoscopic ultrasound-guided fine needle aspiration using targeted amplicon sequencing. Clin Transl Gastroenterol. 2019;10(3):e00022. https://doi.org/10.14309/ctg.0000000000000022.

Itsuki H, Serikawa M, Sasaki T, Ishii Y, Tsushima K, Furukawa Y, Murakami Y, Arihiro K, Chayama K. Indication and usefulness of bile juice cytology for diagnosis of gallbladder cancer. Gastroenterol Res Pract. 2018;2018:5410349. https://doi.org/10.1155/2018/5410349. eCollection 2018.

Iwashita Y, Inomata M. Laparoscopic narrowband imaging for intraoperative diagnosis of the depth of invasion of gallbladder carcinoma: a preliminary study. J Hepatobiliary Pancreat Sci. 2019;26(2):82–3. https://doi.org/10.1002/jhbp.603. Epub 2019 Jan 21.

Jarnagin WR, Bodniewicz J, Dougherty E, Conlon K, Blumgart LH, Fong Y. A prospective analysis of staging laparoscopy in patients with primary and secondary hepatobiliary malignancies. J Gastrointest Surg. 2000;4(1):34–43.

Kalayarasan R, Javed A, Puri AS, Puri SK, Sakhuja P, Agarwal AK. A prospective analysis of the preoperative assessment of duodenal involvement in gallbladder cancer. HPB (Oxford). 2013;15(3):203–9. https://doi.org/10.1111/j.1477-2574.2012.00539.x. Epub 2012 Aug 1.

Kapoor VK, Singh R, Behari A, Sharma S, Kumar A, Prakash A, Singh RK, Kumar A, Saxena R. Anticipatory extended cholecystectomy: the 'Lucknow' approach for thick walled gall bladder with low suspicion of cancer. Chin Clin Oncol. 2016;5(1):8. https://doi.org/10.3978/j.issn.2304-3865.2016.02.07.

Kapoor VK. Peep before you enter – laparoscopy in gall bladder cancer. J Gastrointest Cancer Stromal Tumors. 2017;2:1000116.

Khan MR, Begum S. Extended resection for xanthogranulomatous cholecystitis mimicking gallbladder carcinoma: cases and review of diagnostic approach. J Pak Med Assoc. 2019;69(2):256–60.

Kinugasa H, Nouso K, Ako S, Dohi C, Matsushita H, Matsumoto K, Kato H, Okada H. Liquid biopsy of bile for the molecular diagnosis of gallbladder cancer. Cancer Biol Ther. 2018;19(10):934–8. https://doi.org/10.1080/15384047.2018.1456604. Epub 2018 May 4.

Kishore R, Nundy S, Mehrotra S, Metha N, Mangla V, Lalwani S. Strategies for differentiating gallbladder carcinoma from xanthogranulomatous cholecystitis-a tertiary care centre experience. Indian J Surg Oncol.

2017;8(4):554–9. https://doi.org/10.1007/s13193-017-0677-7. Epub 2017 Jul 27.

Kitazume Y, Taura S, Nakaminato S, Noguchi O, Masaki Y, Kasahara I, Kishino M, Tateishi U. Diffusion-weighted magnetic resonance imaging to differentiate malignant from benign gallbladder disorders. Eur J Radiol. 2016;85(4):864–73. https://doi.org/10.1016/j.ejrad.2016.02.003. Epub 2016 Feb 8.

Kong WT, Shen HY, Qiu YD, Han H, Wen BJ, Wu M. Application of contrast enhanced ultrasound in gallbladder lesion: is it helpful to improve the diagnostic capabilities? Med Ultrason. 2018;20(4):420–6. https://doi.org/10.11152/mu-1626.

Kumar R, Sharma P, Kumari A, Halanaik D, Malhotra A. Role of 18F-FDG PET/CT in detecting recurrent gallbladder carcinoma. Clin Nucl Med. 2012;37(5):431–5. https://doi.org/10.1097/RLU.0b013e31824d24c4.

Lee JW, Kim YT, Lee SH, Son JH, Kang JW, Ryu JK, Jang DK, Paik WH, Lee BS. Tumor marker kinetics as prognosticators in patients with unresectable gallbladder adenocarcinoma undergoing palliative chemotherapy. Gut Liver. 2018;12(1):102–10. https://doi.org/10.5009/gnl16588.

Leem G, Chung MJ, Park JY, Bang S, Song SY, Chung JB, Park SW. Clinical value of contrast-enhanced harmonic endoscopic ultrasonography in the differential diagnosis of pancreatic and gallbladder masses. Clin Endosc. 2018;51(1):80–8. https://doi.org/10.5946/ce.2017.044. Epub 2017 Sep 20.

Leung U, Pandit-Taskar N, Corvera CU, D'Angelica MI, Allen PJ, Kingham TP, DeMatteo RP, Jarnagin WR, Fong Y. Impact of pre-operative positron emission tomography in gallbladder cancer. HPB (Oxford). 2014;16(11):1023–30. https://doi.org/10.1111/hpb.12282. Epub 2014 Jun 4.

Liu F, Hu HJ, Ma WJ, Yang Q, Wang JK, Li FY. Prognostic significance of neutrophil-lymphocyte ratio and carbohydrate antigen 19-9 in patients with gallbladder carcinoma. Medicine (Baltimore). 2019a;98(8):e14550. https://doi.org/10.1097/MD.0000000000014550.

Liu F, Wang JK, Ma WJ, Yang Q, Hu HJ, Li FY. Clinical value of preoperative CA19-9 levels in evaluating resectability of gallbladder carcinoma. ANZ J Surg. 2019b;89(3):E76–80. https://doi.org/10.1111/ans.14893. Epub 2018 Oct 10.

Margonis GA, Gani F, Buettner S, et al. Rates and patterns of recurrence after curative intent resection for gallbladder cancer: a multi-institution analysis from the US extra-hepatic biliary malignancy consortium. HPB (Oxford). 2016;18:872–8.

Min JH, Kang TW, Cha DI, Kim SH, Shin KS, Lee JE, Jang KT, Ahn SH. Apparent diffusion coefficient as a potential marker for tumour differentiation, staging and long-term clinical outcomes in gallbladder cancer. Eur Radiol. 2019;29(1):411–21. https://doi.org/10.1007/s00330-018-5602-0. Epub 2018 Jun 25.

Nagino M, Kamiya J, Nishio H, Ebata T, Arai T, Nimura Y. Two hundred forty consecutive portal vein embolizations before extended hepatectomy for biliary cancer: surgical outcome and long-term follow-up. Ann Surg. 2006;243(3):364–72.

Pandey A, Kumar D, Masood S, Chauhan S, Kumar S. Is final histopathological examination the only diagnostic criteria for xanthogranulomatous cholecystitis? Niger J Surg. 2019;25(2):177–82. https://doi.org/10.4103/njs.NJS_1_19.

Patkar S, Chaturvedi A, Goel M, Rangarajan V, Sharma A, Engineer R. Role of positron emission tomography-contrast enhanced computed tomography in locally advanced gallbladder cancer. J Hepatobiliary Pancreat Sci. 2020;27(4):164–70. https://doi.org/10.1002/jhbp.712.

Rajaguru K, Mehrotra S, Lalwani S, Mangla V, Mehta N, Nundy S. New scoring system for differentiating xanthogranulomatous cholecystitis from gall bladder carcinoma: a tertiary care centre experience. ANZ J Surg. 2018;88(1–2):E34–9. https://doi.org/10.1111/ans.13733. Epub 2016 Sep 6.

Rammohan A, Cherukuri SD, Sathyanesan J, Palaniappan R, Govindan M. Xanthogranulomatous cholecystitis masquerading as gallbladder cancer: can it be diagnosed preoperatively? Gastroenterol Res Pract. 2014;2014:253645. https://doi.org/10.1155/2014/253645. Epub 2014 Oct 27.

Ramos-Font C, Gómez-Rio M, Rodríguez-Fernández A, Jiménez-Heffernan A, Sánchez Sánchez R, Llamas-Elvira JM. Ability of FDG-PET/CT in the detection of gallbladder cancer. J Surg Oncol. 2014;109(3):218–24. https://doi.org/10.1002/jso.23476. Epub 2013 Oct 25.

Rodríguez-Fernández A, Gómez-Río M, Llamas-Elvira JM, Ortega-Lozano S, Ferrón-Orihuela JA, Ramia-Angel JM, Mansilla-Roselló A, Martínez-del-Valle MD, Ramos-Font C. Positron-emission tomography with fluorine-18-fluoro-2-deoxy-D-glucose for gallbladder cancer diagnosis. Am J Surg. 2004;188(2):171–5.

Russolillo N, D'Eletto M, Langella S, Perotti S, Lo Tesoriere R, Forchino F, Ferrero A. Role of laparoscopic ultrasound during diagnostic laparoscopy for proximal biliary cancers: a single series of 100 patients. Surg Endosc. 2016;30(3):1212–8. https://doi.org/10.1007/s00464-015-4333-4. Epub 2015 Jul 3.

Sakamoto K, Takai A, Ueno Y, Inoue H, Ogawa K, Takada Y. Scoring system to predict pt2 in gallbladder cancer based on carcinoembryonic antigen and tumor diameter. Scand J Surg. 2019:1457496919866016. https://doi.org/10.1177/1457496919866016.

Serra C, Felicani C, Mazzotta E, Gabusi V, Grasso V, De Cinque A, Giannitrapani L, Soresi M. CEUS in the differential diagnosis between biliary sludge, benign lesions and malignant lesions. J Ultrasound. 2018;21(2):119–26. https://doi.org/10.1007/s40477-018-0286-5. Epub 2018 Feb 23.

Sharma M, Somani P, Sunkara T. Imaging of gall bladder by endoscopic ultrasound. World J Gastrointest Endosc. 2018;10(1):10–5. https://doi.org/10.4253/wjge.v10.i1.10. Review.

Shirai Y, Sakata J, Wakai T, Hatakeyama K. Full-thickness cholecystectomy with limited lymphadenectomy for gallbladder cancer. Hepatogastroenterology. 2012;59(117):1338–40. https://doi.org/10.5754/hge12276.

Shukla PJ, Barreto G, Kakade A, Shrikhande SV. Revision surgery for incidental gallbladder cancer: factors influencing operability and further evidence for T1b tumours. HPB (Oxford). 2008;10(1):43–7. https://doi.org/10.1080/13651820701867794.

Srikanth G, Kumar A, Khare R, Siddappa L, Gupta A, Sikora SS, Saxena R, Kapoor VK. Should laparoscopic cholecystectomy be performed in patients with thick-walled gallbladder? J Hepatobiliary Pancreat Surg. 2004;11(1):40–4.

Tokumitsu Y, Shindo Y, Matsui H, et al. Laparoscopic total biopsy for suspected gallbladder cancer: a case series. Health Sci Rep. 2020;3(2):e156. https://doi.org/10.1002/hsr2.156.

Tran TB, Norton JA, Ethun CG, Pawlik TM, Buettner S, Schmidt C, Beal EW, Hawkins WG, Fields RC, Krasnick BA, Weber SM, Salem A, Martin RCG, Scoggins CR, Shen P, Mogal HD, Idrees K, Isom CA, Hatzaras I, Shenoy R, Maithel SK, Poultsides GA. Gallbladder cancer presenting with jaundice: uniformly fatal or still potentially curable? J Gastrointest Surg. 2017;21(8):1245–53. https://doi.org/10.1007/s11605-017-3440-z. Epub 2017 May 11.

Weber SM, DeMatteo RP, Fong Y, Blumgart LH, Jarnagin WR. Staging laparoscopy in patients with extrahepatic biliary carcinoma. Analysis of 100 patients. Ann Surg. 2002;235(3):392–9.

Wen Z, Si A, Yang J, Yang P, Yang X, Liu H, Yan X, Li W, Zhang B. Elevation of CA19-9 and CEA is associated with a poor prognosis in patients with resectable gallbladder carcinoma. HPB (Oxford). 2017;19(11):951–6. https://doi.org/10.1016/j.hpb.2017.06.011. Epub 2017 Jul 24.

Yokoyama Y, Nishio H, Ebata T, Igami T, Sugawara G, Nagino M. Value of indocyanine green clearance of the future liver remnant in predicting outcome after resection for biliary cancer. Br J Surg. 2010;97(8):1260–8. https://doi.org/10.1002/bjs.7084.

Yucel O, Uzun MA, Tilki M, Alkan S, Kilicoglu ZG, Goret CC. Xanthogranulomatous cholecystitis: analysis of 108 patients. Indian J Surg. 2017;79(6):510–4. https://doi.org/10.1007/s12262-016-1511-0. Epub 2016 Jun 1.

Zhang L, Hou C, Xu Z, Wang L, Ling X, Xiu D. Laparoscopic treatment for suspected gallbladder cancer confined to the wall: a 10-year study from a single institution. Chin J Cancer Res. 2018;30(1):84–92. https://doi.org/10.21147/j.issn.1000-9604.2018.01.09.

8 Staging of Gall Bladder Cancer

Vinay K. Kapoor

Staging of a cancer is important from the point of view of

1. Selection of treatment
2. Need for neoadjuvant treatment before surgical resection
3. Need for adjuvant treatment after surgical resection
4. Evaluation of effectiveness of various therapies
5. Predict prognosis and outcome
6. Comparison of results from different time periods and between different institutions

Gall bladder cancer (GBC) is an "orphan" (Roa et al. 2016; Nemunaitis et al. 2018) non-western cancer; it has received step-motherly treatment from international bodies also. GBC had been neglected by the International Classification of Diseases (ICD) as it was included in Liver + Biliary Tract in the 6th edition (1950), in Biliary Tract in the 7th edition (1957) and was clubbed with Extrahepatic Bile Duct and Ampulla in the 8th edition (1967). It was only in the 9th edition (1977) that GBC was given its own independent identity as C 156 and later as C 23.9 in the 10th edition (2007) of the ICD. The proposed 11th edition (2018) of the ICD classifies GBC as 2C13.

8.1 Nevin Staging

Nevin et al. (1976) classified GBC into

- Stage 1 = in situ
- Stage 2 = not transmural
- Stage 3 = transmural
- Stage 4 = lymph node metastases
- Stage 5 = distant metastases

Nevin's staging was modified by Donohue et al. (1990) who classified contiguous liver involvement as stage 3 and non-contiguous liver involvement as stage 5. Nevin staging is, however, no longer used.

8.2 Chilean Classification

The Temuco Chile group classified GBC as mucosal (muC), proper muscular (pmC), subserosal (ssC), serosal (seC), and beyond serosa into the adjacent organs (siC) (Roa et al. 2014).

Please also see an Invited Commentary on Staging of Gall Bladder Cancer by Xabier de Aretxabala (pp **–**)

V. K. Kapoor (✉)
Department of Surgical Gastroenterology, Sanjay Gandhi Post-Graduate Institute of Medical Sciences (SGPGIMS), Lucknow, Uttar Pradesh, India
e-mail: vkkapoor.india@gmail.com

V. K. Kapoor (ed.), *A Pictorial Treatise on Gall Bladder Cancer*,
https://doi.org/10.1007/978-981-15-5289-2_8

8.3 Japan Society of Biliary Surgery (JSBS)

The JSBS classification of GBC also follows the TNM system but is different from the most commonly used UICC-AJCC classification. Most Japanese surgeons/centers follow the JSBS classification and report their results using this classification, thus making the interpretation difficult for others.

pT: (primary tumor invasion)

pT1	m, mp	pHinf0	pBinf0	pPV0/PV0	pA0/A0
pT2	ss	pHinf0	pBinf0	pPV0/PV0	pA/A0
pT3	se	pHinf1	pBinf1	pPV0/PV0	pA/A0
pT4	any	pHinf2,3	pBinf2,3p	pPV1,2,3/ PV1,2,3	pA1,2,3/ A1,2,3

m mucosa; *mp* muscularis propria; *ss* subserosa; *se* serosa

pHinf: Liver (direct invasion of the liver parenchyma)

pHinf0	no direct invasion of the liver
pHinf1	<5 mm
pHinf2	5–20 mm
pHinf3	>20 mm

pBinf: Hepatoduodenal ligament invasion

pBinf0	no invasion
pBinf1	invasion of the right margin
pBinf2	invasion of the left margin
pBinf3	invasion through the hepatoduodenal ligament

pPV: Portal veins

pPV0	no invasion
pPV1	adventitia
pPV2	media
pPV3	intima and/or lumen

pA: Hepatic arteries

pA0	no invasion
aA1	adventitia
pA2	media
pA3	intima and/or lumen

N: Lymph Node metastasis

pN0	no lymph node metastasis
pN1	cystic and pericholedochal
pN2	hepatoduodenal ligament, superior retropancreatic, common hepatic
pN3	peripancreatic (except superior retropancreatic), celiac, splenic, superior mesenteric, para-aortic

Stage grouping

	H (liver metastasis) 0, P (peritoneal metastasis) 0, M (any metastasis) (−)				H(+)/P(+) /M(+)
	pN0	pN1	pN2	pN3	
pT1	I	II	III	IVA	IVB
pT2	II	III	III		
pT3	III	III	IVA	IVB	
pT4	IVA IVB		IVB		

T1 and T2 of the JSBS classification are same as those of the UICC classification; T3 and T4 are different in the two classifications. The JSBS classification divides LNs into three stations, viz. N1, N2, and N3, e.g., posterior-superior pancreatic LN (PSPLN) being classified as N2 in the JSBS classification (Sakata et al. 2017b); this is different from the AJCC-UICC classification. Stage I of the JSBS classification is same as that of the UICC classification but stage II of the JSBS classification includes T1N1M0 also (in addition to T2N0M0). Stages III and IV are totally different in the two classifications. In a survival analysis of 224 patients, JSBS staging more clearly stratified the survival curves than UICC staging, mainly because T1/T2N1M0 (stage IIIB) of UICC had better survival than T3N0M0 (stage III A) of UICC (Kishi et al. 2012). In another analysis of 175 patients with GBC, survival was again better (55% vs. 41%) in AJCC-UICC stage IIIB (T2N1M0, n = 23 and T3N1M0, n = 23) than in stage IIIA (T3N0M0, n = 22) (Sakata et al. 2017a).

8.4 AJCC-UICC Staging

Like many other cancers, the most commonly followed staging system for GBC is the American Joint Committee on Cancer (AJCC)–International

Union Against Cancer (UICC) tumor node metastasis (TNM) staging system first published in 1977 and revised every 6–8 years (AJCC-UICC). The timing of TNM classification is indicated as cTNM (clinical), pTNM (pathological), ycTNM (post-therapy clinical), ypTNM (post-therapy pathological), rTNM (recurrence), and aTNM (autopsy). GBC was included in the AJCC-UICC TNM classification and staging system in 1987.

In the 5th edition (1997) of the TNM classification of GBC, the extent of liver infiltration was taken into consideration, i.e., <2 cm was classified as T3 and >2 cm as T4. Similarly, number of organs involved was considered, i.e., invasion of one adjacent organ was classified as T3 and invasion of more than one adjacent organ was classified as T4. Lymph nodes were classified as N1 (cystic, pericholedochal, and hilar) and N2 (peripancreatic, periduodenal, periportal, celiac, and superior mesenteric). This edition of the AJCC-UICC TNM Classification was somewhat similar to the JSBS Classification for LN metastases.

In 1998, the Author (VKK) had proposed some changes in the then existing TNM staging of GBC—some of these proposals were accepted while others are still pending consideration (Kapoor et al. 1998).

In the 6th edition (2002) of the AJCC-UICC staging, T3 and T4 were redefined as T3 (perforates serosa, i.e., visceral peritoneum and/or directly invades liver and/or one adjacent organ) and T4 (invasion of main portal vein or hepatic artery or two or more extrahepatic organs). Most T stages, i.e., T2, T3, and T4 were downstaged from the 5th edition; all regional lymph nodes were placed in a single group (N1) which was staged as IIB (N2 was excluded). T2 was moved from stage II to stage IB, T3 was moved from stage III to IIA, and T4 was moved from stage IV to III. Stage groups were IA (T1 N0 M0), IB (T2 N0 M0), IIA (T3 N0 M0), IIB (T1–3 N1 M0), III (T4 NX M0), and IV (TX NX M1). T3 N1 M0 was moved from stage III of the 5th edition to stage IIB and T4 NX M0 was moved from stage IVA of the 5th edition to stage III. The 6th edition changes were due mainly to the dominance of Japanese data which showed long-term survival even in node-positive patients but no western paper has shown the same results. Fong et al. (2006) observed that the 6th edition of the AJCC-UICC Classification was no better than the 5th edition because it did not discriminate between stage III and stage IV.

In the 7th edition (2010), regional lymph nodes (which were all clubbed as N in the 6th edition) were again segregated into N1 (metastases to the lymph nodes along the cystic duct, CBD, hepatic artery, and portal vein) and N2 (metastases to periaortic, pericaval, superior mesenteric, and/or celiac lymph nodes (peripancreatic and periduodenal LNs were not mentioned). T2 was moved back to stage II, T3 to stage III and T4 was again staged as stage IVA; N1 was staged as IIIB and N2 was staged as IVB. Japanese surgeons objected as they consider peripancreatic and periduodenal LNs as regional vs. aortocaval LNs which are considered as metastatic. Oh et al. (2013) did not find the 7th edition of TNM staging of GBC to be better than the 6th edition and suggested further improvement.

In the 7th edition, peripancreatic LNs were classified as N2 and staged as IVB. Many Japanese surgeons and the Author (VKK), however, do not agree with this and consider that the postero-superior pancreatic LNs should be differentiated from other (e.g., celiac, superior mesenteric, and aortocaval) distant LNs. Five-year survival in patients with involvement of postero-superior pancreatic LNs ($n = 20$) was better (35% vs. 17%) than in patients with involvement of celiac, superior mesenteric, and aortocaval LNs ($n = 46$) (Chaudhary et al. 2019). Higuchi and Yamamoto (2014) could achieve R0 resection status in as many as 44% of 84 patients with postero-superior pancreatic LN involvement with 5-year survival of 20%.

In the 8th edition (2017), the following changes have been made

1. T2 has been subclassified as
   - T2a tumor on the peritoneal side of the GB
   - T2b tumor on the hepatic side of the GB

   This was done based on a report (Shindoh et al. 2015) which showed that tumors on the hepatic side of the GB had more lymph nodal metastases and higher rates of vascular and neural invasion as compared to tumors on the peritoneal side of the GB. In a larger analysis of 1251 patients in the National Cancer Database (NCD) (2009–2012) hepatic-side tumors were more likely to have higher T stage, more node-positive disease and more positive margins (Lafaro et al. 2020).

2. N stage has been changed from location-based to number-based
   - N1: 1–3 positive LNs
   - N2: 4 or more positive LNs

   This was based on the studies (Ito et al. 2011; Negi et al. 2011; Shirai et al. 2012) which showed that the number of LNs harvested (ideal minimum 6), number of positive LNs (Sakata et al. 2010), and LN ratio (LNR) is a stronger predictor of prognosis than the location of the metastatic LNs. Lymph nodes beyond those in the hepatoduodenal ligament (cystic, choledochal, perihepatic, and periportal), i.e., superior mesenteric, celiac, periaortic, and aortocaval LNs were considered as extraregional LNs and classified as distant (M1) and staged as IVB disease. The LN classification of the 8th edition has been questioned. An analysis of 9616 patients in the SEER database and 327 patients in the Fudan University China cohort, stage IIIA patients had poorer survival than stage IIIB patients; the authors have suggested modification of the 8th edition (Wang et al. 2020).

The current TNM staging of GBC as per the 8th edition (2017) is as follows

T (Primary tumor)

- Tx: Primary tumor cannot be assessed
- T0: No evidence of primary tumor
- Tis: Carcinoma in situ
- T1: Tumor invades lamina propria or muscle layer
  - T1a: Tumor invades lamina propria (Fig. 8.1)
  - T1b: Tumor invades muscle layer (Fig. 8.2)
- T2: Tumor invades perimuscular connective tissue (Fig. 8.3); no extension beyond serosal into liver
  - T2a: Tumor invades perimuscular connective tissue on the peritoneal side

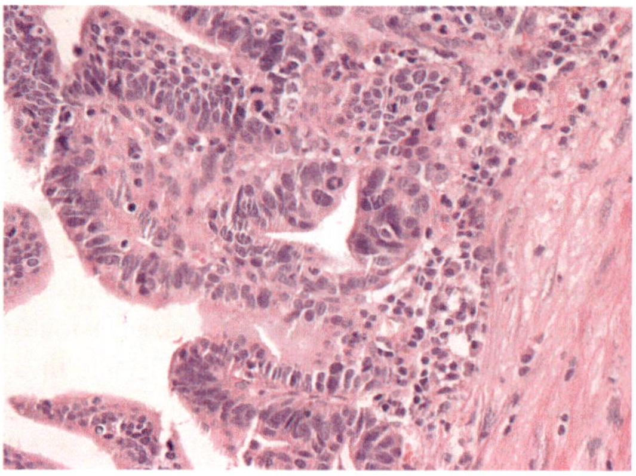

Fig. 8.1 Tumor invading lamina propria (T1a)

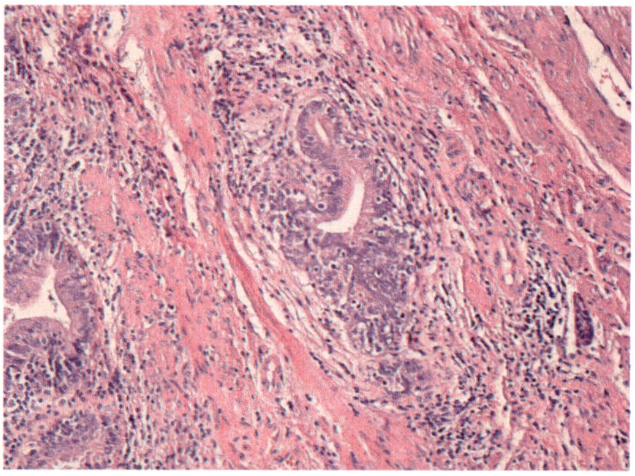

Fig. 8.2 Tumor invading muscle layer (T1b)

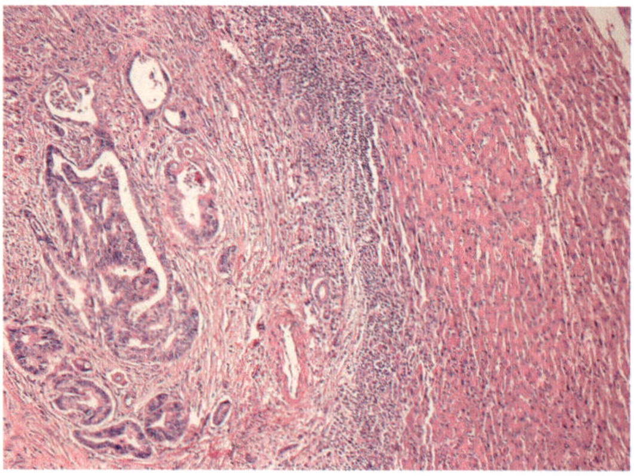

Fig. 8.3 Tumor invading perimuscular connective tissue (T2)

without involvement of serosa (visceral peritoneum)
 - T2b: Tumor invades perimuscular connective tissue on the hepatic side with no extension into liver
- T3: Tumor perforates the serosal (visceral peritoneum) and/or directly invades the liver and/or one other adjacent organ or structure such as the stomach, duodenum (Fig. 8.4), colon, pancreas, omentum, or extrahepatic bile ducts
- T4: Tumor invades the main portal vein (Fig. 8.5) or hepatic artery (Fig. 8.6) or invades two or more extrahepatic organs or structures

N (Regional lymph node)

- NX: Regional lymph nodes cannot be assessed
- N0: No metastasis to regional lymph nodes
- N1: Metastasis to one to three regional lymph nodes (Fig. 8.7)
- N2: Metastasis to four or more regional lymph nodes

M (Metastasis)

- M0: No metastasis
- M1: Distant metastasis, e.g., liver (Fig. 8.8), peritoneum (Fig. 8.9), lungs (Fig. 8.10), bone, and brain.

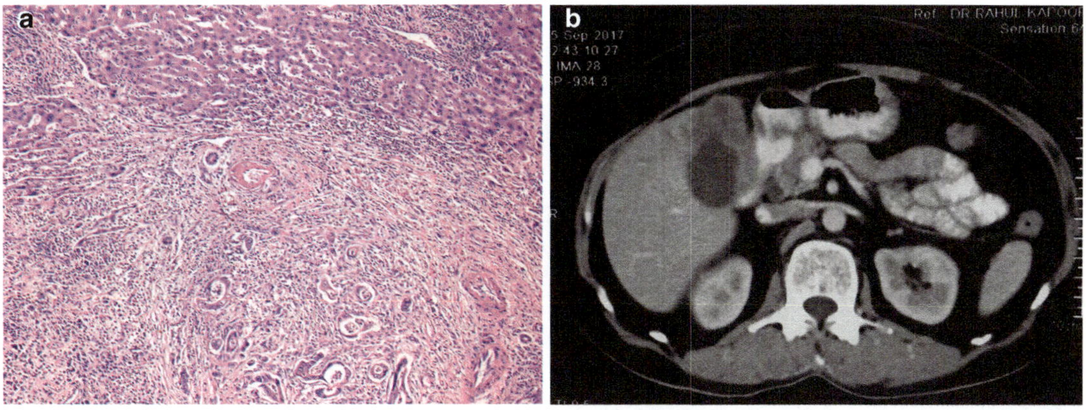

Fig. 8.4 Tumor invading (**a**) liver (T3) (**b**) an adjacent organ, e.g., duodenum (T3)

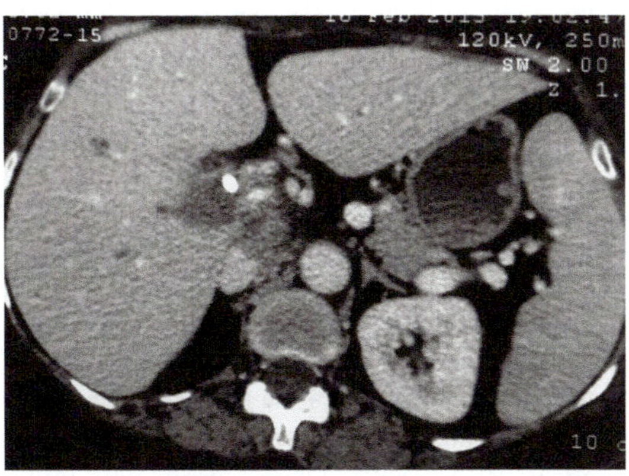

Fig. 8.5 Tumor invading the main portal vein (MPV) (T4) which is reduced to a chink

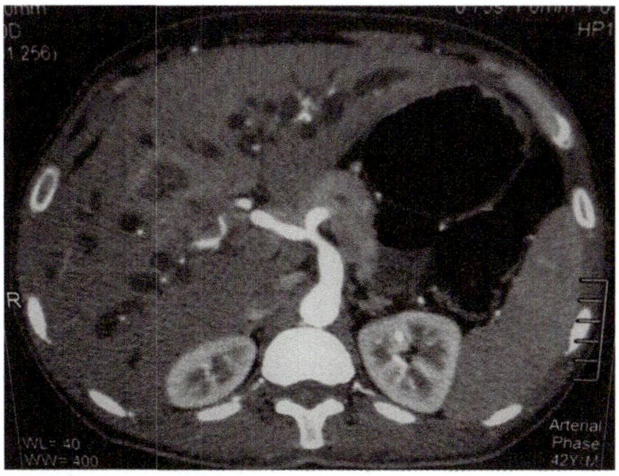

Fig. 8.6 Tumor invading the proper hepatic artery (PHA) (T4)

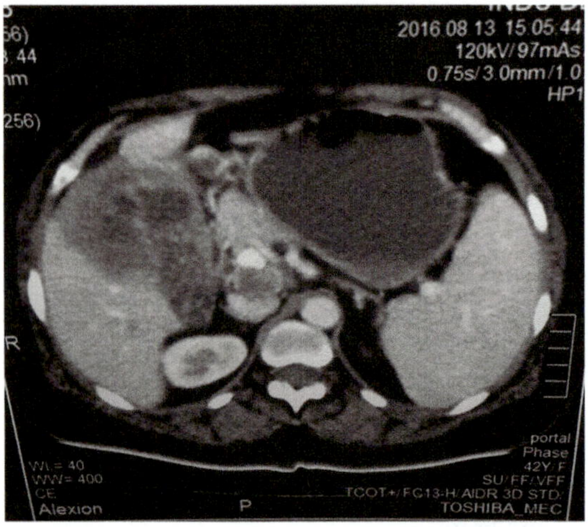

Fig. 8.7 Metastasis to a regional (retroportal) lymph node (N1)

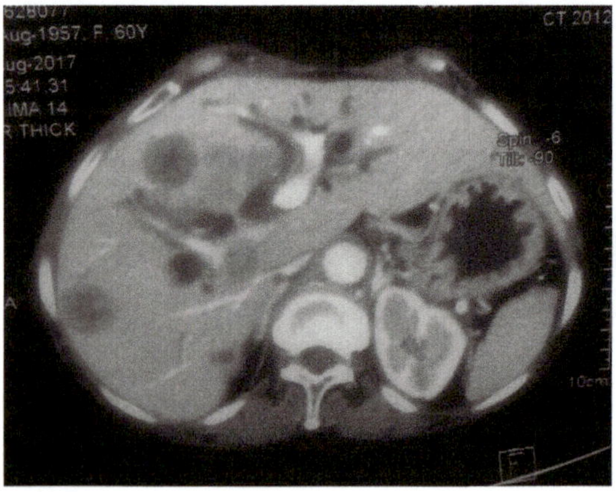

Fig. 8.8 Liver metastases (M1) on CT

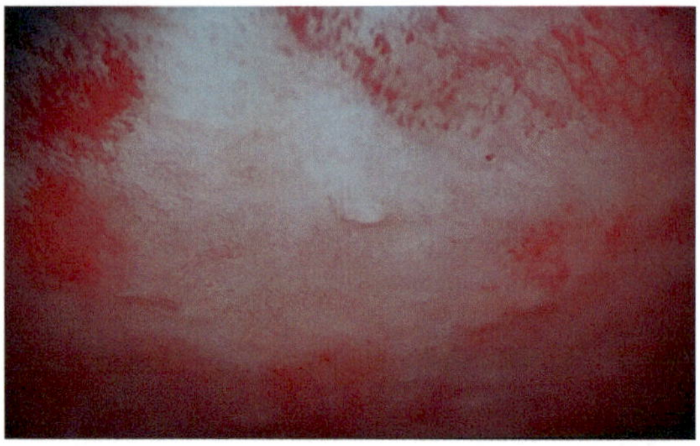

Fig. 8.9 Peritoneal deposit (M1) seen as staging laparoscopy

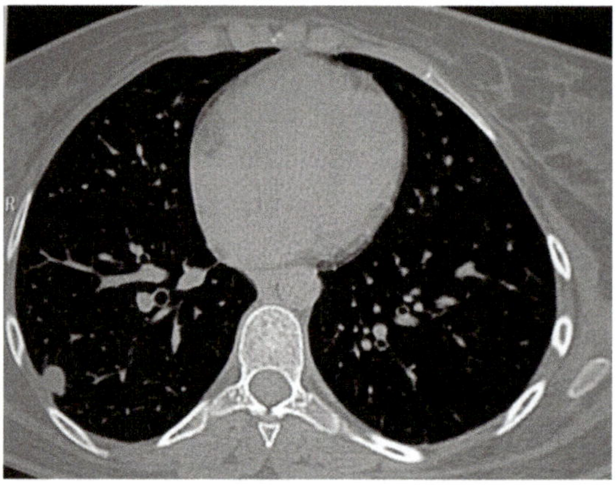

Fig. 8.10 Subpleural nodule (M1) on chest CT

Stage groups

- Tis N0 M0
- I: T1 N0 M0
- IIA: T2a N0 M0
- IIB: T2b N0 M0
- IIIA: T3 N0 M0
- IIIB: T1–3 N1 M0
- IVA: T4 N0–1 M0
- IVB: Any T, N2 or M1

Tis, T1a, and T1b (without nodal spread) are early GBC. T3, T4, and node-positive disease is advanced GBC. Classification of node-negative T2 GBC, whether early or advanced, is debatable. Agarwal et al. (2013) called T2 also early GBC. Higuchi et al. (2014) defined early GBC as limited to the mucosa or muscularis propria (T1) regardless of LN metastasis thus including node-positive disease also; tumors beyond muscularis propria were defined as advanced GBC. Tumor diameter is not mentioned in the TNM staging but Sakamoto et al. (2019) developed a scoring system including tumor diameter and serum CEA level to preoperatively predict pT2. Most reports mention T stage as one of the most important predictors of outcome but Sung et al. (2020) in an analysis of 348 resected cases surprisingly found no significant difference in survival between T1s–T1a, T1a–T1b, and T2a–T2b tumors.

8.5 Proposed Changes

GBC has, unfortunately, received step-motherly treatment at the hands of the AJCC-UICC; frequent changes have been made and then reversed in subsequent editions. The current TNM staging of GBC also has some shortcomings. Wang et al. (2020) analyzed 9616 patients from the SEER database and found that stage IIIA patients had aberrantly poorer survival than stage IIIB. We (Behari and Kapoor 2016) have proposed some changes in the staging of GBC to bring it in conformity with the staging of other GI and HPB cancers.

8.5.1 T Stage

1. In other cancers, e.g., esophagus, stomach, and colon, T1 includes involvement of lamina propria and submucosa only; involvement of muscularis propria is classified as T2. GB has no submucosa; lamina propria includes mucosa only. GBC involving lamina propria (current T1a) has low (<5%) chance of LN spread and can be treated with simple cholecystectomy. GBC involving muscularis propria (current T1b), on the other hand, is associated with LN spread in a significant proportion of cases and requires extended cholecystectomy. In GBC, involvement of lamina propria alone should be classified as T1 and involvement of muscularis propria should be classified as T2 (instead of current T1b) and stage grouped as II (instead of current stage I)
2. In cancer of the pancreas, involvement of unresectable structures, e.g., celiac axis and superior mesenteric artery is classified as T4. Current T3 in GBC includes involvement of the pancreas also which is an unresectable structure (role of pancreato-duodenectomy in GBC is now being questioned—see Chap. 11); involvement of the pancreas should be classified as T4 in GBC.
3. In esophagus, T4 is subclassified as T4a (involvement of resectable adjacent structures, viz. pleura, pericardium, and diaphragm) and T4b (involvement of unresectable adjacent structures, viz. aorta, trachea/bronchus, and vertebra). Current T4 in GBC includes involvement of two or more extrahepatic organs—it does not differentiate easily resectable organs, e.g., colon or duodenum from not-so-easy to resect organs, e.g., pancreas, hepatic artery, and portal vein. It is not the number of organs but the organs involved which is important. T4 in GBC should also be subclassified as T4a (involvement of resectable adjacent structures, viz. liver, CBD, stomach/duodenum, colon, or omentum) and T4b (involvement of unresectable adjacent structures, viz. proper hepatic artery, main portal vein, and pancreas).

8.5.2 N Stage

In esophagus, colon and rectum, non-regional LNs are classified as M1a and staged as stage IVA. The Author (VKK) prefers to support the Japan Society of Biliary Surgery (JSBS) classification of LNs into three echelons

- N1: Hepatoduodenal ligament (HDL) LNs (Fig. 8.11)
- N2: Regional nodes beyond the hepatoduodenal ligament, i.e., along the common hepatic artery (CHA), behind the pancreas (peripancreatic) (Fig. 8.12) and duodenum (periduode-

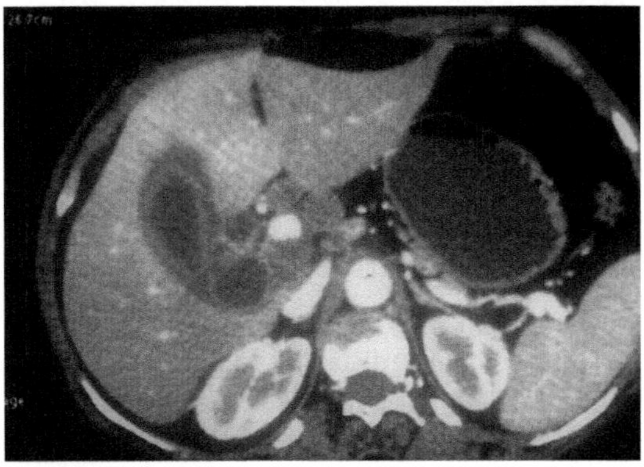

Fig. 8.11 Hepatoduodenal ligament lymph node; the Author (VKK) proposes that the involvement of hepatoduodenal ligament lymph nodes should be classified as N1

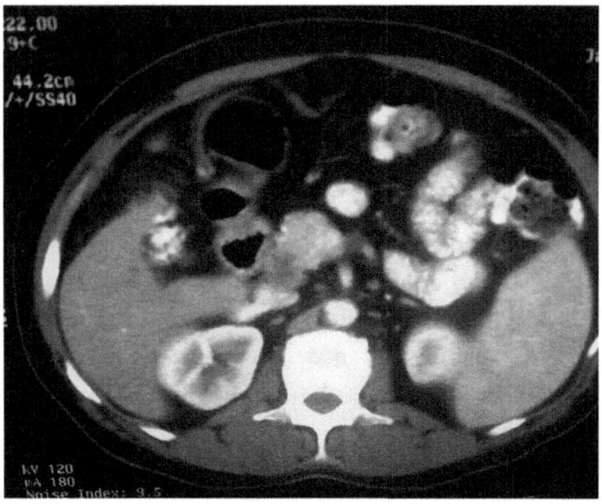

Fig. 8.12 Retropancreatic lymph node; the Author (VKK) proposes that the involvement of retropancreatic lymph nodes should be classified as N2

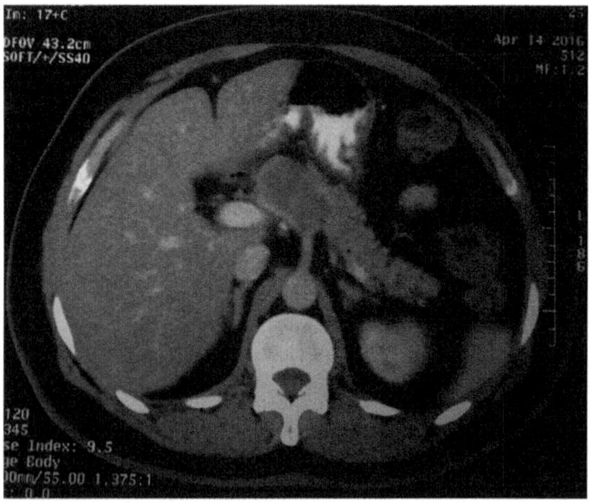

Fig. 8.13 Celiac lymph node; the Author (VKK) proposes that the involvement of distant (non-regional) lymph nodes, e.g., celiac, superior mesenteric, and aortocaval should be classified as M1a and stage grouped as IVA

nal) but which are included in a standard lymphadenectomy during extended cholecystectomy

- Non-regional (distant) LNs, e.g., celiac (Fig. 8.13), superior mesenteric (Fig. 8.14), and aortocaval (Fig. 8.15) which are beyond the standard lymphadenectomy during extended cholecystectomy. Their outcome is poor—as bad as metastasis—even if an extended retroperitoneal LN dissection is per-

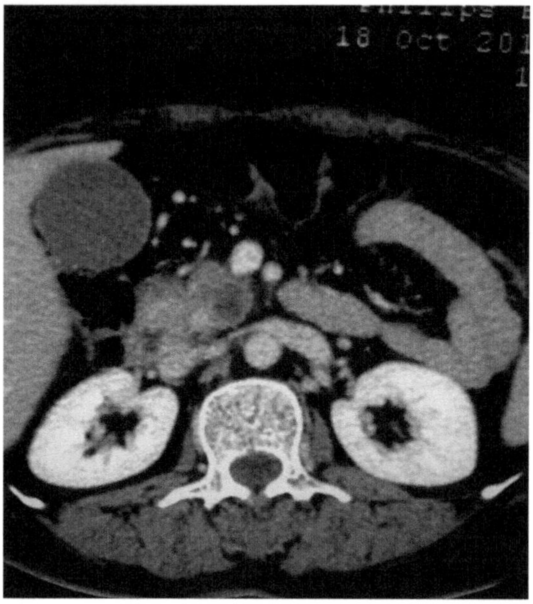

Fig. 8.14 Superior mesenteric lymph node; the Author (VKK) proposes that the involvement of distant (non-regional) lymph nodes, e.g., superior mesenteric, celiac, and aortocaval should be classified as M1a and stage grouped as IVA

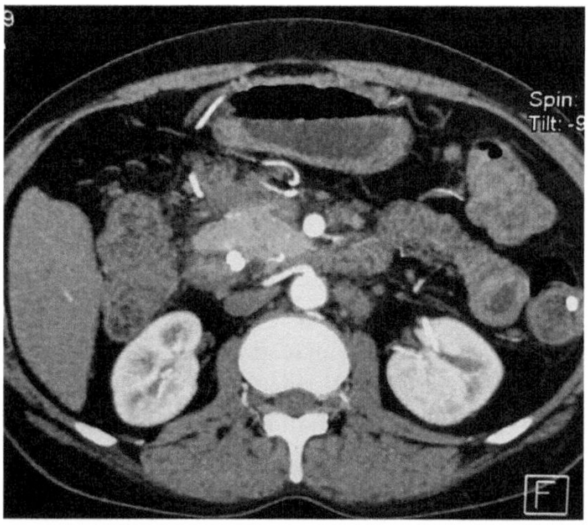

Fig. 8.15 Para-aortic lymph node; the Author (VKK) proposes that the involvement of distant (non-regional) lymph nodes, e.g., aortocaval, celiac, and superior mesenteric should be classified as M1a and stage grouped as IVA

formed (Shimada et al. 1997; Kondo et al. 2000). Involvement of these LNs should be classified as distant metastasis (M1a) and stage grouped as stage IVA. Kishi et al. (2018)

classified LNs in the hepatoduodenal ligament as Na, postero-superior pancreatic LNs as Nb and celiac and superior mesenteric LNs as Nc—5-year disease-free survival (DFS) was 36%, 34%, and 0% in Na, Nb, and Nc, respectively.

The Author (VKK) proposes that

1. Hepatoduodenal ligament LNs should be classified as N1 and stage grouped as stage III
2. Peripancreatic, periduodenal, and CHA LNs should be classified as N2 and stage grouped as IVA

8.5.3 M Stage

In esophagus, stomach and colon, non-regional (distant) LNs are classified as metastasis (M1a) and stage grouped as IVA and non-nodal metastases are classified as M1b and stage grouped as IVB. In GBC also, distant (non-regional) LNs, e.g., celiac, superior mesenteric, and aortocaval should be classified as M1a and stage grouped as IVA and non-nodal distant metastases should be classified as M1b and stage grouped as IVB.

The Author (VKK) proposes stage grouping of GBC (based on the proposed TNM classification *vide supra*) as follows.

- I: T1 N0 M0
- II: T2 N0 M0
- III: T3 N0 M0, T1–T3 N1 M0
- IVA: T4a Any N M0
  - Any T N2 M0
  - Any T Any N M1a
- IVB: T4b Any N M0
  - Any T Any N M1b

In some other cancers, various factors other than TNM have been added to staging, e.g., Gleason score in prostate. C (CEA) stage has been proposed to be added to TNM staging of colo-rectal cancers (Thirunavukarasu et al. 2011). The location of the tumor, whether peritoneal or hepatic side on the GB, has been shown to predict the prognosis of T2 GBC (Shindoh et al. 2015). This has been included in the 8th edition of TNM staging. In GBC, the site of the tumor in the GB, viz. fundus, body, or neck is also important for management and outcome. Kawahara et al. (2017) classified T2 tumors as

1. P-type—tumor in the GB fundus (Gf) or body (Gb) and on the free peritoneal side—managed by full-thickness cholecystectomy (FTC) and regional LN dissection.
2. H-type—tumor in the GB fundus (Gf) or body (Gb) and in contact with the liver in the Gb bed—managed by GB bed resection and regional LN dissection.
3. N-type—tumor located in the GB neck (Gn) (Fig. 8.16)—managed by GB bed resection, bile duct resection and regional LN dissection.

The presence or absence of surgical obstructive jaundice (SOJ) also guides the management and predicts the prognosis in GBC (Kapoor 2015). Tata Memorial Hospital (TMH) Mumbai India group proposed a TMH staging system including the presence of jaundice and CA 19.9 level which provided excellent treatment plan and reduced unnecessary non-resectional surgical explorations in patients with GBC (Shukla et al. 2008). The Author (VKK) has proposed that these two non-TNM factors, viz. the site of tumor in the GB, viz. fundus, body, or neck and surgical

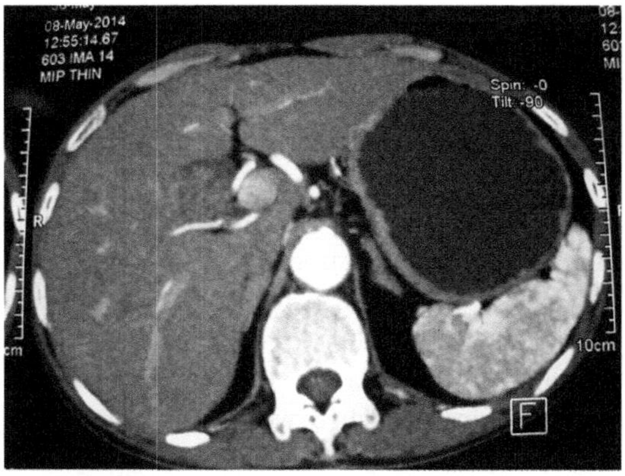

Fig. 8.16 Gall bladder cancer at neck carries a poorer outcome than gall bladder cancer at fundus or body; the Author (VKK) proposes that the location of the tumor in the gall bladder, viz. fundus, body, or neck should also be taken into account in staging of gall bladder cancer

obstructive jaundice (SOJ) should also be included in the staging of GBC (Behari and Kapoor 2016).

The "stage" for GBC is not set, yet!

Invited Commentary on Staging of Gall Bladder Cancer

Xabier de Aretxabala

I would like to thank Professor VK Kapoor for the privilege of commenting on this chapter.

Such as Professor Kapoor pointed out, gallbladder cancer (GBC) was not considered as a separate entity for a long period. In spite of corresponding to a different organ with biological and anatomical differences, GBC was classified together with the ampulla and the biliary tract tumors. Nevin classification was one of the first attempts to classify the disease; however, after beginning to use the classification, it became possible to realize its lack of utility and the need for a new classification.

Since that time until now, numerous classifications for this disease have been published. An important point to consider at the moment of designing a classification should be its simplicity and good correlation with the prognosis. Traditionally, anatomical landmarks have been employed to divide patients into different categories. Of the above, the employment of the depth of gall bladder wall invasion is probably the easier way of classifying the patients. Besides having a very good correlation with the prognosis, the information is obtained only from the gallbladder without the necessity of requiring additional samples from different places. With the information obtained from the gallbladder, it is possible to divide patients into well-defined groups with different prognosis.

Lymph node invasion is another important point to consider when we need to classify a patient. Lymph node invasion is an early step during the tumor dissemination and its presence is considered the most important prognostic factor in GBC. In comparison with the level of gallbladder wall invasion, lymph node invasion seems to be better correlated with the potential biologic behavior of the tumor. However, a formal lymphadenectomy is necessary to obtain the information.

Concerning liver infiltration, numerous attempts were done to include this fact in the previous classifications. Differentiation based on the size of the tumor infiltration was performed, but finally and possibly due to the difficulty to measure the size of infiltration this value has not been included in the last classifications.

Professor Kapoor performs some interesting suggestions to modify the present classifications. Concerning the depth of wall infiltration and due to its higher lymph node compromise rate, he suggests classifying muscle infiltration as T2 instead of T1b. In the same way and as it is employed in the classification of other tumors, he thinks that potential resectability of involved organs instead of the number should be considered to define the stage of the disease. According to Professor Kapoor, lymph node compromise could be divided according to its location into two categories: compromise of the hepatic ligament and regional lymph nodes. Both groups can be resected in a formal lymphadenectomy. On the other hand, non-regional lymph nodes (i.e., para-aortic) should be classified as metastasis.

Finally, until now, classifications have employed anatomical landmarks to categorize the patients. However, in future classifications, we should consider biological characteristics to allow a more complete definition of the patients' prognosis. In this sense, the contribution of molecular biology should add information to perform a more complete classification of patients harboring a GBC.

References

Agarwal AK, Kalayarasan R, Javed A, Gupta N, Nag HH. The role of staging laparoscopy in primary gall bladder cancer—an analysis of 409 patients: a prospective study to evaluate the role of staging laparoscopy in the management of gallbladder cancer. Ann Surg. 2013;258(2):318–23. https://doi.org/10.1097/SLA.0b013e318271497e.

AJCC-UICC classification. 2017. www.cancerstaging.org.

Behari A, Kapoor VK. Gall bladder cancer—is the stage set? Yet! J Gastrointest Cancer Stromal Tumors. 2016;1:1000107.

Chaudhary RK, Higuchi R, Yazawa T, Uemura S, Izumo W, Furukawa T, Kiyohara K, Yamamoto M. Surgery in node-positive gallbladder cancer: the implication of an involved superior retropancreatic lymph node. Surgery. 2019;165(3):541–7. https://doi.org/10.1016/j.surg.2018.09.003. Epub 2018 Oct 19.

Donohue JH, Nagorney DM, Grant CS, Tsushima K, Ilstrup DM, Adson MA. Carcinoma of the gallbladder. Does radical resection improve outcome? Arch Surg. 1990;125(2):237–41.

Fong Y, Wagman L, Gonen M, Crawford J, Reed W, Swanson R, Pan C, Ritchey J, Stewart A, Choti M. Evidence-based gallbladder cancer staging: changing cancer staging by analysis of data from the National Cancer Database. Ann Surg. 2006;243(6):767–71; discussion 771–4.

Higuchi R, Yamamoto M. Aggressive surgical management and treatment outcomes of gallbladder cancer. In: Agarwal A, Fong Y, editors. Carcinoma of the gall bladder. New Delhi: Elsevier; 2014. p. 175–83.

Higuchi R, Ota T, Araida T, Kajiyama H, Yazawa T, Furukawa T, Yoshikawa T, Takasaki K, Yamamoto M. Surgical approaches to advanced gallbladder cancer: a 40-year single-institution study of prognostic factors and resectability. Ann Surg Oncol. 2014;21(13):4308–16. https://doi.org/10.1245/s10434-014-3885-1. Epub 2014 Jul 15.

Ito H, Ito K, D'Angelica M, Gonen M, Klimstra D, Allen P, DeMatteo RP, Fong Y, Blumgart LH, Jarnagin WR. Accurate staging for gallbladder cancer: implications for surgical therapy and pathological assessment. Ann Surg. 2011;254(2):320–5. https://doi.org/10.1097/SLA.0b013e31822238d8.

Japanese Society of Biliary Surgery (JSBS). Classification of biliary tract carcinomas. 2nd ed. Tokyo: Kanehara; 2004.

Kapoor VK. Gall bladder cancer and jaundice—the yellow signal. Clin Med Rev Oncol. 2015;5:1–3.

Kapoor VK, Sonawane RN, Haribhakti SP, Sikora SS, Saxena R, Kaushik SP. Gall bladder cancer: proposal for a modification of the TNM classification. Eur J Surg Oncol. 1998;24(6):487–91. Review.

Kawahara R, Shirahama T, Arai S, Muroya D, Nomura Y, Fukutomi S, Shirahama N, Takagi K, Goto Y, Akashi M, Maruyama Y, Sakai H, Ishikawa H, Hisaka T, Yasunaga M, Horiuchi H, Okuda K, Akagi Y, Tanaka H. Evaluation of surgical procedures for T2 gallbladder cancer in terms of recurrence and prognosis. Kurume Med J. 2017;63(1.2):15–22. https://doi.org/10.2739/kurumemedj.MS65005. Epub 2017 Mar 22.

Kishi Y, Shimada K, Hata S, Oguro S, Sakamoto Y, Nara S, Esaki M, Hiraoka N, Kosuge T. Definition of T3/4 and regional lymph nodes in gallbladder cancer: which is more valid, the UICC or the Japanese staging system? Ann Surg Oncol. 2012;19(11):3567–73. https://doi.org/10.1245/s10434-012-2599-5. Epub 2012 Aug 14.

Kishi Y, Nara S, Esaki M, Hiraoka N, Shimada K. Extent of lymph node dissection in patients with gallbladder cancer. Br J Surg. 2018;105(12):1658–64. https://doi.org/10.1002/bjs.10913. Epub 2018 Jul 11.

Kondo S, Nimura Y, Hayakawa N, Kamiya J, Nagino M, Uesaka K. Regional and para-aortic lymphadenectomy in radical surgery for advanced gallbladder carcinoma. Br J Surg. 2000;87(4):418–22.

Lafaro K, Blakely AM, Melstrom LG. et al, Prognostic impact of tumor location in resected gallbladder cancer: a national cohort analysis. J Surg Oncol. 2020; https://doi.org/10.1002/jso.26107.

Negi SS, Singh A, Chaudhary A. Lymph nodal involvement as prognostic factor in gallbladder cancer: location, count or ratio? J Gastrointest Surg. 2011;15(6):1017–25. Epub 2011 Apr 13.

Nemunaitis JM, Brown-Glabeman U, Soares H, Belmonte J, Liem B, Nir I, Phuoc V, Gullapalli RR. Gallbladder cancer: review of a rare orphan gastrointestinal cancer with a focus on populations of New Mexico. BMC Cancer. 2018;18(1):665. https://doi.org/10.1186/s12885-018-4575-3. Review.

Nevin JE, Moran TJ, Kay S, King R. Carcinoma of the gallbladder: staging, treatment, and prognosis. Cancer. 1976;37(1):141–8.

Oh TG, Chung MJ, Bang S, Park SW, Chung JB, Song SY, Choi GH, Kim KS, Lee WJ, Park JY. Comparison of the sixth and seventh editions of the AJCC TNM classification for gallbladder cancer. J Gastrointest Surg. 2013;17(5):925–30. https://doi.org/10.1007/s11605-012-2134-9. Epub 2013 Jan 9.

Roa I, Ibacache G, Muñoz S, de Aretxabala X. Gallbladder cancer in Chile: pathologic characteristics of survival and prognostic factors: analysis of 1,366 cases. Am J Clin Pathol. 2014;141(5):675–82. https://doi.org/10.1309/AJCPQT3ELN2BBCKA.

Roa I, Garcia H, Game A, de Toro G, de Aretxabala X, Javle M. Somatic mutations of PI3K in early and advanced gallbladder cancer: additional options for an orphan cancer. J Mol Diagn. 2016;18(3):388–94. https://doi.org/10.1016/j.jmoldx.2015.12.003. Epub 2016 Mar 3.

Sakamoto K, Takai A, Ueno Y, Inoue H, Ogawa K, Takada Y. Scoring system to predict pt2 in gallbladder cancer based on carcinoembryonic antigen and tumor diameter. Scand J Surg. 2019;2019:1457496919866016. https://doi.org/10.1177/1457496919866016. [Epub ahead of print].

Sakata J, Shirai Y, Wakai T, Ajioka Y, Hatakeyama K. Number of positive lymph nodes independently determines the prognosis after resection in patients with gallbladder carcinoma. Ann Surg Oncol. 2010;17(7):1831–40. Epub 2010 Jan 15.

Sakata J, Kobayashi T, Ohashi T, Hirose Y, Takano K, Takizawa K, Miura K, Ishikawa H, Toge K, Yuza K, Soma D, Ando T, Wakai T. Prognostic heterogeneity of the seventh edition of UICC Stage III gallbladder carcinoma: which patients benefit from surgical resection? Eur J Surg Oncol. 2017a;43(4):780–7. https://doi.org/10.1016/j.ejso.2017.01.001. Epub 2017 Jan 19.

Sakata J, Kobayashi T, Tajima Y, Ohashi T, Hirose Y, Takano K, Takizawa K, Miura K, Wakai T. Relevance of dissection of the posterior superior pancreaticoduodenal lymph nodes in gallbladder carcinoma. Ann Surg Oncol. 2017b;24(9):2474–81. https://doi.org/10.1245/s10434-017-5939-7. Epub 2017 Jun 26.

Shimada H, Endo I, Togo S, Nakano A, Izumi T, Nakagawara G. The role of lymph node dissection in the treatment of gallbladder carcinoma. Cancer. 1997;79(5):892–9.

Shindoh J, de Aretxabala X, Aloia TA, Roa JC, Roa I, Zimmitti G, Javle M, Conrad C, Maru DM, Aoki T, et al. Tumor location is a strong predictor of tumor progression and survival in T2 gallbladder cancer: an international multicenter study. Ann Surg. 2015;261(4):733–9. https://doi.org/10.1097/SLA.0000000000000728.

Shirai Y, Sakata J, Wakai T, Ohashi T, Ajioka Y, Hatakeyama K. Assessment of lymph node status in gallbladder cancer: location, number, or ratio of positive nodes. World J Surg Oncol. 2012;10:87. https://doi.org/10.1186/1477-7819-10-87.

Shukla PJ, Neve R, Barreto SG, Hawaldar R, Nadkarni MS, Mohandas KM, Shrikhande SV. A new scoring system for gallbladder cancer (aiding treatment algorithm): an analysis of 335 patients. Ann Surg Oncol. 2008;15(11):3132–7. https://doi.org/10.1245/s10434-008-9917-y. Epub 2008 May 6.

Sung YN, Song M, Lee JH, et al. Validation of the 8th edition of the American Joint Committee on Cancer staging system for gallbladder cancer and implications for the follow-up of patients without node dissection. Cancer Res Treat. 2020;52(2):455–68. https://doi.org/10.4143/crt.2019.271.

Thirunavukarasu P, Sukumar S, Sathaiah M, Mahan M, Pragatheeshwar KD, Pingpank JF, Zeh H III, Bartels CJ, Lee KK, Bartlett DL. C-stage in colon cancer: implications of carcinoembryonic antigen biomarker in staging, prognosis, and management. J Natl Cancer Inst. 2011;103(8):689–97. https://doi.org/10.1093/jnci/djr078. Epub 2011 Mar 18.

Wang J, Bo X, Shi X, et al. Modified staging classification of gallbladder carcinoma on the basis of the 8th edition of the American Joint Commission on Cancer (AJCC) staging system. Eur J Surg Oncol. 2020;46(4 Pt A):527–33. https://doi.org/10.1016/j.ejso.2019.10.015.

Philosophy of Management of Gall Bladder Cancer

9

Vinay K. Kapoor

Management of gall bladder cancer (GBC) is an astronomical oncologic challenge. It depends largely on the time of diagnosis (preoperative obvious, intraoperative unsuspected, or postoperative incidental) and the stage of the disease. T1 (a and b) is early (resectable and potentially curable) GBC; T2, though resectable, is not early GBC (see Chap. 10). T3/T4 or N+ is advanced GBC where radical operations are of questionable benefit (see Chap. 11). Surgery is the only potentially curative treatment and remains the mainstay of management. With more and more reports of the use of chemotherapy and radiotherapy in neoadjuvant, adjuvant, and definitive/palliative settings, the role of multimodality management is evolving in GBC (see Chap. 14). Advanced unresectable disease indicates palliation, which is largely non-surgical, i.e., endoscopic or percutaneous (see Chap. 12). Multidisciplinary HPB disease management meetings including surgeons, oncologists (medical and radiation), gastroenterologists/endoscopists, and radiologists (diagnostic/interventional) should be held for managing patients with GBC (Patkar et al. 2018).

Because GBC is uncommon/rare in the western world, very little large volume prospective clinical data is available in the published literature. Very few groups from the West such as the Memorial Sloan Kettering Cancer Center (MSKCC), New York, USA, have reported their experiences with GBC. Recently, a 10-institution extrahepatic biliary malignancies consortium in USA has published several reports on a fairly large experience with GBC (see Chap. 18). There is a lack of high-quality data; there is no Level 1 evidence because of no randomized controlled trials (RCT) and no phase III studies. Most reports are based on single-institution retrospective data analyses. Many published studies include all biliary tract cancers (BTCs), i.e., GBC and cholangiocarcinoma. There are not many guidelines for management of GBC—even those that are available, e.g., Korean Association of Hepato-Biliary-Pancreatic Surgery KAHBPS (Lee et al. 2014), Japanese Society of Hepato-Biliary-Pancreatic Surgery JSHBPS (Miyazaki et al. 2015), Indian Council of Medical Research ICMR (Shukla et al. 2015), American Hepato-Pancreatico-Biliary Association AHPBA (Aloia et al. 2015), and National Comprehensive Cancer Network NCCN (Benson et al. 2019) are based mostly on expert opinions.

Please also see an Invited Commentary on Philosophy of Management of Gall Bladder Cancer by Hiroaki Shimizu (pp **–**)

V. K. Kapoor (✉)
Department of Surgical Gastroenterology, Sanjay Gandhi Post-Graduate Institute of Medical Sciences (SGPGIMS), Lucknow, Uttar Pradesh, India
e-mail: vkkapoor.india@gmail.com

V. K. Kapoor (ed.), *A Pictorial Treatise on Gall Bladder Cancer*,
https://doi.org/10.1007/978-981-15-5289-2_9

9.1 Philosophy of Management

Japanese surgeons have an aggressive approach in the form of supra-radical major surgical resections, e.g., extended right hepatectomy (ERH), hepato-pancreato-duodenectomy (HPD), hepato-ligamento-pancreato-duodenectomy (HLPD) (Kondo et al. 2002, Ota et al. 2007; Kaneoka et al. 2015), and right upper quadrantectomy (major hepatectomy, pancreato-duodenectomy, right hemicolectomy, right nephrectomy and right phrenectomy) even in advanced stages of the disease. In a review of 4424 cases from Japan, 5-year survival was 83% for AJCC (5th ed) stage I, 70% for stage II, 45% for stage III, 23% for stage IVA, and 9% for stage IVB (Kayahara et al. 2008). The Japanese Biliary Tract Cancer Statistics Registry enrolled 2067 patients with GBC between 1998 and 2004—resection rate was 69%; overall 5-year survival was 42%—it was 88% for JSBS stage I, 69% for stage II, 42% for stage III, 23% for stage IVA, and 6% for stage IVB (Miyakawa et al. 2009). Overall 5-year survival in 4534 GBC cases in Japan (2008–2013) was 40% (91% in stage I, 71% in stage II, and 30% in stage III) (Ishihara et al. 2016). At the Tokyo Women's Medical University, resection was performed in 382 patients between 1969 and 2012—5-year survival was 99% in AJCC stage I (n = 87), 85% in stage II (n = 32), 40% in stage IIIA (n = 35), 53% in stage IIIB (n = 56), 0% in stage IVA (n = 30), and 18% for stage IVB (n = 141) (Higuchi and Yamamoto 2014). The aggressive Japanese approach is, however, associated with prolonged hospital stay, high morbidity and significant mortality, and repeated hospitalizations and interventions in the follow-up; 5-year actuarial survival estimates look good but actual long-term survivors are very few.

On the other extreme of the spectrum, there has been an overall fatalistic, pessimistic, and nihilistic attitude towards the management of GBC in the West. This is primarily because of the infrequency of the disease—median annual hospital volume in the National Cancer Database (NCDB) USA analysis of 36,067 cases (1998–2012) was as low as 1.4 (IQR 0.87–2.26) cases/hospital (Goussous et al. 2017). This sometimes results in incomplete, inadequate, and inappropriate management of even early GBC—only 9% of 19,139 resections in the USA were radical (extended) cholecystectomy (Goussous et al. 2017). Resection rate in T1–T3, N1, M0 disease was low (37%) (Tran Cao et al. 2018). In another report from the USA, only 4.5% of T1b and 5.6% of T2 tumors underwent adequate resection (Jensen et al. 2009). Out of 6825 T2 and T3 cases in the NCDB (2004–2014) as many as 89% underwent just simple cholecystectomy—inappropriate treatment (Kasumova et al. 2017). Majority of patients with T2 GBC in the USA were not managed according to recommendations (Wright et al. 2007). The MSKCC, New York, USA, reported much lower 5-year survival rates than the Japanese experience, i.e., 54% for AJCC stage II, 28% for stage III, and 25% for stage IV disease in 410 patients (Fong et al. 2000).

The differences in survival in GBC patients between Japan and the West are because of several factors including better patient selection and preparation, differences in pathological staging, aggressive surgical approach and, may be, different biology of the disease.

The Japanese aggressive approach towards advanced GBC comes at a cost in terms of high morbidity and significant (even double digit) mortality, with only anecdotal actual long-term survivors. On the other extreme, the Western pessimism results in inappropriate management and poor survival of even early disease. The Author (Kapoor 2007) has advocated an Indian "Buddhist" (Fig. 9.1) middle path for management of GBC—aggressive surgical approach for early and less advanced (i.e. confined to the GB) GBC (including incidental GBC) and largely non-surgical palliative approach for more advanced (beyond GB) GBC—major surgical resections performed in specialized centers for selected few good risk patients. Even in Japan, there is a recent rethink about the role and place of major supra-radical surgical procedures in advanced GBC. One report from the Tokyo Women's Medical University (TWMU) report observed that extensive surgeries such as major hepatectomy with pancreato-duodenectomy resulted in poor short-term surgical results and high hospital mortality

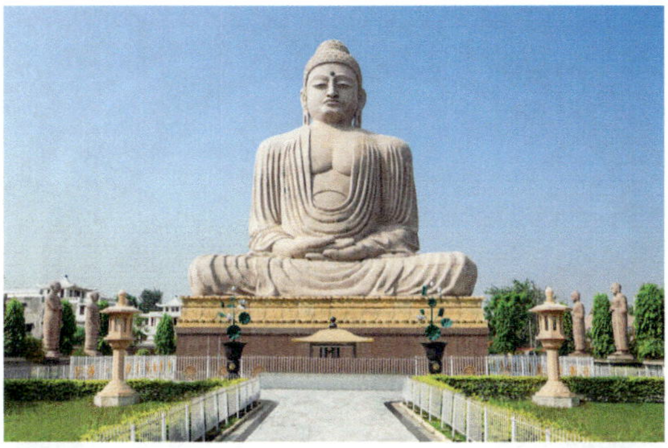

Fig. 9.1 Statue of Lord Buddha at Bodh Gaya, Bihar in north India—Lord Buddha described middle path of moderation between the extremes of sensual indulgence and self-mortification; the Author (VKK) has proposed an Indian "Buddhist" middle path between the Japanese aggressivism and the Western pessimism for management of gall bladder cancer

and such procedures are being avoided since 1997 (Higuchi et al. 2014). A recent publication from the Nagoya University Japan group observed that advanced GBC (requiring HPD) may be technically resectable but is oncologically unresectable (Mizuno et al. 2019a).

9.2 Surgery

9.2.1 Preparation for Surgery

Most patients with GBC are elderly and may have coexisting morbidities—they need detailed systematic organ/system, especially cardio-respiratory, functional evaluation for fitness for general anesthesia and major surgery; in addition, some time may be required for optimization of the patients before they can be operated. They may be malnourished because of anorexia, cancer cachexia, and gastric outlet obstruction/malignant gastroparesis and need nutritional support. The patients may have coagulopathy due to obstructive jaundice; this needs correction with vitamin K and, may be, fresh frozen plasma (FFP). They may be in sepsis because of cholangitis caused by biliary obstruction. Control of cholangitis can be tried with oral or parenteral antibiotics but if there is no response within 24–48 h, biliary drainage (of all segments of liver) may be required to control cholangitis. Blood should be grouped and cross-matched as liver parenchymal resection can sometimes cause massive bleeding. Prophylactic antibiotics should be administered at the time of induction of anesthesia; the choice of antibiotics could be based on previous bile (obtained at endoscopic naso-biliary drainage (ENBD) or percutaneous transhepatic biliary drainage (PTBD)) culture sensitivity report. In patients with a large bulky tumor close to the colon, the bowel should be prepared (mechanical and antibiotics) in anticipation of a colonic resection. Venous thrombo-embolism (VTE) prophylaxis is recommended because of the presence of cancer, the extent of proposed surgery and because majority of the patients will be middle age/old.

In patients with jaundice but without cholangitis, preoperative biliary drainage (PBD) is not required if only extended cholecystectomy (see Chap. 10) is planned, but it should be done if a major liver resection (see Chap. 11) is anticipated. The part of the liver which is going to be retained, i.e., the left lateral segment in case of extended right hepatectomy (ERH), should be drained. Percutaneous transhepatic biliary drainage (PTBD) (Fig. 9.2) used to be performed for PBD earlier by the Japanese surgeons, but it was associated with a significant risk of complications, e.g., intrahepatic vascular injury and bile leak, and tumor seeding along the catheter tract. The choice

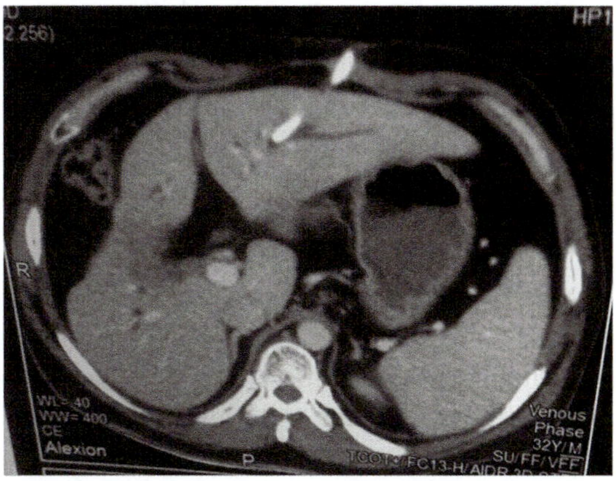

Fig. 9.2 CT shows Percutaneous Transhepatic Biliary Drainage (PTBD) in situ in the left lateral segment of liver—PTBD used to be performed for preoperative biliary drainage (PBD) earlier but is not favored now; endoscopic biliary drainage is preferred

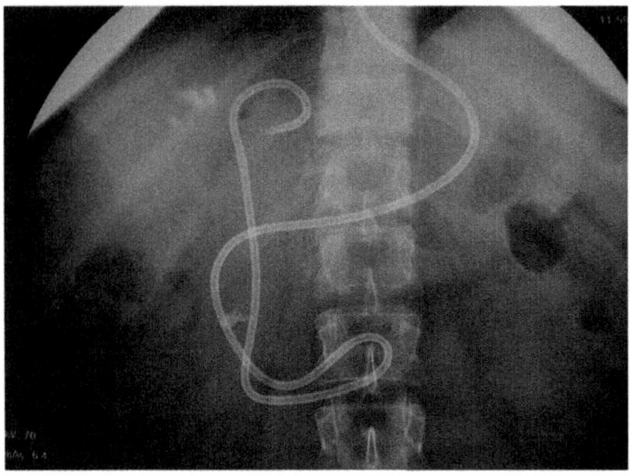

Fig. 9.3 X-ray shows endoscopic naso-biliary drainage (ENBD) in situ—ENBD (or stent) has become the preferred method of preoperative biliary drainage (PBD) now

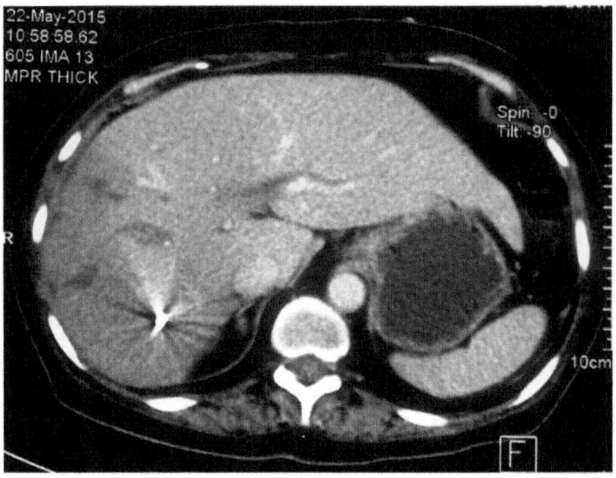

Fig. 9.4 CT shows steel coils used for portal vein embolization (PVE) in the right lobe and hypertrophy of the left lateral segment of the liver—PVE induces atrophy hypertrophy to increase the functional residual volume (FRV) before a major liver resection

of PBD has recently shifted from PTBD to endoscopic naso-biliary drainage (ENBD) (Fig. 9.3). At the Tokyo Women Medical University (TWMU), Japan, PTBD was mainly performed for PBD between 1968 and 2002 but the use of endoscopic PBD gradually increased after 2002 (Higuchi et al. 2014). ENBD is preferred over endoscopic biliary stenting (EBS) as it can be easily flushed to avoid a block but has the disadvantage of external biliary drainage. Endoscopic biliary stenting (EBS) has the advantage of internal (enteral) drainage but is liable to block requiring an exchange. External biliary drainage in the form of PTBD or ENBD has the disadvantage of bile loss which, over a prolonged period of time, may cause chronic dehydration, malabsorption, and malnutrition resulting in protein and vitamin deficiency. Bile refeeding can replace bile loss but is not acceptable to many patients.

If an ERH is anticipated and the functional residual volume (FRV) is less than 30%, which is usually the case, preoperative right portal vein embolization (PVE) (Fig. 9.4) should be performed (after the serum bilirubin has been brought down to <3 mg by PBD) to induce ipsilateral (right) atrophy and contralateral (left) hypertrophy to augment the FRV. In addition to the right portal vein (RPV), the segment IV branch of the left portal vein (LPV) also needs to be embolized; otherwise, segment IV will also hypertrophy and make ERH technically difficult.

Concurrent PBD and PVE in patients with GBC/perihilar CC with jaundice has been reported (Nilsson et al. 2015). One has to wait for 4–6 weeks for atrophy hypertrophy to occur but the disease can progress during this waiting time.

EPASS (Estimation of Physiologic Ability and Surgical Stress) model has been used to predict major morbidity and mortality after major resections for GBC (Haga et al. 2016). Estimates of risk of surgical site infection, reoperation, death, and readmission using the American College of Surgeons (ACS) National Surgical Quality Improvement Program (NSQIP) risk calculator were, however, inaccurate following operation for GBC and extrahepatic cholangiocarcinoma (Beal et al. 2017).

9.2.2 Surgical Management

Surgery, in the form of complete resection, is the only definitive treatment that offers chances of long-term survival and, rarely, cure in GBC. The aim should be a complete intent-to-cure (R0) resection, i.e., tumor-free microscopic margin, but resectability rates of preoperatively diagnosed (i.e. obvious) GBC are low—less than 10% of cases with a preoperative diagnosis of GBC are suitable for surgical resection. Only

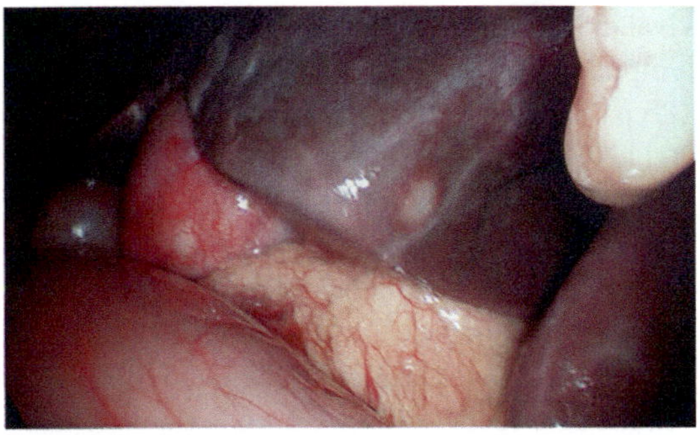

Fig. 9.5 Staging laparoscopy shows a small surface deposit in liver—staging laparoscopy to detect surface deposits is strongly recommended before laparotomy in ALL patients with gall bladder cancer

those with potentially resectable disease should be operated—this selection can be done by judicious use of preoperative investigations, e.g., US, CT, MRI, PET, EUS, and UGIE; staging laparoscopy (Fig. 9.5) before laparotomy is strongly recommended (see Chap. 7). The optimal extent of surgical resection, however, is not well defined. The terminology of surgical procedures performed for GBC is also not well defined, and there is no consensus on the terms used. Different groups use different terms to describe the same surgical procedure or mean different surgical procedures though using the same term. The term "radical cholecystectomy" was first proposed by Glenn and Hays (1954) to describe an operation which comprised of enbloc resection of the GB along with the GB fossa in the liver and the hepatoduodenal ligament lymph nodes. Shirai et al. (2012) included CBD excision and referred the operation as "extended" radical cholecystectomy. In order to avoid confusion, the Author (VKK) suggests that the operation performed for GBC should be called extended cholecystectomy rather than radical cholecystectomy (Fig. 9.6); he has proposed a standard terminology of surgical procedures performed for GBC (Kapoor and Behari 2017).

Resection rates are much higher (69%, Miyakawa et al. 2009 and 292/485, 64% Igami et al. 2014) in reports from Japan than in Europe (25% Cubertafond et al. 1994) and in the USA (53% Fong et al. 2000). At the MSKCC, New York, USA (1995–2005), potentially curative surgery was possible in only 123/435 (28%) patients—94/123 underwent hepatic resection (segments IV and V in 59 and ERH in 35) (Duffy et al. 2008). Agarwal et al. (2014a) reported a high (327/569, 58%) resectability rate from India, probably because of liberal use of EUS (to detect aorto-caval lymph nodes LNs), staging laparoscopy, and laparoscopic aorto-caval LN biopsy. Curative resection was possible in 154/385 (40%) patients in another large series from India—resectability was 1 out of 7 in patients with jaundice vs. 1 out of 2 without jaundice (Mishra et al. 2017). Another report from India (Singh et al. 2015), however, showed a low (21/106, 20%) resectability rate.

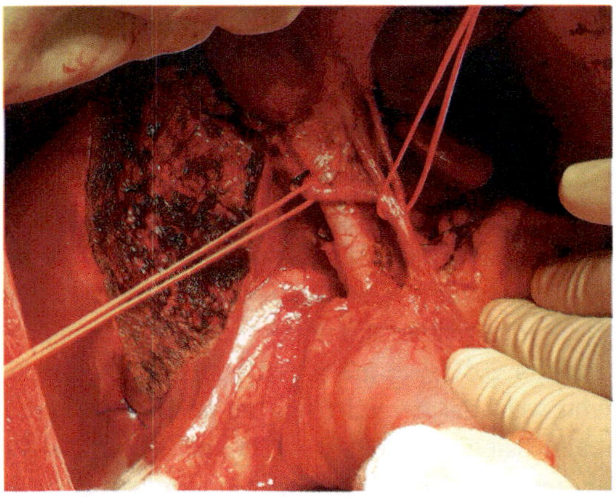

Fig. 9.6 Picture shows the liver bed after liver wedge resection and skeletonized common bile duct and hepatic artery branches (in sling) after extended cholecystectomy—extended cholecystectomy is removal of the gall bladder with a 2 cm non-anatomical wedge of the liver and regional lymphadenectomy

For some unknown reasons, mortality of the same procedures when performed for GBC is higher than when performed for other cancers, e.g., mortality of major hepatectomy was 16% for GBC vs. 4% for cholangiocarcinoma (Ebata et al. 2012), mortality of HPD was 20% for GBC (Ebata et al. 2007) vs. 2.4% for cholangiocarcinoma (Ebata et al. 2012). Mortality of HPD for GBC was 1/5 (20%) vs. 0/14 (0%) for cholangiocarcinoma (Sakamoto et al. 2013). Mortality in 274 patients with advanced (beyond muscularis propria) GBC operated at the TWMU Japan between 1969 and 2002 was 34/274 (12.4%)

(Higuchi et al. 2014). Like other major surgical procedures, e.g., esophagectomy and pancreato-duodenectomy, 90-day mortality is important as it is higher than 30-day mortality in GBC also. In the NCDB (1998–2012) analysis, 19,139 (53%) out of 36,067 patients underwent resection; 90-day mortality (17.1%) was much higher than 30-day mortality (7.4%) (Goussous et al. 2017). Thirty-day readmission rates are high after operations for GBC—as many as 20 out of 239 patients who were discharged from the hospital required readmission within 30 days (Higuchi et al. 2014). Surgery for GBC, like other major procedures, e.g., hepatectomy, pancreato-duodenectomy, esophagectomy, should preferably be performed at a high-volume center. In an analysis of 1524 cases from the NCDB (2010–2012), LN yield was better when surgery was performed at a high-volume center (Ong et al. 2018). Higher hospital volume is also associated with improved overall survival (OS) (Beal et al. 2019).

Patient selection for operation (to achieve high resectability rate) and for resection (to achieve high survival rates) is important. In addition to the stage of the disease, patient selection for surgery should be based on age, comorbidities, and nutritional and performance status of the patient. Factors which predict unresectability need to be identified to avoid performing an unnecessary operation in these patients. There is a need to identify patients who will not benefit from the major resections which are anyway associated with high morbidity and unacceptable mortality; jaundice, significant anorexia and weight loss, palpable GB lump, nodal (especially distant lymph nodes LNs) disease, and adjacent organ involvement are some of these factors. Surgical resection is difficult due to the anatomical complexity of the region—resection in GBC, therefore, remains a surgical challenge. High recurrence rates are seen even after complete R0 resection. Seventy-two patients with stage IV GBC were operated at the Nagoya University Japan—mortality was 14 (19%) and only 11 patients survived >3 years (Kondo et al. 2003). In a later report from Nagoya, 166 stage IV patients were operated with 14% mortality and 15 (12%) 5-year survivors (Nishio et al. 2007). In a report from South Korea, there was no 5-year survival in N2 disease even after HPD and aorto-caval lymphadenectomy (Lim et al. 2013). Mortality in 185 patients with advanced, i.e., T3, T4 GBC was 20 (12%) (Igami et al. 2014).

Unlike obvious/suspected GBC, incidental GBC is more likely to be resectable. All patients with a diagnosis of incidental GBC should be investigated and, unless a distant metastasis is found on the investigations, should be offered the benefit of a reoperation for completion extended cholecystectomy (CEC) (see Chap. 14).

The first step at laparotomy (after a negative staging laparoscopy) should be a thorough exploration of the abdomen and pelvis to look for any distant metastases, e.g., on the surface of liver, on the undersurface of diaphragm, falciform ligament, peritoneal, omental, pelvic, or ovarian deposits which could have been missed on staging laparoscopy. Distant LNs, i.e., celiac, superior mesenteric, and aorto-caval (Fig. 9.7) should be looked for. Outcome in patients with aorto-caval LN involvement is as poor as in those with metastatic disease (Kondo et al. 2000). Aorto-caval LNs are frequently missed on CT (sensitivity only 13%); EUS (and guided fine needle aspiration cytology FNAC) is better—it avoided unnecessary laparotomy in 58%

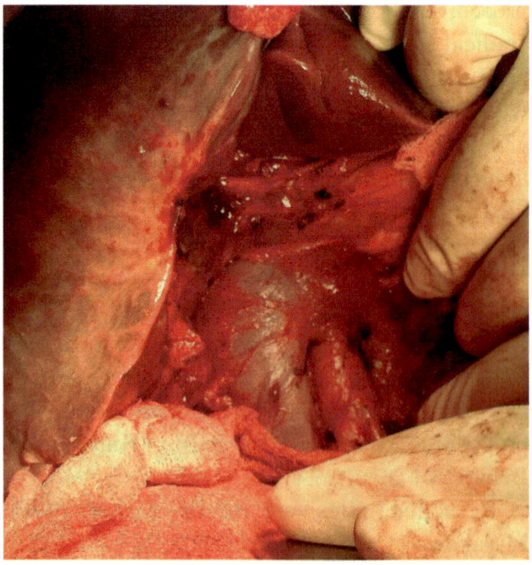

Fig. 9.7 Picture shows exposure of the aorto-caval area after kocherization of the duodenum—at laparotomy, enlarged aorto-caval lymph nodes should be looked for and biopsied

patients in whom aorto-caval LN was suspected on imaging (Agarwal et al. 2014b). Operative evaluation of the inter aorto-caval LN requires kocherization of the duodenum. Any enlarged LNs should be removed for frozen section histopathological examination. Even if no obvious enlarged LN is seen, the aorto-caval areolar fibrofatty tissue below the left renal vein (LRV) should be removed and sent for frozen section histopathological examination. Routine aorto-caval LN (16b1) biopsy was positive in 34/183 (19%) potentially resectable GBC—this was more frequent in T3 and T4 lesions but was seen in even T1 and T2 patients (Agarwal et al. 2014b). Another report showed that para-aortic LNs were involved in 19% of pT2 and pT3 patients (Murakami et al. 2011). Most groups consider the involvement of aorto-caval LNs as a contraindication for surgery/resection. Some groups, however, go ahead with resection even in the presence of the aorto-caval LNs (Murakami et al. 2011) though the Author (VKK) does not agree with this approach.

9.2.3 Contraindications for Surgery

Patients who are unfit (because of old age, uncontrolled comorbidities, and poor nutritional/performance/physiological status) for general anesthesia/major operation and those with distant (e.g., hepatic Fig. 9.8, peritoneal or extra-abdominal) metastases, malignant ascites (Fig. 9.9) (proven by fluid cytology), involvement of distant (celiac, superior mesenteric Fig. 9.10 and aorto-caval Fig. 9.11) lymph nodes, main portal vein, or proper hepatic artery (Fig. 9.12) and bilateral secondary biliary ductal confluence block (in GBC neck) are not candidates for surgery and should not be operated.

NOTE Some earlier reports (Bartlett et al. 1996; Benoist et al. 1998) reported no long-term survival in node-positive patients and questioned the role of operation in such cases but that does not hold true today as most series report 5-year survival in even node-positive patients.

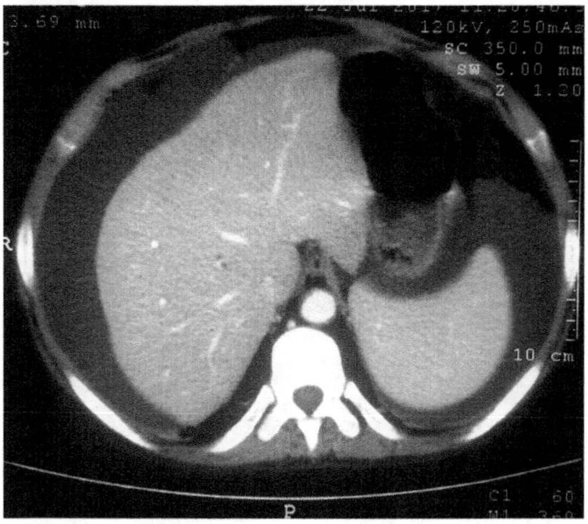

Fig. 9.9 CT shows perihepatic and perisplenic fluid—ascites; if positive on fluid cytology, it is a contraindication for surgery

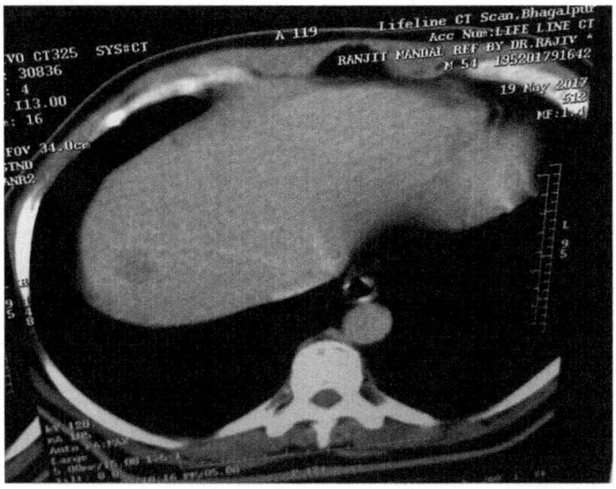

Fig. 9.8 CT shows a solitary hypodense space-occupying lesion suggestive of liver metastasis—this should be targeted for FNAC

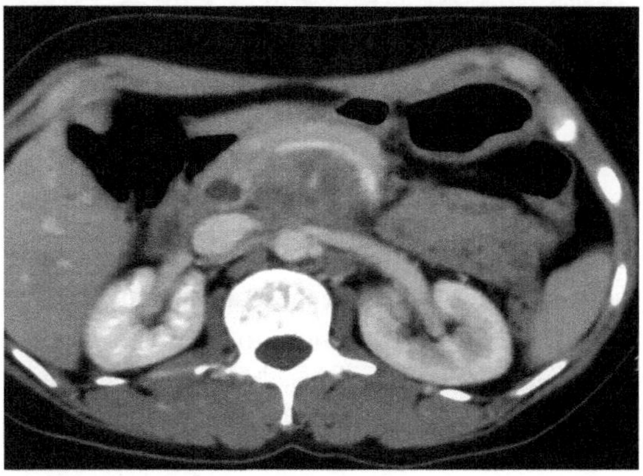

Fig. 9.10 Large superior mesenteric artery lymph nodes—these are distant lymph nodes which, if positive on FNAC, are contraindication for surgery

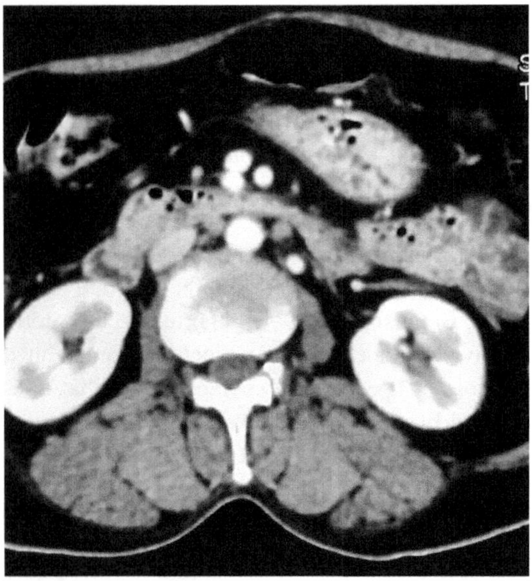

Fig. 9.11 CT shows large aorto-caval lymph node and left para-aortic lymph node—these can be targeted on US, CT, or EUS for FNAC

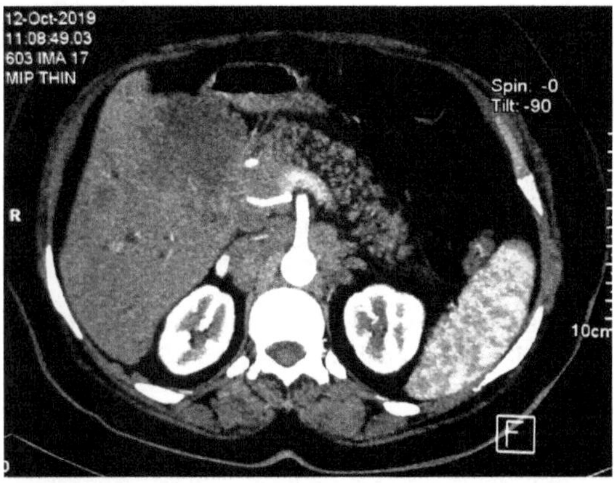

Fig. 9.12 Involvement of proper hepatic artery (as also of main portal vein) is a contraindication for surgery

Periduodenal and peripancreatic (Fig. 9.13) LNs are also a matter of great controversy. Most western centers consider these as distant LNs and do not advocate resection in the presence of involvement of these LNs. Most Japanese centers, however, consider these LNs as regional and recommend resection even if they are involved. Five-year survival in patients with metastasis to postero-superior pancreatic LNs (n = 20) was better (35% vs. 17%) than those with metastasis beyond these LNs (n = 46) (Kishi et al. 2012). In a recent report, 5-year survival in patients with metastasis to postero-superior pancreatic LNs was 56% vs. 15% in those with metastasis beyond these LNs (Sakata et al. 2017). The Author (VKK), and other Indian groups, tend to agree with the Japanese philosophy and consider the periduodenal/peripancreatic LNs as regional and recommend resection even if they are involved although outcome in terms of survival in these cases is not very good.

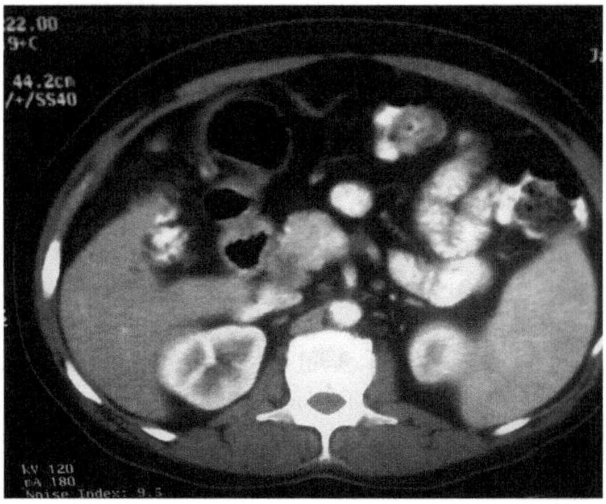

Fig. 9.13 CT shows a large retropancreatic lymph node behind the duodenum and pancreas—retropancreatic lymph nodes are a matter of debate between the AJCC–UICC and JSBS classifications of gall bladder cancer; AJCC–UICC considers them to be distant nodes while JSBS considers them to be regional nodes

Every attempt must be made to find out a reason "not to operate" upon a patient with GBC because if such a reason is present and it is missed, neglected, or ignored and the patient is still operated upon the outcome will be poor and the operation will prove to be futile.

9.3 Non-surgical Management

Adjuvant therapy (chemotherapy with or without radiotherapy) after surgical resection has a role in high-risk (for recurrence) patients with GBC. Neoadjuvant therapy and targeted therapy with biologicals are being evaluated (see Chap. 13). Non-surgical (endoscopic and percutaneous radiological) interventions play a major role in the palliation of unresectable cases (see Chap. 12).

Just like its incidence, the philosophy of management of GBC also varies from region to region. The Author (VKK) advocates an Indian Buddhist "Middle" path.

Invited Commentary on Philosophy of Management of Gall Bladder Cancer

Hiroaki Shimizu

The contents of this chapter include a review of the surgical indications and operative procedures for gallbladder cancer (GBC) (early and advanced stage) in the West and Japan, and clearly show the differences in philosophy and surgical management for GBC between the two. Comparing the two different approaches, the Author (VKK) has established his own philosophy of surgical management (the Indian approach) for GBC, taking good points from each, which seems to be in the middle of Japanese aggressive and Western pessimistic approaches.

The majority of GBC is diagnosed at advanced stage. Surgical complete resection (R0 resection) is the only potentially curative treatment and remains mainstay of management to achieve long-term survival in patients with GBC, but postoperative prognosis is closely correlated with the stage of the disease. In pT1 GBC, lymph node metastasis has almost never been found in Japan; therefore, good prognosis can be achieved even after simple cholecystectomy. As to pT2 GBC, the appropriate surgical strategy can achieve a prognostic improvement, but standard surgical procedure remains controversial in Japan; gallbladder bed resection or resection of liver segments IVA + V (subsegment IVB is called IVA in Japan), and combined with or without extrahepatic bile duct resection for lymph node dissection. There is still no definitive conclusion as to the most preferable surgical procedures for pT2 GBC.

On the other hand, the prognosis is quite poor in pT3 and pT4 GBC, even after complete resection of the tumor. In 1980s, Japanese hepatobiliary surgeons aggressively challenged to perform extended surgical procedures, such as extended right hepatectomy (ERH), hepato-pancreatico-duodenectomy (HPD) or hepato-ligamento-pancreatico-duodenectomy (HLPD) to increase resectability (Takasaki et al. 1980; Nimura et al. 1991). These ultimate procedures carried a high risk of postoperative morbidity and subsequent mortality. In spite of this, very few patients could be cured. Therefore, surgeons in the West have criticized these procedures.

At present, with improvement of surgical techniques and perioperative patient care, including preoperative biliary drainage (PBD) and portal vein embolization (PVE), mortality rate after extended surgical procedures, such as HPD have gradually decreased in Japan. Higher hospital volume is also associated with lower morbidity and mortality rates. However, recent reports have shown still extremely poor survival in patients with locally spreading GBC requiring HPD. The Nagoya group in Japan clearly stated that the indication for HPD for advanced GBC is not recommended from an oncological viewpoint (Mizuno et al. 2019a). That is, advanced GBC requiring HPD, represents technically resectable but oncologically unresectable disease, because of aggressive tumor biology. At present, the role and indication for extended resections such as HPD to achieve complete resection of the tumor in patients with locally spreading GBC should be reconsidered.

References

Chapter References

Agarwal AK, Javed A, Raja K, Sakhuja P. Surgical techniques in the management of primary gall bladder cancer. In: Agarwal A, Fong Y, editors. Carcinoma of the gall bladder. New Delhi: Elsevier; 2014a. p. 106–29.

Agarwal AK, Kalayarasan R, Javed A, Sakhuja P. Role of routine 16b1 lymph node biopsy in the management of gallbladder cancer: an analysis. HPB (Oxford). 2014b;16(3):229–34. https://doi.org/10.1111/hpb.12127. Epub 2013 Jul 22.

Aloia TA, Járufe N, Javle M, Maithel SK, Roa JC, Adsay V, Coimbra FJ, Jarnagin WR. Gallbladder cancer: expert consensus statement. HPB (Oxford). 2015;17(8):681–90. https://doi.org/10.1111/hpb.12444.

Bartlett DL, Fong Y, Fortner JG, Brennan MF, Blumgart LH. Long-term results after resection for gallbladder cancer. Implications for staging and management. Ann Surg. 1996;224(5):639–46.

Beal EW, Lyon E, Kearney J, Wei L, Ethun CG, Black SM, Dillhoff M, Salem A, Weber SM, Tran TB, Poultsides G, Shenoy R, Hatzaras I, Krasnick B, Fields RC, Buttner S, Scoggins CR, Martin RCG, Isom CA, Idrees K, Mogal HD, Shen P, Maithel SK, Pawlik TM, Schmidt CR. Evaluating the American College of Surgeons National Surgical Quality Improvement project risk calculator: results from the U.S. Extrahepatic Biliary Malignancy Consortium. HPB (Oxford). 2017;19(12):1104–11. https://doi.org/10.1016/j.hpb.2017.08.009. Epub 2017 Sep 7.

Beal EW, Mehta R, Tsilimigras DI, Hyer JM, Paredes AZ, Merath K, Dillhoff ME, Cloyd JM, Ejaz A, Pawlik TM. Travel to a high volume hospital to undergo resection of gallbladder cancer: does it impact quality of care and long-term outcomes? HPB (Oxford). 2019; https://doi.org/10.1016/j.hpb.2019.05.004. pii: S1365-182X(19)30543-X.

Benoist S, Panis Y, Fagniez PL. Long-term results after curative resection for carcinoma of the gallbladder. French University Association for Surgical Research. Am J Surg. 1998;175(2):118–22.

Benson AB, D'Angelica MI, Abbott DE, Abrams TA, Alberts SR, Anaya DA, Anders R, Are C, Brown D, Chang DT, Cloyd J, Covey AM, Hawkins W, Iyer R, Jacob R, Karachristos A, Kelley RK, Kim R, Palta M, Park JO, Sahai V, Schefter T, Sicklick JK, Singh G, Sohal D, Stein S, Tian GG, Vauthey JN, Venook AP, Hammond LJ, Darlow SD. Guidelines insights: hepatobiliary cancers, Version 2.2019. J Natl Compr Cancer Netw. 2019;17(4):302–10. https://doi.org/10.6004/jnccn.2019.0019.

Cubertafond P, Gainant A, Cucchiaro G. Surgical treatment of 724 carcinomas of the gallbladder carcinoma: long term results. Ann Surg. 1994;219:275–80.

Duffy A, Capanu M, Abou-Alfa GK, Huitzil D, Jarnagin W, Fong Y, D'Angelica M, Dematteo RP, Blumgart LH, O'Reilly EM. Gallbladder cancer (GBC): 10-year experience at Memorial Sloan-Kettering Cancer Centre (MSKCC). J Surg Oncol. 2008;98(7):485–9. https://doi.org/10.1002/jso.21141.

Ebata T, Nagino M, Nishio H, Arai T, Nimura Y. Right hepatopancreatoduodenectomy: improvements over 23 years to attain acceptability. J Hepatobiliary Pancreat Surg. 2007;14(2):131–5. Epub 2007 Mar 27.

Ebata T, Yokoyama Y, Igami T, Sugawara G, Takahashi Y, Nimura Y, Nagino M. Hepatopancreatoduodenectomy for cholangiocarcinoma: a single-center review of 85 consecutive patients. Ann Surg. 2012;256(2):297–305. https://doi.org/10.1097/SLA.0b013e31826029ca.

Fong Y, Jarnagin W, Blumgart LH. Gallbladder cancer: comparison of patients presenting initially for definitive operation with those presenting after prior noncurative intervention. Ann Surg. 2000;232(4):557–69.

Glenn F, Hays DM. The scope of radical surgery in the treatment of malignant tumors of the extrahepatic biliary tract. Surg Gynecol Obstet. 1954;99(5):529–41.

Goussous N, Hosseini M, Sill AM, Cunningham SC. Minimally invasive and open gallbladder cancer resections: 30- vs 90-day mortality. Hepatobiliary Pancreat Dis Int. 2017;16(4):405–11. https://doi.org/10.1016/S1499-3872(17)60025-0.

Haga Y, Miyamoto A, Wada Y, Takami Y, Takeuchi H. Value of E-PASS models for predicting postoperative morbidity and mortality in resection of perihilar cholangiocarcinoma and gallbladder carcinoma. HPB (Oxford). 2016;18(3):271–8. https://doi.org/10.1016/j.hpb.2015.09.001. Epub 2015 Nov 18.

Higuchi R, Yamamoto M. Aggressive surgical management and treatment outcomes of gallbladder cancer. In: Agarwal A, Fong Y, editors. Carcinoma of the gall bladder. New Delhi: Elsevier; 2014. p. 175–83.

Higuchi R, Ota T, Araida T, Kajiyama H, Yazawa T, Furukawa T, Yoshikawa T, Takasaki K, Yamamoto M. Surgical approaches to advanced gallbladder cancer: a 40-year single-institution study of prognostic factors and resectability. Ann Surg Oncol. 2014;21(13):4308–16. https://doi.org/10.1245/s10434-014-3885-1. Epub 2014 Jul 15.

Igami T, Ebata T, Yokoyama Y, Sugawara G, Nagino M. Advanced resectable gallbladder cancer: diagnosis and surgical approach. In: Agarwal A, Fong Y, editors. Carcinoma of the gall bladder. New Delhi: Elsevier; 2014. p. 89–105.

Ishihara S, Horiguchi A, Miyakawa S, Endo I, Miyazaki M, Takada T. Biliary tract cancer registry in Japan from 2008 to 2013. J Hepatobiliary Pancreat Sci. 2016;23(3):149–57. https://doi.org/10.1002/jhbp.314. Epub 2016 Jan 26.

Jensen EH, Abraham A, Habermann EB, Al-Refaie WB, Vickers SM, Virnig BA, Tuttle TM. A critical analysis of the surgical management of early-stage gallbladder cancer in the United States. J Gastrointest Surg. 2009;13(4):722–7. https://doi.org/10.1007/s11605-008-0772-8. Epub 2008 Dec 13.

Kaneoka Y, Maeda A, Isogai M. En bloc resection of the hepatoduodenal ligament for advanced biliary malignancy. J Gastrointest Surg. 2015;19(4):708–14. https://doi.org/10.1007/s11605-014-2731-x. Epub 2015 Jan 6.

Kapoor VK. Advanced gallbladder cancer: Indian "middle path". J Hepatobiliary Pancreat Surg. 2007;14(4):366–73. Epub 2007 Jul 30. PMID:17653634

Kapoor VK, Behari A. Surgical procedures for gall bladder cancer. BAOJ Cancer Res Ther. 2017;3:037.

Kasumova GG, Tabatabaie O, Najarian RM, Callery MP, Ng SC, Bullock AJ, Fisher RA, Tseng JF. Surgical management of gallbladder cancer: simple versus extended cholecystectomy and the role of adjuvant therapy. Ann Surg. 2017;266(4):625–31. https://doi.org/10.1097/SLA.0000000000002385.

Kayahara M, Nagakawa T, Nakagawara H, Kitagawa H, Ohta T. Prognostic factors for gallbladder cancer in Japan. Ann Surg. 2008;248(5):807–14. https://doi.org/10.1097/SLA.0b013e31818a1561.

Kishi Y, Shimada K, Hata S, Oguro S, Sakamoto Y, Nara S, Esaki M, Hiraoka N, Kosuge T. Definition of T3/4 and regional lymph nodes in gallbladder cancer: which is more valid, the UICC or the Japanese staging system? Ann Surg Oncol. 2012;19(11):3567–73. https://doi.org/10.1245/s10434-012-2599-5. Epub 2012 Aug 14.

Kondo S, Nimura Y, Hayakawa N, Kamiya J, Nagino M, Uesaka K. Regional and para-aortic lymphadenectomy in radical surgery for advanced gallbladder carcinoma. Br J Surg. 2000;87(4):418–22.

Kondo S, Nimura Y, Hayakawa N, Kamiya J, Nagino M, Uesaka K. Extensive surgery for carcinoma of the gallbladder. Br J Surg. 2002;89(2):179–84.

Kondo S, Nimura Y, Kamiya J, Nagino M, Kanai M, Uesaka K, Yuasa N, Sano T, Hayakawa N. Factors influencing postoperative hospital mortality and long-term survival after radical resection for stage IV gallbladder carcinoma. World J Surg. 2003;27(3):272–7. Epub 2003 Feb 27.

Lee SE, Kim KS, Kim WB, Kim IG, Nah YW, Ryu DH, Park JS, Yoon MH, Cho JY, Hong TH, et al. Practical guidelines for the surgical treatment of gallbladder cancer. J Korean Med Sci. 2014;29(10):1333–40. https://doi.org/10.3346/jkms.2014.29.10.1333.

Lim H, Seo DW, Park DH, Lee SS, Lee SK, Kim MH, Hwang S. Prognostic factors in patients with gallbladder cancer after surgical resection: analysis of 279 operated patients. J Clin Gastroenterol. 2013;47(5):443–8. https://doi.org/10.1097/MCG.0b013e3182703409.

Mishra PK, Saluja SS, Prithiviraj N, Varshney V, Goel N, Patil N. Predictors of curative resection and long term survival of gallbladder cancer - a retrospective analysis. Am J Surg. 2017;214(2):278–86. https://doi.org/10.1016/j.amjsurg.2017.02.006. Epub 2017 Feb 9.

Miyakawa S, Ishihara S, Horiguchi A, Takada T, Miyazaki M, Nagakawa T. Biliary tract cancer treatment: 5,584 results from the Biliary Tract Cancer Statistics Registry from 1998 to 2004 in Japan. J Hepatobiliary Pancreat Surg. 2009;16(1):1–7. https://doi.org/10.1007/s00534-008-0015-0. Epub 2008 Dec 26.

Miyazaki M, Yoshitomi H, Miyakawa S, Uesaka K, Unno M, Endo I, Ota T, Ohtsuka M, Kinoshita H, Shimada K, Shimizu H, Tabata M, Chijiiwa K, Nagino M, Hirano S, Wakai T, Wada K, Isayama H, Okusaka T, Tsuyuguchi T, Fujita N, Furuse J, Yamao K, Murakami K, Yamazaki H, Kijima H, Nakanuma Y, Yoshida M, Takayashiki T, Takada T. Clinical practice guidelines for the management of biliary tract cancers 2015: the 2nd English edition. J Hepatobiliary Pancreat Sci. 2015;22(4):249–73. https://doi.org/10.1002/jhbp.233. Epub 2015 Mar 18.

Mizuno T, Ebata T, Yokoyama Y, Igami T, Yamaguchi J, Onoe S, Watanabe N, Ando M, Nagino M. Major hepatectomy with or without pancreatoduodenectomy for advanced gallbladder cancer. Br J Surg. 2019;106(5):626–35. https://doi.org/10.1002/bjs.11088. Epub 2019 Feb 14.

Murakami Y, Uemura K, Sudo T, Hashimoto Y, Nakashima A, Kondo N, Sakabe R, Kobayashi H, Sueda T. Is para-aortic lymph node metastasis a contraindication for radical resection in biliary carcinoma? World J Surg. 2011;35(5):1085–93. https://doi.org/10.1007/s00268-011-1036-4.

Nilsson J, Eriksson S, Nørgaard Larsen P, Keussen I, Christiansen Frevert S, Lindell G, Sturesson C. Concurrent biliary drainage and portal vein embolization in preparation for extended hepatectomy in patients with biliary cancer. Acta Radiol Open. 2015;4(5):2058460115579121. https://doi.org/10.1177/2058460115579121. eCollection 2015 May.

Nishio H, Nagino M, Ebata T, Yokoyama Y, Igami T, Nimura Y. Aggressive surgery for stage IV gallbladder carcinoma; what are the contraindications? J Hepatobiliary Pancreat Surg. 2007;14(4):351–7. Epub 2007 Jul 30.

Ong CT, Leung K, Nussbaum DP, Sun Z, Gloor B, Blazer DG III, Worni M. Open versus laparoscopic portal lymphadenectomy in gallbladder cancer: is there a difference in lymph node yield? HPB (Oxford). 2018;20(6):505–13. https://doi.org/10.1016/j.hpb.2017.10.015. Epub 2018 Feb 19.

Ota T, Araida T, Yamamoto M, Takasaki K. Operative outcome and problems of right hepatic lobectomy with pancreatoduodenectomy for advanced carcinoma of the biliary tract. J Hepatobiliary Pancreat Surg. 2007;14(2):155–8. Epub 2007 Mar 27.

Patkar S, Ostwal V, Ramaswamy A, Engineer R, Chopra S, Shetty N, Dusane R, Shrikhande SV, Goel M. Emerging role of multimodality treatment in gall bladder cancer: outcomes following 510 consecutive resections in a tertiary referral center. J Surg Oncol. 2018;117(3):372–9. https://doi.org/10.1002/jso.24837. Epub 2017 Sep 20.

Sakamoto Y, Nara S, Kishi Y, Esaki M, Shimada K, Kokudo N, Kosuge T. Is extended hemihepatectomy plus pancreaticoduodenectomy justified for advanced bile duct cancer and gallbladder cancer? Surgery. 2013;153(6):794–800. https://doi.org/10.1016/j.surg.2012.11.024. Epub 2013 Feb 13.

Sakata J, Kobayashi T, Tajima Y, Ohashi T, Hirose Y, Takano K, Takizawa K, Miura K, Wakai T. Relevance of dissection of the posterior superior pancreaticoduodenal lymph nodes in gallbladder carcinoma. Ann Surg Oncol. 2017;24(9):2474–81. https://doi.org/10.1245/s10434-017-5939-7. Epub 2017 Jun 26.

Shirai Y, Sakata J, Wakai T, Ohashi T, Hatakeyama K. "Extended" radical cholecystectomy for gallbladder cancer: long-term outcomes, indications and limitations. World J Gastroenterol. 2012;18(34):4736–43.

Shukla HS, Sirohi B, Behari A, Sharma A, Majumdar J, Ganguly M, Tewari M, Kumar S, Saini S, Sahni P, Singh T, Kapoor VK, Sucharita V, Kaur T, Shukla DK, Rath GK. Indian Council of Medical Research consensus document for the management of gall bladder cancer. Indian J Med Paediatr Oncol. 2015;36(2):79–84. https://doi.org/10.4103/0971-5851.158829.

Singh SK, Talwar R, Kannan N, Tyagi AK, Jaiswal P, Kumar A. Aggressive surgical approach for gallbladder cancer: a single-center experience from northern

India. J Gastrointest Cancer. 2015;46(4):399–407. https://doi.org/10.1007/s12029-015-9766-4.

Tran Cao HS, Zhang Q, Sada YH, Chai C, Curley SA, Massarweh NN. The role of surgery and adjuvant therapy in lymph node-positive cancers of the gallbladder and intrahepatic bile ducts. Cancer. 2018;124(1):74–83. https://doi.org/10.1002/cncr.30968. Epub 2017 Aug 25.

Wright BE, Lee CC, Iddings DM, Kavanagh M, Bilchik AJ. Management of T2 gallbladder cancer: are practice patterns consistent with national recommendations? Am J Surg. 2007;194(6):820–5; discussion 825–6.

References for Commentary Notes

Nimura Y, Hayakawa N, Kamiya J, Maeda S, Kondo S, Yasui A, et al. Hepatopancreatoduodenectomy for advanced carcinoma of the biliary tract. Hepatogastroenterology. 1991;38:170–5.

Takasaki K, Kobayashi S, Mutoh H, Akimoto S, Toda K, Asado S, et al. Our experiences (5 cases) of extended right lobectomy combined with pancreatoduodenectomy for the carcinoma of the gall bladder (in Japanese). Tan to Sui. 1980;1:923–32.

Extended Cholecystectomy for Gall Bladder Cancer

10

Vinay K. Kapoor

Radical cholecystectomy, i.e., removal of the gall bladder (GB) with a rim of liver tissue and lymphatic tissue within the hepatoduodenal ligament (HDL) for gall bladder cancer (GBC) was first reported by Glenn and Hays (1954). The terms radical and extended cholecystectomy (EC) have been used as synonyms; the term extended radical cholecystectomy has also been used (Sakata et al. 2010a). "Radical" denotes the oncological adequacy of a procedure, which depends on the stage of the tumor and the extent of surgical resection. Radicality of an operation can be decided only after histopathological examination of the specimen showing R0 resection status, i.e., negative margins. Thus, while a simple cholecystectomy alone is radical for a T1aN0 lesion, a major operation such as hepato-pancreato-duodenectomy (HPD) with combined resection of adjacent organs (CRAO) will be required to achieve radicality in a locoregionally advanced T4N2 tumor. Extended cholecystectomy, on the other hand, is a well-defined surgical procedure independent of the stage of the tumor. The Author (VKK) prefers to use the term extended cholecystectomy. According to the author (Kapoor and Behari 2017a), EC should be defined as removal of the GB, a non-anatomical 2 cm wedge of the liver in segments IVB and V around the GB bed and regional lymphadenectomy (Fig. 10.1). There is, however, hardly any evidence in favor of a 2 cm liver wedge—it could be less (i.e., 1 cm) or more (i.e., 3 cm); just 1 cm liver wedge may also be

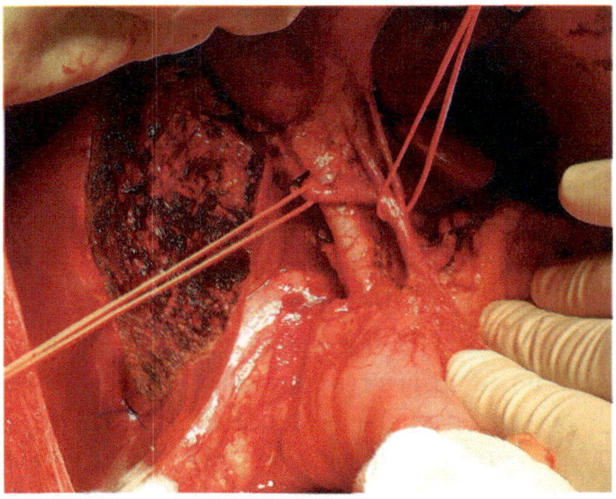

Fig. 10.1 Operative picture shows liver bed after wedge resection and skeletonized common bile duct and hepatic artery (right hepatic artery in right sling and proper hepatic artery in left sling; note that there are three branches of the proper hepatic artery—right, middle, and left). Extended cholecystectomy is removal of the gall bladder, a non-anatomical 2 cm wedge of the liver in segments IVB and V around the gall bladder bed and regional lymphadenectomy

Please also see the Invited Commentaries on Extended Cholecystectomy for Gall Bladder Cancer by Prasoon Pankaj and Toshifumi Wakai (pp **–**) and Yoo-Seok Yoon (pp **–**)

V. K. Kapoor (✉)
Department of Surgical Gastroenterology, Sanjay Gandhi Post-Graduate Institute of Medical Sciences (SGPGIMS), Lucknow, Uttar Pradesh, India
e-mail: vkkapoor.india@gmail.com

V. K. Kapoor (ed.), *A Pictorial Treatise on Gall Bladder Cancer*,
https://doi.org/10.1007/978-981-15-5289-2_10

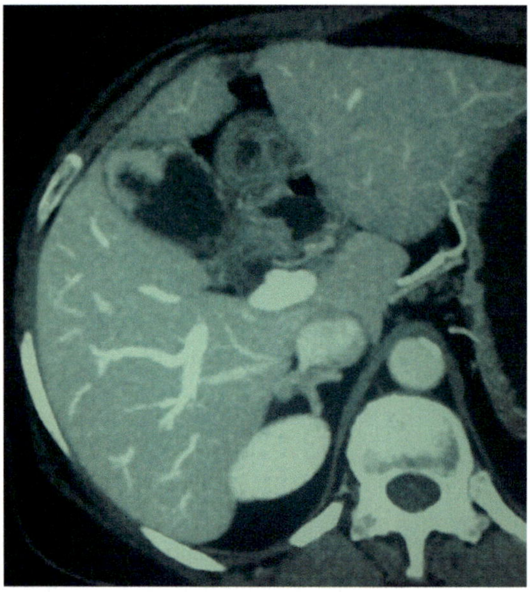

Fig. 10.2 CT shows focal thickening of the gall bladder wall with no liver infiltration, i.e., a clear fat plane is seen between the GB wall and the liver parenchyma—extended cholecystectomy can be performed for gall bladder cancer, which is confined to the gall bladder wall

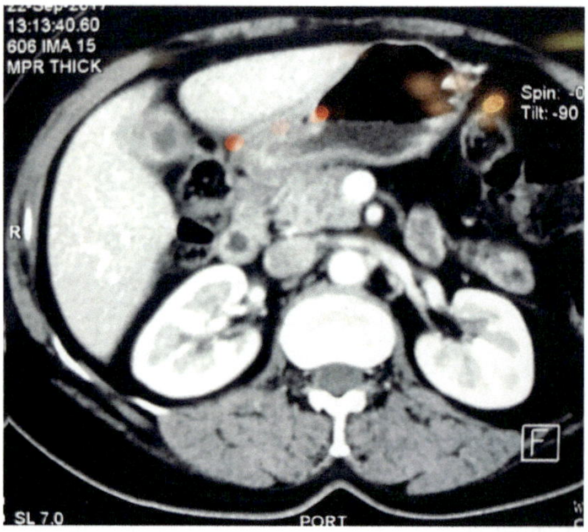

Fig. 10.3 CT shows diffuse thickening of the GB wall with minimal liver infiltration, i.e., no fat plane is seen between the GB wall and the liver parenchyma—extended cholecystectomy can be performed for gall bladder cancer with minimal (i.e., <1 cm) liver infiltration if the tumor is in the gall bladder fundus/body

adequate if there is no liver infiltration or in patients with significant liver infiltration, even >2 cm liver wedge or even a formal liver resection may be required. The trend these days is towards a moderate liver resection but more aggressive lymphadenectomy.

EC can be

1. Primary extended cholecystectomy (PEC) when performed for a preoperative/intraoperative diagnosis/suspicion of GBC which is confined to the GB wall (Fig. 10.2), and there is no adjacent organ invasion. It can also be performed in the presence of minimal (i.e., <1 cm) liver infiltration (Fig. 10.3) if the tumor is in the GB fundus/body (but not in the GB neck where a major hepatectomy will be required if there is any amount of liver infiltration *vide infra*). EC is curative for early GBC confined to the GB wall (T1, T2) and lymph nodes confined to the hepatoduodenal ligament (HDL).
2. Completion extended cholecystectomy (CEC) when performed for a postoperative/histopathological diagnosis of an incidental GBC.

10.1 Tissue Diagnosis

Tissue diagnosis is not mandatory for performing PEC. This would, however, mean that some patients who undergo EC with a suspicion of GBC will finally turn out to have a benign disease. Twelve out of 30 patients who were taken up for laparoscopic EC with an imaging diagnosis of early GBC were found to have a benign disease (Cho et al. 2010). Sixteen out of 77 patients who underwent radical (extended) cholecystectomy with a suspicion of GBC finally turned out to have xantho-granulomatous cholecystitis (XGC) (Rammohan et al. 2014). As many as 100 out of 164 patients who were taken up for laparoscopic EC for suspected GBC confined to the GB wall were finally found to have benign lesions (xanthogranulomatous cholecystitis XGC $n = 31$, adenomyomatosis $n = 29$, adenoma $n = 27$, and cholesterol polyps $n = 13$) (Zhang et al. 2018).

10.2 Contraindications

EC cannot (should not) be performed in patients with

1. Significant (>1 cm) liver infiltration (Fig. 10.4)—segments IVB + V or a major liver resection, e.g., extended right hepatectomy (ERH) will be required in such cases.
2. GB neck tumor with any amount of liver infiltration (Fig. 10.5) because the right portal pedicle is so close (2–9 mm) to the GB neck bed that an adequate oncological margin cannot be achieved without sacrificing the right portal pedicle thus necessitating an extended right hepatectomy (ERH).

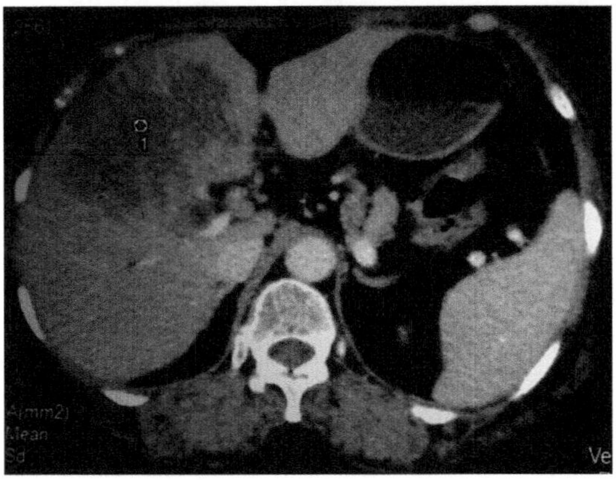

Fig. 10.4 CT shows a large necrotic mass involving segments IV and V—extended cholecystectomy cannot be performed if there is significant (>1 cm) liver infiltration; segments IVB + V resection or a major liver resection, e.g., extended right hepatectomy (ERH) will be required in such cases

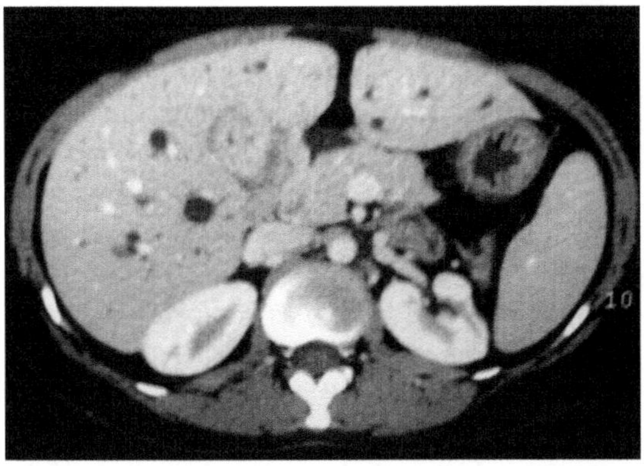

Fig. 10.5 Extended cholecystectomy (EC) cannot be performed in gall bladder cancer at neck with any amount of liver infiltration because the right portal pedicle lies very close (2–9 mm) to the gall bladder neck bed; extended right hepatectomy (ERH) will be required in such cases

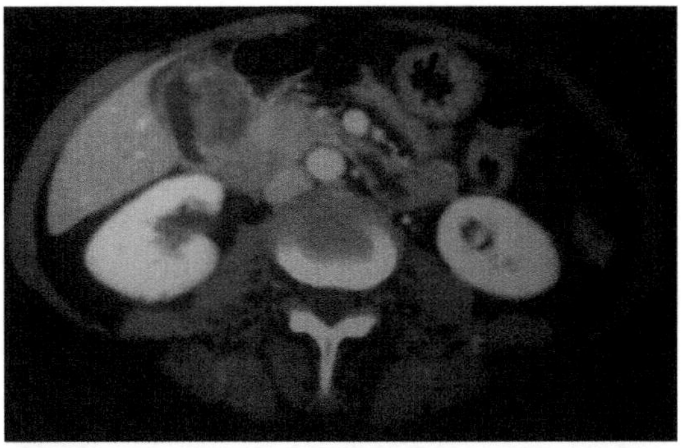

Fig. 10.6 CT shows gall bladder cancer infiltrating duodenum and pancreas—extended cholecystectomy (EC) cannot be performed in gall bladder cancer with involvement of the duodenum/pancreas; this will require pancreato-duodenectomy in addition

3. Involvement of the common bile duct (CBD) which will require CBD excision in addition to EC.

   NOTE *The Author (VKK) does not consider CBD excision as a part of EC.*
4. Involvement of the duodenum (Fig. 10.6)/pancreas (which will require pancreato-duodenectomy PD).

10.3 Open Extended Cholecystectomy

The patient is placed supine with a roll under the right lower rib cage and arms by the side and is administered general (+ epidural, for postoperative pain relief) anesthesia. In anticipation of liver parenchymal transection, excessive infusion of crystalloids should be avoided to achieve and maintain a low central venous pressure (CVP). A staging laparoscopy (Fig. 10.7) is strongly recommended before laparotomy in ALL patients with GBC to pick up any small peritoneal, omental, or liver surface deposits which were missed on preoperative imaging. The choice of incision depends on the body habitus of the patient. A generous long right subcostal incision with extension upwards in the midline towards the xiphisternum or a bilateral incision, i.e., right subcostal incision extended across the midline to the left can be used. Ligamentum teres (round ligament)

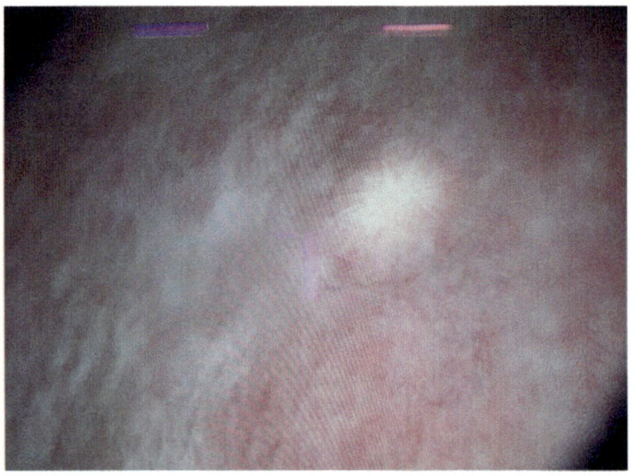

Fig. 10.7 Picture shows a small surface liver deposit on staging laparoscopy—staging laparoscopy is strongly recommended before laparotomy in ALL patients with gall bladder cancer to pick up any small peritoneal, omental, or liver surface deposits

is divided between clamps/ligatures and its cephalad stump is retracted upwards. Falciform ligament is separated from the anterior parietes and the undersurface of the diaphragm. A table mounted self-retaining retractor is applied for the right costal margin. A thorough exploration of the abdomen and pelvis is done to look for any peritoneal metastasis on the surface of liver, undersurface of the diaphragm, omentum, or peritoneum, which could have been missed on staging laparoscopy. Celiac and superior mesenteric lymph nodes (LN) should be looked for and any enlarged LNs should be removed for frozen section histopathological examination. Hepatic flexure and proximal (right) transverse colon are mobilized and the second part of the duodenum is kocherized. Aortocaval (para-aortic) LN (Fig. 10.8) is looked for between the celiac axis and the inferior mesenteric artery (IMA) and, if present, is removed for biopsy. If no obvious enlarged LN is seen in the aortocaval area, the aortocaval areolar fibro-fatty tissue below the left renal vein (LRV) should be sampled and sent for frozen section histopathological examination. Following para-aortic LN sampling, the anterior surfaces of the aorta, inferior vena cava (IVC), and the left renal vein should be exposed without any areolar (fatty) tissue covering them. Routine sampling biopsy and frozen section of the aortocaval LNs revealed metastases in 34 (19%) of 183 potentially resectable GBC; this was more likely in advanced (T3, T4) lesions but was seen in early (T1, T2) cases also (Agarwal et al. 2014).

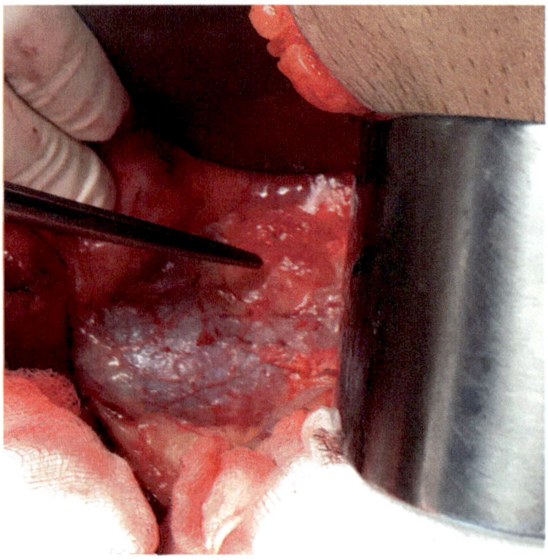

Fig. 10.8 Picture shows enlarged lymph nodes in the aortocaval region after kocherization of the duodenum—aortocaval (as also celiac and superior mesenteric) lymph nodes should be looked for and, if present, removed for frozen section histopathological examination; if they are positive, resection should not be performed

EC has two major components—GB with a non-anatomical liver wedge in segments IVB and V (called marginal hepatectomy in some reports) and lymphadenectomy. The sequence could be GB + liver wedge first followed by lymphadenectomy later or vice versa. The advantage of the former approach is that the liver cut surface can be packed/compressed with gauze or sponge while lymphadenectomy is being done—this helps in compression hemostasis and allows time to look for any bile leak (yellow staining of the gauze); the Author (VKK) prefers this approach.

In EC, the cystic duct is divided close to the common bile duct (CBD) as compared to simple cholecystectomy for gall stones where it is advised to stay away from the CBD to avoid an inadvertent bile duct injury; cystic duct margin is sent for frozen section histopathological examination (if the cystic duct margin is positive, CBD excision will be required).

Liver wedge is marked (scored) with electrocautery in segments IVB and V at a distance of

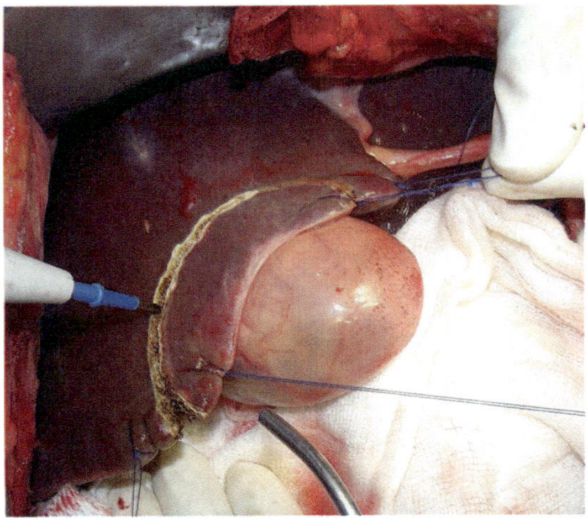

Fig. 10.9 Liver wedge is marked (scored) with electro-cautery in segments IVB and V at a distance of 2 cm from the edges of the gall bladder; Prolene sutures have been taken at the two corners of the liver wedge for retraction

2 cm from the edges of the GB (Fig. 10.9). Caution should be exercised on the under (inferior) surface of the liver; the liver wedge has to stay away from the hepatic hilum—it should remain 1–2 cm away from the porta hepatis to avoid injury to the right main or right anterior sectoral portal pedicle which lies at a depth of a few (2–9) mm from the GB bed near the GB neck. Prolene sutures (ties) may be taken at the liver edge on either side of the marking of the wedge for retraction of the liver during parenchymal dissection. Inflow control may be obtained with intermittent portal clamping (the Pringle maneuver). Liver parenchyma is divided using electro-cautery (at high wattage) for the first few (about 5) mm from the surface (Fig. 10.10), and then using a combination of clamp crush (Fig. 10.11) with ligatures/clips, Harmonic scalpel (Fig. 10.12) and cavitron ultrasonic aspirator (CUSA) (Fig. 10.13) with bipolar cautery (Fig. 10.14). Caution has to be exercised that the thickness (depth) of the liver wedge remains uniform (i.e., 2 cm) all through and it does not become less (too superficial) or more (too deep). The only major vessel encountered during liver wedge resection is the terminal part of the middle hepatic vein (MHV) between segments IVB and V (Fig. 10.15). Any brisk bleeding (arterial) or venous bleed is controlled with fine (5-0 or 6-0)

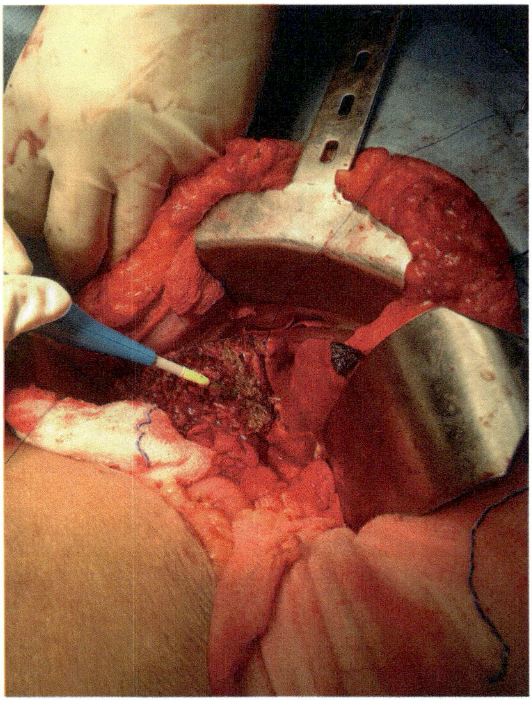

Fig. 10.10 Liver parenchyma is divided using electro-cautery (at high wattage) for the first few (about 5) mm from the surface

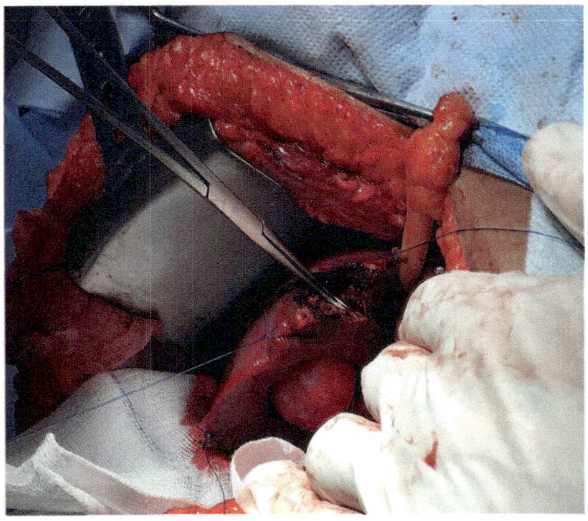

Fig. 10.11 Deeper liver parenchyma is divided using clamp crush with ligatures/clips

monofilament (Prolene) sutures. Diffuse ooze can be controlled with argon beam coagulator (ABC), if available. Local (topical) hemostatic agents, e.g., Surgicel, fibrin glue may be used. Pressure is applied with a gauze or sponge pack

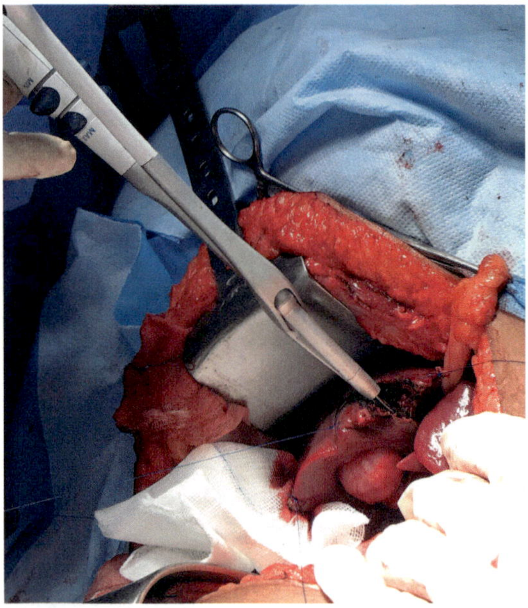

Fig. 10.12 Harmonic (ultrasonic) scalpel can be used to divide deeper liver parenchyma

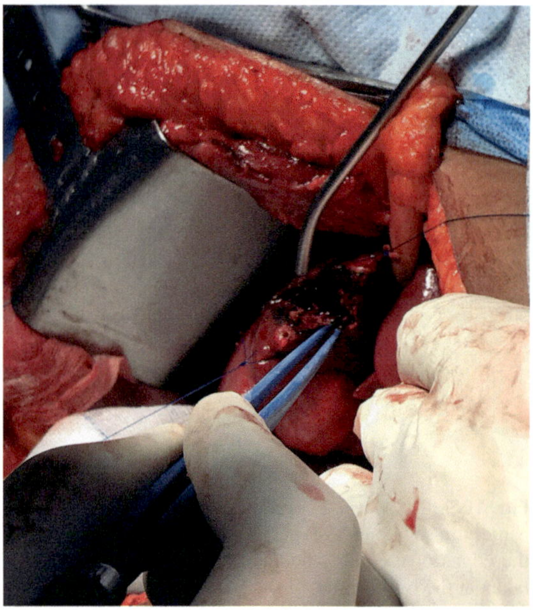

Fig. 10.14 Bipolar cautery is a useful instrument for achieving hemostasis during liver parenchyma transection

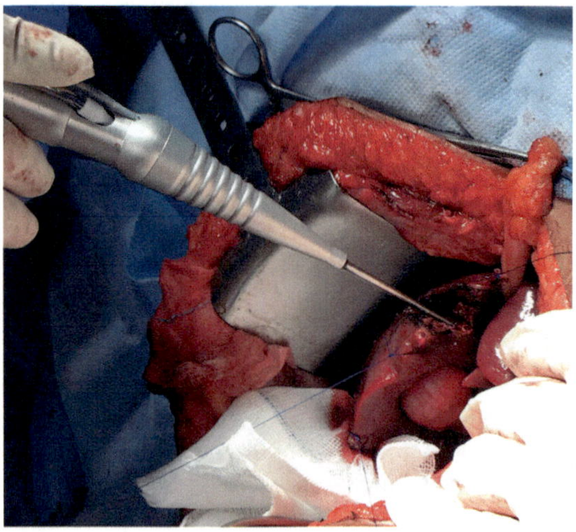

Fig. 10.13 Cavitron ultrasonic aspirator (CUSA) can be used to divide deeper liver parenchyma

to achieve hemostasis (this also helps to detect any bile leak causing yellow staining of the gauze). Bile leak, if any, is controlled with fine monofilament absorbable (polydioxanone PDS) sutures.

Lymphadenectomy for GBC includes en bloc removal of fibro-areolar tissues containing the cystic (12c), superior and inferior pericholedochal

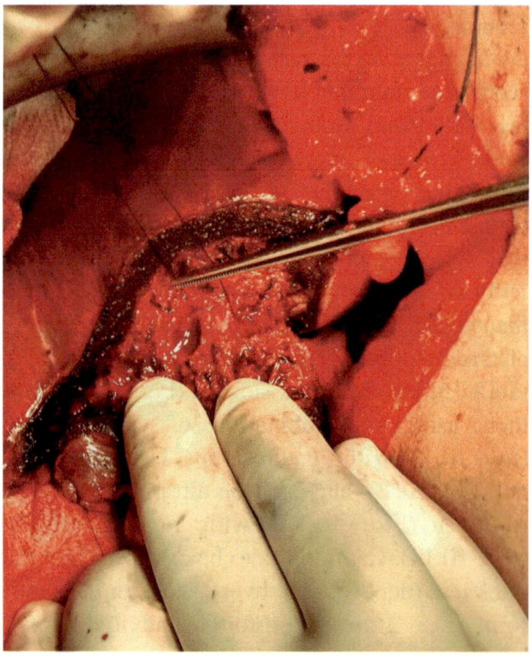

Fig. 10.15 The terminal part of the middle hepatic vein (MHV) lying between segments IVB and V of the liver is the only major vessel encountered during a liver wedge resection; note the superficial few millimeters of the liver wedge divided using electrocautery and the deeper parts of the liver wedge divided using CUSA

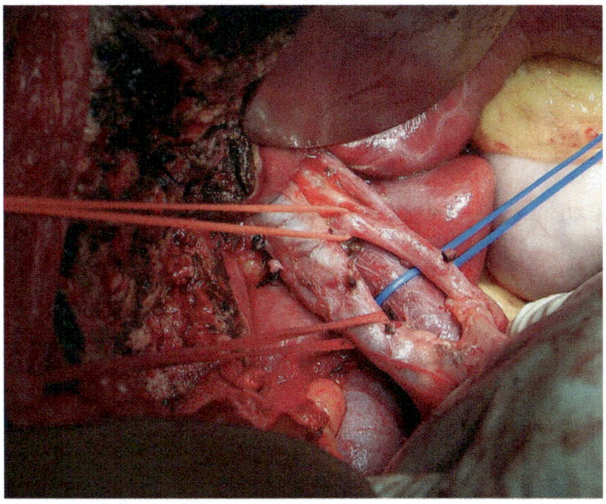

Fig. 10.16 Lymphadenectomy for gall bladder cancer includes en bloc removal of fibro-areolar tissues in the hepatoduodenal ligament containing the pericholedochal, perihepatic arterial, periportal, and porta hepatis lymph nodes so that the common bile duct (umbilical tape), hepatic arteries (red sling around the right hepatic artery), and portal vein (blue sling) are left bare (skeletonized); note that the proper hepatic artery has three branches—right, middle, and left hepatic arteries; posterior pancreatico-duodenal lymph nodes are also removed

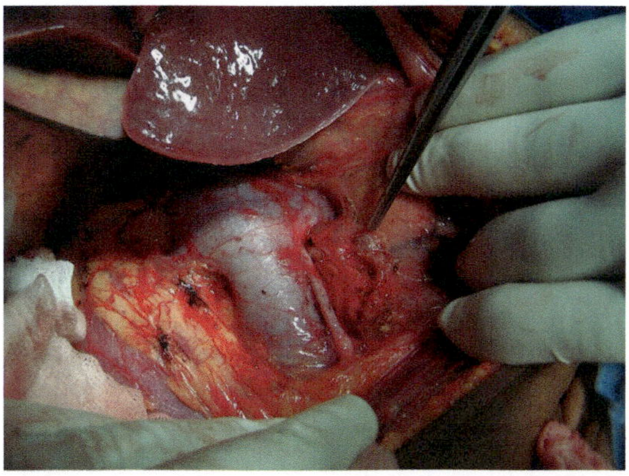

Fig. 10.17 Picture shows an enlarged retroduodenal/retropancreatic lymph node after kocherization of the duodenum; inferior vena cava and both renal veins are also seen—lymphadenectomy for gall bladder cancer includes en bloc removal of the fibro-areolar tissues in the retroduodenal/retropancreatic region containing the posterior pancreatico-duodenal lymph nodes

(12b), superior and inferior periportal and retroportal (12p), around the proper hepatic artery (12a) and porta hepatis or hilum of liver (12h) LNs in the hepatoduodenal ligament (Fig. 10.16). Peritoneum covering the hepatoduodenal ligament (HDL) is incised. All loose fibro-areolar tissue around, in between and behind the CBD, proper hepatic artery (PHA) and its branches (right hepatic artery RHA, middle hepatic artery MHA, and left hepatic artery LHA), main portal vein (MPV) and its branches (right portal vein RPV and left portal vein LPV) from porta hepatis above to the first part of the duodenum below is removed leaving these structures bare (skeletonized), i.e., exposed circumferentially without any fibro-areolar tissue covering them. There is no significant branch of the portal vein in the hepatoduodenal ligament (except a cholecystic vein which drains directly from the GB into the portal vein). An aberrant (accessory or replaced) right hepatic artery (RHA) from the superior mesenteric artery (SMA), which should have been identified on the preoperative contrast enhanced CT (CECT), should be looked for behind and to the right of the CBD and protected during the dissection in the hepatoduodenal ligament. Retroduodenal/retropancreatic, retroportal, periduodenal (C loop), and peripancreatic (head) fibro-areolar tissue containing the posterior pancreato-duodenal (13) LNs (Fig. 10.17) is dissected. Postero-superior pancreato-duodenal vein (PSPDV) joins on the right lateral border of the portal vein immediately above the pancreas and may get injured. Sharp (scissors) or energy (bipolar, harmonic) dissection is used for lymphadenectomy. Small vessels are controlled with electro-cautery (preferably bipolar), ligature, or clips. Fibro-areolar tissues in the lesser omentum from right to left along the common hepatic artery (CHA) running on the superior border of the pancreas to the right of the celiac axis containing the common hepatic artery (8a) LNs should be removed (Fig. 10.18). Right gastric artery and vein and the left gastric (coronary) vein may have to be divided. An aberrant (accessory or replaced) left hepatic artery (LHA) from the left gastric artery (LGA), which should have been identified on the preoperative CECT, should be looked for and protected during the dissection in the gastro-hepatic omentum. Complete celiac lymphadenectomy is NOT done (only LNs lying along the CHA to the right of the celiac axis are removed); superior mesenteric and aortocaval LNs are not removed (except for biopsy, *vide supra*).

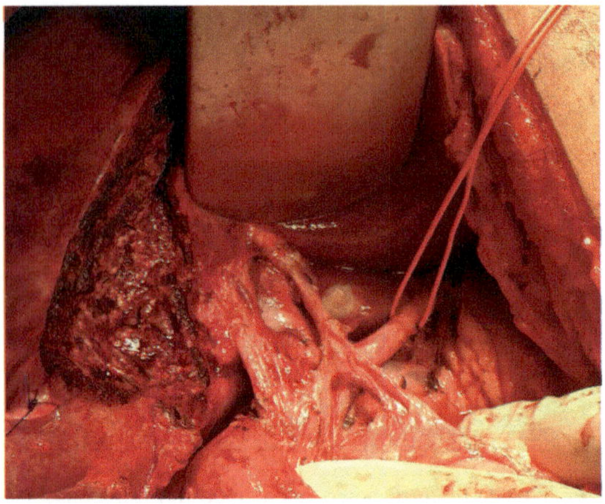

Fig. 10.18 Lymphadenectomy for gall bladder cancer includes en bloc removal of fibro-areolar tissues in the lesser omentum from right to left along the common hepatic artery (seen here in red sling) running on the superior border of the pancreas to the right of the celiac axis containing the common hepatic artery lymph nodes

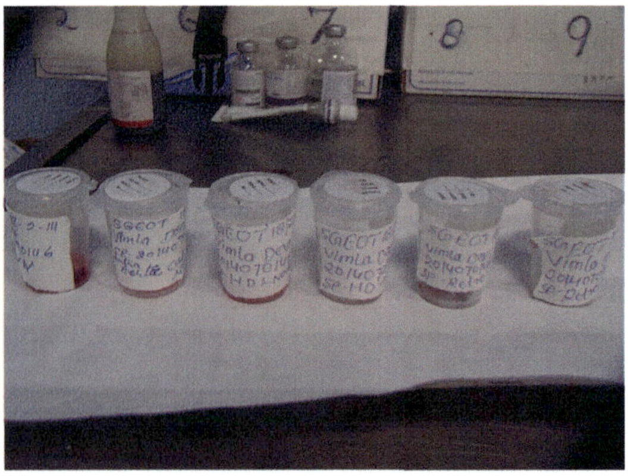

Fig. 10.19 Lymph nodes at various stations (groups) should be packed and labeled separately; this, however, is not of much importance now because the new nodal classification in the TNM staging (8th edition) is based on the number and NOT on the site of the lymph nodes involved

After achieving hemostasis, a drain (24–28 F closed tube drain or 16–18 F suction drain) is placed in the subhepatic fossa and the abdomen is closed.

Lymph nodes at various stations (groups) should be packed and labeled separately (Fig. 10.19) (this, however, is not of much importance now because the new nodal classification in the TNM staging is based on the number and NOT on the site of the lymph nodes involved).

10.4 Liver Resection in Extended Cholecystectomy

Liver can be involved in GBC by direct infiltration or lymphatic and hematogenous spread. Any extent of liver resection is adequate as long as it achieves R0 resection status. The extent of liver resection is decided based on the location of the primary tumor (viz. fundus, body, or neck) in the GB, T stage, extent of liver involvement and whether CBD and/or vessels (hepatic artery and portal vein) are involved (Ogura et al. 1998). Kondo et al. (2002) classified liver involvement as hepatic bed type (GB fundus/body tumor) (Fig. 10.20) and hepatic hilum type (GB body/neck tumor) (Fig. 10.21). Kondo et al. (2011) described two types of liver resection depending on the type of spread—hepatectomy alone for the hepatic bed type and hepatectomy with biliary resection for the hepatic hilum type. While all GB neck tumors with liver infiltration will require ERH (because of the proximity or the involvement of the right portal pedicle in the bed of the GB neck), the extent of liver resection in GB fundus/body tumors will depend on the extent of liver infiltration.

Subsegment IVB is the lower (inferior, caudal) part of segment IV of the liver; Japanese sur-

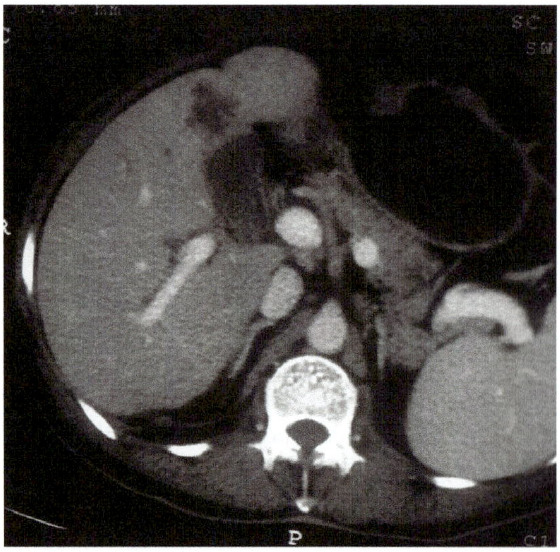

Fig. 10.20 CT shows gall bladder cancer at fundus with liver infiltration—hepatectomy alone is required for the hepatic bed type of tumor in gall bladder fundus/body

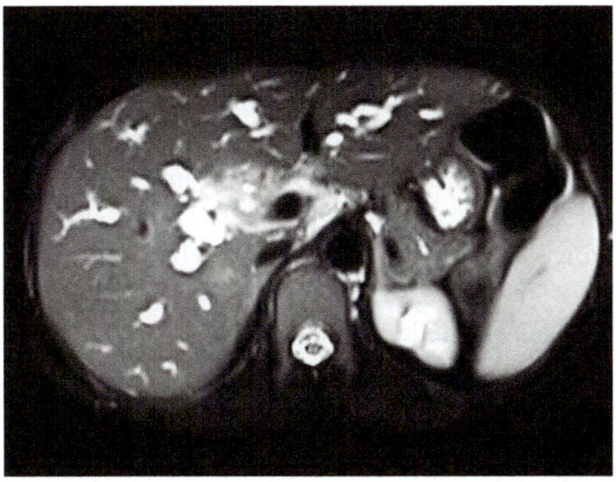

Fig. 10.21 MRI shows a hilar mass in gall bladder cancer at neck—hepatectomy with biliary resection is required for the hepatic hilum type tumor in gall bladder neck

geons, however, call it segment IVA (Miyazaki et al. 2012). Formal segments IVB + V resection (Fig. 10.22), also called bisegmental resection or bisubsegmentectomy (Yoshikawa et al. 1998), central inferior subsegmentectomy (Sasaki et al. 2004), or anatomic hepatectomy (Yu et al. 2019) is an anatomical procedure which is associated with less blood loss and bile leak than non-anatomical liver wedge resection. A variable (2–20) number of cholecysto-hepatic veins drain the GB into the branches of the portal vein. Segments IVB + V resection is supposed to take care of the micro-metastases to the liver through these cholecysto-hepatic veins (Kondo et al. 2002) but why should micro-metastases through the cholecysto-hepatic veins have a specific predilection for segments IVB and V only and not involve the rest of the liver? Venous drainage from the GB to the liver may extend 2–5 cm from the GB bed—wedge resection of liver cannot cover this hence segments IVB + V liver resection is required (Goetze and Paolucci 2012). Some surgeons/groups perform segments IVB + V resection as a routine in all patients with GBC or in T2 tumors (Yi et al. 2013) and then term the procedure as EC.

Segments IVB + V resection was found to be superior to wedge resection in 201 patients with liver infiltration <2 cm (Yoshikawa et al. 1998). On the other hand, in 450 patients with T2, T3

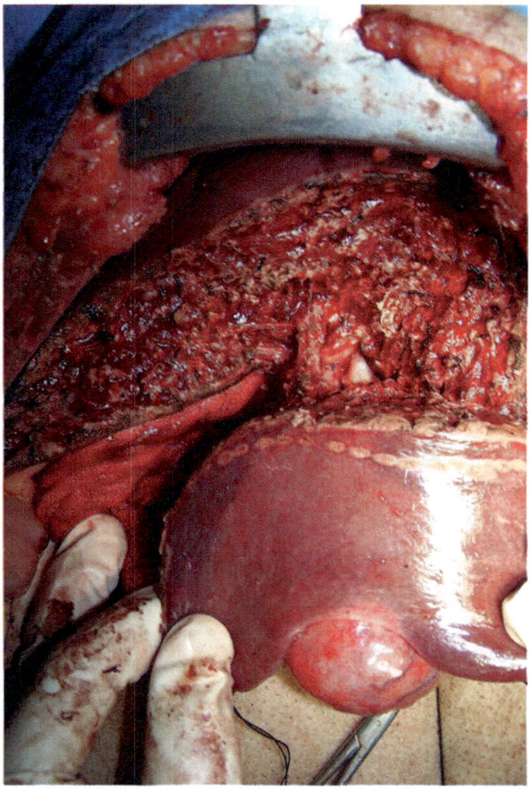

Fig. 10.22 Segment IVB + V resection. (Image courtesy Dr. Biju Pottakkat JIPMER Puducherry)

GBC, no difference was found in recurrence or survival between liver wedge resection and segments IVB + V resection as long as a curative resection is done (Araida et al. 2009a). A review of 85 T2N0 patients found no difference in survival between liver wedge resection ($n = 55$) and segments IVB + V resection (Horiguchi et al. 2013a). Segmentectomy IVB + V ($n = 37$) did not improve the prognosis as compared to those who underwent wedge resection ($n = 57$) in T3 GBC (Chen et al. 2016). Tata Memorial Hospital (TMH) Mumbai India group reported 97 patients in whom radical (extended) cholecystectomy with 2.5–3.0 cm liver wedge was performed (2010–2015)—3-year overall survival (OS) was 86% for stage II and 60% for stage III; 11 patients had locoregional and 22 had distant recurrence. The authors observed that liver wedge resection was equivalent to segments IVB + V resection (Patkar et al. 2019). Yu et al. (2019) did not find any difference in survival between wedge hepatectomy (wedge resection) and anatomic hepatectomy (segment IVB + V resection).

There is, thus, no strong evidence to favor segments IVB + V resection over liver wedge resection in all cases and the Author (VKK) believes that a liver wedge resection, i.e., EC is suitable for T1, T2 GBC, i.e., tumor confined to the GB wall with no liver infiltration or T3 with minimal (<1 cm) liver infiltration. Segments IVB + V resection should be performed if there is moderate (>1 cm) liver infiltration in the GBC fundus or body. As mentioned earlier, a GB neck tumor with liver infiltration will require ERH. EC, in the opinion of the Author (VKK), includes a 2 cm non-anatomical wedge of the liver (*vide supra*) and if segments IVB + V resection is performed, it should be mentioned as such and not called EC.

10.4.1 Technique

Many surgeons actually perform just a larger (>2 cm) liver wedge resection and then call it segments IVB + V resection. The technique of segments IVB + V resection has been best described by Miyazaki et al. (2012). The left hepatic artery (LHA) supplies the segment IV (Fig. 10.23) before it divides into branches to segments II and III. The left portal vein (LPV) gives off 2–3 branches to segment IV (Fig. 10.24) from its right (upper) border; these branches should be divided in the umbilical fissure. They usually supply subsegment IVB and their division demarcates subsegment IVB from IVA but they may be supplying subsegment IVA also; in such a scenario, their division may inadvertently devascularize subsegment IVA also (in addition to subsegment IVB). Injection of indigo carmine blue dye into these branches delineates the area of segment IV of the liver supplied by them. If the left portal vein branch is found to be supplying both subsegments IVB and IVA, the Glissonian sheath supplying subsegment IVB can be identified inside the liver parenchyma after

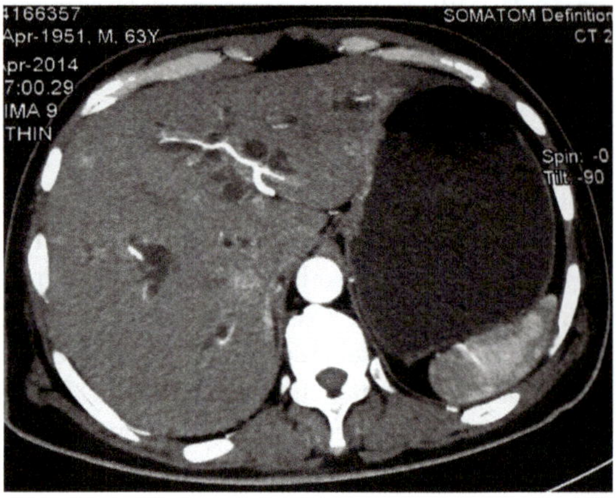

Fig. 10.23 CT (arterial phase) shows left hepatic artery lying in the umbilical fissure with a major branch to segment IV and a small twig to segment III—left hepatic artery supplies segment IV before it divides into branches to segments II and III

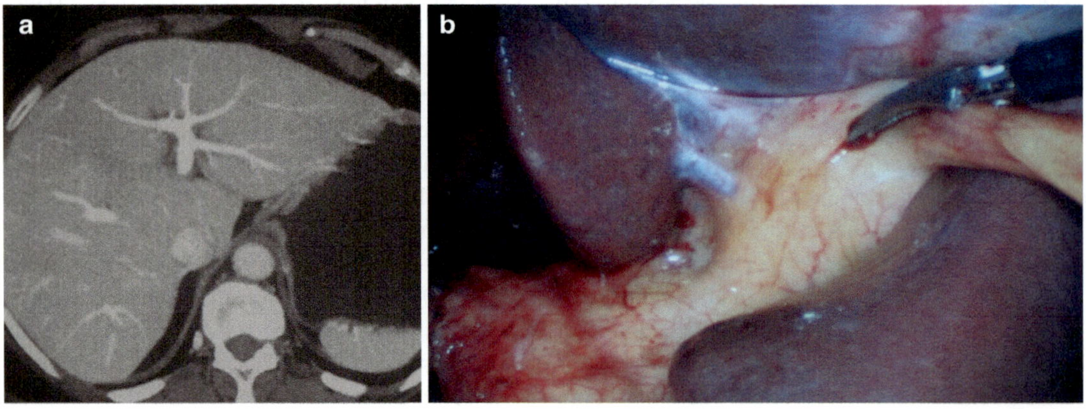

Fig. 10.24 (**a**) CT shows the left portal vein in the umbilical fissure with branches to segment IV (to the right) and to segments II and III (to the left) (**b**) branch of the left portal vein to segment IV in the umbilical fissure

making a hepatotomy to the right of the falciform ligament. Clamping (with a vascular clamp) of this pedicle demarcates subsegment IVB from IVA. This line of demarcation is marked on the surface of the liver with cautery. An inadvertent injury can occur to the left portal vein and the left hepatic duct (LHD) during division of the left portal vein branches to subsegment IVB; left portal vein and left hepatic duct should be carefully protected. Right portal pedicle (Fig. 10.25) is then identified and followed into the hepatic hilum to delineate the right anterior and right posterior sectoral pedicles—clamping of the right posterior sectoral pedicle demarcates segment VI (and VII) posteriorly from V (and VIII) anteriorly. The line of demarcation between segments IVB and IVA is then extended horizontally to meet the vertical line of demarcation between segments V and VI—this horizontal line roughly marks the demarcation between segment V inferiorly (caudally) and segment VIII superiorly (cranially). When the liver parenchymal transection reaches the hepatic hilum, the right anterior sectoral Glisson sheath is encountered. Branches to segment V from the right anterior sectoral Glissonian sheath are divided. The branches of the right anterior sectoral portal pedicle to segment VIII, the right posterior sectoral pedicle, and the right main portal pedicle may get inadvertently injured during the division of the portal pedicle to segment V; they should be carefully protected.

Intermittent inflow occlusion can be performed using a Pringle maneuver. Intraoperative US (IOUS) can be used (in addition to rule out occult liver metastases) to evaluate the extent of liver infiltration, delineate intrahepatic vascular anatomy (especially the middle hepatic vein) and perform a controlled liver resection. Chiba et al. (2019) described indo-cyanine green (ICG) navigation for hepatic resection in GBC—ICG is injected into the cholecystic artery and ICG fluorescence illumination is visualized with Hyper Eye Medical System.

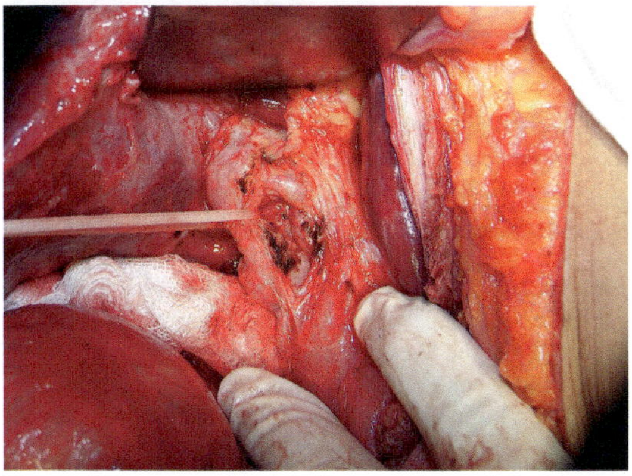

Fig. 10.25 Right portal pedicle dissected and looped

Major (>2 anatomical segments) hepatic resection, e.g., central (segments IV, V, and VIII) hepatectomy will be required for liver infiltration beyond segments IVB and V. Parenchyma preserving central (segments IV, V, and VIII) hepatectomy may be done in a patient with GBC and jaundice due to involvement of the bile duct when the right portal pedicle is free (not a common situation, however)—frozen section of the right duct margin (as is done in hilar cholangiocarcinoma) should be done. Extensive liver infiltration into segments VI, VII, or VIII will require ERH. Involvement of the biliary ductal confluence or the right portal pedicle by a GBC neck will also necessitate ERH (see Chap. 11)

10.5 Lymphadenectomy During Extended Cholecystectomy

GBC has a high propensity for LN spread; LN involvement is very common in GBC. Frequency of LN involvement increases with T stage—it is virtually absent (<5%) in T1a, 5–10% in T1b, 40–60% in T2, and 80–90% in T3, T4.

There are three prominent lymphatic pathways from the GB

1. Cholecysto-retropancreatic pathway, i.e., cystic (12c) LN—pericholedochal (12b) LN—perihepatic (12a) and periportal and retroportal (12p) LN—retroduodenal/pancreatic LN (13a); this is the principal pathway present in large majority of cases.
2. Cholecysto-celiac pathway, i.e., cystic LN—common hepatic artery (CHA) and celiac LNs (through the gastro-hepatic ligament).
3. Cholecysto-mesenteric pathway, i.e., periportal LNs and LNs at the root (origin) of the superior mesenteric artery (SMA).

Lymphadenectomy is an important and essential part of surgical management of GBC (except in T1aN0 disease where simple cholecystectomy alone without lymphadenectomy is adequate). Several reports call it portal lymphadenectomy (Ong et al. 2018), hilar lymphadenectomy, or hepatoduodenal ligament lymphadenectomy but the extent of lymphadenectomy is much beyond the porta hepatis, hepatic hilum, or hepatoduodenal ligament. Birnbaum et al. (2015) classified LN dissection in GBC as D1 (hepatic pedicle) and D2 (hepatic pedicle + celiac and retropancreatic); D2 dissection identified skip LN metastases that would have been missed on D1 dissection in 5/87 (6%) patients in whom it was done. Kokudo et al. (2003) proposed that if N12c, N12b, and N13a are negative no further LN dissection is required; if N12c and N12b are positive but N13a is negative, complete dissection of N1 LNs should be done; if N13a is positive, N2 dissection with or without pancreato-duodenectomy is recommended.

LN involvement is one of the most important predictors of prognosis in GBC. LN yield, i.e., total number of LNs examined (TNLE) is important but only 3% of patients who underwent lymphadenectomy had more than three LNs excised (Coburn et al. 2008). A SEER database analysis revealed that patients with 5 or more excised LNs had better survival than those with 1–4 LNs but only 3.6% of patients had 5 or more LNs harvested (Downing et al. 2011). For an adequate lymphadenectomy, a minimum of 6 LNs should be excised to declare a patient having node-negative disease. Attempt, therefore, should be to remove at least 6 LNs as that is the minimum number of LNs required for accurate staging (Ito et al. 2011; Negi et al. 2011). This, however, is not always achieved. Only 12% of patients who underwent surgical resection in the National Cancer Database (NCDB) (2004–2014) had >6 LNs resected (Lee et al. 2018). Only 21% of 6531 patients with GBC who were identified from the National Cancer Database (NCDB) between 2004 and 2015 had 6 or more LNs evaluated (Tsilimigras et al. 2019). In a report from the USA, a total lymph node count (TLNC) of 6 or more was achieved in only 20% of 92 patients who underwent portal lymphadenectomy (Leigh et al. 2019). Total lymph node count (TLNC) predicts the outcome also—patients classified as N0 based on TLNC <6 had poorer survival (median recurrence-free survival RFS 22 months vs. not reached, median overall survival OS 41 months vs. not reached) than those classified as N0 based on TLNC >6 (Ito et al. 2011).

The highest superior retropancreatic LN (13a) (Fig. 10.26) is the transition between N1 and N2 LNs; its involvement predicts recurrence and survival (Kelly et al. 2014). According to the Western philosophy of management of GBC, LN involvement beyond the hepatoduodenal ligament, i.e., involvement of retroduodenal/retropancreatic (13a) LNs, is not resectable for cure as long-term (>5 year) survival in node-positive patients is very rarely reported from the West, but most Japanese surgeons consider retroduodenal/retropancreatic (13a) as regional LNs and go ahead with resection even in the presence of these LNs. In a report of 148 patients who underwent radical resection, patients with involvement of the posterior superior pancreatico-duodenal LNs had similar survival as those with involvement of regional LNs; both these groups had better survival than those with involvement of distant nodes (Sakata

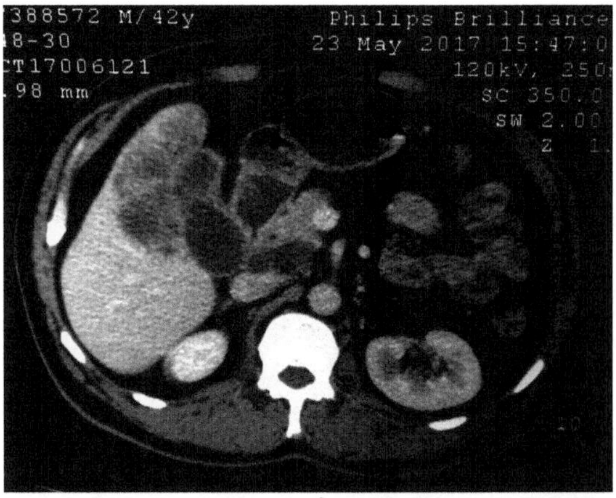

Fig. 10.26 CT shows a large necrotic retropancreatic lymph node lying in front of the inferior vena cava—according to the Western philosophy of management of gall bladder cancer, involvement of retroduodenal/retropancreatic lymph nodes is not resectable for cure but the Japanese surgeons consider retroduodenal/retropancreatic lymph nodes as regional lymph nodes

et al. 2017). Five-year survival of patients with positive 13a (superior retropancreatic) LNs was similar to that of those with N1 disease—40% and 33%, respectively (Chaudhary et al. 2019). The Author (VKK), and other Indian groups, tend to agree with the Japanese philosophy in this regard and considers retroduodenal/retropancreatic (13a) as regional LNs.

Some groups advocate CBD excision as a routine to facilitate and ensure complete lymphadenectomy but CBD excision does not increase the LN yield and increases the morbidity (Nigri et al. 2016). The Author (VKK) does not perform CBD excision for this indication, i.e., to ensure complete lymphadenectomy.

Extensive retroperitoneal LN dissection between the origins of the celiac axis (CA) and the inferior mesenteric artery (IMA) is not recommended in GBC. Sixty patients underwent routine extended, i.e., regional plus retroperitoneal para-aortic lymphadenectomy—aortocaval LN metastases were present in 38% of cases but para-aortic lymphadenectomy offered no survival benefit and prognosis was as poor as that of metastatic (hepatic or peritoneal) disease. The authors recommended sampling biopsy of the para-aortic LN before a radical surgical procedure (Kondo et al. 2000). In another report, no patient with aortocaval LN metastasis survived more than 2 years (Kaneoka et al. 2003). There are a few anecdotal reports of long-term survival in patients with positive para-aortic LN but, by and large, para-aortic LN metastasis is as bad as a distant (liver or peritoneal) metastasis and contraindicates resection in GBC. The Nagoya University Japan group, which used to perform these periaortic LN dissections earlier as a routine, has abandoned it since 2005 (Mizuno et al. 2019).

Lymphadenectomy, like in any other cancer, offers the following benefits in GBC:

1. Better staging, thus resulting in improved stage-wise survival (Will Roger phenomenon).
2. It guides selection of cases for adjuvant therapy—all node-positive patients should receive adjuvant therapy.
3. It prognosticates the outcome of the disease, being worse in node positive than in node-negative patients.
4. It may improve survival, which, of course, is dependent on several other factors also. In a SEER database of 4614 patients, lymphadenectomy improved survival from 22 to 123 months in T1b and T2 GBC; it did not, however, have much impact in T3 lesions (10 vs. 6 months) (Jensen et al. 2009).

10.6 Laparoscopic Extended Cholecystectomy

Traditionally, even a suspicion of GBC used to be a contraindication for laparoscopic cholecystectomy for gall stone disease because of several reports of port site metastases due to peritoneal dissemination of the disease due to inadvertent iatrogenic GB perforation/opening and bile (tumor) spill during laparoscopic procedure which can potentially convert an eminently curable disease into peritoneal dissemination. Laparoscopic resection has been used and advocated for many cancers including colo-rectal, stomach, liver, and pancreas but GBC is one of the last abdominal cancers to be resected laparoscopically.

Laparoscopic EC (Fig. 10.27) has been done for preoperatively diagnosed early, i.e., T1/T2, no liver infiltration, no CBD involvement GBC, confirmed by computed tomography (CT) and endoscopic ultrasonography (EUS). EUS is strongly recommended for selection of cases for laparoscopic EC; the presence of liver infiltration on EUS is a contraindication for laparoscopic EC.

The technique of laparoscopic EC has been very beautifully demonstrated in a video by Kim et al. (2018a). Patient is positioned supine in low lithotomy position with a reverse Trendelenburg and left lateral tilt, the surgeon standing between the patient's separated legs (French position). Five ports are used—infraumbilical 10 mm camera port, 10 mm left pararectal main working port, 5 mm right pararectal, 5 mm epigastric, and 5 mm left midclavicular port. A 30° telescope or a flex-

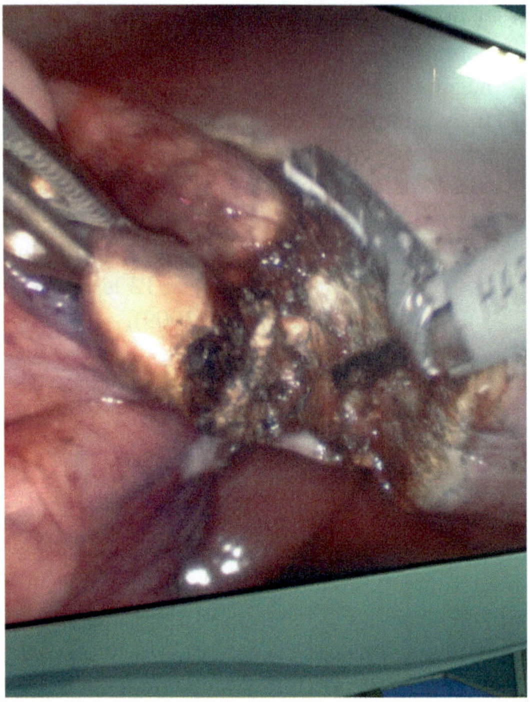

Fig. 10.27 Extended cholecystectomy can be performed laparoscopically also

ible laparoscope is preferred. Staging laparoscopy is done as a routine; in addition to visual staging, laparoscopic US (using 7.5 MHz probe) should be used to evaluate liver infiltration and for detection of any missed intraparenchymal liver metastases. If liver infiltration is found on laparoscopic US, laparoscopic approach should be abandoned and open approach should be used. Laparoscopic celiac (Palanisamy 2016) and aortocaval (Agarwal et al. 2014) LN biopsy may also be done. Minimal handling of the GB should be done; liver retraction is done without holding the GB to avoid inadvertent GB perforation and bile spill. Self-locking clips (Hem-o-lok^R Weck) are preferred on the cystic duct to avoid bile spill; cystic duct margin is sent for frozen section histopathological examination. Cystic plate and a thin (2 mm) rim of liver tissue are resected with the GB (Han et al. 2019a)—mainly to avoid GB perforation and bile spill. Laparoscopic Harmonic shears, CUSA, and bipolar cautery are used for liver parenchymal transection. The specimen is placed and extracted in a retrieval bag to avoid contamination of the extraction port site with tumor, which could cause port site metastases (PSM).

Laparoscopic EC was first reported as completion EC (CEC) for incidental GBC (Gumbs and Hoffman 2010; Belli et al. 2011). Agarwal et al. (2015) compared 24 patients who underwent laparoscopic radical cholecystectomy with 46 matched controls who had undergone open radical cholecystectomy – while operating time was longer blood loss was less; LN yield was comparable and recurrences during a follow up of 18 (6–33) months were equal. Yoon et al. (2015) reported a large experience of 83 patients with suspected early-stage GBC who were taken up for laparoscopic surgery between 2004 and 2014—45 were finally confirmed on histology to have GBC. EC was performed in 32 of these 45 GBC patients and 13 had simple cholecystectomy alone. After a median follow-up of 60 months, recurrence occurred in 4 patients; all were distant metastases. Disease-specific 5-year survival of all 45 patients was 94% (100% for pT1a and T1b and 90% for pT2); in 26 patients who had follow-up of >5 years, it was 92%. Surprisingly, no liver resection was performed in any patient (including 8 T1b and 25 T2 patients)—only a thin (2 mm) rim of liver tissue was removed along with the GB. Zhang et al. (2018) reported laparoscopic EC in 164 patients (2006–2015) with suspected GBC confined to the GB wall—5 had unresectable disease and 12 were converted to open surgery. de Aretxabala et al. (2018) reported 51 patients with incidental GBC (2006–2016) who were reoperated laparoscopically—17 underwent only laparoscopy because of the presence of tumor dissemination; 10 were converted to open operation while 24 underwent laparoscopic resection. A recent report of 102 patients with Tis–T3 GBC who underwent either laparoscopic (n = 41) or open (n = 61) resections in China showed similar survival with no increase in incision metastasis rate after laparoscopic resection (Feng et al. 2019). Jang et al. (2019) reported no difference in survival (5-year 73% vs. 66% after laparoscopic (n = 55) or open (n = 44) surgery in patients with T2 GBC; no port site metastasis was seen in patients who underwent laparoscopic surgery. Piccolo (2019) reported laparoscopic radical cholecystectomy in 18 cases (primary GBC $n = 7$ and incidental GBC $n = 11$); they included cases with liver infiltration (T3) also but this resulted in high conversion rate (29%) and liver recurrence (27%).

A review of 13 articles including 152 patients who underwent laparoscopic EC reported a conversion rate of 10% (Zimmitti et al. 2016). Conversion rate was 20% in an NCDB review (2010–2012) of 792 patients who were intended to undergo laparoscopic surgery for GBC (Ong et al. 2018). Piccolo and Piozzi (2017) reviewed 9 articles including 129 patients (including 13 incidental GBC) who underwent laparoscopic surgery—majority, i.e., 63% were pT2; hospital stay was 5 days, there was no mortality but major complications, e.g., portal vein/branch injury and bile leak were reported. In a meta-analysis of 20 studies including 1217 patients, laparoscopic EC was associated with less blood loss, less postoperative complications, and shorter hospital stay; scar recurrence rates were higher (7%. vs. 4%) but overall recurrence rate was similar (45% vs. 42%) and 5-year survival was better 48% vs. 39% in the laparoscopic group (Zhao et al. 2018). In an analysis of the NCDB (2010–2012) database of 1524 patients, LN yield was lower in laparoscopic than in open surgery—only 34% patients undergoing laparoscopic surgery had >3 LNs cf. 47% of those undergoing open surgery (Ong et al. 2018).

Totally, laparoscopic hepatic bisegmentectomy (segments IVB + V) with hilar lymphadenectomy for incidental GBC (Machado et al. 2015), laparoscopic hepatic bisegmentectomy (segments IVB + V) with regional lymphadenectomy (Nag et al. 2018), laparoscopic radical cholecystectomy with CBD resection (Navarro and Kang 2019), and robotic radical cholecystectomy (n = 27) (Goel et al. 2019a, b) have also been reported. Nag et al. (2019) reported that the oncological outcome and survival after laparoscopic EC with bisegmentectomy (n = 30) was not inferior to that after open EC (n = 38).

Most reports of laparoscopic EC have a significant number of patients viz. 3/6 (Gumbs and Hoffman 2010), 12/30 (Cho et al. 2010), 3/19 (Itano et al. 2015), 2/14 (Palanisamy et al. 2016) and 3/12 (Nag et al. 2018), finally turning out to be benign (non-malignant) on histopathology of the specimen.

Laparoscopic EC is technically feasible, has been shown to be safe (in expert hands) and is oncologically equal to open EC. It should, however, be performed in patients with early GBC by those with expertise in both hepatobiliary and minimally invasive surgery and in high-volume specialized centers. Laparoscopic resection for GBC is still in the early phase of adoption curve and more evidence is required (Han et al. 2019a).

The Author (VKK), however, is still not convinced about the role and place of laparoscopic EC in the management of early GBC. Moreover, accurate preoperative diagnosis of early (T1, T2 N0) GBC may be difficult and what is thought as early GBC on imaging may turn out to be advanced GBC. The comment made by Jeffrey B Mathews in Cho et al. (2010) "in the zeal to offer laparoscopic surgery to patients with early GBC, surgeons should balance the risk of rendering a potentially curable situation incurable" remains valid even today.

10.7 CBD Excision in Extended Cholecystectomy

CBD excision (Fig. 10.28), also called bile duct resection (BDR) or excision of the extrahepatic bile duct (EBD) or extrahepatic bile duct resection (EHBDR) or choledochectomy, as a routine during EC is a matter of debate. Some Japanese groups (Todoroki et al. 1999; Shimizu et al. 2004) advocate CBD excision as a routine during EC in patients with advanced (T2 or more) GBC even in the absence of jaundice or obvious CBD involvement on the grounds that CBD excision facilitates adequate and complete lymphadenectomy in the hepatoduodenal ligament (HDL) and takes care of occult metastases in the CBD wall and in the areolar connective tissue around the CBD and the perineural tissue invasion in the hepatoduodenal ligament. Kosuge et al. (1999) reported improved survival following routine CBD excision in stage IV GBC. Hundred and nine resections were performed for GBC at the Memorial Sloan Kettering

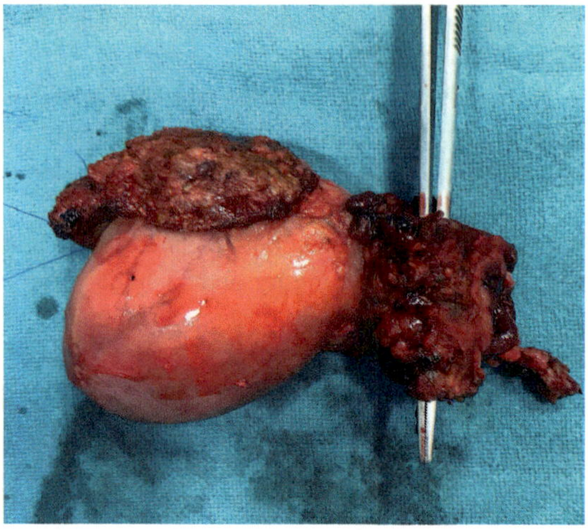

Fig. 10.28 Operative specimen of extended cholecystectomy with common bile duct excision

Cancer Center (MSKCC), New York, USA—68 bile duct resections (BDR) were done (36 in whom the CBD wall was involved and 32 empirical); bile duct resection resulted in higher morbidity but there was no increase in survival (D'Angelica et al. 2009). In a large national study of 4243 patients treated at 114 Japanese institutions over 9 years, EHBDR was performed in 2897 (68%) patients (R0 resection was achieved in 1443, 50% of these)—there was no significant difference in recurrence or survival with or without prophylactic bile duct resection for achieving better LN dissection as long as R0 resection is achieved (Araida et al. 2009b). In a study of 48 patients with T2 GBC, Gwark et al. (2012) did not find any survival advantage after EHBDR in 16 patients. Choi et al. (2013) did not find any difference in survival after EHBDR in 71 T2/T3 GBCs operated between 2000 and 2001; yet the authors went on to recommend EHBDR. The Nagoya University Japan group performed EHBDR in 52 GBC patients without extrahepatic bile duct invasion—8 (15%) of these were found to have micro-vessel invasion (MVI), i.e., lymphatic, venous, and/or perineural invasion on histopathological examination. No patient with micro-vessel invasion survived for 2 years (Igami et al. 2015). CBD resection, done in 41/112 patients did not increase the number of retrieved LNs (Birnbaum et al. 2015). In a consortium report of 449 GBCs, CBD resection in 27% patients did not yield a higher LN count and was not associated with improved survival. The authors observed that routine CBD resection is unwarranted; it should be performed selectively (Gani et al. 2016). Sixty-seven T2 or more GBC patients underwent segments IVB (called segment IVA in Japan) + V resection with (n = 33) or without (n = 34) bile duct resection (BDR)—there was no significant difference in overall survival (OS) and disease-free survival (DFS) between the two groups (Fujii et al. 2018). Lim et al. (2018) reported 149 T2 and T3 GBC operated in Korea (2000–2011)—54 underwent bile duct resection and 95 did not—LN retrieval was more (15 vs. 5) but survival was less (43% vs. 57%) after bile duct resection; there was minimal increase in the morbidity. The authors still recommended that bile duct resection should be actively considered.

A systematic review of 7 papers including 424 patients who underwent routine extrahepatic bile duct resection without bile duct infiltration showed that CBD excision was not associated with better lymph node harvest or improved survival but was associated with higher morbidity (Nigri et al. 2016). Gavriilidis et al. (2017) reviewed 24 articles including 12,251 patients who were operated out of which 6722 (55%) had EHBDR, and recommended EHBDR selectively for tumors involving (macroscopically or microscopically) the GB neck and/or the cystic duct. A review of 42 observational studies and 7 case series showed that it was uncertain whether routine bile duct resection improved survival in patients with T2–T4 GBC (Sternby Eilard et al. 2017).

If CBD excision is done, CBD should be divided as low as possible in the pancreatic parenchyma below and at the biliary ductal confluence in the hepatic hilum above. Both the ends (lower and upper) should be sent for frozen section histopathological examination to ensure negative (clear) margins. If the lower end is positive pancreato-duodenectomy may be required; if the upper (proximal) margin is positive, hepatectomy may be required. Reconstruction is done with end-to-side Roux-en-Y hepatico-jejunostomy at the biliary ductal confluence

CBD is frequently involved in GBC by

1. Direct infiltration from GBC neck.
2. LNs in the hepatoduodenal ligament adherent to/infiltrating the CBD.
3. Intraductal spread (tumor embolization) from a papillary tumor in the GB.
4. Micro-vessel invasion (MVI), i.e., lympho-vascular and perineural invasion leading to microscopic involvement of the CBD wall (Igami et al. 2015).

Most groups/surgeons follow a policy of selective excision of the CBD, which is performed in following cases:

1. Direct involvement of the CBD (in GB neck tumor) (Fig. 10.29) or a GBC neck or cystic duct tumor, which is close to the CBD.
2. Gross/heavy/bulky lymph nodal involvement in the hepatoduodenal ligament, fatty (fat laden), or inflamed hepatoduodenal ligament making lymphadenectomy difficult.
3. LNs adherent to the CBD (Fig. 10.30).
4. Cystic duct margin positive on frozen section histopathological examination (in GB neck tumor); cystic duct stump positive on frozen section histopathological examination in incidental GBC.
5. Associated choledochal cyst (Fig. 10.31).
6. Papillary tumors with a high propensity for intraductal embolic spread (Fig. 10.32).

Routine CBD excision is not recommended in the Korean Guidelines (Lee et al. 2014) for the management of GBC. The Author (VKK) does not perform routine CBD excision as a part of EC; it is done on a selective basis (mainly 1,4 and 5 *vide supra*).

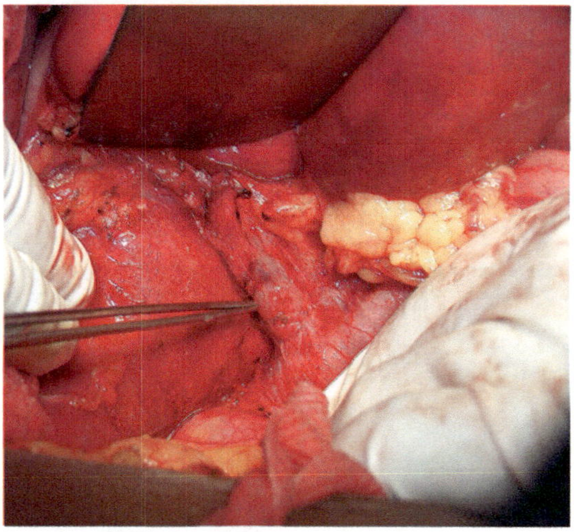

Fig. 10.30 Lymph nodes densely adherent to the common bile duct (CBD) may necessitate CBD excision along with extended cholecystectomy

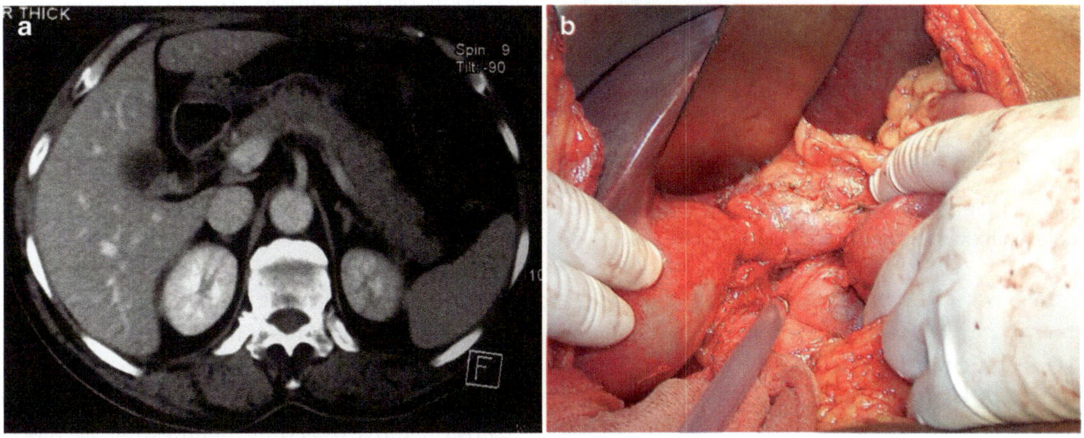

Fig. 10.29 (**a**) CT shows a small tumor in the gall bladder neck involving the common bile duct (**b**) operative picture shows gall bladder cancer at neck involving the common bile duct (the suction tip points to the portal vein lying behind the common bile duct)—direct involvement of the common bile duct (CBD) (in gall bladder neck tumor) requires CBD excision along with extended cholecystectomy

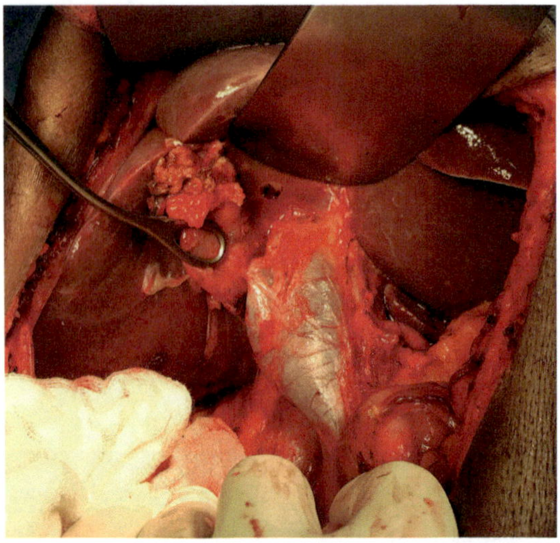

Fig. 10.31 Gall bladder cancer with coexisting choledochal cyst may necessitate common bile duct excision along with extended cholecystectomy

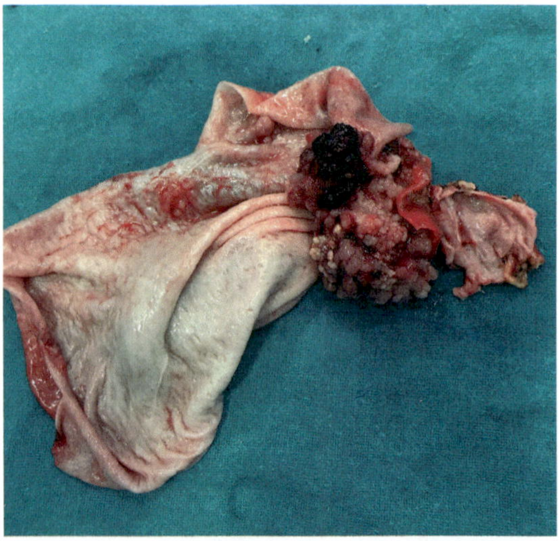

Fig. 10.32 A papillary tumor in the gall bladder may be associated with multicentric deposits in the common bile duct (CBD); some surgeons perform a CBD excision along with extended cholecystectomy in such patients

10.8 Complications of Extended Cholecystectomy

Anatomical variations (aberrations) of biliary, e.g., aberrant right segmental, sectoral, or even main duct in the Calot's triangle and vascular,

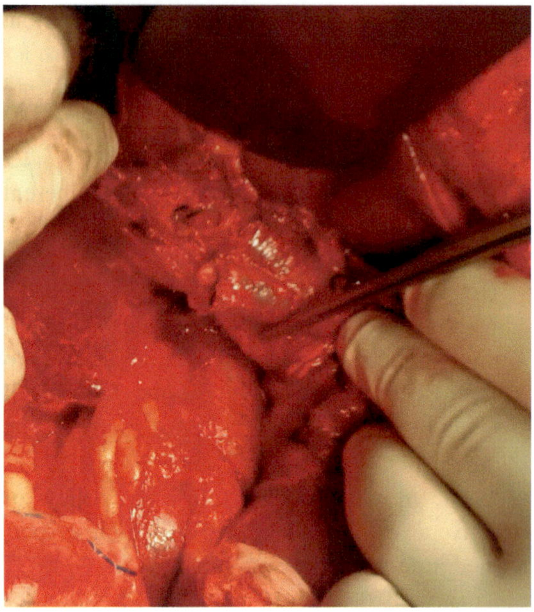

Fig. 10.33 An aberrant (accessory or replaced) right hepatic artery (pointed by the forceps) lies to the right of the common bile duct and may get injured during lymphadenectomy in the hepatoduodenal ligament

e.g., aberrant right hepatic artery (RHA) anatomy are very common and should be kept in mind to avoid an inadvertent biliary or arterial injury during EC. An aberrant (accessory or replaced) right hepatic artery (RHA) lies in the hepatoduodenal ligament to the right of the CBD (Fig. 10.33) and can get injured during lymphadenectomy in the hepatoduodenal ligament. An aberrant (accessory or replaced) left hepatic artery (LHA) lies in the gastro-hepatic ligament and can get injured during lymphadenectomy in the gastro-hepatic ligament. Injury can occur to the right main or right anterior sectoral portal pedicle if the liver wedge is extended too close to the porta hepatis (hepatic hilum) (Fig. 10.34). Bile leak from an injured bile duct should be looked for in the GB bed (Fig. 10.35)—if the duct is small (i.e., <3 mm) it can be suture ligated but if it is large (i.e., >3 mm) the defect should be repaired with a fine long-lasting absorbable suture.

Postoperative bleeding manifesting as blood in the drain is usually mild and small in amount and invariably stops on its own; if large, it may require reoperation for control. A hematoma may

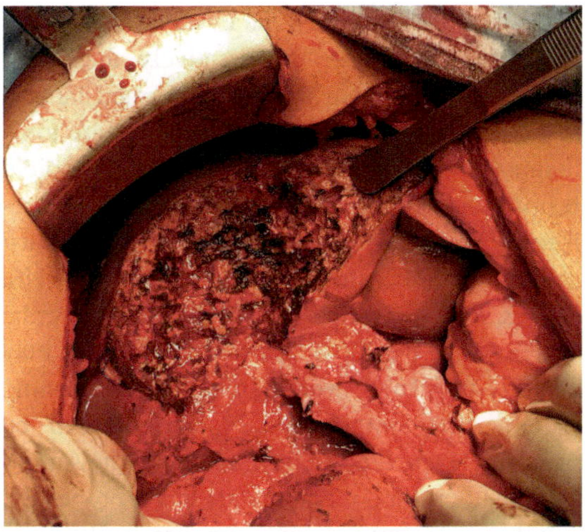

Fig. 10.34 If the liver wedge is taken too close to the hepatic hilum, the right main or anterior sectoral portal pedicle may get injured; the medial edge of the liver wedge should remain short of the hepatic hilum

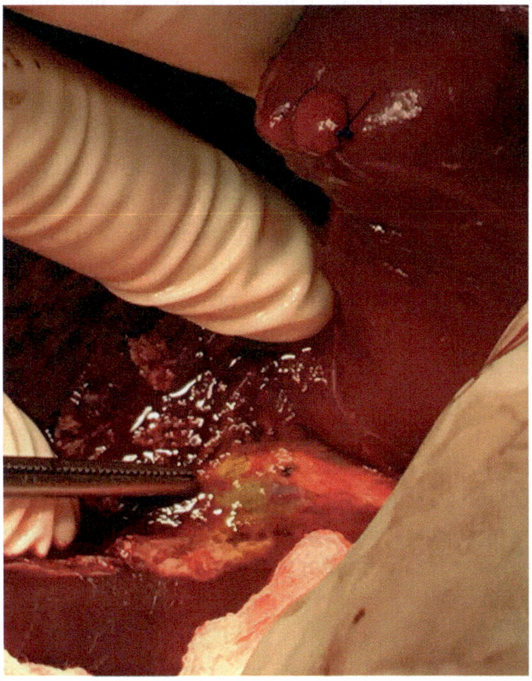

Fig. 10.35 Picture shows a drop of bile (pointed by the forceps) in the liver bed—at the end of the liver wedge resection, the liver bed should be carefully examined for any bile leak

form in the GB bed (Fig. 10.36), which may get infected to form an intra-abdominal abscess.

Bile leak can occur from the cut surface of the liver. If drain shows bile (Fig. 10.37), imaging

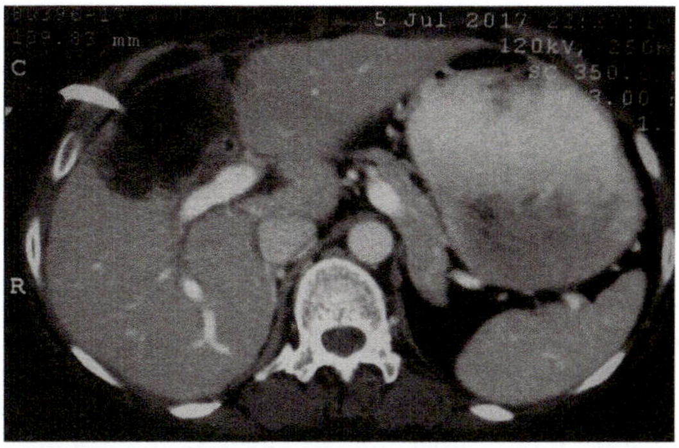

Fig. 10.36 CT shows percutaneous catheter drain (PCD) in liver to drain an infected hematoma after extended cholecystectomy—a hematoma may form in the liver following a wedge resection; it can get infected and form an abscess which then requires percutaneous catheter drainage (PCD)

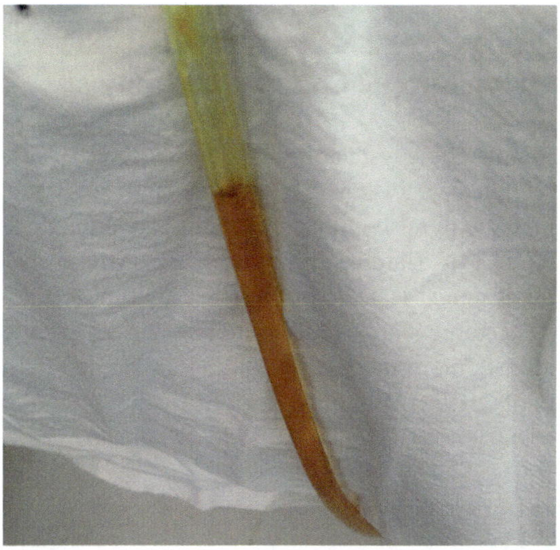

Fig. 10.37 Bile in the drain after extended cholecystectomy indicates bile leak from the gall bladder bed (or an injury to an aberrant duct in the Calot's triangle)

(US and/or CT) should be done to look for any bile collection, which, if present, should be drained by percutaneous catheter drainage (PCD). Small bile leaks will stop on their own or after PCD; if the bile leak is large or persists in spite of the PCD, placement of an endoscopic biliary stent will usually stop it. Lymphorrhea manifesting as high drain output settles on its own over a period of time.

Skeletonization of the CBD may damage the peribiliary (periductal) vascular plexus so that blood supply to the CBD from the proper hepatic artery, postero-superior pancreato-duodenal artery (PSPDA) and 3 and 9 O'clock arteries along the CBD is disrupted resulting in ischemia of the CBD with a risk of long-term stricture but no report of EC mentions an ischemic CBD stricture during the follow-up.

CBD resection is usually associated with increased (as compared to EC alone) morbidity in the form of anastomotic leak causing biliary and peritoneal sepsis in the postoperative period and leading to bilio-enteric anastomotic stricture and recurrent cholangitis in the long term.

In a report of 218 incidental GBCs, 148 out of whom were reoperated, EHBDR was performed in 63/148 (43%)—it was associated with higher (60% vs. 23%) morbidity as compared to when EHBDR was not performed (Fuks et al. 2011).

10.9 Simple Cholecystectomy

Simple cholecystectomy where the plane of dissection is between the GB wall and the cystic plate, without lymphadenectomy is adequate for only T1a (lamina propria) GBC where LN involvement is seen in <5% cases; simple cholecystectomy can be performed laparoscopically also. Some groups (Kinoshita et al. 2001; Shirai et al. 2012a) recommend a full thickness cholecystectomy (FTC) (Fig. 10.38) where the plane of dissection is between the cystic plate and the liver parenchyma in preoperatively diagnosed T1a GBC; FTC also can be performed laparoscopically. T1a GBC is, however, very rare to be diagnosed preoperatively (except in a polypoidal lesion) and simple cholecystectomy will, therefore, be very rarely performed for an obvious/suspected GBC. The accuracy of imaging (US, EUS, CT, or MRI) for T and N stage can never be 100%, i.e., what looks like a T1aN0 tumor may actually be T1b or even higher and N+ meaning thereby that simple cholecystectomy will be incomplete and inadequate treatment. The Author (VKK), therefore, recommends that a proper EC should be performed for a preoperatively diagnosed/suspected GBC, irrespective of the imaging T and N stage. If the pathological stage turns out to be T1aN0, it may appear to be an overkill but that is acceptable. This is the Indian "Buddhist" Middle Path advocated by the Author (Kapoor 2007)—aggressive approach towards early GBC so that no opportunity of potential cure is missed. The only clinical application of this knowledge is in the management of an incidental GBC, where if it is T1a disease AND the cystic duct margin is negative AND the cystic LN included in the specimen is negative AND there was no GB perforation and bile spill during the index cholecystectomy – no more intervention (i.e., reoperation or adjuvant therapy) is indicated in such a case and only follow-up is required.

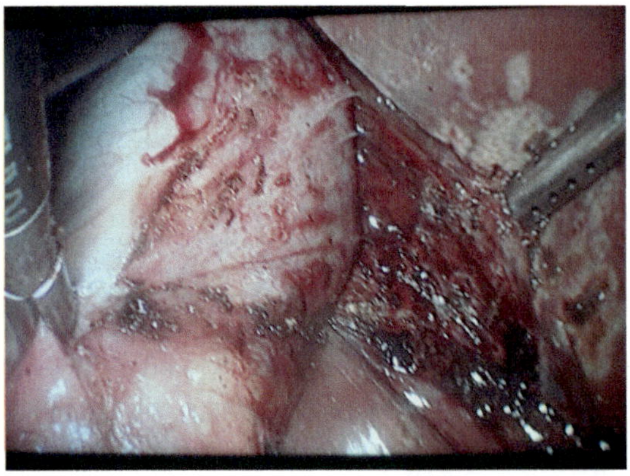

Fig. 10.38 Full-thickness cholecystectomy (FTC) including the cystic plate is recommended by some surgeons for an early gall bladder cancer; the Author (VKK) however, disagrees and recommends a proper extended cholecystectomy

A less (than EC) invasive procedure in the form of full-thickness (with cystic plate) cholecystectomy with limited (first echelon only, i.e., in the hepatoduodenal ligament) lymphadenectomy has been described in patients with advanced age and/or comorbid diseases (Shirai et al. 2012a).

10.10 Non-curative Resection

If preoperative imaging indicates that an intended R0 resection is not possible and only R2 resection can be performed, e.g., GBC with duodeno-pancreatic involvement and pancreato-duodenectomy is not planned or the primary tumor in the GB is technically resectable but distant LNs, e.g., celiac, superior mesenteric, or aortocaval are present and extended retroperitoneal lymphadenectomy is not planned, laparotomy is not recommended. Non-curative (R2) resection leaving gross residual disease is not recommended to be performed but most large reports include a significant number of patients who, for various reasons, ended up having a non-curative (R2) resection. Todoroki et al. (1999) reported that 12 out of 135 resections performed between 1976 and 1998 were non-curative. In another recent report, 58 out of 94 stage IV patients who were operated underwent palliative cholecystectomy (Kang et al. 2012). Thirteen out of 165 resections for T3, T4 GBC at Nagoya University Japan were (non-curative) simple cholecystectomy (Igami et al. 2014). These are probably patients in whom preoperative imaging suggested that R0 resection is possible but at laparotomy distant disease, mainly in the distant lymph nodes or metastases, is found.

Non-curative (R2) resection can be subclassified as

1. Leaving residual disease in the distant LNs or metastases but primary tumor is resected without violating oncological principles, i.e., not going through the tumor.
2. Violating oncological principles, i.e., dissection through a locally advanced tumor with infiltration of an adjacent organ.

While the former may be performed, the latter is not recommended. Non-curative simple cholecystectomy, if and when performed

1. May relieve/reduce pain
2. Reduces tumor burden so that adjuvant therapy works better on the minimal residual metastatic disease
3. Prevents future local complications, e.g., acute cholecystitis, empyema
4. May prolong survival. Tewari et al. (2008) reported median survival of 7 months in 30 patients with T3,T4; N0,N1; M0 GBC who underwent a non-curative cholecystectomy. Palliative resection provided better survival than non-surgical treatment in stage IVB (He et al. 2015). No patient, however, survived >2 years after a non-curative (R2) resection (Igami et al. 2014).

The Author (VKK) does not recommend operating upon a patient with GBC with an aim to perform a non-curative (R2) resection but does perform it occasionally in the situations described above.

Extended (also called radical) cholecystectomy is the standard surgical procedure for early GBC; more extensive surgical procedures are required for advanced GBC.

Invited Commentary on Extended Cholecystectomy for Gall Bladder Cancer

Prasoon Pankaj and Toshifumi Wakai

Gall bladder cancer (GBC) may be diagnosed preoperatively, intraoperatively at the time of surgical exploration for abdominal symptoms attributed to another disease process, or postoperatively upon examination of the gall bladder (GB) specimen, typically removed for symptomatic cholelithiasis. In contemporary series, only approximately 50% of GBCs are recognized before surgery (Duffy et al. 2008; Löhe et al. 2009).

According to the Author (VKK), EC should be defined as removal of the GB, a non-anatomical 2 cm wedge of the liver in segments IVB and V around the GB bed and lymphadenectomy. There is, however, hardly any evidence in favor of a 2 cm liver wedge as it could be less than 1 cm or more than 3 cm; just 1 cm may also be adequate if there is no liver infiltration or in patients with significant liver infiltration, >2 cm, including a formal liver resection, may be required (Kapoor and Behari 2017a). Direct liver invasion, portal tract invasion, and intrahepatic lymphatic invasion, are the main modes of hepatic spread from resectable GBC. The mode of hepatic spread independently predicts long-term survival after resection for patients with GBC (Wakai et al. 2010).

Primary extended cholecystectomy (PEC) is performed for a preoperative or intraoperative diagnosis and suspicion of GBC which is confined to the GB wall, and there is no adjacent organ invasion. It can also be performed in the presence of minimal (i.e., <1 cm) liver infiltration if the tumor is in the GB fundus/body (but not in the GB neck where a major hepatectomy will be required) (Kapoor and Behari 2017a). However, regarding the role and outcomes of tissue diagnosis in primary extended cholecystectomy (PEC), substantial studies from tertiary centers would be more informative.

According to the Author (VKK), lymphadenectomy for GBC includes en bloc removal of fibro-areolar tissues containing the cystic (12c), superior and inferior pericholedochal (12b), superior and inferior periportal (12p), retroportal, around the proper hepatic artery (12a) and porta hepatis or hilum of liver (12h) LNs in the hepatoduodenal ligament (Kapoor and Behari 2017a). An aberrant right hepatic artery, which should have been identified on the preoperative CECT, should be looked for behind and to the right of the CBD and protected during the dissection in the hepatoduodenal ligament.

Our study revealed that tumor location in patients with pT2 GBC can predict the presence or absence of regional lymph node metastasis but not the number and anatomical distribution of positive regional lymph nodes (Toge et al. 2019). The extent of regional lymphadenectomy should not be changed even in patients with pT2a (peritoneal side) tumors, provided that they are fit enough for surgery (Toge et al. 2019). In a retrospective analysis of 135 patients with GBC who underwent a radical resection with regional lymphadenectomy, we witnessed that the number of positive lymph nodes better predicts patient outcome after resection than either the location of positive lymph nodes or lymph node ratio (LNR) in GBC (Shirai et al. 2012b). Dividing the number of positive lymph nodes into three categories (0, 1 to 3, or ≥4) is valid for stratifying patients based on the prognosis after resection (Shirai et al. 2012b).

The Author (VKK) recommends that while all GB neck tumors with liver infiltration will require extended right hepatectomy (ERH) because of the proximity or the involvement of the right portal pedicle in the bed of the GB neck, the extent of liver resection in GB fundus/body tumors will depend on the extent of liver infiltration. There is, thus, no strong evidence to favor segments IVB + V over wedge resection in all cases and the Author (VKK) is of the opinion that a liver wedge, i.e., extended cholecystectomy (EC) is suitable for T1, T2 GBC, i.e., tumor confined to the GB wall with no liver infiltration or T3 with minimal (<1 cm) liver infiltration. Segments IVB + V resection should be performed if there is moderate (>1 cm) liver infiltration in the GBC fundus or body. A GB neck tumor with liver infiltration will require extended right hepatectomy. EC, in the opinion of the Author (VKK), includes a 2 cm non-anatomical wedge of the liver and if segment IVB + V resection is performed, it should be mentioned as such and not called EC (Kapoor and Behari 2017a). In a study of nationwide data from the Japanese Biliary Tract Cancer Registry and a questionnaire survey for pT2 GBC, comparing hepatectomy of segments 4a and 5 (S4a + 5) versus GB bed resection, S4a + 5 hepatectomy was not superior to GB bed resection (Horiguchi et al. 2013a).

Extensive retroperitoneal lymph node (LN) dissection between the origins of the celiac axis (CA) and the inferior mesenteric artery (IMA) is not recommended (Kapoor and Behari 2017a). We retrospectively analyzed 116 consecutive patients who underwent an R0 radical resection for GBC. Our findings revealed that, the number, not the location, of positive lymph nodes independently determines the prognosis after resection in GBC (Sakata et al. 2010a). No nodal disease or a single positive node indicates a favorable outcome after resection, whereas radical lymph node dissection is effective for selected patients with multiple positive nodes, provided that an R0 resection is feasible (Sakata et al. 2010a). Shindoh et al. revealed that in T2 GBC hepatic side tumors have a higher tendency for early metastasis, the anatomic location of tumors in the GB could be a predictor of microscopic tumor progression and surgical outcomes. Tumor location predicts survival after curative resection of T2 GBC (Shindoh et al. 2015).

Laparoscopic EC has been done for preoperatively diagnosed early, i.e., T1/T2, no liver infiltration, no common bile duct (CBD) involvement GBC, confirmed by computed tomography (CT) and endoscopic ultrasonography (EUS). EUS is strongly recommended for selection of cases for laparoscopic EC; the presence of liver infiltration on EUS is a contraindication for laparoscopic EC. The Author (VKK) is still not convinced about the role and place of laparoscopic EC in the management of early GBC (Kapoor and Behari 2017a). Moreover, accurate preoperative diagnosis of early (T1, T2 N0) GBC may be difficult and what is thought as early GBC on imaging may turn out to be advanced GBC. Diagnostic dilemma persists till operative measures ensue.

T1a GBC is, on the other hand, rare to get clinically determined preoperatively except for a polypoidal lesion and simple cholecystectomy will, consequently, be hardly ever carried out with an apparent or assumed GBC. The precision of imaging modalities for T and N stage cannot be 100%, i.e., what appears like a T1aN0 tumor might actually be T1b or perhaps higher and N+ meaning that simple cholecystectomy will probably be imperfect and insufficient treatment method. For this reason, the Author (VKK), and we advocate that the proper EC ought to be carried out for any preoperatively diagnosed GBC, irrespective of imaging T and N stage (Wakai et al. 2010).

An international multicenter study of 14 specialized tertiary hospitals concluded that simple cholecystectomy (SC) including laparoscopic cholecystectomy (LC) showed similar outcomes in terms of recurrence and survival as EC; therefore, extended cholecystectomy (EC) is not needed for the treatment of T1b GBC (Kim et al. 2018b).

If preoperative imaging indicates that an intended R0 resection is not possible and only R2 resection can be performed in case of GBC with duodeno-pancreatic involvement and pancreatoduodenectomy is not planned or the primary tumor in the GB is technically resectable but distant LNs, e.g., celiac, superior mesenteric, or aortocaval are present and extended retroperitoneal lymphadenectomy is not planned, laparotomy is not recommended (Kapoor and Behari 2017a). These are generally most likely patients in whom preoperative imaging suggested that R0 resection was achievable but at laparotomy distant disease, predominantly within the lymph nodes or metastases, tend to be found. Non-curative simple cholecystectomy is usually considered to lessen the tumor burden to ensure that adjuvant therapy works more effectively within the minimal residual metastatic disease, inhibits potential regional complications such as acute cholecystitis and empyema. Palliative resection offered better survival than non-surgical treatment in stage IVB, nevertheless. The survival advantage is, however, marginal.

To conclude, the number, not the location, of positive regional lymph nodes separately ascertains the prognosis following resection for patients with GBC. The lack of nodal disease or a single positive lymph node results in an advantageous result after resection, in contrast to radical lymph node dissection which is most effective for selected patients with multiple positive lymph nodes, given that R0 resection is achievable. Pancreato-duodenectomy plays a part in the surgical treatment for GBC with peripancreatic (head only) nodal disease, possibly due to much better clearance of regional nodal disease.

Invited Commentary on Extended Cholecystectomy for Gall Bladder Cancer (Laparoscopic Approach)

Yoo-Seok Yoon

In this book, Prof. VK Kapoor, an expert surgeon in the field of gall bladder surgery, has extensively reviewed the current evidence of surgery for gall bladder cancer (GBC), a topic faced with much controversy. Prof. Kapoor offers suggestions that are based on the results of a literature review and his clinical experience. His comprehensive description and strong focus on the optimal extent of resection will be helpful for surgeons establishing surgical strategies for patients with GBC and a variety of clinical manifestations. This book also suggests the need for more research in this field, because most of the suggestions are not based on a high level of evidence.

Regarding the application of laparoscopic surgery in patients with GBC, the Author (VKK) has described the favorable outcomes reported by several experts. He has also raised some concerns that laparoscopic surgery may worsen the prognosis of patients. For many years, laparoscopic surgery was contraindicated in patients with GBC, even those with suspected early GBC, out of fear of tumor dissemination following bile spillage. However, this negative view was based largely on older studies that included patients in whom GBC was incidentally detected during/after laparoscopic cholecystectomy for gall stones. If GBC was not suspected, the surgeons were unlikely to adhere to the oncologic principles and this might explain the worse survival outcomes of laparoscopic surgery. Therefore, the index of suspicion for GBC should be considered when interpreting the oncologic outcomes of laparoscopic surgery for GBC in prior studies. With preoperative diagnosis of GBC and careful manipulation to avoid bile spillage, recent reports have shown that laparoscopic surgery does not compromise the oncologic outcomes of patients with early GBC (Han et al. 2019). The Author (VKK) describes two advantages of laparoscopic surgery for GBC based on the current evidence. First, unnecessary laparotomy could be avoided in a significant number of patients with suspected GBC if they are diagnosed with a benign lesion postoperatively. Second, if laparoscopic-extended cholecystectomy is selected carefully for patients with overt GBC and is performed by experienced surgeons, it provides rapid postoperative recovery and less blood loss compared with open surgery without compromising the survival outcomes.

However, as described by the Author (VKK), laparoscopic surgery for GBC is still in an early phase of the adoption curve. Most of the favorable outcomes of laparoscopic surgery for GBC have been reported by a small number of experts and there is no consensus regarding its indications or surgical techniques. A recent survey of experts revealed that laparoscopic surgery is performed only in very selective cases of GBC, and the indications and surgical techniques vary amongst experienced surgeons (Yoon et al. 2019). I agree with the Author's (VKK) opinion that laparoscopic surgery should be selected carefully, even for patients with early-stage GBC, and its advantages should be balanced with the risk of rendering a potentially curable situation incurable. For wider acceptance of laparoscopic surgery in the treatment of GBC, standardization of the procedure and the accumulation of more experience and high-quality evidence are required.

References

Chapter References

Agarwal AK, Kalayarasan R, Javed A, Sakhuja P. Role of routine 16b1 lymph node biopsy in the management of gallbladder cancer: an analysis. HPB (Oxford). 2014;16(3):229–34. https://doi.org/10.1111/hpb.12127. Epub 2013 Jul 22.

Agarwal AK, Javed A, Kalayarasan R, Sakhuja P. Minimally invasive versus the conventional open surgical approach of a radical cholecystectomy for gallbladder cancer: a retrospective comparative study. HPB (Oxford). 2015;17(6):536–41. https://doi:10.1111/hpb.12406. Epub 2015 Feb 28. PMID: 25727091; PMCID: PMC4430785.

Araida T, Higuchi R, Hamano M, Kodera Y, Takeshita N, Ota T, Yoshikawa T, Yamamoto M, Takasaki K. Hepatic resection in 485 R0 pT2 and pT3 cases of advanced carcinoma of the gallbladder: results of a Japanese Society of Biliary Surgery survey—a multicenter study. J Hepatobiliary Pancreat Surg. 2009a;16(2):204–15. https://doi.org/10.1007/s00534-009-0044-3. Epub 2009 Feb 14.

Araida T, Higuchi R, Hamano M, Kodera Y, Takeshita N, Ota T, Yoshikawa T, Yamamoto M, Takasaki K. Should the extrahepatic bile duct be resected or preserved in R0 radical surgery for advanced gallbladder carcinoma? Results of a Japanese Society of Biliary Surgery Survey: a multicenter study. Surg Today. 2009b;39(9):770–9. https://doi.org/10.1007/s00595-009-3960-6. Epub 2009 Sep 24.

Belli G, Cioffi L, D'Agostino A, Limongelli P, Belli A, Russo G, Fantini C. Revision surgery for incidentally detected early gallbladder cancer in laparoscopic era. J Laparoendosc Adv Surg Tech A. 2011;21(6):531–4. https://doi.org/10.1089/lap.2011.0078. Epub 2011 May 25.

Birnbaum DJ, Viganò L, Russolillo N, Langella S, Ferrero A, Capussotti L. Lymph node metastases in patients undergoing surgery for a gallbladder cancer. Extension of the lymph node dissection and prognostic value of the lymph node ratio. Ann Surg Oncol. 2015;22(3):811–8. https://doi.org/10.1245/s10434-014-4044-4. Epub 2014 Sep 9.

Chaudhary RK, Higuchi R, Yazawa T, Uemura S, Izumo W, Furukawa T, Kiyohara K, Yamamoto M. Surgery in node-positive gallbladder cancer: the implication of an involved superior retropancreatic lymph node. Surgery. 2019;165(3):541–7. https://doi.org/10.1016/j.surg.2018.09.003. Epub 2018 Oct 19.

Chen C, Geng Z, Shen H, Song H, Zhao Y, Zhang G, Li W, Ma L, Wang L. Long-term outcomes and prognostic factors in advanced gallbladder cancer: focus on the advanced T stage. PLoS One. 2016;11(11):e0166361. https://doi.org/10.1371/journal.pone.0166361. eCollection 2016.

Chiba N, Shimazu M, Ochiai S, Yokozuka K, Gunji T, Okihara M, Sano T, Tomita K, Tsutsui R, Oshima G, Takano K, Abe Y, Hirano H, Kawachi S. Resection of hepatic lesions perfused by the cholecystic vein using indocyanine green navigation in patients with cT2 gallbladder cancer. World J Surg. 2019;43(2):608–14. https://doi.org/10.1007/s00268-018-4810-8.

Cho JY, Han HS, Yoon YS, Ahn KS, Kim YH, Lee KH. Laparoscopic approach for suspected early-stage gallbladder carcinoma. Arch Surg. 2010;145(2):128–33. https://doi.org/10.1001/archsurg.2009.261.

Choi SB, Han HJ, Kim WB, Song TJ, Suh SO, Choi SY. Surgical strategy for T2 and T3 gallbladder cancer: is extrahepatic bile duct resection always necessary? Langenbecks Arch Surg. 2013;398(8):1137–44. https://doi.org/10.1007/s00423-013-1120-3. Epub 2013 Sep 21.

Coburn NG, Cleary SP, Tan JC, Law CH. Surgery for gallbladder cancer: a population-based analysis. J Am Coll Surg. 2008;207(3):371–82. https://doi.org/10.1016/j.jamcollsurg.2008.02.031. Epub 2008 May 12.

D'Angelica M, Dalal KM, DeMatteo RP, Fong Y, Blumgart LH, Jarnagin WR. Analysis of the extent of resection for adenocarcinoma of the gallbladder. Ann Surg Oncol. 2009;16(4):806–16.

de Aretxabala X, Oppliger F, Solano N, Rencoret G, Vivanco M, Carvajal D, Hepp J, Roa I. Laparoscopic management of incidental gallbladder cancer. Surg Endosc. 2018;32(10):4251–5. https://doi.org/10.1007/s00464-018-6173-5. Epub 2018 Jun 20.

Downing SR, Cadogan KA, Ortega G, Oyetunji TA, Siram SM, Chang DC, Ahuja N, Leffall LD Jr, Frederick WA. Early-stage gallbladder cancer in the Surveillance, Epidemiology, and End Results database: effect of extended surgical resection. Arch Surg. 2011;146(6):734–8. https://doi.org/10.1001/archsurg.2011.128.

Feng JW, Yang XH, Liu CW, Wu BQ, Sun DL, Chen XM, Jiang Y, Qu Z. Comparison of laparoscopic and open approach in treating gallbladder cancer. J Surg Res. 2019;234:269–76. https://doi.org/10.1016/j.jss.2018.09.025. Epub 2018 Oct 16.

Fujii Y, Nanashima A, Hiyoshi M, Imamura N, Yano K, Hamada T. Significance of bile duct resection for advanced gallbladder cancer without biliary infiltration. Am J Surg. 2018;216(6):1122–6. https://doi.org/10.1016/j.amjsurg.2018.07.014. Epub 2018 Jul 21.

Fuks D, Regimbeau JM, Le Treut YP, Bachellier P, Raventos A, Pruvot FR, Chiche L, Farges O. Incidental gallbladder cancer by the AFC-GBC-2009 Study Group. World J Surg. 2011;35(8):1887–97. https://doi.org/10.1007/s00268-011-1134-3.

Gani F, Buettner S, Margonis GA, Ethun CG, Poultsides G, Tran T, Idrees K, Isom CA, Fields RC, Krasnick B, Weber SM, Salem A, Martin RC, Scoggins C, Shen P, Mogal HD, Schmidt C, Beal E, Hatzaras I, Shenoy R, Maithel SK, Pawlik TM. Assessing the impact of common bile duct resection in the surgical management of gallbladder cancer. J Surg Oncol. 2016;114(2):176–80. https://doi.org/10.1002/jso.24283. Epub 2016 May 20.

Gavriilidis P, Askari A, Azoulay D. To resect or not to resect extrahepatic bile duct in gallbladder cancer? J Clin Med Res. 2017;9(2):81–91. https://doi.org/10.14740/jocmr2804w. Epub 2016 Dec 31. Review.

Glenn F, Hays DM. The scope of radical surgery in the treatment of malignant tumors of the extrahepatic biliary tract. Surg Gynecol Obstet. 1954;99(5):529–41.

Goel M, Kurunkar SR, Kanetkar A, Patkar S. Outcome of robot-assisted radical cholecystectomy in a high-volume tertiary cancer center in India. J Laparoendosc Adv Surg Tech B Videoscop. 2019a;29(3):vor.2018.0539. https://doi.org/10.1089/vor.2018.0539.

Goel M, Khobragade K, Patkar S, Kanetkar A, Kurunkar S. Robotic surgery for gallbladder cancer: operative technique and early outcomes. J Surg Oncol. 2019b;119(7):958–63. https://doi.org/10.1002/jso.25422. Epub 2019 Feb 25.

Goetze TO, Paolucci V. The prognostic impact of positive lymph nodes in stages T1 to T3 incidental gallbladder carcinoma: results of the German Registry. Surg Endosc. 2012;26(5):1382–9. https://doi.org/10.1007/s00464-011-2044-z. Epub 2011 Nov 17.

Gumbs AA, Hoffman JP. Laparoscopic completion radical cholecystectomy for T2 gallbladder cancer. Surg Endosc. 2010;24(12):3221–3. Epub 2010 May 25.

Gwark SC, Hwang S, Kim KH, Lee YJ, Park KM, Ahn CS, Moon DB, Ha TY, Song GW, Jung DH, Park GC, Lee SG. Extent of resection for T2N0 gallbladder carcinoma regarding concurrent extrahepatic bile duct resection. Korean J Hepatobiliary Pancreat Surg. 2012;16(4):142–6. https://doi.org/10.14701/kjhbps.2012.16.4.142. Epub 2012 Nov 30.

Han HS, Yoon YS, Agarwal AK, Belli G, Itano O, Gumbs AA, Yoon DS, Kang CM, Lee SE, Wakai T, Troisi RI. Laparoscopic surgery for gallbladder cancer: an expert consensus statement. Dig Surg. 2019a;36(1):1–6. https://doi.org/10.1159/000486207. Epub 2018 Jan 16.

He XD, Li JJ, Liu W, Qu Q, Hong T, Xu XQ, Li BL, Wang Y, Zhao HT. Surgical procedure determination based on tumor-node-metastasis staging of gallbladder cancer. World J Gastroenterol. 2015;21(15):4620–6. https://doi.org/10.3748/wjg.v21.i15.4620.

Horiguchi A, Miyakawa S, Ishihara S, Miyazaki M, Ohtsuka M, Shimizu H, Sano K, Miura F, Ohta T, Kayahara M, Nagino M, Igami T, Hirano S, Yamaue H, Tani M, Yamamoto M, Ota T, Shimada M, Morine Y, Kinoshita H, Yasunaga M, Takada T. Gallbladder bed resection or hepatectomy of segments 4a and 5 for pT2 gallbladder carcinoma: analysis of Japanese registration cases by the study group for biliary surgery of the Japanese Society of Hepato-Biliary-Pancreatic Surgery. J Hepatobiliary Pancreat Sci. 2013a;20(5):518–24. https://doi.org/10.1007/s00534-012-0584-9. Erratum in: J Hepatobiliary Pancreat Sci. 2014;21(1):86.

Igami T, Ebata T, Yokoyama Y, Sugawara G, Nagino M. Advanced resectable gallbladder cancer: diagnosis and surgical approach. In: Agarwal A, Fong Y, editors. Carcinoma of the gall bladder. New Delhi: Elsevier; 2014. p. 89–105.

Igami T, Ebata T, Yokoyama Y, Sugawara G, Mizuno T, Yamaguchi J, Shimoyama Y, Nagino M. Combined extrahepatic bile duct resection for locally advanced gallbladder carcinoma: does it work? World J Surg. 2015;39(7):1810–7. https://doi.org/10.1007/s00268-015-3011-y.

Itano O, Oshima G, Minagawa T, Shinoda M, Kitago M, Abe Y, Hibi T, Yagi H, Ikoma N, Aiko S, Kawaida M, Masugi Y, Kameyama K, Sakamoto M, Kitagawa Y. Novel strategy for laparoscopic treatment of pT2 gallbladder carcinoma. Surg Endosc. 2015;29(12):3600–7. https://doi.org/10.1007/s00464-015-4116-y. Epub 2015 Mar 5.

Ito H, Ito K, D'Angelica M, Gonen M, Klimstra D, Allen P, DeMatteo RP, Fong Y, Blumgart LH, Jarnagin WR. Accurate staging for gallbladder cancer: implications for surgical therapy and pathological assessment. Ann Surg. 2011;254(2):320–5. https://doi.org/10.1097/SLA.0b013e31822238d8.

Jang JY, Han HS, Yoon YS, Cho JY, Choi Y. Retrospective comparison of outcomes of laparoscopic and open surgery for T2 gallbladder cancer—thirteen-year experience. Surg Oncol. 2019;29:142–7. https://doi.org/10.1016/j.suronc.2019.05.007. Epub 2019 May 13.

Jensen EH, Abraham A, Jarosek S, Habermann EB, Al-Refaie WB, Vickers SA, Virnig BA, Tuttle TM. Lymph node evaluation is associated with improved survival after surgery for early stage gallbladder cancer. Surgery. 2009;146(4):706–11.; ; discussion 711–3. https://doi.org/10.1016/j.surg.2009.06.056.

Kaneoka Y, Yamaguchi A, Isogai M, Harada T, Suzuki M. Hepatoduodenal ligament invasion by gallbladder carcinoma: histologic patterns and surgical recommendation. World J Surg. 2003;27(3):260–5. https://doi.org/10.1007/s00268-002-6702-0.

Kang MJ, Song Y, Jang JY, Han IW, Kim SW. Role of radical surgery in patients with stage IV gallbladder cancer. HPB (Oxford). 2012;14(12):805–11. https://doi.org/10.1111/j.1477-2574.2012.00544.x. Epub 2012 Aug 20.

Kapoor VK. Advanced gallbladder cancer: Indian "middle path". J Hepatobiliary Pancreat Surg. 2007;14(4):366–73. Epub 2007 Jul 30.

Kapoor VK, Behari A. Surgical procedures for gall bladder cancer. BAOJ Cancer Res Ther. 2017a;3:037.

Kelly KJ, Dukleska K, Kuk D, Kingham TP, D'Angelica MI, DeMatteo RP, Allen PJ, Jarnagin WR, Fong Y. Prognostic significance of the highest peripancreatic lymph node in biliary tract adenocarcinoma. Ann Surg Oncol. 2014;21(3):979–85. https://doi.org/10.1245/s10434-013-3352-4. Epub 2013 Nov 9.

Kim S, Yoon YS, Han HS, Cho JY, Choi Y. Laparoscopic extended cholecystectomy for T3 gallbladder cancer. Surg Endosc. 2018a;32(6):2984–5. https://doi.org/10.1007/s00464-017-5952-8. Epub 2017 Dec 7.

Kinoshita H, Hashino K, Hashimoto M, Kodama T, Nishimura K, Kawabata M, Furukawa S, Tamae T, Nagashima J, Hara M, Imayama H, Aoyagi S. Clinicopathological evaluation of surgical treatment for early gallbladder cancer. Kurume Med J. 2001;48(4):267–71.

Kokudo N, Makuuchi M, Natori T, Sakamoto Y, Yamamoto J, Seki M, Noie T, Sugawara Y, Imamura H, Asahara S, Ikari T. Strategies for surgical treatment of gallbladder carcinoma based on information available before resection. Arch Surg. 2003;138(7):741–50; discussion 750.

Kondo S, Nimura Y, Hayakawa N, Kamiya J, Nagino M, Uesaka K. Regional and para-aortic lymphadenectomy in radical surgery for advanced gallbladder carcinoma. Br J Surg. 2000;87(4):418–22.

Kondo S, Nimura Y, Kamiya J, Nagino M, Kanai M, Uesaka K, Hayakawa N. Mode of tumor spread and surgical strategy in gallbladder carcinoma. Langenbecks Arch Surg. 2002;387(5–6):222–8. Epub 2002 Oct 2.

Kondo S, Hirano S, Tanaka E, Tsuchikawa T, Kato K, Matsumoto J, Nasu Y, Shichinohe T. Two types of extended liver resection for advanced gallbladder cancer: how to do it. Dig Surg. 2011;28(2):148–53. https://doi.org/10.1159/000323826. Epub 2011 Apr 29.

Kosuge T, Sano K, Shimada K, Yamamoto J, Yamasaki S, Makuuchi M. Should the bile duct be preserved or removed in radical surgery for gallbladder cancer? Hepatogastroenterology. 1999;46(28):2133–7.

Lee SE, Kim KS, Kim WB, Kim IG, Nah YW, Ryu DH, Park JS, Yoon MH, Cho JY, Hong TH, et al. Practical guidelines for the surgical treatment of gallbladder cancer. J Korean Med Sci. 2014;29(10):1333–40. https://doi.org/10.3346/jkms.2014.29.10.1333.

Lee AJ, Chiang YJ, Lee JE, Conrad C, Chun YS, Aloia TA, Vauthey JN, Tzeng CD. Validation of American Joint Committee on Cancer eighth staging system for gallbladder cancer and its lymphadenectomy guidelines. J Surg Res. 2018;230:148–54. https://doi.org/10.1016/j.jss.2018.04.067. Epub 2018 May 31.

Leigh NL, Solomon D, Feingold D, Hiotis SP, Labow DM, Magge DR, Sarpel U, Golas BJ. Staging gallbladder cancer with lymphadenectomy: the practical application of new AHPBA and AJCC guidelines. HPB (Oxford). 2019; https://doi.org/10.1016/j.hpb.2019.03.372. pii: S1365-182X(19)30498-8.

Lim JH, Chong JU, Kim SH, Park SW, Choi JS, Lee WJ, Kim KS. Role of common bile duct resection in T2 and T3 gallbladder cancer patients. Ann Hepatobiliary Pancreat Surg. 2018;22(1):42–51. https://doi.org/10.14701/ahbps.2018.22.1.42. Epub 2018 Feb 26.

Machado MA, Makdissi FF, Surjan RC. Totally laparoscopic hepatic bisegmentectomy (s4b+s5) and hilar lymphadenectomy for incidental gallbladder cancer. Ann Surg Oncol. 2015;22(Suppl 3):S336–9. https://doi.org/10.1245/s10434-015-4650-9. Epub 2015 Jun 10.

Miyazaki M, Shimizu H, Ohtsuka M, Yoshidome H, Kato A, Yoshitomi H, Furukawa K, Kimura F. Hepatic S4a + S5 and bile duct resection for gallbladder carcinoma. J Hepatobiliary Pancreat Sci. 2012;19(3):225–9. https://doi.org/10.1007/s00534-011-0500-8.

Mizuno T, Ebata T, Yokoyama Y, Igami T, Yamaguchi J, Onoe S, Watanabe N, Ando M, Nagino M. Major hepatectomy with or without pancreatoduodenectomy for advanced gallbladder cancer. Br J Surg. 2019;106(5):626–35. https://doi.org/10.1002/bjs.11088. Epub 2019 Feb 14.

Nag HH, Raj P, Sisodia K. The technique of laparoscopic hepatic bisegmentectomy with regional lymphadenectomy for gallbladder cancer. J Minim Access Surg. 2018;14(2):124–9. https://doi.org/10.4103/jmas.JMAS_181_16.PMID:28928327.

Nag HH, Sachan A, Nekarakanti PK. Laparoscopic versus open extended cholecystectomy with bisegmentectomy (s4b and s5) in patients with gallbladder cancer. J Minim Access Surg. 2019; https://doi.org/10.4103/jmas.JMAS_98_19.

Navarro JG, Kang CM. Laparoscopic radical cholecystectomy with common bile duct resection for T2 gallbladder cancer. Ann Hepatobiliary Pancreat Surg. 2019;23(1):69–73. https://doi.org/10.14701/ahbps.2019.23.1.69. Epub 2019 Feb 28.

Negi SS, Singh A, Chaudhary A. Lymph nodal involvement as prognostic factor in gallbladder cancer: location, count or ratio? J Gastrointest Surg. 2011;15(6):1017–25. Epub 2011 Apr 13.

Nigri G, Berardi G, Mattana C, Mangogna L, Petrucciani N, Sagnotta A, Aurello P, D'Angelo F, Ramacciato G. Routine extra-hepatic bile duct resection in gallbladder cancer patients without bile duct infiltration: a systematic review. Surgeon. 2016;14(6):337–44. https://doi.org/10.1016/j.surge.2016.06.004. Epub 2016 Jul 6. Review.

Ogura Y, Tabata M, Kawarada Y, Mizumoto R. Effect of hepatic invasion on the choice of hepatic resection for advanced carcinoma of the gallbladder: histologic analysis of 32 surgical cases. World J Surg. 1998;22(3):262–6; discussion 266–7.

Ong CT, Leung K, Nussbaum DP, Sun Z, Gloor B, Blazer DG III, Worni M. Open versus laparoscopic portal lymphadenectomy in gallbladder cancer: is there a difference in lymph node yield? HPB (Oxford). 2018;20(6):505–13. https://doi.org/10.1016/j.hpb.2017.10.015. Epub 2018 Feb 19.

Palanisamy S, Patel N, Sabnis S, Palanisamy N, Vijay A, Palanivelu P, Parthasarthi R, Chinnusamy P. Laparoscopic radical cholecystectomy for suspected early gall bladder carcinoma: thinking beyond convention. Surg Endosc. 2016;30(6):2442–8. https://doi.org/10.1007/s00464-015-4495-0. Epub 2015 Sep 28.

Patkar S, Patil V, Acharya MR, Kurunkar S, Goel M. Achieving margin negative resection-doing less is justified: oncological outcomes of wedge excision of liver in gallbladder cancer (GBC) surgery. Chin Clin Oncol. 2019;8(4):38. https://doi.org/10.21037/cco.2019.07.07. Epub 2019 Aug 7.

Piccolo G, Piozzi GN. Laparoscopic radical cholecystectomy for primary or incidental early gallbladder cancer: the new rules governing the treatment of gallbladder cancer. Gastroenterol Res Pract. 2017;2017:8570502. https://doi.org/10.1155/2017/8570502. Epub 2017 Jun 11. Review.

Piccolo G, Ratti F, Cipriani F, Catena M, Paganelli M, Aldrighetti L. Totally Laparoscopic Radical Cholecystectomy for Gallbladder Cancer: A Single Center Experience. J Laparoendosc Adv Surg Tech A. 2019;29(6):741–46. https://doi:10.1089/lap.2019.0227. Epub 2019 May 10. PMID: 31074684.

Rammohan A, Cherukuri SD, Sathyanesan J, Palaniappan R, Govindan M. Xanthogranulomatous cholecystitis masquerading as gallbladder cancer: can it be diagnosed preoperatively? Gastroenterol Res Pract. 2014;2014:253645. https://doi.org/10.1155/2014/253645. Epub 2014 Oct 27.

Sakata J, Shirai Y, Wakai T, Ajioka Y, Hatakeyama K. Number of positive lymph nodes independently determines the prognosis after resection in patients with gallbladder carcinoma. Ann Surg Oncol. 2010a;17(7):1831–40. Epub 2010 Jan 15.

Sakata J, Kobayashi T, Tajima Y, Ohashi T, Hirose Y, Takano K, Takizawa K, Miura K, Wakai T. Relevance of dissection of the posterior superior pancreaticoduodenal lymph nodes in gallbladder carcinoma. Ann Surg Oncol. 2017;24(9):2474–81. https://doi.org/10.1245/s10434-017-5939-7. Epub 2017 Jun 26.

Sasaki R, Takeda Y, Hoshikawa K, Takahashi M, Funato O, Nitta H, Murakami M, Kawamura H, Suto T, Yaegashi Y, Kanno S, Saito K. Long-term results of central inferior (S4a + S5) hepatic subsegmentectomy and pancreatoduodenectomy combined with extended lymphadenectomy for gallbladder carcinoma with subserous or mild liver invasion (pT2–3) and nodal involvement: a preliminary report. Hepatogastroenterology. 2004;51(55):215–8.

Shimizu Y, Ohtsuka M, Ito H, Kimura F, Shimizu H, Togawa A, Yoshidome H, et al. Should the extrahepatic bile duct be resected for locally advanced gallbladder cancer? Surgery. 2004;136(5):1012–1017; discussion 1018. https://doi.org/10.1016/j.surg.2004.04.032.

Shirai Y, Sakata J, Wakai T, Hatakeyama K. Full-thickness cholecystectomy with limited lymphadenectomy for gallbladder cancer. Hepatogastroenterology. 2012a;59(117):1338–40. https://doi.org/10.5754/hge12276.

Sternby Eilard M, Lundgren L, Cahlin C, Strandell A, Svanberg T, Sandström P. Surgical treatment for gallbladder cancer—a systematic literature review. Scand J Gastroenterol. 2017;52(5):505–14. https://doi.org/10.1080/00365521.2017.1284895. Epub 2017 Feb 9. Review.

Tewari M, Kumar V, Mishra RR, Kumar M, Shukla HS. Is there a role for cholecystectomy in gallbladder carcinoma discovered to be unresectable for cure at laparotomy? World J Surg. 2008;32(12):2683–7. https://doi.org/10.1007/s00268-008-9763-x.

Todoroki T, Kawamoto T, Takahashi H, Takada Y, Koike N, Otsuka M, Fukao K. Treatment of gallbladder cancer by radical resection. Br J Surg. 1999;86(5):622–7.

Tsilimigras DI, Hyer JM, Paredes AZ, Moris D, Beal EW, Merath K, Mehta R, Ejaz A, Cloyd JM, Pawlik TM. The optimal number of lymph nodes to evaluate among patients undergoing surgery for gallbladder cancer: correlating the number of nodes removed with survival in 6531 patients. J Surg Oncol. 2019;119(8):1099–107. https://doi.org/10.1002/jso.25450. Epub 2019 Mar 12.

Yi X, Long X, Zai H, Xiao D, Li W, Li Y. Unsuspected gallbladder carcinoma discovered during or after cholecystectomy: focus on appropriate radical re-resection according to the T-stage. Clin Transl Oncol. 2013;15(8):652–8. https://doi.org/10.1007/s12094-012-0988-7. Epub 2013 Jan 29.

Yoon YS, Han HS, Cho JY, Choi Y, Lee W, Jang JY, Choi H. Is laparoscopy contraindicated for gallbladder cancer? A 10-year prospective cohort study. J Am Coll Surg. 2015;221(4):847–53. https://doi.org/10.1016/j.jamcollsurg.2015.07.010. Epub 2015 Jul 20.

Yoshikawa T, Araida T, Azuma T, Takasaki K. Bisubsegmental liver resection for gallbladder cancer. Hepatogastroenterology. 1998;45(19):14–9.

Yu LH, Yuan B, Fu XH, Yu WL, Liu J, Zhang YJ. Does anatomic resection get more benefits than wedge hepatectomy on the prognosis for pT3 unsuspected gallbladder cancer? J Laparoendosc Adv Surg Tech A. 2019; https://doi.org/10.1089/lap.2018.0690.

Zhang L, Hou C, Xu Z, Wang L, Ling X, Xiu D. Laparoscopic treatment for suspected gallbladder cancer confined to the wall: a 10-year study from a single institution. Chin J Cancer Res. 2018;30(1):84–92. https://doi.org/10.21147/j.issn.1000-9604.2018.01.09.

Zhao X, Li XY, Ji W. Laparoscopic versus open treatment of gallbladder cancer: a systematic review and meta-analysis. J Minim Access Surg. 2018;14(3):185–91. https://doi.org/10.4103/jmas.JMAS_223_16. PMID:28782743.

Zimmitti G, Manzoni A, Guerini F, Ramera M, Bertocchi P, Aroldi F, Zaniboni A, Rosso E. Current role of minimally invasive radical cholecystectomy for gallbladder cancer. Gastroenterol Res Pract. 2016;2016:7684915. Epub 2016 Nov 3.

References for Commentary Notes by Prasoon Pankaj and Toshifumi Wakai

Duffy A, Capanu M, Abou-Alfa GK, Huitzil D, Jarnagin W, Fong Y, D'Angelica M, Dematteo RP, Blumgart LH, O'Reilly EM. Gallbladder cancer (GBC): 10-year experience at Memorial Sloan-Kettering Cancer Centre (MSKCC). J Surg Oncol. 2008;98(7):485–9. https://doi.org/10.1002/jso.21141.

Kim HS, Park JW, Kim H, Han Y, Kwon W, Kim SW, Hwang YJ, Kim SG, Kwon HJ, Vinuela E, Járufe N, Roa JC, Han IW, Heo JS, Choi SH, Choi DW, Ahn KS, Kang KJ, Lee W, Jeong CY, Hong SC, Troncoso A, Losada H, Han SS, Park SJ, Yanagimoto H, Endo I, Kubota K, Wakai T, Ajiki T, Adsay NV, Jang JY. Optimal surgical treatment in patients with T1b gallbladder cancer: an international multicenter study. J Hepatobiliary Pancreat Sci. 2018b;25(12):533–43.

Löhe F, Meimarakis G, Schauer C, Angele M, Jauch KW, Schauer RJ. The time of diagnosis impacts surgical management but not the outcome of patients with gallbladder carcinoma. Eur J Med Res. 2009;14(8):345–51.

Shindoh J, de Aretxabala X, Aloia T, Roa J, Roa I, Zimmitti G, Javle M, Conrad C, Maru D, Aoki T, Vigano L, Ribero D, Kokudo N, Capussotti L, Vauthey J-N. Tumor location is a strong predictor of tumor progression and survival in T2 gallbladder cancer: an international multicenter study. Ann Surg. 2015;261(4):733–9.

Shirai Y, Sakata J, Wakai T, Ohashi T, Ajioka Y, Hatakeyama K. Assessment of lymph node status in gallbladder cancer: location, number, or ratio of positive nodes. World J Surg Oncol. 2012b;10:87. https://doi.org/10.1186/1477-7819-10-87.

Toge K, Sakata J, Hirose Y, Yuza K, Ando T, Soma D, Katada T, Miura K, Takizawa K, Kobayashi T, Wakai T. Lymphatic spread of T2 gallbladder carcinoma: regional lymphadenectomy is required independent of tumor location. Eur J Surg Oncol. 2019;45(8):1446–52. https://doi.org/10.1016/j.ejso.2019.03.038. Epub 2019 Mar 30.

Wakai T, Shirai Y, Sakata J, Nagahashi M, Ajioka Y, Hatakeyama K. Mode of hepatic spread from gallbladder carcinoma: an immunohistochemical analysis of 42 hepatectomized specimens. Am J Surg Pathol. 2010;34(1):65–74. https://doi.org/10.1097/PAS.0b013e3181c467d4.

References for Commentary Notes by Yoo-Seok Yoon

Han HS, Yoon YS, Agarwal AK, Belli G, Itano O, Gumbs AA, et al. Laparoscopic surgery for gallbladder cancer: an expert consensus statement. Dig Surg. 2019b;36(1):1–6.

Yoon YS, Han HS, Agarwal A, Belli G, Itano O, Gumbs AA, et al. Survey results of the expert meeting on laparoscopic surgery for gallbladder cancer and a review of relevant literature. Dig Surg. 2019;36(1):7–12.

11 Major Resections for Gall Bladder Cancer

Vinay K. Kapoor

Extended cholecystectomy (EC) is the standard surgical procedure for gall bladder cancer (GBC), but very few patients with a preoperative (clinical or imaging) diagnosis of GBC are suitable for EC. EC can (should) be performed in patients with GBC confined to the GB wall (T1 or T2) or T3 with minimal (<1 cm) liver infiltration (please see Chap. 10). Most patients with GBC have advanced (T3, T4, or N+ or with jaundice) disease and require a more major resection than EC, e.g., major hepatectomy, hepato-pancreatoduodenectomy (HPD), combined resection of adjacent organs (CRAO), vascular resection, and even hepato-ligamento-pancreato-duodenectomy (HLPD) (Ota et al. 2007; Kaneoka et al. 2015). PET scan (Fig. 11.1) should preferably be obtained before a major resection is planned so as to ensure that there is no distant disease beyond the limits of the proposed major resection. Threshold for the use of neoadjuvant therapy (NAT) should be low in patients who would require a major resection; this may decrease the extent of resection and, more importantly, buys time to observe the biology and aggressiveness of the disease so that poor-biology aggressive tumors opt out of resection and only good-biology favorable tumors are resected. These procedures are, however, associated with high morbidity and significant mortality. Extensive surgical resections were performed at Nagoya University Japan in 68 T3, T4 GBC—morbidity was 50% and mortality was 18% (Kondo et al. 2000a). Mortality of resection in 79 stage IV GBC patients was 11% (Shimizu et al. 2007). For some unknown reasons, however, mortality of the same procedures when performed for GBC is higher than when performed for other cancers, e.g., mortality of major hepatectomy was 16% for GBC versus 4% for cholangiocarcinoma (CC) (Ebata et al. 2012b), mortality of HPD was only 2.4% for CC, much lower than that for GBC which is 10–20% (Ebata et al. 2012a). Mortality of HPD for GBC was 1/5, 20% versus 0/14 for CC (Sakamoto et al. 2013). Like other major surgical procedures, e.g., esophagectomy and pancreatoduodenectomy, 90-day mortality is important as it is higher than 30-day mortality in GBC also. In the National Cancer Database (NCDB) USA (1998–2012), 19,139 (53%) out of 36,067 GBC patients underwent resection; 90-day mortality (17.1%) was much higher than 30-day mortality (7.4%) (Goussous et al. 2017a).

The philosophy of management of GBC varies from region to region. The Japanese aggressive approach toward advanced GBC comes at a cost in

Please also see an Invited Commentary on Major Resections for Gall Bladder Cancer by Junichi Kaneko and Kiyoshi Hasegawa (pp **–**)

V. K. Kapoor (✉)
Department of Surgical Gastroenterology, Sanjay Gandhi Post-Graduate Institute of Medical Sciences (SGPGIMS), Lucknow, Uttar Pradesh, India
e-mail: vkkapoor.india@gmail.com

V. K. Kapoor (ed.), *A Pictorial Treatise on Gall Bladder Cancer*,
https://doi.org/10.1007/978-981-15-5289-2_11

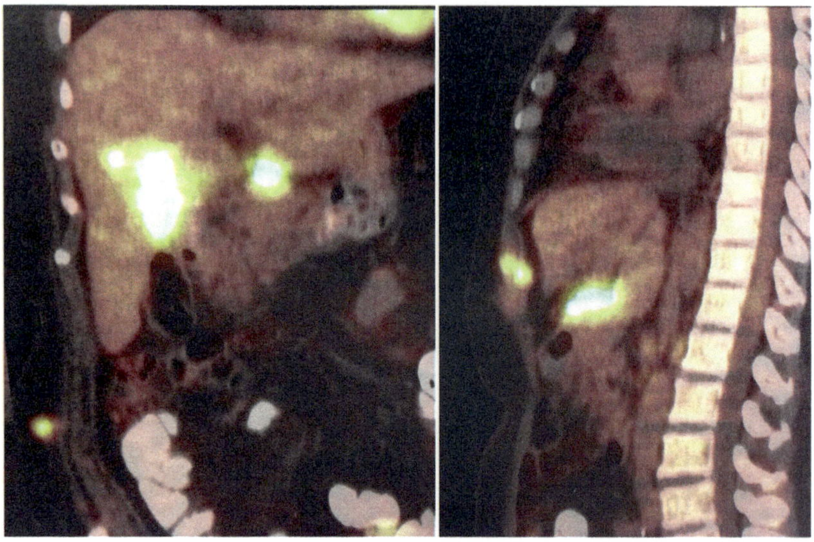

Fig. 11.1 PET shows the primary gall bladder tumor and a large lymph node deposit; PET scan should be obtained before a major resection to ensure that there is no distant disease beyond the limits of the proposed major resection

terms of high morbidity and significant (even double-digit) mortality with only anecdotal long-term survivors. On the other extreme of the spectrum, the Western pessimism toward GBC sometimes results in inappropriate management of even early disease. The Author (Kapoor 2007) has advocated an Indian "Buddhist" middle path for management of GBC—aggressive surgical approach for early and less advanced (confined to the GB) GBC (including incidental GBC) and largely nonsurgical palliative approach for more advanced (beyond GB) GBC; major surgical resections being performed in specialized centers for selected few good-risk patients (see Chap. 9).

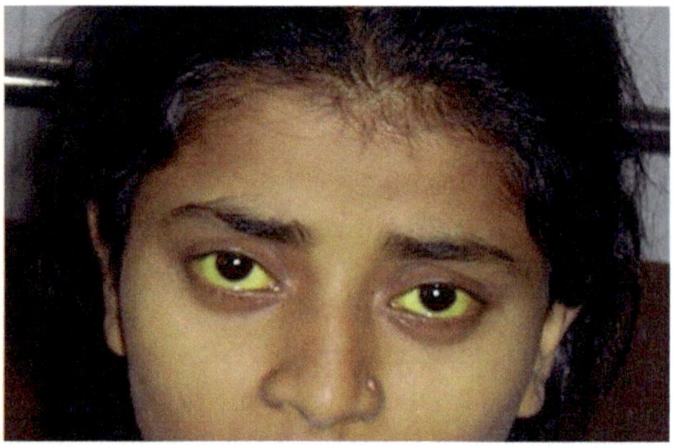

Fig. 11.2 Jaundice is frequently present in patients with advanced (clinically obvious) gall bladder cancer; majority of the patients with jaundice are unresectable; the ones which are resectable will require a major liver resection

11.1 Jaundice

Jaundice (Fig. 11.2) is frequently present in patients with advanced (clinically obvious) GBC—82/240, 34% (Hawkins et al. 2004), 110/429, 26% (Regimbeau et al. 2011) and 62/120, 52% (Varma et al. 2009). Bile duct infiltration (BDI) is a predictor of poor outcome—3-year survival in patients with BDI was less (6% with LN involvement and 14% without LN involvement) versus in patients without BDI (35% with LN involvement and 66% without LN involvement) (Kaneoka et al. 2003). Jaundice in GBC is an ominous sign; it indicates advanced, usually unresectable disease, and predicts poor outcome. Eighty-two out of 240 GBC patients treated at the Memorial Sloan Kettering Cancer Center (MSKCC) New York USA had jaundice—79 (96%) had advanced (stage III + IV) disease; 55 were operated but only 6 (7%) out of 82 could be resected—R0 resection status was achieved in only 4 (5%) (cf. R0 resection status in 39% non-jaundiced patients). Median disease-specific survival (DSS) in patients with jaundice was only 6 months (cf. 16 months in GBC without jaundice); there was no 2-year survival in patients with jaundice (cf. 21% in GBC without jaundice) (Hawkins et al. 2004). Agarwal et al. (2007a) could perform resection in 14 (27%) of 51 patients with jaundice with mortality of 1/14 (7%); median survival was 26 months and 7 patients survived for >2 years. None of the 32 patients with CBD involvement survived for 5 years (D'Angelica et al. 2009). A retrospective multicenter analysis of 110 GBC patients with jaundice treated in France (1998–2008) had mortality of 16% and overall 3-year survival was 15%—only four patients survived for 5 years. Median survival after R0 resection in N0 patients was 20 months (cf. 6 months in N+ patients). The authors recommended resection in highly selected (N0) patients with jaundice (Regimbeau et al. 2011). Extrahepatic bile duct invasion (EBI; another term for bile duct infiltration BDI), however, is a predictor of poor survival (5-year 23% vs. 54% and median 1.5 years vs. 15.4 years in those with and without EBI) (Nishio et al. 2011). At a university hospital in Shanghai China, 192 resections were performed for GBC from 2003 to 2012—47 of these 192 patients had jaundice. Patients with jaundice more frequently (23.4% vs. 2.8%) required combined resection of adjacent organs (CRAO) resulting in longer operative time and more intraoperative bleeding and had more (34% vs. 12%) postoperative complications. Survival in 47 patients with jaundice was poorer as compared to those without jaundice (5-year 6% vs. 37%; median 14 vs. 43 months) (Yang et al. 2014). In one report, however, equal (27% vs. 31%) 5-year overall survival was achieved after surgical resection in GBC with jaundice ($n = 37$) and without jaundice ($n = 28$) (Nasu et al. 2016). Hundred and eight (27%) out of 400 GBC patients operated at a 10-institution consortium in the United States between 2000 and 2014 had jaundice. Curative intent resection was possible much less often ($n = 33$, 30%) in jaundiced patients than in non-jaundiced patients ($n = 218$, 75%). Postoperative morbidity (69% vs. 38%) and reoperation rates (12% vs. 1%) were higher in jaundiced patients than in non-jaundiced patients. Ninety-day mortality was higher (6.5% vs. 3.6%) and overall median survival was worse (14 vs. 32 months) in jaundiced patients. However, among the jaundiced patients, survival was longer (40 vs. 12 months) in patients with CA 19-9 <50 (Tran et al. 2017). In a large series from India, resectability rate in patients with jaundice (1 out of 7) was much lower than that in those without jaundice (1 out of 2). Median survival in 234 patients without jaundice was much longer (61 vs. 12 months) than in 151 patients with jaundice. GBC patients with jaundice were more likely to have metastatic (48% vs. 37%) and unresectable (25% vs. 10%) disease than those without jaundice. One, 2 and 5-year survival was less (49%, 32%, and 0% vs. 80%, 65%, and 53%) in jaundiced patients (Mishra et al. 2017).

A recent systematic review and meta-analysis revealed that patients with jaundice were less likely (OR 0.27) to have resectable disease. Odds for postoperative morbidity, e.g., bile leak and liver failure were higher in jaundiced patients. Overall survival was shorter. The authors concluded that jaundiced patients with advanced GBC may be considered for surgical resection but after careful evaluation and proper counseling (Dasari et al. 2018). The Author (Kapoor 2015) considers the presence of jaundice in GBC akin to the yellow light on a traffic signal, i.e., stop, look (investigate), and proceed but with caution.

An uncommon but favorable scenario is associated CBD stones causing jaundice in a patient with GBC. Endoscopic stone removal can be followed by EC.

11.2 Major Liver Resections

Pack et al. (1955) reported total right hepatic lobectomy (right trisectionectomy of today) for GBC in three cases, one of whom survived for more than 2 years.

A major hepatic resection (defined as resection of >2 segments of liver) may be required for

1. GBC fundus/body with extensive liver infiltration (Fig. 11.3) where EC or even segment IVB + V resection cannot achieve R0 resection status.
2. GBC neck with liver infiltration (of any extent) (Fig. 11.4) because the right portal pedicle lies at a depth of 2–9 mm from the GB bed and an adequate margin cannot be obtained without sacrificing it.

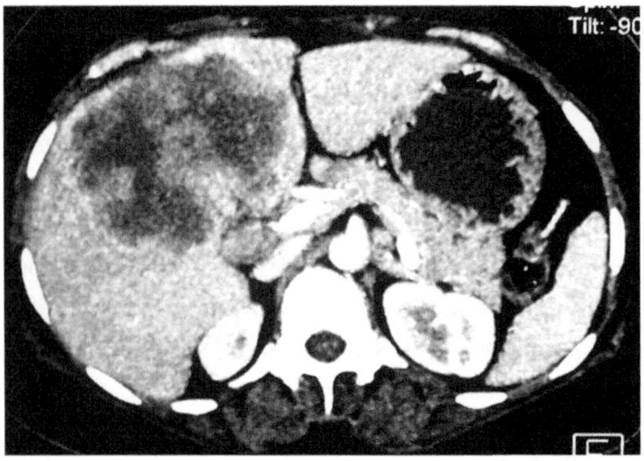

Fig. 11.3 CT shows extensive invasion of segments V and IV; note that the tumor falls short of the falciform ligament—this will require a major hepatic resection in the form of an extended right hepatectomy (ERH)

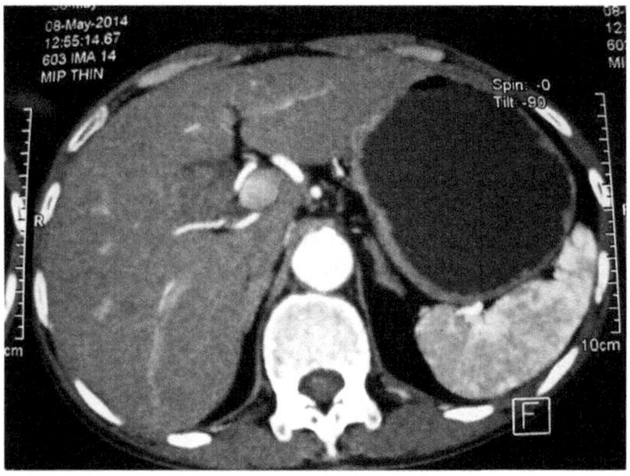

Fig. 11.4 CT shows a gall bladder neck mass with liver infiltration; right hepatic artery (RHA) lying anterior to the portal vein is running close to the tumor and an accessory RHA lying posterior to the common bile duct and the portal vein is also present—a major hepatic resection may be required for gall bladder cancer at neck with any amount of liver infiltration

3. GBC neck with hilar (biliary ductal confluence) block (Fig. 11.5).
4. Involvement of the right portal vein (RPV) (Fig. 11.6) and right hepatic artery (RHA) (Fig. 11.7).

GB lies on the undersurface of the liver straddling segments IV and V (Fig. 11.8). Hepatectomy in GBC (cf. in hilar cholangiocarcinoma) is never right hepatectomy alone; it is always combined with resection of segment IV, i.e., extended right hepatectomy (ERH) (Fig. 11.9) (also called right

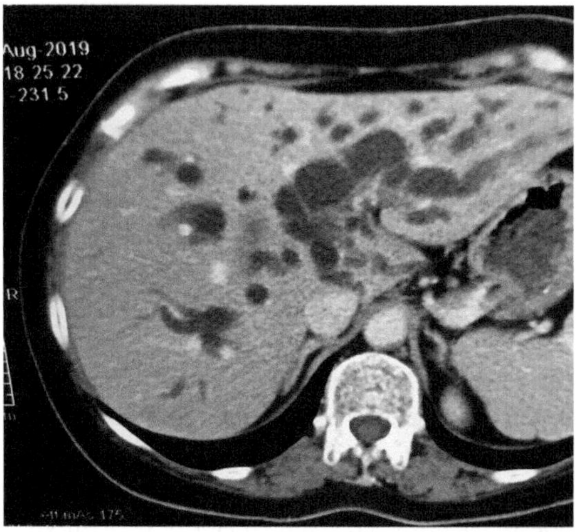

Fig. 11.5 CT shows a hilar mass with bilateral intrahepatic biliary radical dilatation—a major hepatic resection may be required for gall bladder cancer at neck with hilar (biliary ductal confluence) block

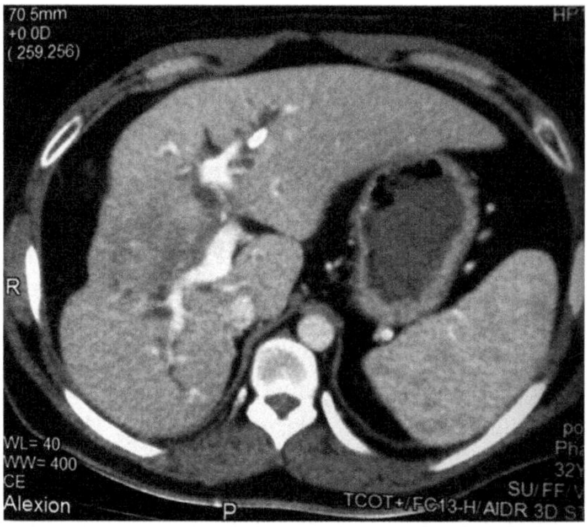

Fig. 11.6 CT shows a large gall bladder mass with partial compression of the lumen of the right portal vein—a major hepatic resection may be required for gall bladder cancer with involvement of the right portal vein

trisectionectomy). Caudate lobe (segment I) resection is not required in GBC (cf. in hilar cholangiocarcinoma).

Chances of achieving R0 resection status increase with a major liver resection but at the cost of high mortality and morbidity. The commonest cause of postoperative mortality after a major liver resection, e.g., extended right hepa-

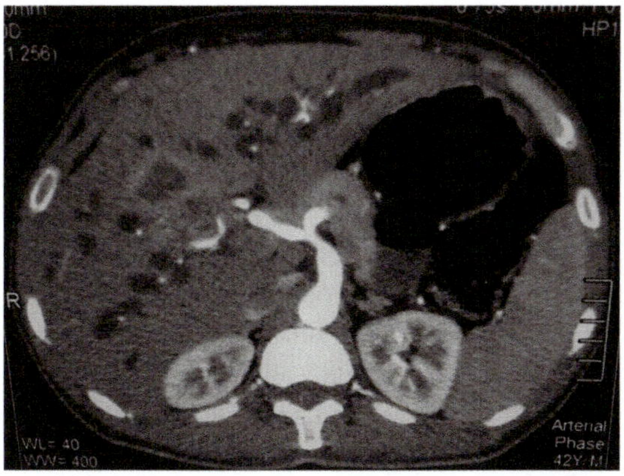

Fig. 11.7 CT shows a large gall bladder mass with invasion of the right hepatic artery (RHA)—a major hepatic resection may be required for gall bladder cancer with involvement of the RHA

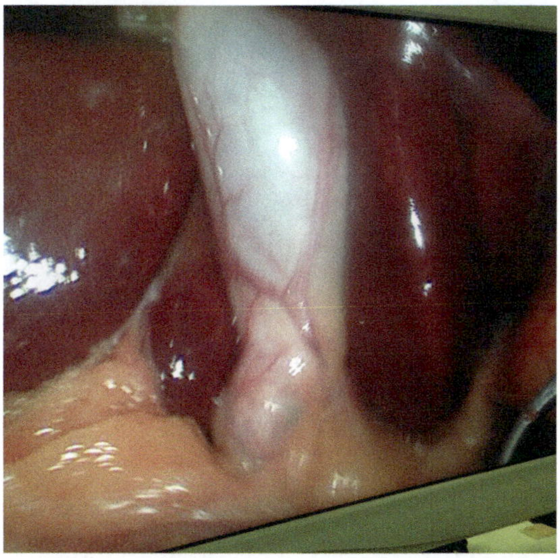

Fig. 11.8 Gall bladder lies on the undersurface of the liver straddling segments IV and V; that is why any resection for gall bladder cancer involves parts of segments IV and V

tectomy (ERH), is hepatic failure because of inadequate functional residual volume (FRV), also called future liver remnant (FLR). Preoperative estimation of FRV with CT (Fig. 11.10), MRI, or isotope scintigraphy is essential before a major hepatectomy. Indocyanine green (ICG) plasma clearance rate of the FLR is a good predictor of the surgical outcome of a major hepatectomy; ICG retention >10–15%

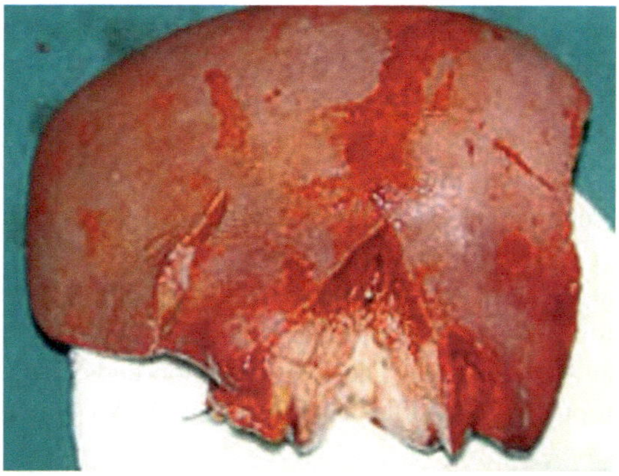

Fig. 11.9 Extended right hepatectomy (right hepatectomy + segment IV resection) for gall bladder cancer

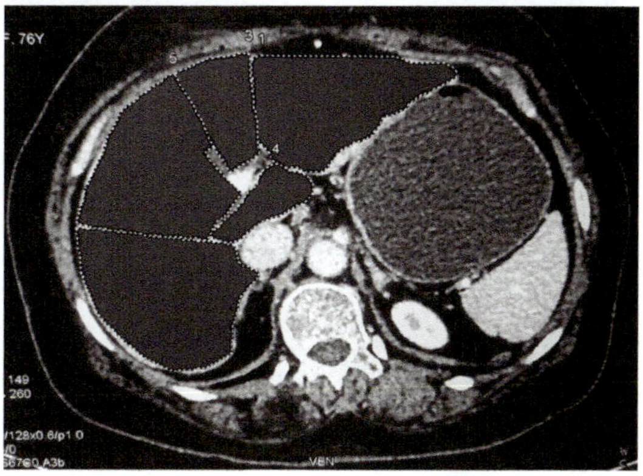

Fig. 11.10 CT volumetry for estimation of the remnant liver volume (RLV) is essential before extended right hepatectomy; RLV can be estimated using MRI or isotope scintigraphy also

at 15 min predicts a high risk of postoperative liver failure (Yokoyama et al. 2010). If an ERH is anticipated and the FRV of the left lateral segment is <30% (Fig. 11.11), which is usually the case, preoperative portal vein embolization (PVE) should be performed to induce ipsilateral atrophy and contralateral hypertrophy (Fig. 11.12) to augment the FRV. This is done with transhepatic ipsilateral approach using fibrin glue or steel coils with absolute alcohol. In addition to the right portal vein (RPV), the segment IV branch of the left portal vein (LPV) also needs to be embolized; otherwise segment IV will also hypertrophy and make ERH technically difficult. Modified ERH (removing only segment IVB and preserving IVA in order to have more FRV) is an option; in such cases however, the segment IV branch of the LPV should not be embolized. A "Taj Mahal" resection including segments IVB + V with total resection of the caudate lobe (segment I) has been described by Kawarada et al. (1999). The procedure is so called because at the end of the resection, the remaining liver looks like the dome of the Taj Mahal (Fig. 11.13) at Agra in India. The liver resection ends at the root of the middle hepatic vein (MHV) which then lies exposed at the pinnacle of the dome-shaped resected liver. The limits of the dome are B2 + 3 (bile ducts to segment II and III) bifurcation and the right margin of the umbilical portion of the LPV on the left side and B8 of the right anterior sectoral branch and B6 + 7 bifurcation of the right posterior sectoral branch on the right side. Taj Mahal resection requires multiple intrahepatic biliary-enteric anastomoses in the form of intrahepatic cholangio-jejunostomy. Taj Mahal resection is suitable for GBC at neck involving

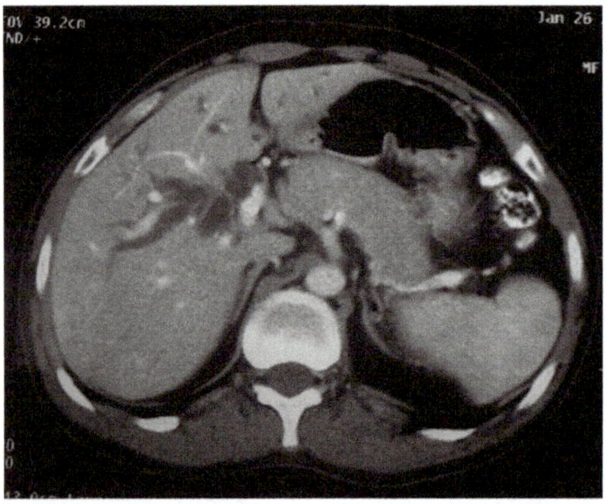

Fig. 11.11 A small left lateral segment before portal vein embolization (PVE)

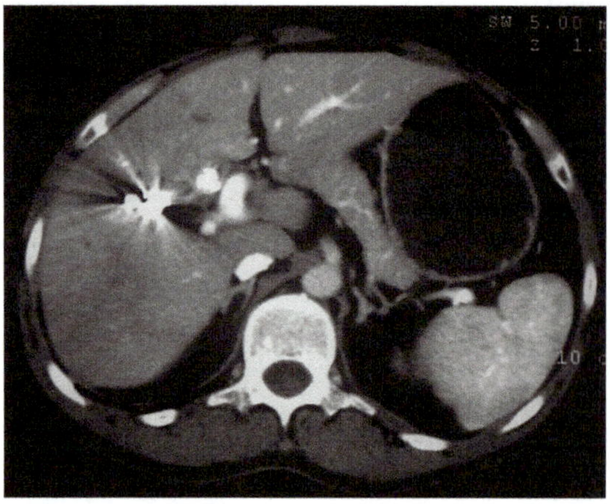

Fig. 11.12 Hypertrophied left lateral segment after portal vein embolization (PVE); coils of PVE can be seen in the right lobe

Fig. 11.13 Taj Mahal at Agra in Uttar Pradesh India—one of the most beautiful buildings in the world; a central liver parenchyma preserving liver resection has been named as Taj Mahal resection because the residual defect in the liver resembles the dome of the Taj Mahal

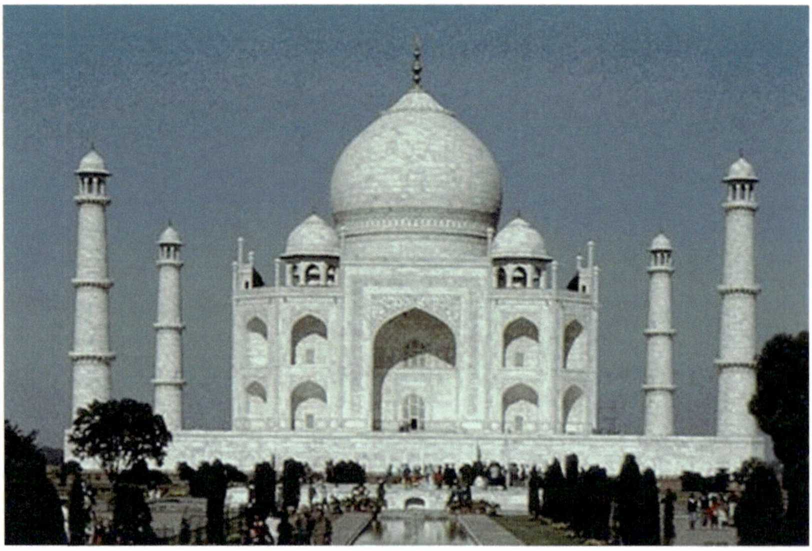

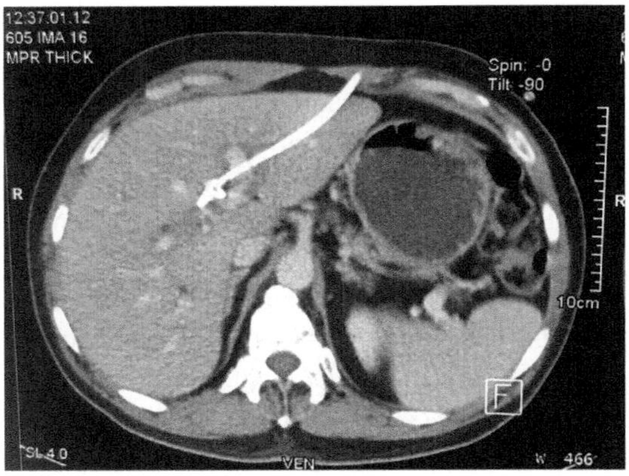

Fig. 11.14 Percutaneous transhepatic biliary drainage (PTBD) in situ in the left lateral segment of liver for preoperative biliary drainage (PBD) before a major liver resection—PTBD used to be performed earlier for PBD but has been replaced by endoscopic naso-biliary drainage (ENBD) now

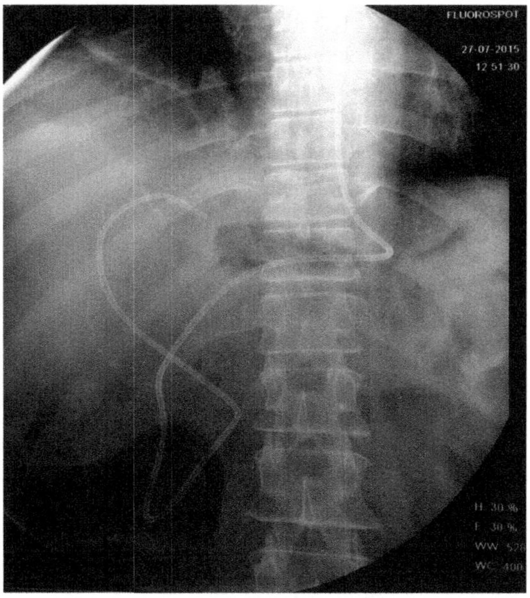

Fig. 11.15 Endoscopic naso-biliary drainage (ENBD) for preoperative biliary drainage (PBD) before a major liver resection—ENBD (and endoscopic stent) has replaced percutaneous transhepatic biliary drainage (PTBD) as the method of choice for PBD

the biliary ductal confluence only but without involvement of the right hepatic artery (RHA) or right portal vein (RPV), not a common situation though in GBC. It has not become very popular, probably because of technical difficulties. Also, it cannot be performed if RHA and/or RPV are involved.

In patients with jaundice, preoperative biliary drainage (PBD) is required for normalization of serum bilirubin before PVE. There has been a change in strategy in Japan from percutaneous transhepatic biliary drainage (PTBD) (Fig. 11.14) to endoscopic naso-biliary drainage (ENBD) (Fig. 11.15) as the method of choice for PBD in GBC. At the Tokyo Women's Medical University (TWMU) Japan, PTBD was performed for biliary drainage in all patients during 2000–2001, but in 2008–2009, PTBD was performed in only 41% and ENBD was preferred for biliary drainage in 59% patients with jaundice (Higuchi and Yamamoto 2014). Endoscopic biliary drainage in 72 patients was associated with less postoperative major morbidity than PTBD in 99 patients undergoing major hepatectomy for biliary tract cancers (BTC) i.e., GBC and cholangiocarcinoma (Kishi et al. 2016). Incidence of tumor dissemination was lower (14.6% vs. 35.9%) in the ENBD group ($n = 76$) than in the PTBD group ($n = 87$) when performed for perihilar cholangiocarcinoma (Higuchi et al. 2017). These highly invasive interventional procedures, i.e., PBD and PVE, are associated with complications and the disease usually progresses, while these preoperative interventions are being done. PVE was done in 141 GBC patients but as many as 61 (43%) did not finally undergo hepatectomy (Ebata et al. 2012b).

Associating liver partition with portal vein ligation for staged hepatectomy ALPPS has been described as an alternative to PVE to increase the FLR in patients requiring major/multiple liver resections for colorectal liver metastases (CRLM). Access to the hilum of liver may, however, be technically difficult in patients with GBC neck with hilar involvement—the very patients in whom a major liver resection is usually required. Tsui et al. (2016) described double ALPPS where central segments, i.e., I, IV, V, and VIII were split and right anterior sectoral portal vein was ligated thus inducing rapid hypertrophy of the right posterior sector (segments VI and VII) and the left lateral segment (segments II and III) for a future mesohepatectomy after 7–9 days in two patients with advanced GBC; one patient, however, died (from severe ARDS attributed to neoadjuvant chemotherapy). Schmelzle et al. (2019) reported partial ALPPS, preserving a 1 cm paranchymal bridge between the left lateral and left medial segments; left pedicle was maintained in continuity but segment IV vessels were divided, PVE of segments V–VIII was performed on day 1—this achieved hypertrophy of segments I–III and ERH was performed later.

There are very few reports of major liver resection for GBC from the West. Ten ERH were reported from the University of Hamburg Germany (Bloechle et al. 1995). Thirty-five major hepatectomies were performed at the MSKCC New York USA (1990–2002) (D'Angelica et al. 2009). French University Association for Surgical Research reported 177 resections for GBC performed at 25 centers—these included only two ERH (Benoist et al. 1998). University of Toronto Canada performed nine ERH over a period of 12 years (1990–2002) (Dixon et al. 2005). In the American College of Surgeons (ACS)—National Surgical quality Improvement Program (NSQIP) database (2005–2009), mortality of extended hepatectomy in 424 patients who underwent curative resection at 243 hospitals was 16% (Jin et al. 2013). A multi-institutional consortium database (2000–2014) of 449 patients with GBC from the United States included only 16 hepatectomies and 5 pancreatoduodenectomies out of 217 curative intent resections (Margonis 2016).

Most reports of major liver resections for GBC are from Japan but mortality after major (right) hepatectomy for GBC has remained high—12.5% (Nishio et al. 2011), 13/80 (16%) (Ebata et al. 2012b), 29/102 (28%) (Higuchi 2014), and 6/26 (23%) (Haga et al. 2016). Only 10 out of 80 patients who underwent major hepatectomy survived for 5 years—at the same time 13 (16%) patients had died in the hospital after the operation (Ebata et al. 2012b). Kishi et al. (2012) reported 65 (extended) hemiliver resections in an experience of 277 patients who underwent laparotomy with curative intent at Tokyo Cancer Center Japan between 1974 and 2011. Sixteen out of 94 patients with stage IV GBC underwent resection with curative intent—4 had ERH (3 died at 7, 16, and 22 months and 1 was alive at 39 months) (Kang et al. 2012). Twenty-nine out of 96 patients with stage II, III, and IV GBC underwent major hepatectomy—there was no mortality but morbidity was 55% (higher than 27% in 67 patients who underwent minor hepatectomy). Median survival was 17.7 months cf. 11.4 months in unresectable cases. If liver metastasis was present or the hepatic artery was involved, survival even after major hepatectomy was the same as in unresectable cases (Yamamoto et al. 2017). The Nagoya University Japan group reported its experience with major hepatectomy (1996–2016) in 117 patients with GBC—79 major hepatectomy alone and 38 with pancreatoduodenectomy, i.e., HPD. PBD was performed in 101 (86%) and PVE in 102 (87%). Mortality was 11/117 (9.4%) and only 13 patients survived >5 years (Mizuno et al. 2019). In an analysis of 7732 hepatectomies performed at 987 hospitals in 2011 from the National Clinical Database (NCD) in Japan, 90-day mortality after hepatectomy for GBC (n = 107) was 13% (Kenjo et al. 2014).

Very few reports from India mention ERH for GBC. We reported major hepatic resection in nine patients (median sectorectomy in two, modified ERH i.e. with segment IVB only in three and modified HPD i.e. with segments IVB + V only in four patients) (Pottakkat et al. 2013). Agarwal et al. (2007b) reported only three hepatectomies (two ERH and one HPD) in 252 resections for GBC over a 5-year period. Only 5 out of 154 resections in another series from India were ERH (Mishra et al. 2017).

11.3 Hepato-Pancreato-Duodenectomy (HPD)

Duodenum/pancreas may be involved in GBC by

1. Direct infiltration of duodenum (Fig. 11.16)/ pancreas (Fig. 11.17).
2. Intrapancreatic extension of involvement of the CBD.

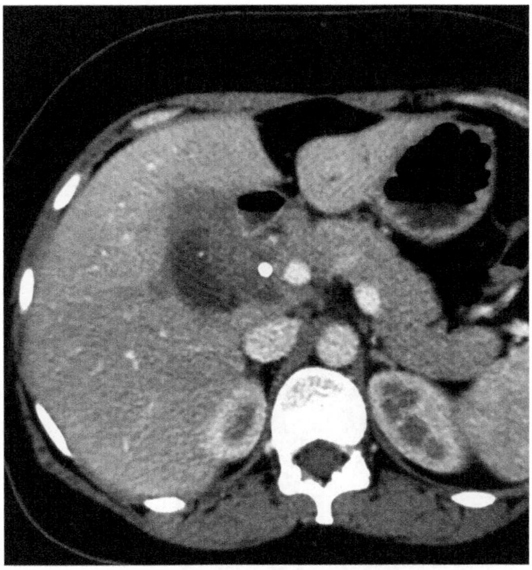

Fig. 11.16 CT shows gall bladder cancer involving the duodenum—this may require pancreatoduodenectomy

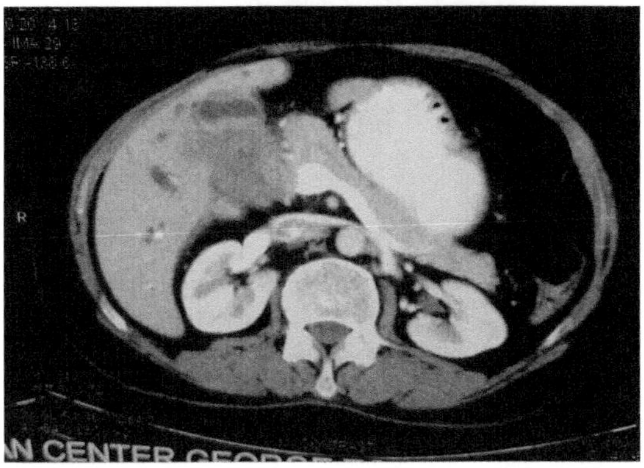

Fig. 11.17 CT shows gall bladder cancer involving the head of the pancreas—this may require pancreatoduodenectomy

3. Involvement of the hepato-duodenal ligament (HDL) in a GBC neck tumor.
4. Large periduodenal/peripancreatic LNs densely adherent to or even infiltrating duodenum/pancreas (Fig. 11.18).

Duodenal involvement is suspected clinically when symptoms of gastric outlet obstruction (GOO) or gastroparesis are present. Patients may have upper GI bleed also. US has poor sensitivity to detect gastroduodenal or pancreatic involvement; it can be suspected on CT (with oral contrast) or EUS (mural thickening or mucosal irregularity) and confirmed on UGIE (mucosal infiltration) or at operation.

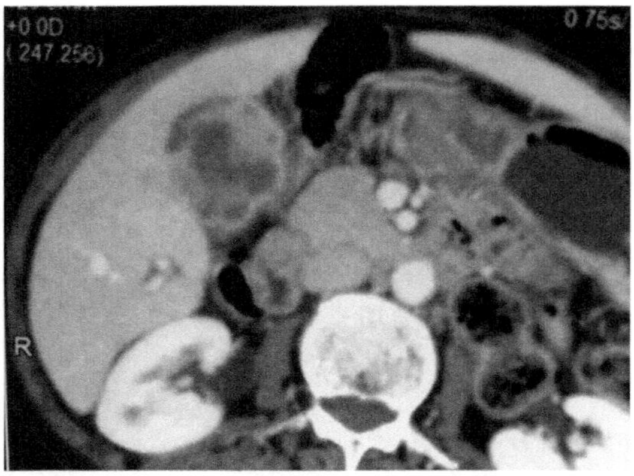

Fig. 11.18 CT shows a large retro-pancreatic lymph node medial to the duodenum; note the primary gall bladder tumor involving the duodenum—retro-pancreatic lymph nodes densely adherent to the pancreas may require pancreatoduodenectomy

Indications for PD in GBC include

1. Involvement of duodenum (Fig. 11.16)/pancreas (Fig. 11.17).
2. Extensive bulky densely adherent retroduodenal/retropancreatic lymph nodes (Fig. 11.18) which cannot be adequately cleared without PD—PD is required to facilitate complete excision of the lymph nodes densely adherent to the pancreas or duodenum.
3. Biliary involvement (in a papillary tumor) in the intrapancreatic part.
4. Synchronous GBC and pancreatic/periampullary cancer.

Hepato-pancreatoduodenectomy (HPD) is a major (>2 segments) hepatectomy combined with PD (Fig. 11.19); EC with PD (Fig. 11.20) does not qualify to be called HPD. Yamamoto et al. (2016) performed 21 PDs in 96 patients who underwent resections for GBC but only 9 of these 21 were HPDs.

HPD was first described by Takasaki et al. (1980) who performed it in five patients with locally advanced GBC—three died within 30 days; two survived but only for 5 and

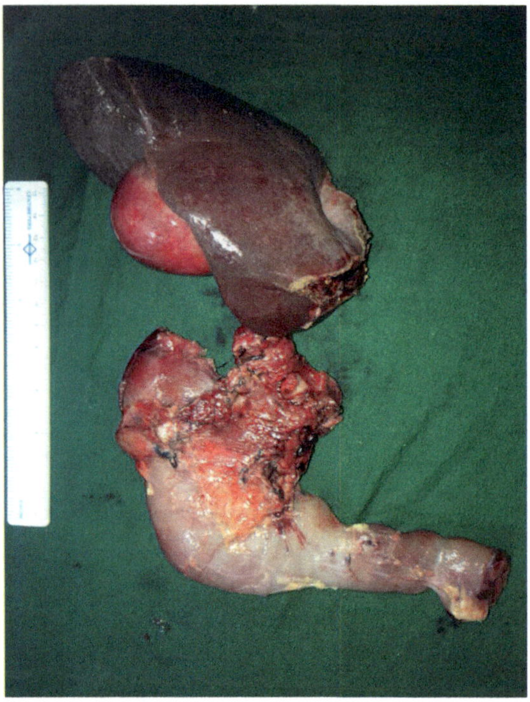

Fig. 11.19 Hepato-pancreatoduodenectomy (HPD) is a major (>2 segments) hepatectomy combined with pancreatoduodenectomy. (Image courtesy Prof Vikas Gupta, Postgraduate Institute of Medical Education and Research PGIMER Chandigarh)

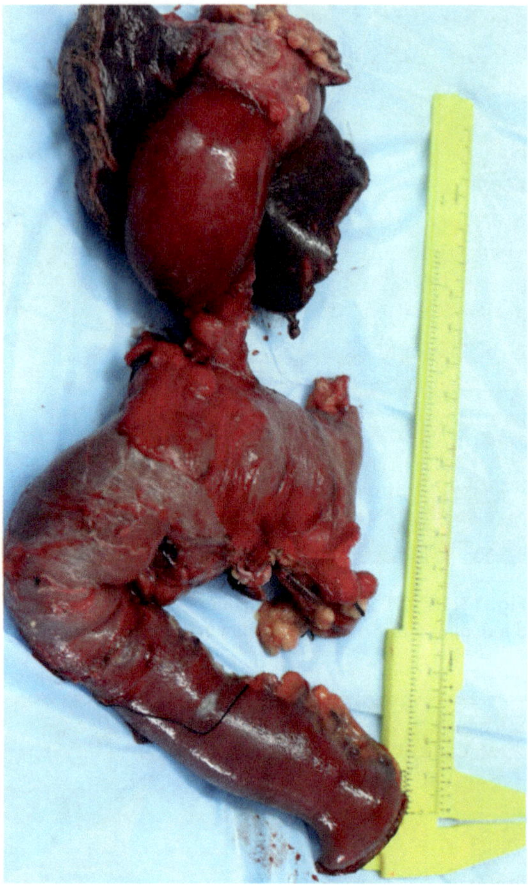

Fig. 11.20 Extended cholecystectomy (liver wedge resection or segments IVB + V resection, shown here) with pancreato-duodenectomy does not qualify to be called hepato-pancreato-duodenectomy (HPD). (Image courtesy Prof TD Yadav, Postgraduate Institute of Medical Education and Research PGIMER Chandigarh)

16 months. Nagoya University Japan group reported 24 HPDs (14 for GBC)—complications occurred in 22 (92%) patients and 3 patients died in the hospital; 2-year survival was 21% and median survival was 12 months for GBC. The longest survivor died of recurrence at 5 years 7 months (Nimura et al. 1991b). Miyagawa et al. (1996) reported HPD in ten patients with no mortality; late-stage pancreatico-jejunostomy was performed in all cases—median survival was 32 months. Todoroki et al. (1999) reported 32 HPDs out of 135 resections for GBC (1976–1998). The Nagoya University Japan group did not report survival advantage of PD performed in 15 out of 37 patients with N2 disease—mortality of PD was, however, 20% (Kokudo et al. 2003a). Fifty-eight HPDs were performed in Nagoya over a period of 23 years—33 were for GBC. Median operating time was 840 (583–1210) min; median blood loss was 3450 (683–39,000) g. Mortality was 12/58 (20%); the authors observed "our results are not satisfactory" (Ebata et al. 2007). Ota et al. (2007) performed HPD in 32 patients between 1979 and 1996—morbidity was seen in 29 (91%) and mortality in 15 (47%) patients; 1-, 3-, and 5-year survival was 12%, 6%, and 3%. Miwa (2007) reported 26 HPDs (GBC $n = 9$) performed between 1990 and 2005—morbidity was 31% and there was no mortality; 2 patients with GBC survived >5 years. Wakai et al. (2008) reported 28 HPDs (11 for GBC)—morbidity was 82% and mortality 21%; 5-year survival was 11% and median survival 9 months; only 1 GBC patient survived for 5 years. Sakamoto et al. (2013) reported 19 HPDs (5 for GBC)—pancreatic fistula formed in 18/19; hospital stay was 47 days. Mortality of major hepatectomy with

pancreatoduodenectomy was 15/31 (48%) in a report from Tokyo Women's Medical University (TWMU) Japan (Higuchi and Yamamoto 2014). Largest experience of HPD for GBC comes from Nagoya—38 HPDs were performed for GBC between 1996 and 2016, i.e., <2 HPDs per year. Mortality was 7/38 (18%) and overall median survival was only 10 (6–14) months cf. 6 (6–10) months in those who did not undergo resection; only three patients survived for >5 years after HPD. The authors observed that though HPD may eradicate locally advanced GBC, its indication from an oncological viewpoint is questionable and it should not be indicated as the first-line treatment for advanced GBC (Mizuno et al. 2019).

HPD has been reported from South Korea also. Twenty-three HPDs were performed in stage IV GBC (R0 resection was achieved in 17/23, 74%) at the Seoul National University South Korea from 1995 to 2007—morbidity was 91% and mortality 13%. Five-year survival in GBC (n = 10) was only 10% (vs. 32% for bile duct cancer BDC i.e. cholangiocarcinoma); all patients with stage III GBC died within 2 years. The authors observed that its adoption in patients with adjacent organ invasion or lymph node metastasis cannot be recommended (*but which other patient with GBC will need HPD?*) (Lim et al. 2012). Sixteen out of 94 patients with stage IV GBC underwent resection with curative intent—5 of these 16 had HPD (4 died within 12 months and 1 was alive at 11 months) (Kang et al. 2012). At the Asan Medical Center Seoul South Korea, 103 patients with GBC underwent R0 resection between 1996 and 2009—these included 12 HPDs (Hwang et al. 2015).

HPD is known as the "Japanese operation" in the West; there are very few cases of HPD in reports on GBC from the West. Out of 1280 resections performed at the MSKCC New York USA (1994–2000) for hepatobiliary cancers only 17 were HPDs (only 8 were with PD and 9 were with distal pancreatectomy only 1 of these 17 HPDs was for GBC)—morbidity was 47% and mortality 18% (D'Angelica et al. 2009). Forty HPDs (GBC n = 9) were performed at the University of California at San Diego (UCSD), United States from 1996 to 2009 but liver resection was segmental in 12 and pancreatectomy was distal in 14; there was no mortality (Hemming et al. 2010). Fernandes Ede et al. (2016) reported the largest western experience with HPD—35 HPDs (18 for GBC) were performed in three institutions in Rio De Janeiro Brazil (2004–2014)—morbidity was 97%, 30-day mortality was 12 (34%)—mortality was higher 7/10 (70%) in those who underwent right hepatectomy; out of 23 surviving patients, 11 were lost to follow-up, 4 died of recurrence; only 3 had >5-year survival. The European African Hepato-Pancreato-Biliary Association reported 66 HPDs performed for GBC and bile duct cancer at 19 centers between 2003 and 2018—90-day mortality was 13% and 3-year survival (after excluding 90-day mortality) was 30% (D'Souza et al. 2019).

We performed a modified HPD (segments IVB + V and PD) in four patients (Pottakkat et al. 2013). Agarwal et al. (2014) reported 6 HPDs in 327 resections for GBC in India. Another large Indian series of 154 resections in 385 patients included only 5 HPDs (Mishra et al. 2017).

Ogura et al. (1991) reviewed 150 HPDs performed in 172 hospitals in Japan—major complication rate was 54%. Zhou et al. (2016) performed a systematic review of 18 studies (1991–2014), all except one each from Korea and United States, were from Japan. HPD was done in 397 patients (GBC n = 152) with morbidity of 79%, mortality of 41/397 (10%); median 5-year survival in GBC was 10%.

Mortality of HPD is high (6–30%) because of combination of liver failure due to inadequate liver remnant after a major liver resection and pancreatic anastomotic leak leading to fistula, collection, abscess, and sepsis. The risk of pancreatic anastomotic leak is high because the pancreas is always normal, i.e., soft with undilated duct. Moreover, majority of patients soon develop recurrence and long-term survival is anecdotal. Various options have been described to reduce the complications of PD.

1. Omental flap wrapped around the pancreatic anastomosis to cover the vessels, especially the GDA (Kapoor et al. 2016).
2. External drainage of the pancreatic duct (controlled external pancreatic fistula) and second-stage pancreaticojejunostomy. Miwa (2007)

attributed the good results (no mortality in 26 HPDs) to PBD, PVE, and external drainage of the pancreatic stump. Tokyo University reported 52 HPDs (for GBC and BDC) with 0% 90-day mortality—two-stage pancreaticojejunostomy was used in all cases (Aoki et al. 2018a).

HPD involves invasive preoperative preparation including preoperative biliary drainage (PBD) to improve liver function and preoperative portal vein embolization (PVE) to induce ipsilateral atrophy and contralateral hypertrophy. It is a complex challenging operation associated with high morbidity and mortality and actual long-term survivals are very few. Ebata et al. (2007) described HPD as a "demanding" procedure and observed "our results are not satisfactory, much more remains to be achieved." HPD *may* be performed in highly and carefully selected patients with definite expected oncological benefit, i.e., only if R0 resection status can be achieved. It should be performed by experienced surgeons in high volume specialized hepatobiliary centers. In a recent review, the Nagoya group observed that HPD, which can be performed for CC, remains controversial for GBC (Ebata et al. 2014).

Segmental/sleeve duodenal resection (Fig. 11.21a, b) and pancreatic wedge excision have been reported as alternatives to PD in patients with minimal/limited duodenal/pancreatic involvement. Kondo et al. (2002) performed sleeve resection of duodenum in patients with minimal duodenal involvement. Hirano et al. (2007) performed wedge resection of pancreas in nine patients with minimal pancreatic involvement—there was no difference in recurrence or survival versus eight patients in whom PD was performed. Ota et al. (2007) changed their policy from HPD to right hepatectomy + partial pancreatectomy and partial duodenectomy—42 such procedures were performed between 1997 and 2004—morbidity reduced to 13 (41%) and there was no mortality. Agarwal et al. (2014) reported duodenal sleeve resection (n = 27) or distal gastrectomy with proximal duodenectomy followed by gastro-jejunostomy (GJ) (n = 36) in 63 patients with gastro-duodenal (but without pancreatic) involvement; wedge resection of pancreas was performed in 7 patients and HPD in 6. Mishra et al. (2017) reported 14 gastroduodenal resections (cf. 5 HPDs) in a series of 154 resections for GBC.

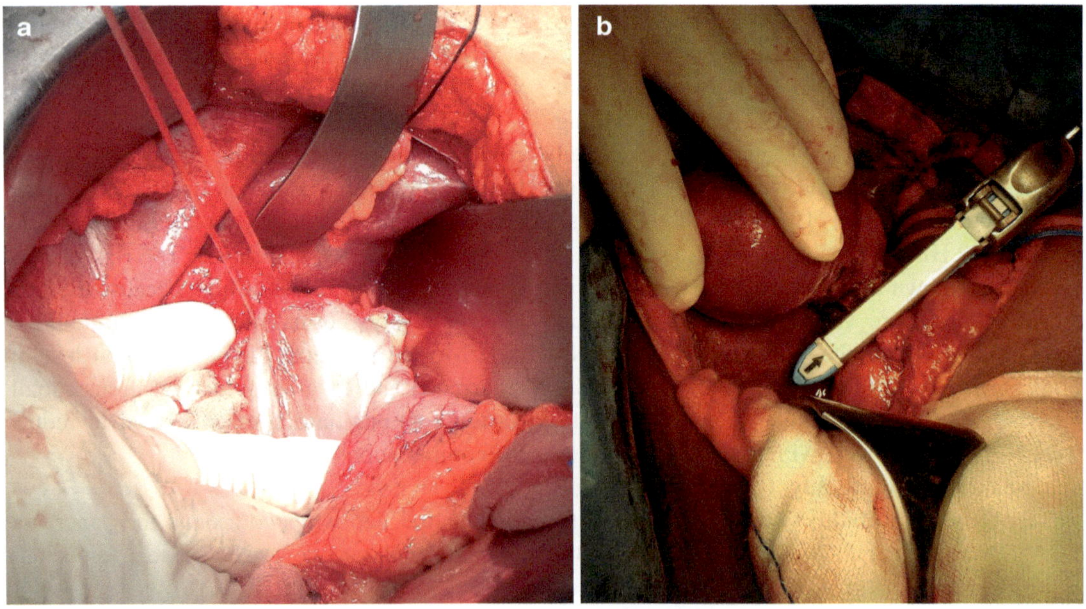

Fig. 11.21 (**a**) Minimal infiltration of the duodenum by a gall bladder cancer at operation. (**b**) Duodenal sleeve resection using a stapler (not the same patient as in Fig. 11.21a)

11.4 Combined Resection of Adjacent Organs (CRAO)

GB is an anatomically "busy" organ. Adjacent organs which can get involved in GBC are liver, omentum, duodenum, pancreas, colon, and structures in the hepato-duodenal ligament viz. CBD, proper hepatic artery (PHA) and main portal vein (MPV). Involvement of any of these organs requires adjacent organ resection to achieve R0 resection status. Minor (<2 segments) liver resection, i.e., wedge or segments IVB + V is an integral component of extended cholecystectomy; CBD excision, either as a routine in all cases or selective, i.e., as and when indicated, is also a part of extended cholecystectomy (please see Chap. 10). Major (>2 segments) hepatectomy and pancreatoduodenectomy have been discussed above. Todoroki et al. (1999) reported 27 patients with stage IV disease who underwent resection—combined resection of adjacent organs (CRAO, e.g., stomach, duodenum, colon, abdominal wall was done in as many 17 of these patients. CRAO was required in 113 out of 327 resections reported by Agarwal et al. (2014). The Nagoya University Japan group reported CRAO (other than liver and CBD) in 88/165 (53%) patients with advanced (T3 and T4) GBC (Igami et al. 2014).

Miyazaki et al. (1996) classified involvement of adjacent organs as follows

- Type I: a: hepatic involvement
  - b: hepatic involvement + gastrointestinal (gastroduodenal, colonic) involvement
- II: a: bile duct involvement
  - b: bile duct involvement + gastrointestinal (gastroduodenal, colonic) involvement
- III: a: both hepatic and bile duct involvement
  - b: both hepatic and bile duct involvement + gastrointestinal (gastroduodenal, colonic) involvement
- IV: gastrointestinal (gastroduodenal, colonic) involvement alone (without hepatic or bile duct involvement)

This classification, however, does not mention pancreatic involvement, which is important for deciding resectability of the lesion.

Hepatic involvement needs liver resection, the extent of which depends on the extent of liver infiltration. Bile duct involvement necessitates CBD excision. If the bile duct involvement extends proximally into the hilum, hepatectomy may be required. If the bile duct involvement extends distally into the intrapancreatic part of the CBD, PD will be required. Involvement of the pyloric antrum (Fig. 11.22) may require a distal gastrectomy. Most reports mention duodeno-pancreatic involvement as unresectable disease; the other option is to combine EC with PD which is an acceptable option. Patients who would oth-

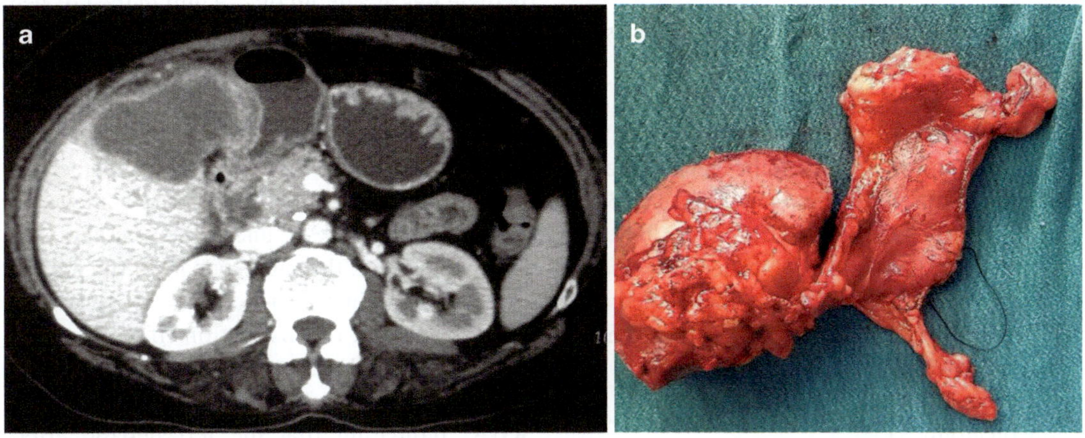

Fig. 11.22 CT shows gall bladder cancer involving the pyloric antrum—this may require distal gastrectomy; (**b**) Extended cholecystectomy with distal gastrectomy for gall bladder cancer infiltrating the pylorus (not the same patient as in Fig. 11.22a) (Image courtesy Dr Ajit Mishra, Ramkrishna Care Hospital Raipur)

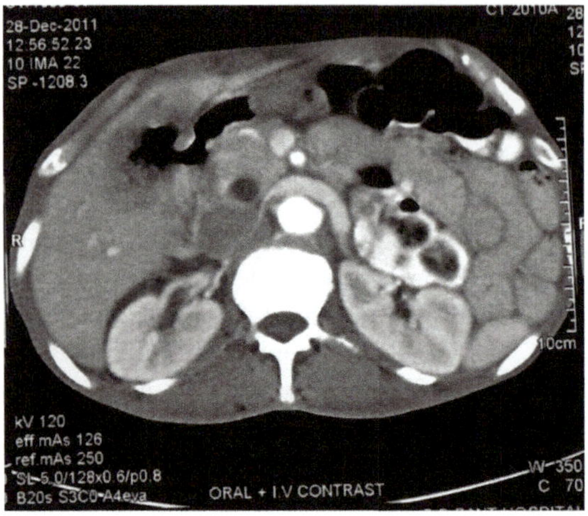

Fig. 11.23 CT shows a fistula between the GB and colon in GBC. (Image courtesy Dr. Amit Javed, GB Pant Hospital New Delhi)

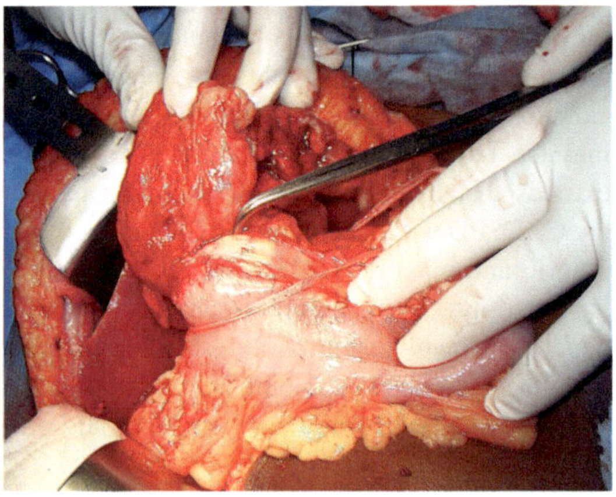

Fig. 11.24 Gall bladder cancer involving the transverse colon may require segmental colonic resection

erwise require a major hepatectomy would then need HPD. Involvement of the hepatic flexure and proximal transverse colon (Figs. 11.23 and 11.24) is fairly common in GBC; it can be easily handled by combining EC with sleeve/segmental resection of colon or right hemicolectomy. Agarwal et al. (2014) reported 327 resections for GBC (2006–2012)—colonic resection was performed in 33 patients (sleeve/segment 25, right hemicolectomy 8).

Need for CRAO is a predictor for poor survival; even after R0 resection, 5-year and median survival were lower (16% vs. 36% and 0.8 years vs. 3.8 years) in patients who required CRAO than in those who did not (Nishio et al. 2011).

11.5 Vascular Resection

Structures in the hepato-duodenal ligament (HDL) viz. CBD, PHA and MPV are frequently involved in GBC neck.

Shimizu et al. (2004) defined four types of invasion of the hepato-duodenal ligament in GBC

1. Direct extramural spread
2. Continuous intramural spread
3. Distant spread separate from the primary tumor
4. Spread of cancer cells from metastatic LNs

While involvement of the CBD alone is manageable with CBD excision, involvement of the proper hepatic artery (PHA) (Fig. 11.25) or main portal vein (MPV) (Fig. 11.26) is a contraindication for resection.

Technically speaking, R0 resection status can still be achieved by vascular (PHA and MPV) resection and reconstruction, as is done in cholangiocarcinoma, but outcome in GBC is poor cf. cholangiocarcinoma, where vascular (especially portal venous) resection is a justified procedure and is recommended.

In the region of the GB neck, the right portal pedicle lies at a depth of 2–9 mm in the GB bed. GB neck tumor with even minimal liver infiltration may, therefore, involve the right portal pedicle even though MPV and PHA are free. Involvement of the right portal pedicle in the GB neck bed necessitates a right hepatectomy (with segment IV, i.e., ERH) to achieve R0 resection status. An uncommon situation is involvement of the right hepatic artery alone (portal vein being free)—excision of RHA with or even without reconstruction (if the right PV is free) can be done, especially if there is backflow of blood from the divided distal end of the RHA, indicating that the left hepatic artery (LHA) is supplying blood to the right lobe via interlobar arterial communications (Miyazaki et al. 2000; Sakamoto et al. 2006). Higuchi

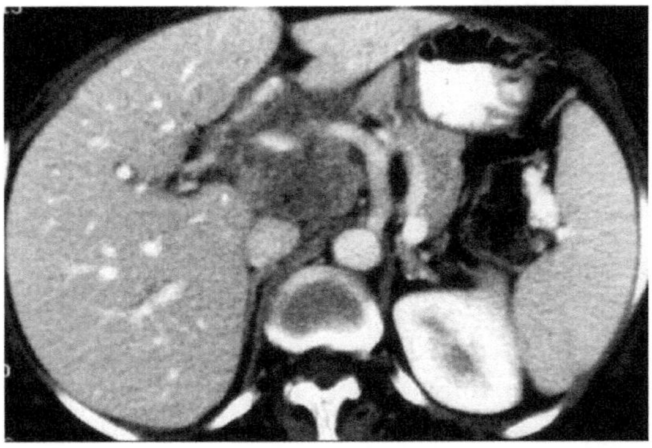

Fig. 11.25 CT shows a large hepato-duodenal ligament mass encircling the proper hepatic artery (PHA)—gall bladder cancer involving the PHA is a contraindication for resection

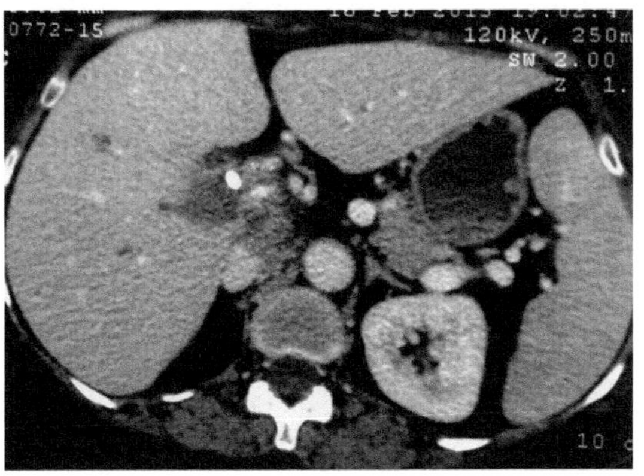

Fig. 11.26 CT shows a gall bladder tumor infiltrating the hepato-duodenal ligament; the main portal vein (MPV) is reduced to a chink—gall bladder cancer involving the MPV is a contraindication for resection

(2014) reported 56 vascular resections in 274 patients with advanced GBC—hepatic artery was resected but not reconstructed in 10 patients.

Segmental resection or wedge (sleeve) resection of PV wall was described by Nimura et al. (1991a). The Nagoya University Japan group reported resection in 72 patients with stage IV GBC—mortality was 14 (19%)—portal vein resection was an independent risk factor for hospital death (Kondo et al. 2003). Shimizu et al. (2007) reported 79 resections for stage IV GBC—major vascular resections were performed in 17 patients. Kurosaki et al. (2008) reported median survival of only 6.8 months in GBC (vs. 37 months in hilar CC and 20 months in pancreatic cancer); vascular resection was accompanied by dismal outcome in GBC and should not be recommended. The Nagoya University Japan group recommends portal vein resection but says that hepatic artery resection is not justified for GBC (Igami et al. 2014).

Shimada et al. (2003) reported both PV and HA resection in GBC. In presence of hepatic arterial invasion, survival after resection is as poor as in unresectable disease (Yamamoto et al. 2017). Fukami et al. (2016) reported 38 HPDs with HA resection in 12 patients—they recommended hepatic artery resection for BDC only but cautioned that it should not be performed for GBC because of poor outcome.

11.6 Metastatic GBC

Unlike many other cancers, e.g., colorectal, breast, genitourinary, where cure is possible even in presence of metastases and surgical resection of the primary (and even metastases) is recommended, presence of a distant metastasis, including a distant LN, is an absolute contraindication for surgical resection in GBC.

Four hundred and twenty-one GBCs were operated at the Seoul National University Hospital (SNUH) South Korea from 1996 to 2010—94 had stage IV (16 stage IVA and 78 stage IVB) disease. Benefit of resection was seen in patients with isolated liver metastasis near (within 3 cm of) the GB bed ($n = 4$, median survival 32 vs. 9 months after no resection $n = 16$) or limited (<3) number of small (2–3 mm) peritoneal implantations ($n = 5$, median survival 20 months vs. 6 months in those with large peritoneal implantations $n = 31$). Three-stage IVb patients survived for 39, 57, and 109 months, respectively. The authors recommended surgical resection in carefully selected subset of patients with distant metastases (stage IVb) (Kang et al. 2012). Many Japanese centers/surgeons have an aggressive approach towards advanced, even metastatic GBC. As many as 141 out of 382 patients operated at the Tokyo Women's Medical University (TWMU) Japan (1969–2012) had stage IVB disease—5-year survival was as high as 19% (Higuchi and Yamamoto 2014).

The Nagoya University Japan group (Amemiya 2008) reported 13-year recurrence-free survival after central hepatic bisectionectomy and para-aortic lymphadenectomy followed by percutaneous ethanol injection (PEI) and transcatheter arterial chemoembolization (TACE) of liver metastases followed by dissection of LNs around and resection of external iliac artery followed by radiotherapy of paraesophageal LNs. Long-term (>7 years after initial surgery and >3 years after resection of the peritoneal metastasis) survival was reported in a patient who underwent resection (along with chemotherapy) of a peritoneal recurrence after initial surgery (Tomita et al. 2016). Kuga et al. (2017) reported long-term (6 years) survival after neoadjuvant chemotherapy and right hepatectomy, extrahepatic bile duct resection (EHBDR), partial duodenectomy, and partial colectomy in a patient with T3N0M1 Stage IVB GBC. The authors, in these reports, claimed the long survival to the aggressive treatment but the Author (VKK) feels these are anecdotal examples probably due to the good biology of the tumor.

Liver can be involved in GBC in two ways

1. Direct infiltration of liver parenchyma (Fig. 11.27) which can be handled by liver resection, the extent of which, i.e., liver wedge, segments IVB + V or ERH will depend on the extent of liver infiltration.
2. Metastases to liver (Fig. 11.28) through hematogenous spread via cholecysto-hepatic veins—these metastases are usually away from the GB bed but can be close to the GB (satellite nodules).

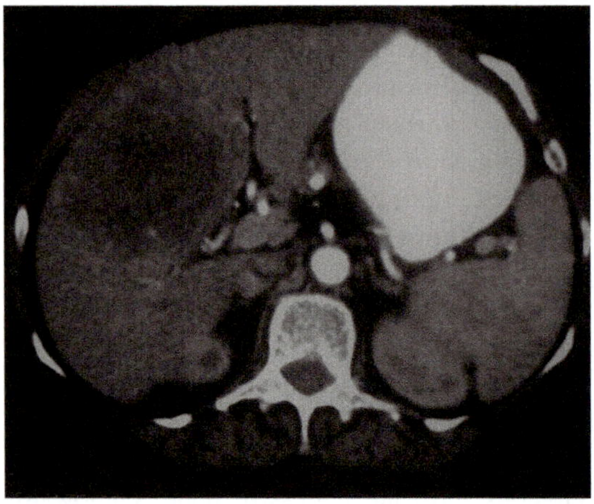

Fig. 11.27 CT shows a large necrotic mass involving segments V and IV (falciform ligament is free); this will require extended right hepatectomy—direct infiltration of the liver (of any extent) can be treated with a major liver resection

Some students/surgeons have a misconception that the satellite nodules are local spread and are not metastases and should be resected. Also, it is very tempting to think that if the metastases are located in the part of the liver that will be resected

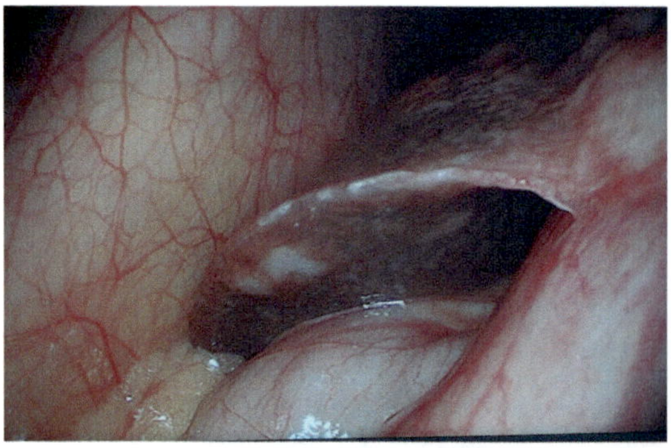

Fig. 11.28 Liver metastasis, irrespective of site, number, and size, is a contraindication for resection

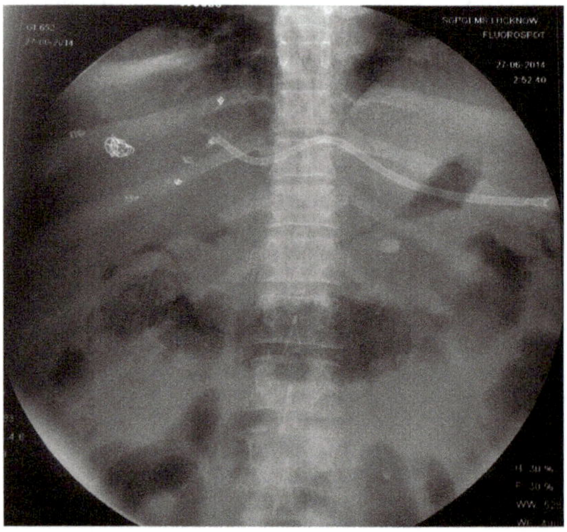

Fig. 11.29 X-ray shows coils of portal vein embolization (PVE) in the right lobe of liver and percutaneous transhepatic biliary drainage (PTBD) in situ—major hepatic resections for gall bladder cancer require extensive invasive preoperative preparation including PTBD or ENBD and PVE

i.e. wedge, segment IVB + V or ERH, an R0 resection can be achieved and survival can be prolonged. But this, in the opinion of the Author (VKK), is not true; a liver metastasis is a metastasis irrespective of its site, size, and number.

Unlike hepatocellular carcinoma (HCC), cholangiocarcinoma (CC) and neuroendocrine tumors (NET) where total hepatectomy and liver transplant are an option in presence of liver metastases, there is no place for liver transplant in GBC.

Major resections including extended right hepatectomy (ERH), hepato-pancreato-duodenectomy (HPD), and combined resection of adjacent organs (CRAO) are required in advanced GBC but these procedures require extensive invasive preoperative preparations including PTBD or ENBD and PVE (Fig. 11.29)*; the morbidity and mortality of these procedures remain high, while the benefits in term of long-term survival are anecdotal.*

Invited Commentary on Major Resections for Gall Bladder Cancer

Junichi Kaneko and Kiyoshi Hasegawa

Gall bladder cancer (GBC) is difficult to diagnose in the early stage due to the absence of specific signs or symptoms. As for advanced GBC, no appropriate treatment has been established. Prof. Kapoor has covered one of the important clinical topics of GBC in full detail. We congratulate him on his valuable review. We agree with him that the surgical indications for advanced GBC must be cautiously considered due to the poor postoperative outcomes. On the other hand, no other effective treatment choices provide better outcomes than surgery. Here we discuss our views concerning the optimal treatments for advanced GBC.

Radical cholecystectomy for T1 or T2 GBC is the standard procedure for achieving an R0 resection, but the appropriate operative procedures for T3 or T4 GBC and/or GBC with lymph node metastasis remain under debate. Goussous and colleagues reported a 90-day mortality rate of 17% according to a national cancer database of the United States (Goussous et al. 2017b), in which 59% of patients were T1 or T2 and the remaining 41% were T3 or T4. Although a 90-day mortality rate of 17% is high, we stress that treatment-related and disease-related deaths must be considered separately when evaluating the effects of each treatment choice. Because the presence of lymph node metastasis is clearly a poor prognostic factor, GBC with extensive lymph node metastasis is not a good indication for surgery. Accurately diagnosing the extent of GBC is important for deciding the optimal choice. An intraoperative step-by-step regional lymph node dissection would be helpful, as we have advocated (Kokudo et al. 2003b). On the other hand, an aggressive surgical strategy against locally advanced GBC may be justified because of the poor efficacy of nonsurgical treatments, such as chemotherapy and radiotherapy, if zero or very low postoperative mortality is achieved.

Although hepato-pancreatoduodenectomy (HPD) is a highly invasive procedure, it may be applicable for advanced GBC. Generally, GBC directly invades in two directions: the liver bed in contact with the gallbladder and lymphatic metastasis alongside the pancreas head. Pancreatoduodenectomy is required for lymphatic metastasis (Clavien et al. 2007). For example, in the distribution of positive lymph nodes in pN2 cases, the posterosuperior peripancreatic nodes (N13a) were the most prevalent metastatic sites (79% positive rate) (Kokudo et al. 2003b). In addition, HPD can achieve R0 resection for locally advanced GBC invading the right side of the hepatoduodenal ligament. Thus, HPD has a potential oncologic advantage for obtaining an R0 resection for T3 or T4 GBC (Manterola et al. 2019).

Major and extensive surgical resection, including HPD, for advanced T3 or T4 GBC remains a challenging procedure, however, because of the high-mortality rate of extensive surgical resections (13–17%) (Nimura et al. 1991; Kondo et al. 2000b). A decade after introduction of HPD for advanced T3 or T4 GBC, the Japanese Society of Hepato-Biliary-Pancreatic Surgery reported an HPD-associated in-hospital mortality rate of 8% (Aoki et al. 2018b). Although there are very few reports of major liver resection for GBC from the West, nationwide data from the United States indicate that the mortality rate of hemihepatectomy plus pancreatoduodenectomy is still relatively high—a

30-day mortality rate of 8% and an in-hospital mortality rate of 18% (Tran et al. 2015). Considering that these high mortality rates are due to the invasiveness of HPD procedures, HPD may not be a good choice, as mentioned by Prof. Kapoor.

Recently, however, we reported zero 90-day mortality in 52 HPDs for GBC ($n = 13$) and bile duct cancer ($n = 39$), suggesting that nearly zero-mortality is no longer unrealistic (Aoki et al. 2018b). The majority of GBC patients (85%) had a T classification of pT3 or T4. Among the 52 patients, 54% underwent combined resection including the portal vein ($n = 2$), hepatic artery ($n = 1$), and/or colon ($n = 6$). Among the 13 GBC patients, an R0 resection was achieved in 8 (62%) and an R1 resection was achieved in the remaining 5 (38%) patients. Thirty-eight percent of all the patients were UICC stage III and 54% were stage IV. In our report, the 1, 3, and 5-year overall survival rate for all 52 patients was 79%, 48%, and 45%, respectively.

Our strategy of using HPD to treat GBC has five essential elements. First, to relieve jaundice before surgery, an endoscopic approach is preferred (Aoki et al. 2018b). Second, preoperative portal vein embolization should be performed. Third, the future remnant liver volume must be precisely estimated by virtual hepatectomy using surgical planning software during pre- and post-portal vein embolization (Mise et al. 2018). Fourth, a quantitative liver-function test should be performed preoperatively using indocyanine green (ICG) dye (i.e., the rate of retention of indocyanine green determined at 15 min) (Clavien et al. 2007). Lastly, a two-stage pancreaticojejunostomy should be performed to avoid a postoperative pancreatic fistula from the anastomosis (Aoki et al. 2018b; Hasegawa et al. 2008). Certainly, although complicated preoperative preparations and procedures are required, up-to-date interventional radiology and an operating room equipped with information technology may provide the required support for confident medical specialists. HPD should only be performed with adequate preparation and in limited institutions with well-trained staff.

Further studies are required to determine the type of GBC patient that should undergo an extensive operation like HPD to obtain long-term survival. With the recent progress in chemotherapy, extensive surgery together with chemotherapy may provide satisfactory outcomes for advanced GBC patients in the near future. The development of safer surgical techniques and more effective chemotherapy is eagerly anticipated for patients with advanced GBC.

References

Chapter References

Agarwal AK, Mandal S, Singh S, Bhojwani R, Sakhuja P, Uppal R. Biliary obstruction in gall bladder cancer is not sine qua non of inoperability. Ann Surg Oncol. 2007a;14(10):2831–7.

Agarwal AK, Mandal S, Singh S, Sakhuja P, Puri S. Gallbladder cancer with duodenal infiltration: is it still resectable? J Gastrointest Surg. 2007b; 11(12):1722–7. Epub 2007 Sep 29.

Agarwal AK, Javed A, Raja K, Sakhuja P. Surgical techniques in the management of primary gall bladder cancer. In: Agarwal A, Fong Y, editors. Carcinoma of the gall bladder. New Delhi: Elsevier; 2014. p. 106–29.

Amemiya T, Yokoyama Y, Oda K, Nishio H, Ebata T, Abe T, Igami T, Nagino M, Nimura Y. A patient with gallbladder cancer with paraaortic lymph node and hepatic metastases who has survived for more than 13 years after the primary extended radical operation. J Hepatobiliary Pancreat Surg. 2008;15(6):648–51. https://doi.org/10.1007/s00534-007-1316-4. Epub 2008 Nov 7. PMID: 18987937.

Aoki T, Sakamoto Y, Kohno Y, Akamatsu N, Kaneko J, Sugawara Y, Hasegawa K, Makuuchi M, Kokudo N. Hepatopancreaticoduodenectomy for biliary cancer: strategies for near-zero operative mortality and acceptable long-term outcome. Ann Surg. 2018a;267(2):332–7. https://doi.org/10.1097/SLA.0000000000002059.

Benoist S, Panis Y, Fagniez PL. Long-term results after curative resection for carcinoma of the gallbladder. French University Association for Surgical Research. Am J Surg. 1998;175(2):118–22.

Bloechle C, Izbicki JR, Passlick B, et al. Is radical surgery in locally advanced gallbladder carcinoma justified? Am J Gastroenterol. 1995;90:2195–200.

D'Angelica M, Dalal KM, DeMatteo RP, Fong Y, Blumgart LH, Jarnagin WR. Analysis of the extent of resection for adenocarcinoma of the gallbladder. Ann Surg Oncol. 2009;16(4):806–16.

D'Souza MA, Valdimarsson VT, Campagnaro T, et al. Hepatopancreatoduodenectomy - a controversial treatment for bile duct and gallbladder cancer from a European perspective. HPB (Oxford). 2019; https://doi.org/10.1016/j.hpb.2019.12.008.

Dasari BVM, Ionescu MI, Pawlik TM, Hodson J, Sutcliffe RP, Roberts KJ, Muiesan P, Isaac J, Marudanayagam R, Mirza DF. Outcomes of surgical resection of gallbladder cancer in patients presenting with jaundice: a systematic review and meta-analysis. J Surg Oncol. 2018;118(3):477–85. https://doi.org/10.1002/jso.25186. Review.

Dixon E, Vollmer CM Jr, Sahajpal A, Cattral M, Grant D, Doig C, Hemming A, Taylor B, Langer B, Greig P, Gallinger S. An aggressive surgical approach leads to improved survival in patients with gallbladder cancer: a 12-year study at a North American Center. Ann Surg. 2005;241(3):385–94.

Ebata T, Nagino M, Nishio H, Arai T, Nimura Y. Right hepatopancreatoduodenectomy: improvements over 23 years to attain acceptability. J Hepatobiliary Pancreat Surg. 2007;14(2):131–5. Epub 2007 Mar 27.

Ebata T, Yokoyama Y, Igami T, Sugawara G, Takahashi Y, Nimura Y, Nagino M. Hepatopancreatoduodenectomy for cholangiocarcinoma: a single-center review of 85 consecutive patients. Ann Surg. 2012a;256(2):297–305. https://doi.org/10.1097/SLA.0b013e31826029ca.

Ebata T, Yokoyama Y, Igami T, Sugawara G, Takahashi Y, Nagino M. Portal vein embolization before extended hepatectomy for biliary cancer: current technique and review of 494 consecutive embolizations. Dig Surg. 2012b;29(1):23–9. https://doi.org/10.1159/000335718. Epub 2012 Mar 15.

Ebata T, Yokoyama Y, Igami T, Sugawara G, Mizuno T, Nagino M. Review of hepatopancreatoduodenectomy for biliary cancer: an extended radical approach of Japanese origin. J Hepatobiliary Pancreat Sci. 2014;21(8):550–5. https://doi.org/10.1002/jhbp.80. Epub 2014 Jan 27. Review.

Fernandes Ede S, Mello FT, Ribeiro-Filho J, Monte-Filho AP, Fernandes MM, Coelho RJ, Matos MC, Souza AA, Torres OJ. The largest western experience with hepatopancreatoduodenectomy: lessons learned with 35 cases. Arq Bras Cir Dig. 2016;29(1):17–20. https://doi.org/10.1590/0102-6720201600010005. English, Portuguese.

Fukami Y, Kaneoka Y, Maeda A, Takayama Y, Onoe S. Major hepatopancreatoduodenectomy with simultaneous resection of the hepatic artery for advanced biliary cancer. Langenbecks Arch Surg. 2016;401(4):471–8. https://doi.org/10.1007/s00423-016-1413-4. Epub 2016 Mar 29.

Goussous N, Hosseini M, Sill AM, Cunningham SC. Minimally invasive and open gallbladder cancer resections: 30- vs 90-day mortality. Hepatobiliary Pancreat Dis Int. 2017a;16(4):405–11. https://doi.org/10.1016/S1499-3872(17)60025-0.

Haga Y, Miyamoto A, Wada Y, Takami Y, Takeuchi H. Value of E-PASS models for predicting postoperative morbidity and mortality in resection of perihilar cholangiocarcinoma and gallbladder carcinoma. HPB (Oxford). 2016;18(3):271–8. https://doi.org/10.1016/j.hpb.2015.09.001. Epub 2015 Nov 18.

Hawkins WG, DeMatteo RP, Jarnagin WR, Ben-Porat L, Blumgart LH, Fong Y. Jaundice predicts advanced disease and early mortality in patients with gallbladder cancer. Ann Surg Oncol. 2004;11(3):310–5.

Hemming AW, Magliocca JF, Fujita S, Kayler LK, Hochwald S, Zendejas I, Kim RD. Combined resection of the liver and pancreas for malignancy. J Am Coll Surg. 2010;210(5):808–14, 814–6. https://doi.org/10.1016/j.jamcollsurg.2009.12.007.

Higuchi R, Yamamoto M. Aggressive surgical management and treatment outcomes of gallbladder cancer. In: Agarwal A, Fong Y, editors. Carcinoma of the gall bladder. New Delhi: Elsevier; 2014. p. 175–83.

Higuchi R, Ota T, Araida T, Kajiyama H, Yazawa T, Furukawa T, Yoshikawa T, Takasaki K, Yamamoto M. Surgical approaches to advanced gallbladder cancer: a 40-year single-institution study of prognostic factors and resectability. Ann Surg Oncol. 2014;21(13):4308–16. https://doi.org/10.1245/s10434-014-3885-1. Epub 2014 Jul 15.

Higuchi R, Yazawa T, Uemura S, Izumo W, Chaudhary RJ, Furukawa T, Yamamoto M. ENBD is associated with decreased tumor dissemination compared to PTBD in perihilar cholangiocarcinoma. J Gastrointest Surg. 2017;21(9):1506–14. https://doi.org/10.1007/s11605-017-3492-0. Epub 2017 Jul 18.

Hirano S, Tanaka E, Shichinohe T, Saitoh K, Takeuchi M, Senmaru N, Suzuki O, Kondo S. Feasibility of en-bloc wedge resection of the pancreas and/or the duodenum as an alternative to pancreatoduodenectomy for advanced gallbladder cancer. J Hepatobiliary Pancreat Surg. 2007;14(2):149–54. Epub 2007 Mar 27.

Hwang KY, Yoon YI, Hwang S, Ha TY, Ahn CS, Kim KH, Moon DB, Song GW, Jung DH, Lee YJ, Park KM, Lee SG. Survival analysis following resection of AJCC stage III gallbladder carcinoma based on different combinations of T and N stages. Korean J Hepatobiliary Pancreat Surg. 2015;19(1):11–6. https://doi.org/10.14701/kjhbps.2015.19.1.11. Epub 2015 Feb 28

Igami T, Ebata T, Yokoyama Y, Sugawara G, Nagino M. Advanced resectable gallbladder cancer: diagnosis and surgical approach. In: Agarwal A, Fong Y, editors. Carcinoma of the gall bladder. New Delhi: Elsevier; 2014. p. 89–105.

Jin LX, Pitt SC, Hall BL, Pitt HA. Aggressive surgical management of gallbladder cancer: at what cost? Surgery. 2013;154(2):266–73. https://doi.org/10.1016/j.surg.2013.04.022. Epub 2013 Jul 2.

Kaneoka Y, Yamaguchi A, Isogai M, Harada T, Suzuki M. Hepatoduodenal ligament invasion by gallbladder carcinoma: histologic patterns and surgical recommendation. World J Surg. 2003;27(3):260–5. https://doi.org/10.1007/s00268-002-6702-0.

Kaneoka Y, Maeda A, Isogai M. En bloc resection of the hepatoduodenal ligament for advanced biliary malignancy. J Gastrointest Surg. 2015;19(4):708–14. https://doi.org/10.1007/s11605-014-2731-x. Epub 2015 Jan 6.

Kang MJ, Song Y, Jang JY, Han IW, Kim SW. Role of radical surgery in patients with stage IV gallbladder cancer. HPB (Oxford). 2012;14(12):805–11. https://doi.org/10.1111/j.1477-2574.2012.00544.x. Epub 2012 Aug 20.

Kapoor VK. Advanced gallbladder cancer: Indian "middle path". J Hepatobiliary Pancreat Surg. 2007;14(4):366–73. Epub 2007 Jul 30.

Kapoor VK. Gall bladder cancer and jaundice – the yellow signal. Clin Med Rev Oncol. 2015;5:1–3.

Kapoor VK, Gupta N, Behari A, Sharma S, Kumar A, Prakash A, Singh RK, Kumar A, Saxena R. Omental flap to protect gastro-duodenal artery stump from pancreatic anastomotic leak in pancreato-duodenectomy. J Pancreas. 2016;17:289–93.

Kawarada Y, Isaji S, Taoka H, Tabata M, Das BC, Yokoi H. S4a + S5 with caudate lobe (S1) resection using the Taj Mahal liver parenchymal resection for carcinoma of the biliary tract. J Gastrointest Surg. 1999;3(4):369–73.

Kenjo A, Miyata H, Gotoh M, Kitagawa Y, Shimada M, Baba H, Tomita N, Kimura W, Sugihara K, Mori M. Risk stratification of 7,732 hepatectomy cases in 2011 from the National Clinical Database for Japan. J Am Coll Surg. 2014;218(3):412–22. https://doi.org/10.1016/j.jamcollsurg.2013.11.007. Epub 2013 Nov 16.

Kishi Y, Shimada K, Hata S, Oguro S, Sakamoto Y, Nara S, Esaki M, Hiraoka N, Kosuge T. Definition of T3/4 and regional lymph nodes in gallbladder cancer: which is more valid, the UICC or the Japanese staging system? Ann Surg Oncol. 2012;19(11):3567–73. https://doi.org/10.1245/s10434-012-2599-5. Epub 2012 Aug 14.

Kishi Y, Shimada K, Nara S, Esaki M, Kosuge T. The type of preoperative biliary drainage predicts short-term outcome after major hepatectomy. Langenbecks Arch Surg. 2016;401(4):503–11. https://doi.org/10.1007/s00423-016-1427-y. Epub 2016 Apr 13.

Kokudo N, Makuuchi M, Natori T, Sakamoto Y, Yamamoto J, Seki M, Noie T, Sugawara Y, Imamura H, Asahara S, Ikari T. Strategies for surgical treatment of gallbladder carcinoma based on information available before resection. Arch Surg. 2003a;138(7):741–50; discussion 750.

Kondo S, Nimura Y, Hayakawa N, Kamiya J, Nagino M, Uesaka K. Regional and para-aortic lymphadenectomy in radical surgery for advanced gallbladder carcinoma. Br J Surg. 2000a;87(4):418–22.

Kondo S, Nimura Y, Hayakawa N, Kamiya J, Nagino M, Uesaka K. Extensive surgery for carcinoma of the gallbladder. Br J Surg. 2002;89(2):179–84.

Kondo S, Nimura Y, Kamiya J, Nagino M, Kanai M, Uesaka K, Yuasa N, Sano T, Hayakawa N. Factors influencing postoperative hospital mortality and long-term survival after radical resection for stage IV gallbladder carcinoma. World J Surg. 2003;27(3):272–7. Epub 2003 Feb 27.

Kuga D, Ebata T, Yokoyama Y, Igami T, Sugawara G, Mizuno T, Yamaguchi J, Nagino M. Long-term survival after multidisciplinary therapy for residual gallbladder cancer with peritoneal dissemination: a case report. Surg Case Rep. 2017;3(1):76. https://doi.org/10.1186/s40792-017-0351-x. Epub 2017 Jun 14.

Kurosaki I, Hatakeyama K, Minagawa M, Sato D. Portal vein resection in surgery for cancer of biliary tract and pancreas: special reference to the relationship between the surgical outcome and site of primary tumor. J Gastrointest Surg. 2008;12(5):907–18. Epub 2007 Oct 30.

Lim CS, Jang JY, Lee SE, Kang MJ, Kim SW. Reappraisal of hepatopancreatoduodenectomy as a treatment modality for bile duct and gallbladder cancer. J Gastrointest Surg. 2012;16(5):1012–8. https://doi.org/10.1007/s11605-012-1826-5. Epub 2012 Jan 24.

Margonis GA, Gani F, Buettner S, et al. Rates and patterns of recurrence after curative intent resection for gallbladder cancer: a multi-institution analysis from the US Extra-hepatic Biliary Malignancy Consortium. HPB (Oxford). 2016;18:872–8.

Mishra PK, Saluja SS, Prithiviraj N, Varshney V, Goel N, Patil N. Predictors of curative resection and long term survival of gallbladder cancer - a retrospective analysis. Am J Surg. 2017;214(2):278–86. https://doi.org/10.1016/j.amjsurg.2017.02.006. Epub 2017 Feb 9.

Miwa S, Kobayashi A, Akahane Y, Nakata T, Mihara M, Kusama K, Ogawa S, Soeda J, Miyagawa S. Is major hepatectomy with pancreatoduodenectomy justified for advanced biliary malignancy? J Hepatobiliary Pancreat Surg. 2007;14(2):136–41. https://doi.org/10.1007/s00534-006-1107-3. Epub 2007 Mar 27. PMID: 17384903.

Miyagawa S, Makuuchi M, Kawasaki S, Hayashi K, Harada H, Kitamura H, Seki H. Outcome of major hepatectomy with pancreatoduodenectomy for advanced biliary malignancies. World J Surg. 1996;20(1):77–80.

Miyazaki M, Itoh H, Ambiru S, Shimizu H, Togawa A, Gohchi E, Nakajima N, Suwa T. Radical surgery for advanced gallbladder carcinoma. Br J Surg. 1996;83(4):478–81.

Miyazaki M, Ito H, Nakagawa K, Ambiru S, Shimizu H, Yoshidome H, Shimizu Y, Okaya T, Mitsuhashi N, Wakabayashi Y, Nakajima N. Unilateral hepatic artery reconstruction is unnecessary in biliary tract carcinomas involving lobar hepatic artery: implications of interlobar hepatic artery and its preservation. Hepatogastroenterology. 2000;47(36):1526–30.

Mizuno T, Ebata T, Yokoyama Y, Igami T, Yamaguchi J, Onoe S, Watanabe N, Ando M, Nagino M. Major hepatectomy with or without pancreatoduodenectomy for advanced gallbladder cancer. Br J Surg. 2019;106(5):626–35. https://doi.org/10.1002/bjs.11088. Epub 2019 Feb 14.

Nasu Y, Hirano S, Tsuchikawa T, Shichinohe T. Aggressive surgery for locally advanced gallbladder cancer with obstructive jaundice: result of a prospective study. Dig Surg. 2016;33(3):213–9. https://doi.org/10.1159/000443842. Epub 2016 Feb 27.

Nimura Y, Hayakawa N, Kamiya J, Maeda S, Kondo S, Yasui A, Shionoya S. Combined portal vein and liver resection for carcinoma of the biliary tract. Br J Surg. 1991a;78(6):727–31.

Nimura Y, Hayakawa N, Kamiya J, Maeda S, Kondo S, Yasui A, Shionoya S. Hepatopancreatoduodenectomy for advanced carcinoma of the biliary tract. Hepatogastroenterology. 1991b;38(2):170–5.

Nishio H, Ebata T, Yokoyama Y, Igami T, Sugawara G, Nagino M. Gallbladder cancer involving the extrahepatic bile duct is worthy of resection. Ann Surg. 2011;253(5):953–60. https://doi.org/10.1097/SLA.0b013e318216f5f3.

Ogura Y, Mizumoto R, Isaji S, Kusuda T, Matsuda S, Tabata M. Radical operations for carcinoma of the gallbladder: present status in Japan. World J Surg. 1991;15(3):337–43.

Ota T, Araida T, Yamamoto M, Takasaki K. Operative outcome and problems of right hepatic lobectomy with pancreatoduodenectomy for advanced carcinoma of the biliary tract. J Hepatobiliary Pancreat Surg. 2007;14(2):155–8. Epub 2007 Mar 27

Pack GT, Miller TR, Brasfield RD. Total right hepatic lobectomy for cancer of the gallbladder; report of three cases. Ann Surg. 1955;142(1):6–16.

Pottakkat B, Kapoor A, Prakash A, Singh RK, Behari A, Kumar A, Kapoor VK, Saxena R. Evaluation of a prospective surgical strategy of extended resection to achieve R0 status in gall bladder cancer. J Gastrointest Cancer. 2013;44(1):33–40. https://doi.org/10.1007/s12029-012-9432-z.

Regimbeau JM, Fuks D, Bachellier P, Le Treut YP, Pruvot FR, Navarro F, Chiche L, Farges O. Prognostic value of jaundice in patients with gallbladder cancer by the AFC-GBC-2009 study group. Eur J Surg Oncol. 2011;37(6):505–12. https://doi.org/10.1016/j.ejso.2011.03.135. Epub 2011 Apr 21.

Sakamoto Y, Sano T, Shimada K, Kosuge T, Kimata Y, Sakuraba M, Yamamoto J, Ojima H. Clinical significance of reconstruction of the right hepatic artery for biliary malignancy. Langenbecks Arch Surg. 2006;391(3):203–8. Epub 2006 Mar 9

Sakamoto Y, Nara S, Kishi Y, Esaki M, Shimada K, Kokudo N, Kosuge T. Is extended hemihepatectomy plus pancreaticoduodenectomy justified for advanced bile duct cancer and gallbladder cancer? Surgery. 2013;153(6):794–800. https://doi.org/10.1016/j.surg.2012.11.024. Epub 2013 Feb 13.

Schmelzle M, Öllinger R, Gebauer B, Podrabsky P, Pratschke J. [Stage 1-laparoscopy partial PVE-ALPPS followed by step 2-hand-assisted laparoscopic extended right hepatectomy in a patient with gallbladder cancer]. Zentralbl Chir. 2019;144(1):21–3. https://doi.org/10.1055/a-0651-0830. Epub 2018 Oct 22. German.

Shimada H, Endo I, Sugita M, Masunari H, Fujii Y, Tanaka K, Misuta K, Sekido H, Togo S. Hepatic resection combined with portal vein or hepatic artery reconstruction for advanced carcinoma of the hilar bile duct and gallbladder. World J Surg. 2003;27(10):1137–42. Epub 2003 Aug 21

Shimizu Y, Ohtsuka M, Ito H, Kimura F, Shimizu H, Togawa A, Yoshidome H, et al. Should the extrahepatic bile duct be resected for locally advanced gallbladder cancer? Surgery. 2004;136(5):1012–1017; discussion 1018. https://doi.org/10.1016/j.surg.2004.04.032.

Shimizu H, Kimura F, Yoshidome H, Ohtsuka M, Kato A, Yoshitomi H, Nozawa S, Furukawa K, Mitsuhashi N, Takeuchi D, Suda K, Yoshioka I, Miyazaki M. Aggressive surgical approach for stage IV gallbladder carcinoma based on Japanese Society of Biliary Surgery classification. J Hepatobiliary Pancreat Surg. 2007;14(4):358–65. Epub 2007 Jul 30

Takasaki K, Kobayashi S, Mutoh H, et al. Our experience (5 cases) of extended right lobectomy combined with pancreato-duodenectomy for carcinoma of the gall bladder (in Japanese). Tan to Sui. 1980;1:923–32.

Todoroki T, Kawamoto T, Takahashi H, Takada Y, Koike N, Otsuka M, Fukao K. Treatment of gallbladder cancer by radical resection. Br J Surg. 1999;86(5):622–7.

Tomita K, Takano K, Shimazu M, Okihara M, Sano T, Chiba N, Kawachi S. Long-term survival of a recurrent gallbladder carcinoma patient with lymph node and peritoneal metastases after multidisciplinary treatments: a case report. Surg Case Rep. 2016;2(1):12. https://doi.org/10.1186/s40792-016-0135-8. Epub 2016 Feb 11.

Tran TB, Norton JA, Ethun CG, Pawlik TM, Buettner S, Schmidt C, Beal EW, Hawkins WG, Fields RC, Krasnick BA, Weber SM, Salem A, Martin RCG, Scoggins CR, Shen P, Mogal HD, Idrees K, Isom CA, Hatzaras I, Shenoy R, Maithel SK, Poultsides GA. Gallbladder cancer presenting with jaundice: uniformly fatal or still potentially curable? J Gastrointest Surg. 2017;21(8):1245–53. https://doi.org/10.1007/s11605-017-3440-z. Epub 2017 May 11.

Tsui TY, Heumann A, Vashist YK, Izbicki JR. How we do it: double in situ split for staged mesohepatectomy in patients with advanced gall bladder cancer and marginal future liver remnant. Langenbecks Arch Surg. 2016;401(4):565–71. https://doi.org/10.1007/s00423-016-1410-7. Epub 2016 Mar 30.

Varma V, Gupta S, Soin AS, Nundy S. Does the presence of jaundice and/or a lump in a patient with gall bladder cancer mean that the lesion is not resectable? Dig Surg. 2009;26(4):306–11. https://doi.org/10.1159/000231880. Epub 2009 Aug 5.

Wakai T, Shirai Y, Tsuchiya Y, Nomura T, Akazawa K, Hatakeyama K. Combined major hepatectomy and pancreaticoduodenectomy for locally advanced biliary carcinoma: long-term results. World J Surg. 2008;32(6):1067–74. https://doi.org/10.1007/s00268-007-9393-8.

Yamamoto Y, Sugiura T, Okamura Y, Ito T, Ashida R, Uemura S, Miyata T, Kato Y, Uesaka K. Is combined pancreatoduodenectomy for advanced gallbladder cancer justified? Surgery. 2016;159(3):810–20. https://doi.org/10.1016/j.surg.2015.09.009. Epub 2015 Oct 23.

Yamamoto Y, Sugiura T, Ashida R, Okamura Y, Ito T, Uesaka K. Indications for major hepatectomy and combined procedures for advanced gallbladder cancer. Br J Surg. 2017;104(3):257–66. https://doi.org/10.1002/bjs.10401. Epub 2016 Nov 16.

Yang XW, Yuan JM, Chen JY, Yang J, Gao QG, Yan XZ, Zhang BH, Feng S, Wu MC. The prognostic importance of jaundice in surgical resection with curative intent for gallbladder cancer. BMC Cancer. 2014;14:652. https://doi.org/10.1186/1471-2407-14-652.

Yokoyama Y, Nishio H, Ebata T, Igami T, Sugawara G, Nagino M. Value of indocyanine green clearance of the future liver remnant in predicting outcome after resection for biliary cancer. Br J Surg. 2010;97(8):1260–8. https://doi.org/10.1002/bjs.7084.

Zhou Y, Zhang Z, Wu L, Li B. A systematic review of safety and efficacy of hepatopancreatoduodenectomy for biliary and gallbladder cancers. HPB (Oxford). 2016;18(1):1–6. https://doi.org/10.1016/j.hpb.2015.07.008. Epub 2015 Nov 30. Review.

References for Commentary Notes

Clavien PA, Petrowsky H, DeOliveira ML, Graf R. Strategies for safer liver surgery and partial liver transplantation. N Engl J Med. 2007;356(15):1545–59.

Hasegawa K, Kokudo N, Sano K, Seyama Y, Aoki T, Ikeda M, et al. Two-stage pancreatojejunostomy in pancreaticoduodenectomy: a retrospective analysis of short-term results. Am J Surg. 2008;196(1):3–10.

Manterola C, Duque G, Grande L, de Aretxabala X, Conejeros R, Otzen T, et al. A systematic review of the effectiveness of adjuvant therapy for patients with gallbladder cancer. HPB (Oxford). 2019;21(11):1427–35.

Mise Y, Hasegawa K, Satou S, Shindoh J, Miki K, Akamatsu N, et al. How has virtual hepatectomy changed the practice of liver surgery?: experience of 1194 virtual hepatectomy before liver resection and living donor liver transplantation. Ann Surg. 2018;268(1):127–33.

Tran TB, Dua MM, Spain DA, Visser BC, Norton JA, Poultsides GA. Hepato-pancreatectomy: how morbid? Results from the National Surgical Quality Improvement Project. HPB (Oxford). 2015;17(9):763–9.

12 Palliation in Gall Bladder Cancer

Vinay K. Kapoor

Majority of patients with gall bladder cancer (GBC) have locally advanced unresectable or metastatic disease at the time of presentation and diagnosis and are, therefore, candidates for palliative management only. Aim of palliation in such cases is to mainly relieve symptoms such as pain, jaundice, pruritus, gastrointestinal obstruction, etc. in order to improve the quality of life, and, in addition, may be to prolong the survival to some extent. Nonsurgical (endoscopic or percutaneous) palliation is preferred over surgical because these patients with unresectable/metastatic disease usually have a short life span of around 6 months. Surgery, even for bypass (biliary or intestinal), in these patients with advanced disease carries a high risk of morbidity and significant mortality. In a 15-year (2000–2014) multicenter study in the United States, patients who underwent surgical palliation had more postoperative complications and longer hospital stay than those in whom surgery was aborted after laparotomy; overall survival (OS) was comparable (Buettner et al. 2016). The only possible indication for surgical palliation could be non-availability of nonsurgical palliation. Palliation involves a wide array of specialists including gastroenterologists (therapeutic endoscopists), interventional radiologists, oncologists, anesthetists, and surgeons.

While tissue diagnosis is not required for surgical resection, meaning thereby that resection can be done on radiological suspicion alone even without a tissue diagnosis thus resulting in some benign cases, e.g., chronic cholecystitis or xantho-granulomatous cholecystitis (XGC) being resected, confirmation of malignancy by tissue diagnosis is a must before the patient is referred for palliation. This can be obtained with US/CT/EUS guided fine needle aspiration cytology (FNAC). Potential sites from which a tissue diagnosis can be obtained are GB mass, liver metastases, enlarged lymph nodes, ascitic fluid, and rare metastases, e.g., umbilical nodule, left supraclavicular lymph node (LN), etc. FNAC is done using a fine (25–20 G) needle; core biopsy using a thicker (19–14 G) needle is rarely required. Ascitic fluid can be centrifuged to increase the yield of positive cells in fluid cytology. MRI can also be used to guide FNAC using non-ferromagnetic tools; PET CT guidance has also been used. In patients with jaundice, percutaneous transhepatic cholangiography (PTC) guided transabdominal transhepatic FNAC can be done to obtain tissue for diagnosis after a percutaneous transhepatic biliary drainage (PTBD) has been performed. Endoscopic or percutaneous transhepatic

Please also see an Invited Commentary on Palliation in Gall Bladder Cancer by Christopher T. Aquina and Timothy M. Pawlik (pp **–**)

V. K. Kapoor (✉)
Department of Surgical Gastroenterology, Sanjay Gandhi Post-Graduate Institute of Medical Sciences (SGPGIMS), Lucknow, Uttar Pradesh, India
e-mail: vkkapoor.india@gmail.com

V. K. Kapoor (ed.), *A Pictorial Treatise on Gall Bladder Cancer*,
https://doi.org/10.1007/978-981-15-5289-2_12

brush cytology can be obtained in patients with infiltration of the common bile duct (CBD).

12.1 Pain

Pain is present in almost all patients with advanced unresectable GBC. The standard approach to the management of pain is the WHO three-step ladder of nonsteroidal anti-inflammatory drugs (NSAIDs), weak opioids, and strong opioids. Pain not responding to standard analgesics can be relieved/controlled by celiac plexus block or celiac plexus neurolysis (CPN) performed either at operation (after the disease is found to be unresectable on laparotomy) or by an image (US, CT) guided percutaneous posterior approach using an image intensifier (fluoroscopy) with two long (15–20 cm) needles or EUS-guided anterior transgastric approach using 50–75% alcohol 20–30 mL injected on either side of the celiac axis. Bupivacaine may be added for the control of the immediate procedure-related pain. Rai et al. (2020) reported EUS-CPN in 21 patients with GBC.

12.2 Jaundice

Jaundice and associated cholangitis, pruritus, and anorexia, due to biliary obstruction caused by GBC, can be relieved by biliary drainage. Biliary drainage may not increase the survival but definitely improves the quality of life by relieving symptoms of biliary obstruction and preventing complications related to it. Biliary drainage can be

1. Pre-procedure as a preparation for portal vein embolization (PVE).
2. Preoperative as a preparation for surgery, e.g., major liver resection in the form of extended right hepatectomy (ERH).
3. Pre-chemotherapy/radiotherapy (in neoadjuvant or definitive palliative setting).
4. Definitive for palliation of associated symptoms.

Biliary drainage to relieve biliary obstruction can be endoscopic or percutaneous transhepatic. Endoscopic drainage is preferred over percutaneous transhepatic drainage because it is associated with fewer complications and achieves internal (enteric) drainage of bile. An external percutaneous drainage may be preferred if access is required to the bile duct for treatment, e.g., photodynamic therapy (PDT) or intraluminal brachytherapy (ILBT). An automatic temperature controlled endo-biliary radiofrequency ablation (RFA) system has recently been reported (Lee et al. 2019). Unlike in low malignant block, e.g., pancreatic and periampullary cancer, where biliary bypass in the form of choledocho-/hepatico-jejunostomy is technically easy, biliary obstruction in GBC is usually high (hilar). Bilio-enteric anastomosis in the form of intrahepatic segment III cholangio-jejunostomy has been described for relief of high (hilar) obstruction (Kapoor et al. 1996; Jarnagin et al. 1998) but is rarely used now (because of the availability of less invasive non-surgical methods).

In the absence of cholangitis, an internal stent can be placed at the time of the first intervention. If, however, cholangitis is present, it is better to drain the biliary system externally with endoscopic naso-biliary drainage (ENBD) or percutaneous transhepatic biliary drainage (PTBD) in the first go and place the stent later after the cholangitis has been controlled.

Biliary obstruction in GBC can be at the level of mid CBD, biliary ductal confluence (hilar), or even intrahepatic (usually on the right side). MR is better than CT to evaluate the level of biliary obstruction. If the common hepatic duct is blocked but the biliary ductal confluence is intact (patent), i.e., Bismuth type I block, single stent will drain the entire liver—endoscopic drainage is, therefore, preferred. In presence of primary biliary ductal confluence block where right and left hepatic ducts are separated, i.e., Bismuth type II block or in presence of even secondary biliary ductal confluence block where right anterior and posterior sectoral ducts are also separated, i.e., Bismuth type III block, multiple stents can be placed into all the blocked ducts by an expert endoscopist to achieve complete (bilateral) drainage but chances of success with endoscopic drainage are less; moreover, a duct which is not intended to be drained may get canulated and infected. Percutaneous transhepatic biliary drainage (multiple) (Fig. 12.1) is, therefore, preferred in such cases, i.e., Bismuth type II and III block. Even unilateral drainage of one-fourth or one-third of the liver volume can bring the serum bilirubin down and relieve pruritus but in presence of chemotherapy-associated steatohepatitis (CASH) or cirrhosis, larger volume of liver parenchyma may need drainage. Rate of fall of serum bilirubin is variable and it may take a few weeks for the serum bilirubin to fall to near normal. If serum bilirubin does not fall after unilateral biliary drainage, contralateral drainage may also be required. Cholangitis may require bilateral drainage. Unilateral percutaneous puncture can achieve bilateral drainage by passing a catheter from one side to the other across the blocked biliary ductal confluence. Ducts in an atrophic segment or segments with high tumor burden should be avoided for biliary drainage.

Coagulation profile (PT/INR, aPTT) should be checked and coagulopathy, if any, should be corrected using vitamin K and/or fresh frozen plasma (FFP). Periprocedural broad-spectrum antibiotic cover should be used. Bile should be sent for culture sensitivity.

12.2.1 Endoscopic Biliary Drainage

Endoscopic intervention is in the form of placement of a plastic (polyethylene) stent (Fig. 12.2) or self-expandable metal stent (SEMS) (Fig. 12.3) made of an alloy mesh. Plastic stents are available in lengths varying from 5 to 15 cm but are narrow in diameter (5–11 Fr). They can be straight with flaps at both ends or have pigtail ends to reduce the risk of migration. Plastic stents are more likely to get blocked (and cause cholan-

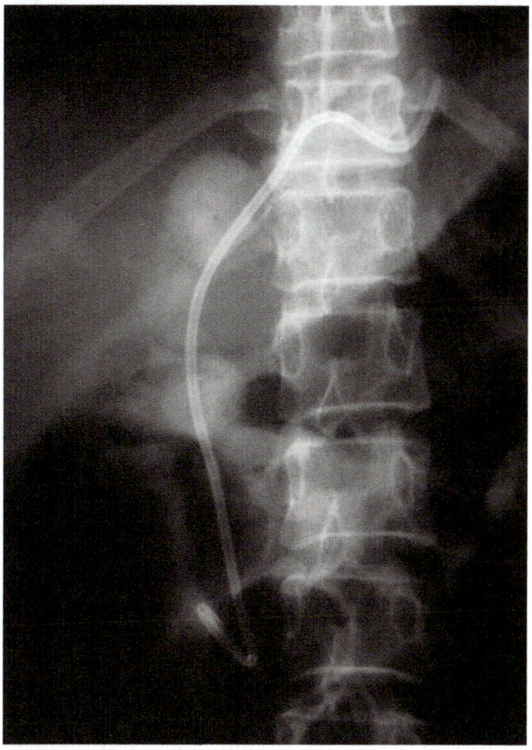

Fig. 12.2 Endoscopic plastic stent in situ in the common bile duct for palliation of jaundice in unresectable gall bladder cancer

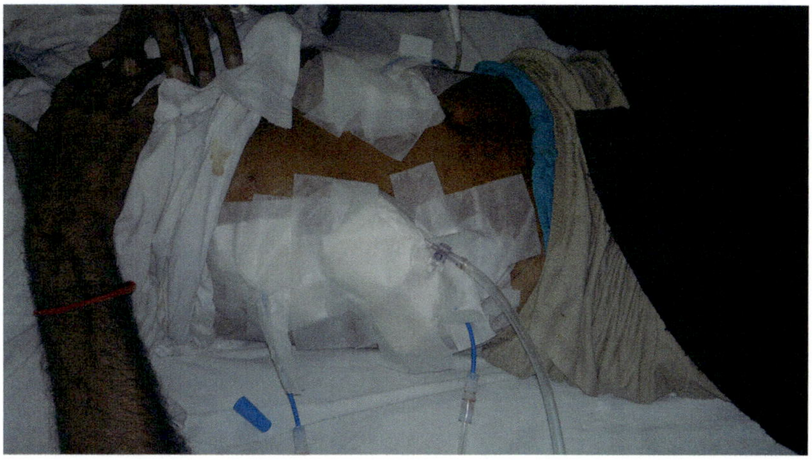

Fig. 12.1 Multiple percutaneous transhepatic biliary drainage (PTBD) in situ—multiple PTBDs may be required to control cholangitis in presence of a high (Bismuth type III) block due to gall bladder cancer at neck

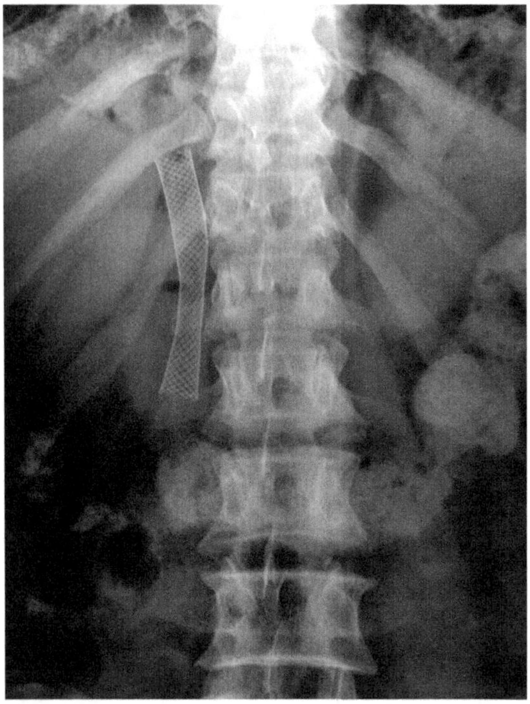

Fig. 12.3 Endoscopic self-expandable metal stent (SEMS) in situ in the common bile duct for palliation of jaundice in unresectable gall bladder cancer

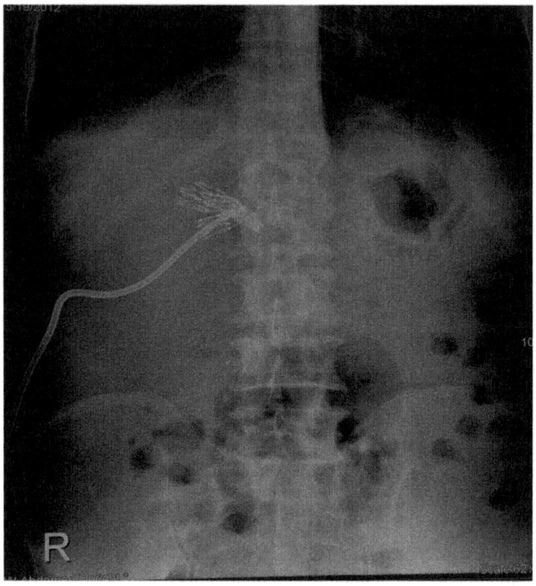

Fig. 12.4 Percutaneous transhepatic biliary drainage (PTBD) in situ (multiple self-expandable metal stents (SEMS) are also seen)

gitis) and need to be changed at an average of about 3 months; even when they remain patent the plastic stents can cause ascending cholangitis. SEMS is wider (6–10 mm) and have longer (6–9 months) patency than plastic stents but have the disadvantage of higher cost. SEMS can also get blocked due to tumor ingrowth or overgrowth but this takes an average of 8–9 months, less than the life expectancy of most of these patients. Covered SEMS have a permalume membrane over the alloy mesh and are resistant to tumor ingrowth. They are, however, more prone to migration and are more likely to cause acute cholecystitis and acute pancreatitis due to blockage of the cystic duct and the pancreatic duct, respectively. SEMS cannot be removed when they get blocked—but another stent can be placed through the blocked SEMS. When a SEMS is placed, its lower end should lie above the papilla in the CBD in order to reduce the risk of reflux of the duodenal contents into the CBD.

12.2.2 Percutaneous Biliary Drainage

Ascites should be looked for (on US) and controlled, as much as possible, before any percutaneous transhepatic intervention on the biliary tract.

Percutaneous drainage can be

1. External (PTBD) (Fig. 12.4)—the catheter tip lies proximal to the obstruction; external drainage is, however, not preferred as it leads to bile loss and is associated with catheter-related problems, e.g., pain, ascitic fluid leak, dislodgement, infection, etc. External drainage is indicated for the control of uncontrolled cholangitis only. It may also be required for obtaining tissue for brush cytology and for therapeutic purpose, e.g., administration of PDT or ILBT. Multiple PTBDs may be required in patients with intrahepatic block involving the secondary biliary ductal confluence, i.e., separation of even right anterior and posterior sectoral ducts, especially when the indication of drainage is cholangitis. Once cholangitis is controlled, external should be changed to internal drainage.

2. Internal–external—the catheter is passed through the malignant obstruction into the common bile duct beyond but the proximal end is exteriorized; this is only temporary—after a few days, when there is no evidence of sepsis (no fever, normal total leucocyte count TLC, and differential leucocyte counts DLC), the external end can be capped and later a pure internal stent is placed. However, if PDT or ILBT is planned, the external catheter is retained.
3. Internal—indwelling stent (plastic or SEMS) placement across the malignant obstruction (no external drainage).

Atrophic segments of liver should be avoided for drainage with the aim of improving liver function (exception being for control of cholangitis). Right liver is accessed through the 11th intercostal space (ICS) in the mid-axillary line (MAL) and the left liver is accessed using a subxiphoid approach. A fine (21 or 22 G) needle and guidewire (0.018″) is used to cross the obstruction; the catheter is placed after using a coaxial dilator (0.035″). A peripheral duct should be targeted to reduce the risk of bleeding from a major vessel and to ensure a long length of the catheter, with multiple holes, positioned inside the bile duct for adequate drainage. The puncture tract may be embolized with gelfoam or coils to reduce the risk of bleed and bile leak.

Empyema of the GB caused by a neck tumor causing obstruction to the cystic duct may necessitate percutaneous cholecystostomy, even though it may become permanent.

Complications of percutaneous transhepatic biliary intervention include

1. Bleeding—upsizing of the catheter can help to control the bleed from the liver parenchyma by achieving a tamponade. A subcapsular hematoma may form at the site of the liver puncture (Fig. 12.5); it may get infected to form an abscess. Late (around 2 weeks) bleed is caused by an arterial injury resulting in a pseudoaneurysm—it manifests as fresh red blood in and around the catheter and hemobilia (biliary colic, jaundice, and melena)—diagnosis is confirmed on angiography—treatment of choice is radiological embolization.
2. Cholangitis—biliary intervention itself may cause cholangitis because of contamination of an obstructed duct, more so if it is not adequately drained. Cholangitis may occur during the follow-up due to stent block or tumor progression causing fresh block of an unstented duct. Adjuvant chemotherapy and/or radiotherapy may decrease the risk of or delay the tumor blocking the stent; ILBT prevents/reduces stent occlusion by tumor ingrowth and prolongs stent patency (Wang et al. 2011). A systematic review and meta-analysis of 12 studies including 641 patients (out of which 340 received ILBT) with malignant obstructive jaundice in whom stent was placed showed that ILBT reduced the risk of stent occlusion and improved survival (Xu et al. 2018).
3. Bile leak and peritonitis.

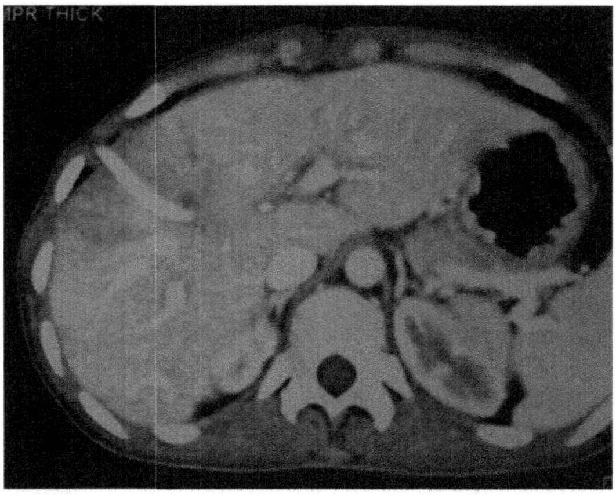

Fig. 12.5 CT shows large subcapsular hematoma in the liver caused by percutaneous transhepatic biliary drainage (PTBD); PTBD in situ

PTBD for malignant biliary obstruction (MBO) has high mortality—it was 10% at 4 weeks and 28% at 8 weeks with a median survival of 4.7 months (Robson et al. 2010).

Endoscopic and percutaneous stenting for Bismuth Type II/III blocks was compared in 54 patients—success rates using 10 F plastic stent were higher (89% vs. 41%), early post procedure cholangitis was less (11% vs. 48%) and stent occlusion was less frequent (30% vs. 50%) and patency was longer (140 vs. 90 days) with percutaneous stenting (Saluja et al. 2008).

Rendezvous combined percutaneous and radiological approach for biliary drainage has also been described.

12.3 Gastrointestinal Obstruction

Patients with advanced unresectable GBC may have symptoms of gastric outlet obstruction (GOO) (Fig. 12.6) viz. early satiety, postprandial fullness, sitophobia, nausea, and vomiting. Obstruction is in the first part of the duodenum. Vomiting is due to GOO caused by gastroduodenal involvement; it is usually non-bilious. UGIE should be performed to make sure that the symptoms of GOO are due to mechanical obstruction and not malignant gastroparesis, i.e., no mechanical obstruction. Patients with advanced disease may have both mechanical obstruction and malignant gastroparesis. Mechanical GOO can be relieved by a gastroduodenal stent (Fig. 12.7) which can be placed endoscopically (Kumar et al. 2018) or radiologically under fluoroscopic guidance. Self-expandable metal stents (SEMS) are used. Stent migration and stent block (due to tumor ingrowth) are common complications. Gastrojejunostomy (GJ) may be performed if unresectable disease is found at laparotomy and mechanical gastroduodenal obstruction is present. Surgical bypass, however, is associated with significant morbidity and even mortality. Moreover, the gastrojejunostomy (GJ) may not function and symptoms of GOO may persist because of malignant gastroparesis (Sikora and Kapoor 1999).

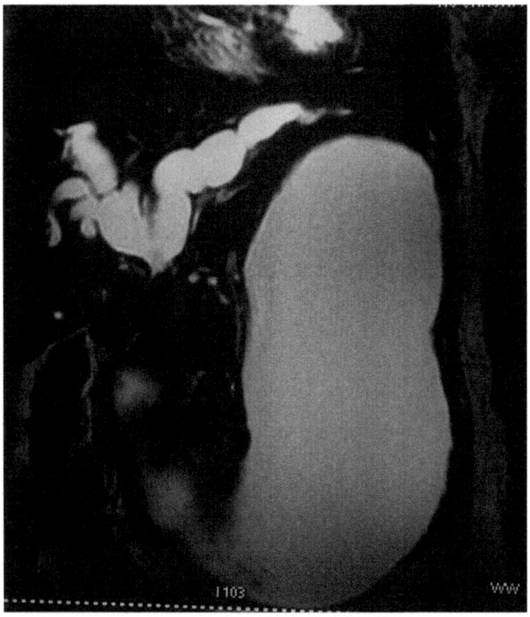

Fig. 12.6 MRC shows hugely distended stomach—gastric outlet obstruction caused by gall bladder cancer; intrahepatic biliary radicle dilatation (IHBRD) with hilar block is also seen

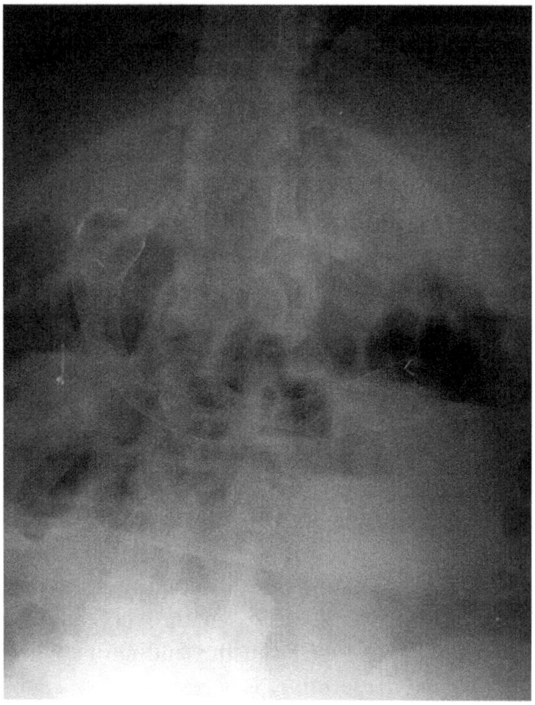

Fig. 12.7 Gastroduodenal self-expandable metal stent (SEMS) in situ to relieve gastric outlet obstruction in unresectable gall bladder cancer infiltrating the duodenum

Colonic (caused by direct infiltration of the hepatic flexure or transverse colon Fig. 12.8) or small bowel (caused by large peritoneal metastatic deposits) obstruction may be present in patients with advanced GBC. Colonic involvement by direct infiltration of a GBC is not a contraindication for resection. In otherwise unre-

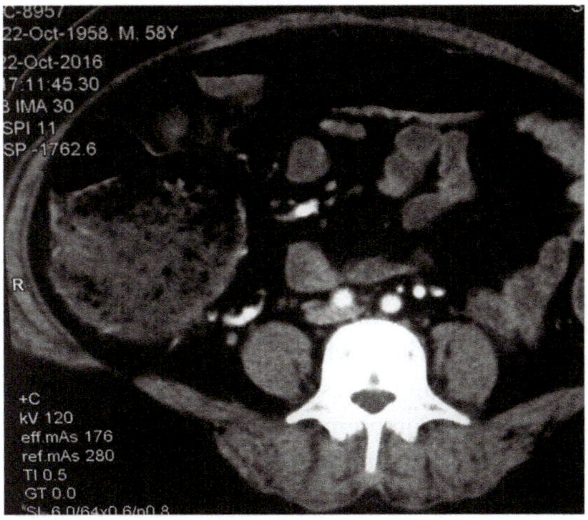

Fig. 12.8 CT shows hugely distended right colon filled with feces due to gall bladder cancer infiltrating and obstructing the transverse colon

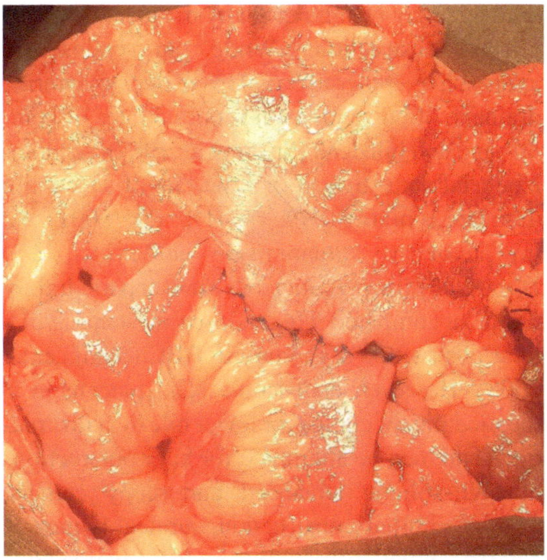

Fig. 12.9 Side-to-side hand sewn ileotransverse colostomy to palliate colonic obstruction in unresectable gall bladder cancer

sectable cases, ileotransverse colostomy (Fig. 12.9) or even terminal ileostomy (for colonic obstruction), segmental small bowel resection, or entero-enteric bypass (to relieve small bowel obstruction) may rarely be performed to palliate intestinal obstruction. This may, however, not be possible in patients with extensive peritoneal dissemination.

12.4 Palliative Chemoradiotherapy

Palliative chemotherapy may be advised in patients with good performance status (ECOG 0–1). In the ABC-02 trial, 148 patients with GBC were randomized to gemcitabine 1000 mg/m^2 + cisplatin 25 mg/m^2 on days 1 and 8 every 3 weeks for 6 cycles versus gemcitabine alone—median survival was 11.7 months versus 8.3 months (Valle et al. 2010). Gemcitabine + oxaliplatin (median overall survival mOS 14.3 months), gemcitabine + capecitabine (mOS 12.7 months), 5FU + cisplatin (mOS 11.5 months), 5 FU + capecitabine (mOS 11.3 months) are other options. Palliative external beam radiotherapy (EBRT), with 5FU as radiosensitizer, has also been used. Less toxic and more tolerable oral capecitabine (mOS 9.9 months) has been used in patients with poor performance status (Gupta et al. 2018). EBRT may also help to control GI bleed in an unresectable GBC. Many patients with advanced GBC, who have very poor performance status, may not be candidates even for a nonsurgical palliation and are offered best supportive care (BSC); expected median survival is 3–6 months (Sharma et al. 2010).

12.5 Palliative Resection

Unlike some other cancers, e.g., colorectal or stomach, where palliative resection if technically feasible, is justified and recommended even in presence of distant metastases, there is no place for a palliative (R2) resection in GBC. The only possible exception could be if a distant metastasis, e.g., liver, peritoneum, or distant LN is found at laparotomy and the primary tumor in the GB fundus or body is easily resectable, i.e., it is confined to the GB wall with no adjacent organ involvement; in such a situation, a non-curative simple cholecystectomy *MAY* be performed if no tumor plane is breached.

Palliation in unresectable GBC is best achieved with non-surgical (endoscopic and/or percutaneous) methods (Fig. 12.10).

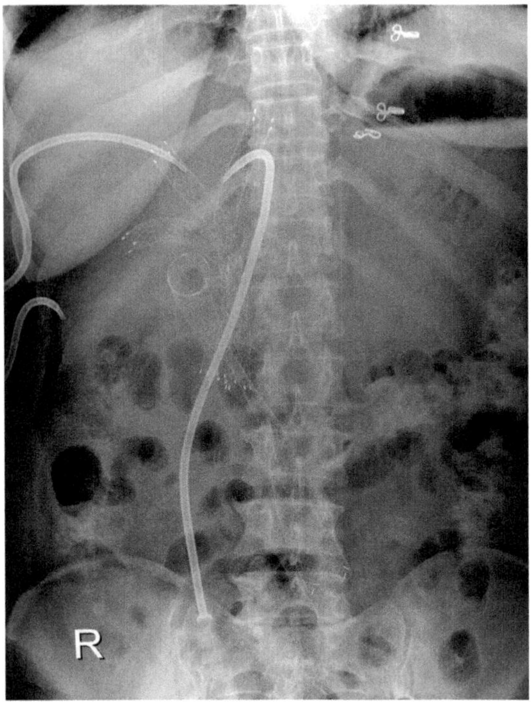

Fig. 12.10 Multiple percutaneous transhepatic biliary drainage (PTBD), multiple biliary self-expandable metal stents (SEMS), and gastro-duodenal SEMS in situ—palliation of biliary and gastro-duodenal obstruction in unresectable gall bladder cancer is largely nonsurgical, i.e., endoscopic and percutaneous

Invited Commentary on Palliation in Gall Bladder Cancer

Christopher T. Aquina and Timothy M. Pawlik

As discussed in this chapter by Dr. VK Kapoor, gallbladder cancer (GBC) is unfortunately often a non-curative, highly fatal disease for the majority of patients due to its propensity for local invasion into critical structures, as well as distant metastasis. Survival following a diagnosis of unresectable GBC is typically around 6 months. Therefore, the goal of therapy is palliation with improvement in quality of life. This chapter nicely highlights the key targets of a palliative approach:

1. Pain relief
2. Resolution of obstructive jaundice
3. Relief of gastrointestinal obstruction
4. Prolongation of life with chemoradiotherapy

Pain is best treated through a multimodal approach including non-narcotic analgesics and opioids. For refractory pain, celiac plexus neurolysis (CPN) has been shown to improve pain while decreasing consumption of opioids (Nagels et al. 2013). The inclusion of dedicated palliative medicine services, where available, may be helpful in managing doses and side effects of various pain medication regimens.

As stressed in this chapter, surgical biliary bypass procedures for biliary obstruction are fraught with high rates of morbidity and mortality in this patient population and should be generally avoided. With respect to the preferred modality of stenting, the success of a percutaneous versus an endoscopic approach to biliary drainage may be influenced by the location of the biliary obstruction. While an endoscopic approach is generally preferred due to internal drainage of bile and lower reported rates of hemorrhage and bile leak (Speer et al. 1987), randomized trial data suggest that the rate of successful drainage is higher (89% vs. 41%; $P < 0.001$) and the rate of early cholangitis lower (11% vs. 48%; $P = 0.002$) for percutaneous transhepatic biliary drainage compared with endoscopic stenting of a hilar obstruction secondary to GBC (Saluja et al. 2008). However, endoscopic stent placement is the modality of choice for lower bile duct obstructions and may be attempted for hilar obstructions at high-volume advanced endoscopy centers. Similar to biliary obstruction, surgical bypass of a gastric outlet obstruction should be avoided due to the high risk of morbidity and mortality. Endoscopic or fluoroscopic-guided gastroduodenal stent placement with a self-expandable metal stent (SEMS) is the modality of choice. However, when this procedure is not technically feasible, venting percutaneous endoscopic gastrostomy (PEG) tube placement remains an option to obviate the need for nasogastric suction.

Finally, prolongation of life with potentially concurrent improved quality of life may be achieved with the use of chemotherapy in appropriately selected patients. Despite the fact that most randomized controlled trials also included patients with other types of biliary tract malignancy, such as cholangiocarcinoma and ampullary cancer, due to the relative rarity of GBC, both the National Comprehensive Cancer Network (NCCN) and European Society for Medical Oncology (ESMO) currently recommend gemcitabine-based combination therapy as first-line chemotherapy for locally advanced and metastatic GBC in patients with good performance status (National Comprehensive Cancer Network (NCCN) n.d.; Valle et al. 2016). These recommendations are based on the aforementioned ABC-02 trial that demonstrated longer median overall survival (11.7 months vs. 8.1 months, $P < 0.001$) and improved median progression-free survival (8.0 months vs. 5.0 months, $P < 0.001$) for cisplatin–gemcitabine therapy versus gemcitabine alone (Valle et al. 2010). In subgroup analysis for GBC, the risk of death was 39% lower for the cisplatin–gemcitabine group compared with gemcitabine alone (hazard ratio = 0.61, 95% confidence interval = 0.42–0.89). Other chemotherapy options currently supported by phase II clinical trials include capecitabine-based and fluorouracil-based combination therapies (National Comprehensive Cancer Network (NCCN) n.d.). For patients with borderline performance status, gemcitabine as a single agent is an appropriate alternative. However, given the poor prognosis associated with advanced GBC, all patients should be encouraged to enroll in clinical trials.

References

Chapter References

Buettner S, Wilson A, Margonis GA, Gani F, Ethun CG, Poultsides GA, Tran T, Idrees K, Isom CA, Fields RC, Krasnick B, Weber SM, Salem A, Martin RC, Scoggins CR, Shen P, Mogal HD, Schmidt C, Beal E, Hatzaras I, Shenoy R, Maithel SK, Pawlik TM. Assessing trends in palliative surgery for extrahepatic biliary malignancies: a 15-year multicenter study. J Gastrointest Surg. 2016;20(8):1444–52. https://doi.org/10.1007/s11605-016-3155-6. Epub 2016 Apr 27.

Gupta R, Anand A, Kumar M, Bhatt M, Singh S, Sonkar AA. Safety and efficacy of low-dose single-agent capecitabine in inoperable gallbladder cancer with jaundice post-single-system single-catheter external biliary drainage: a pilot study from a highly endemic area. Indian J Surg Oncol. 2018;9(4):530–7. https://doi.org/10.1007/s13193-018-0798-7. Epub 2018 Jul 31.

Jarnagin WR, Burke E, Powers C, Fong Y, Blumgart LH. Intrahepatic biliary enteric bypass provides effective palliation in selected patients with malignant obstruction at the hepatic duct confluence. Am J Surg. 1998;175(6):453–60.

Kapoor VK, Pradeep R, Haribhakti SP, Singh V, Sikora SS, Saxena R, Kaushik SP. Intrahepatic segment III cholangiojejunostomy in advanced carcinoma of the gallbladder. Br J Surg. 1996;83(12):1709–11.

Kumar V, Ghoshal UC, Mohindra S, Saraswat VA. Palliation of malignant gastroduodenal obstruction with self-expandable metal stent using side- and forward-viewing endoscope: feasibility and outcome. JGH Open. 2018;3(1):65–70. https://doi.org/10.1002/jgh3.12110. eCollection 2019 Feb.

Lee YN, Jeong S, Choi HJ, Cho JH, Cheon YK, Park SW, Kim YS, Lee DH, Moon JH. The safety of newly developed automatic temperature-controlled endobiliary radiofrequency ablation system for malignant biliary strictures: a prospective multicenter study. J Gastroenterol Hepatol. 2019; https://doi.org/10.1111/jgh.14657.

Rai P, Lokesh CR, Harish KC. Endoscopic ultrasound-guided celiac plexus neurolysis improves pain in gallbladder cancer. Indian J Gastroenterol. 2020;39(2):171–5. https://doi.org/10.1007/s12664-019-01003-z.

Robson PC, Heffernan N, Gonen M, Thornton R, Brody LA, Holmes R, Brown KT, Covey AM, Fleischer D, Getrajdman GI, Jarnagin W, Sofocleous C, Blumgart L, D'Angelica M. Prospective study of outcomes after percutaneous biliary drainage for malignant biliary obstruction. Ann Surg Oncol. 2010;17(9):2303–11. https://doi.org/10.1245/s10434-010-1045-9. Epub 2010 Apr 1.

Saluja SS, Gulati M, Garg PK, Pal H, Pal S, Sahni P, Chattopadhyay TK. Endoscopic or percutaneous biliary drainage for gallbladder cancer: a randomized trial and quality of life assessment. Clin Gastroenterol Hepatol. 2008;6(8):944–950.e3. https://doi.org/10.1016/j.cgh.2008.03.028. Epub 2008 Jun 30.

Sharma A, Dwary AD, Mohanti BK, Deo SV, Pal S, Sreenivas V, Raina V, Shukla NK, Thulkar S, Garg P, Chaudhary SP. Best supportive care compared with chemotherapy for unresectable gall bladder cancer: a randomized controlled study. J Clin Oncol. 2010;28(30):4581–6. https://doi.org/10.1200/JCO.2010.29.3605. Epub 2010 Sep 20

Sikora SS, Kapoor VK. Bypass for malignant duodenal obstruction. Indian J Gastroenterol. 1999; 18:99–100.

Valle J, Wasan H, Palmer DH, Cunningham D, Anthoney A, Maraveyas A, Madhusudan S, Iveson T, Hughes S, Pereira SP, Roughton M, Bridgewater J, ABC-02 Trial Investigators. Cisplatin plus gemcitabine versus gemcitabine for biliary tract cancer. N Engl J Med. 2010;362(14):1273–81. https://doi.org/10.1056/NEJMoa0908721.

Wang SJ, Lemieux A, Kalpathy-Cramer J, Ord CB, Walker GV, Fuller CD, Kim JS, Thomas CR Jr. Nomogram for predicting the benefit of adjuvant chemoradiotherapy for resected gallbladder cancer. J Clin Oncol. 2011;29(35):4627–32. https://doi.org/10.1200/JCO.2010.33.8020. Epub 2011 Nov 7.

Xu X, Li J, Wu J, Zhu R, Ji W. A systematic review and meta-analysis of intraluminal brachytherapy versus stent alone in the treatment of malignant obstructive jaundice. Cardiovasc Intervent Radiol. 2018;41(2):206–17. https://doi.org/10.1007/s00270-017-1827-6. Epub 2017 Oct 26. Review.

References for Commentary Notes

Nagels W, Pease N, Bekkering G, et al. Celiac plexus neurolysis for abdominal cancer pain: a systematic review. Pain Med. 2013;14(8):1140–63.

National Comprehensive Cancer Network (NCCN). NCCN clinical practice guidelines in oncology. https://www.nccn.org/professionals/physician_gls/default.aspx. Accessed 27 August 2019.

Speer AG, Cotton PB, Russell RC, et al. Randomised trial of endoscopic versus percutaneous stent insertion in malignant obstructive jaundice. Lancet. 1987;2(8550):57–62.

Valle JW, Borbath I, Khan SA, et al. Biliary cancer: ESMO clinical practice guidelines. Ann Oncol. 2016;27(suppl 5):v28–37.

13 Incidental Gall Bladder Cancer

Vinay K. Kapoor

Nomenclature and definition of the term incidental gall bladder cancer (GBC) are not well defined. It has been variously called inapparent (Agarwal et al. 2012) and subclinical (Yamaguchi and Tsuneyoshi 1992) GBC also; Goetze (2015) used the term occult GBC. Clemente (2016) called it unexpected and Yu et al. (2019) called it unsuspected GBC. Chen et al. (2016) called GBCs diagnosed during or after cholecystectomy as unsuspected GBC. Many reports include GBC suspected during cholecystectomy also as incidental GBC (Qadan 2016; Zhong et al. 2019).

In the Authors' opinion (Kapoor 2001a), incidental GBC is GBC detected for the first time on histopathological examination of the GB removed (by open or laparoscopic simple cholecystectomy) with a presumed preoperative (clinical and US) diagnosis of gall stone disease (GSD)—even intraoperative diagnosis is GSD, i.e., there are no operative findings to suspect GBC and the GB specimen on gross examination (by the surgeon) does not have any suspicion of cancer.

The operation for incidental GBC has been variously called reoperation, reresection, revision surgery, etc. The Author (Kapoor and Behari 2017) has proposed the term completion extended cholecystectomy (CEC) for the operation for incidental GBC. Cholecystectomy has already been done at the index operation; liver wedge resection and lymphadenectomy are performed at the reoperation to complete the EC.

A careful review of preoperative imaging (US; and CT, if it was done for some reason) in many cases which are labeled by the referring surgeon as "incidental" GBC very often shows that there was some abnormality in the GB, e.g., wall thickening, which should have raised a preoperative suspicion of GBC—they will, therefore, qualify to be called suspected GBC and should not have been treated with a simple cholecystectomy in the first place (Shukla et al. 2007). In such cases, especially when the degree of suspicion of GBC is low, we have described anticipatory extended cholecystectomy (AEC)—the GB is removed with a small wedge of liver and subjected to frozen section histopathological examination (Kapoor et al. 2016).

13.1 Unsuspected GBC

Early stages of GBC are difficult to diagnose preoperatively because the symptoms of early GBC are similar to those of GSD. Moreover, US fails to pick up early GBC, especially in presence of associated GS. Most patients with

Please also see Invited Commentaries on Incidental Gall Bladder Cancer by Thorsten Oliver Goetze (pp **–**) and Shishir K. Maithel (pp **–**)

V. K. Kapoor (✉)
Department of Surgical Gastroenterology, Sanjay Gandhi Post-Graduate Institute of Medical Sciences (SGPGIMS), Lucknow, Uttar Pradesh, India
e-mail: vkkapoor.india@gmail.com

V. K. Kapoor (ed.), *A Pictorial Treatise on Gall Bladder Cancer*,
https://doi.org/10.1007/978-981-15-5289-2_13

early GBC are, therefore, taken up for cholecystectomy with a preoperative diagnosis of gall stones. The Author (VKK) has proposed that unsuspected GBC should be defined as one where the preoperative (i.e., clinical and imaging) diagnosis is GSD but there is some suspicion of GBC at operation, e.g., omentum densely adherent to the GB (Fig. 13.1), thick-walled contracted GB (Fig. 13.2) (which was missed on preoperative imaging, i.e., US), puckering of the liver around the GB (Fig. 13.3), difficult or obliterated Calot's triangle (Fig. 13.4), difficult dissection in the GB bed, or in the GB specimen, e.g., focal, asymmetrical, nonuniform, irregular GB wall thickening (Fig. 13.5), plaque (Fig. 13.6), scar (Fig. 13.7), nodule (Fig. 13.8), ulcer (Fig. 13.9), mass, or polyp (Fig. 13.10). This is different from incidental GBC (where the GB is grossly normal and GBC is detected for the first time on histopathological examination of the GB specimen)

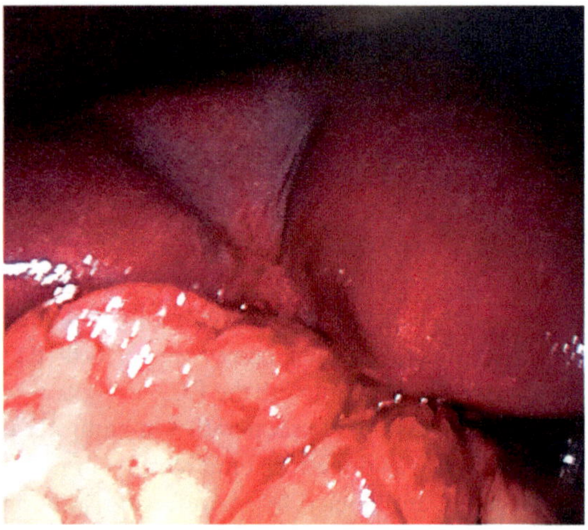

Fig. 13.1 Operative picture shows omentum densely adherent to the gall bladder in a patient operated for gall stones—this should raise an intraoperative suspicion of gall bladder cancer

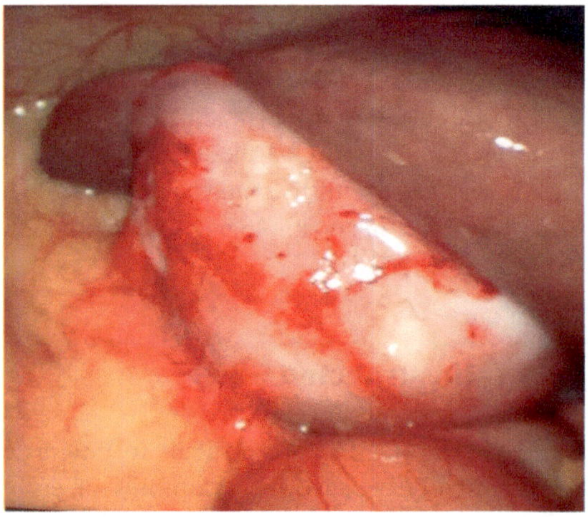

Fig. 13.2 Operative picture shows thick-walled contracted gall bladder (which was missed on preoperative imaging, i.e., US) in a patient operated for gall stones—this should raise an intraoperative suspicion of gall bladder cancer

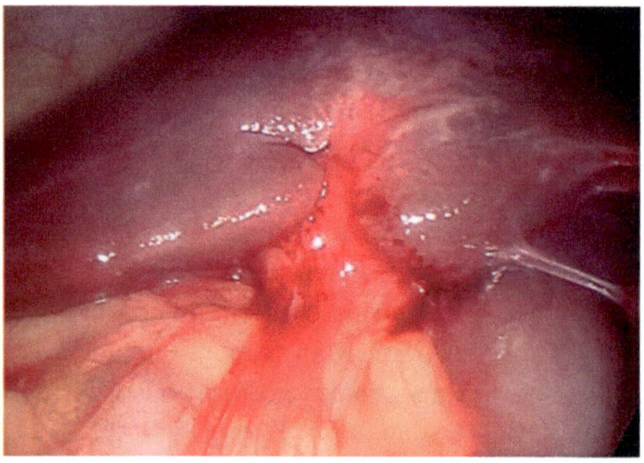

Fig. 13.3 Operative picture shows puckering of liver near the gall bladder bed in a patient operated for gall stones—this should raise an intraoperative suspicion of gall bladder cancer

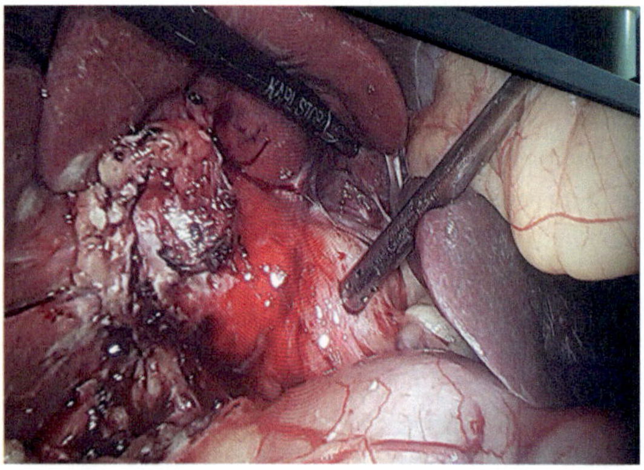

Fig. 13.4 Operative picture shows no Calot's triangle (the suction tip points to the hepatoduodenal ligament) in a patient operated for gall stones—a difficult or obliterated Calot's triangle should raise an intraoperative suspicion of gall bladder cancer

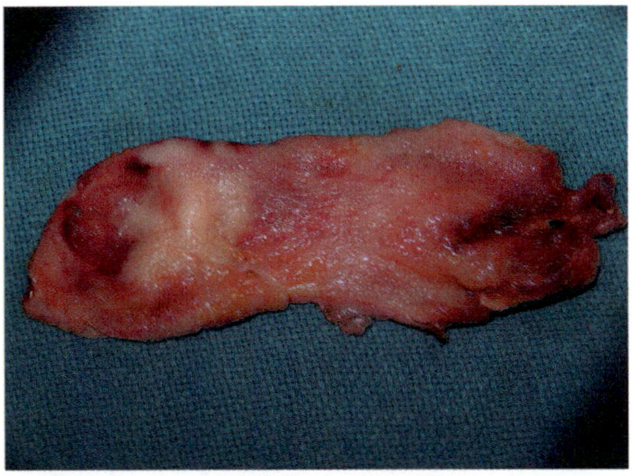

Fig. 13.5 Focal, asymmetrical, nonuniform, irregular wall thickening in the gall bladder specimen—this should raise a suspicion of gall bladder cancer; frozen section histopathological examination should be done

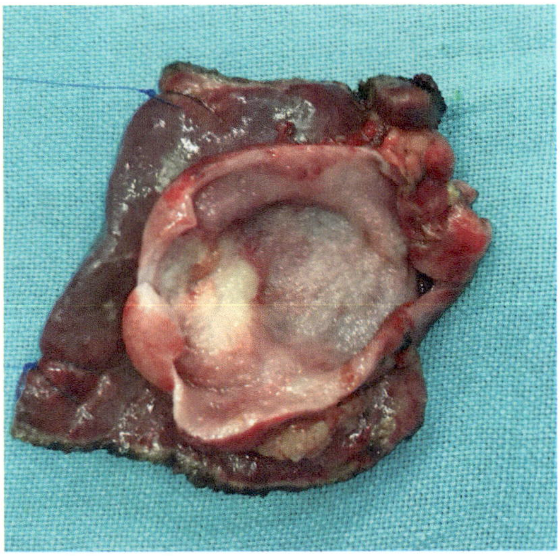

Fig. 13.6 A plaque in the wall in the gall bladder specimen—this should raise a suspicion of gall bladder cancer; in this case an anticipatory extended cholecystectomy (AEC) was performed (liver wedge can be seen attached to the gall bladder)

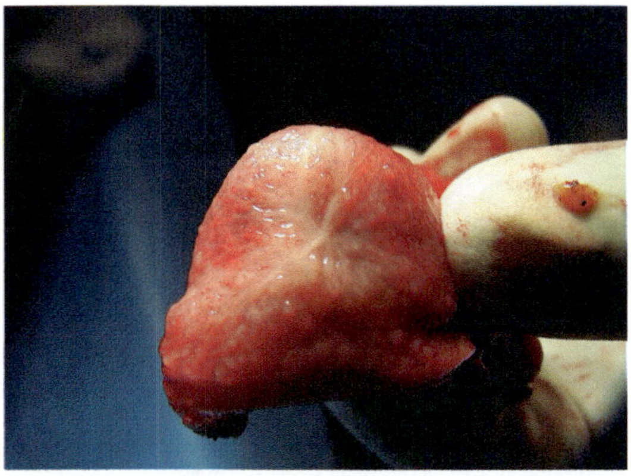

Fig. 13.7 A scar in the wall in the gall bladder specimen—this should raise a suspicion of gall bladder cancer; frozen section histopathological examination should be done

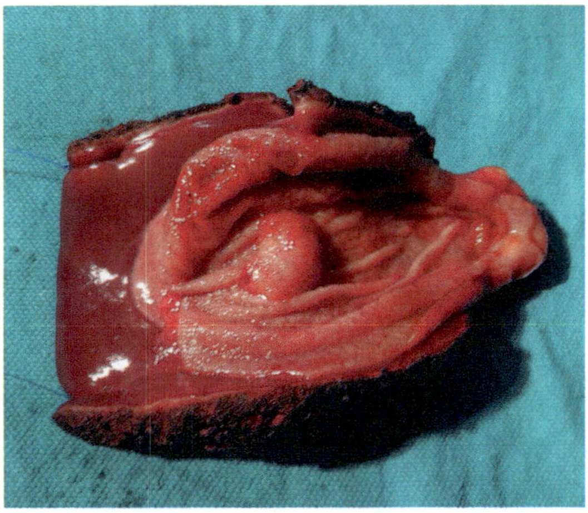

Fig. 13.8 A nodule in the wall in the gall bladder specimen—this should raise a suspicion of gall bladder cancer; in this case an anticipatory extended cholecystectomy (AEC) was performed (liver wedge can be seen attached to the gall bladder)

and such patients should be called unsuspected (unexpected) GBC (Kapoor 2006).

If there is a suspicion of GBC at laparoscopy but expertise and experience for EC are not available, there is no need to convert to open operation - no dissection should be done around the GB, no biopsy should be taken from the GB, omentum, if available, may be placed around the GB, and the patient referred to an HPB/oncology surgeon for further workup and management.

If expertise and experience for EC are available, intraoperative fine needle aspiration cytology (FNAC) may be performed to confirm the diagnosis. If the FNAC is positive, EC will be performed, either laparoscopic or open (after conversion), as per the philosophy and policy of the treating surgeon/unit. It should, however, be kept in mind that FNAC has a low sensitivity, i.e., not all cases will be picked up; this means that even if the FNAC is negative, the patient will still require an EC if the suspicion of GBC is high (some of these cases may finally turn out to have benign

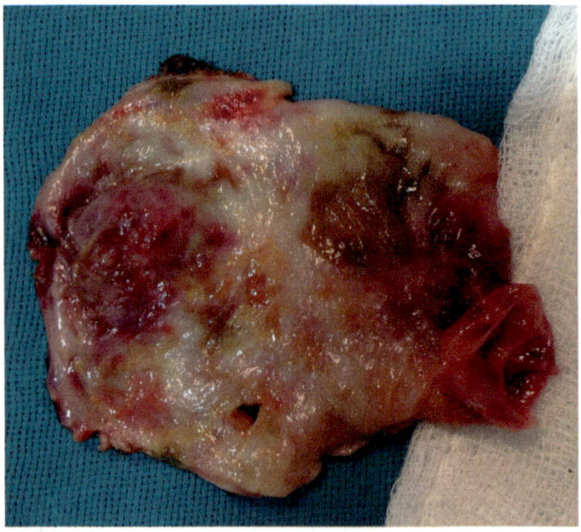

Fig. 13.9 An ulcer in the wall in the gall bladder specimen—this should raise a suspicion of gall bladder cancer; frozen section histopathological examination should be done

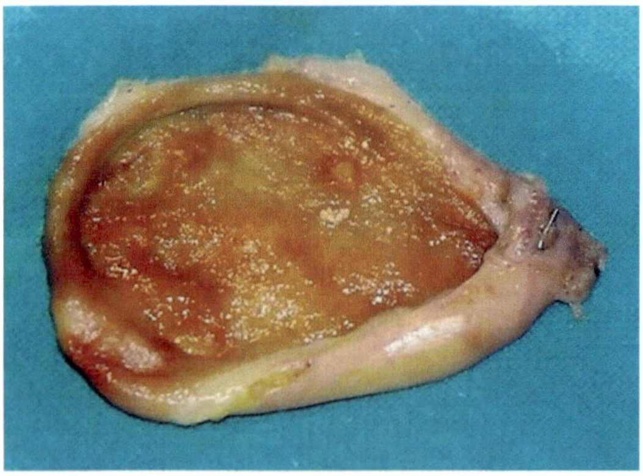

Fig. 13.10 A polyp in the wall in the gall bladder specimen—this should raise a suspicion of gall bladder cancer; frozen section histopathological examination should be done

disease, i.e., chronic cholecystitis or xanthogranulomatous cholecystitis XGC). For this reason, the Author (VKK) usually does not perform FNAC but bases his decision on the degree of suspicion of cancer. A positive FNAC is, however, mandatory if a major resection, e.g., hepatectomy is required in order to avoid doing it (i.e. major resection) in a benign disease, e.g., XGC.

In case there is no obvious lesion from which FNAC can be performed, the management depends on the degree of suspicion of GBC. Qadan and Kingham (2016) advocated resection of the cystic plate to avoid GB perforation and bile spill in case there is a suspicion of malignancy. The Author (VKK) does not agree because this would mean a compromise of the liver margin if the lesion is T1b or T2, for which liver wedge resection is required. In patients with low suspicion of GBC, we have described anticipatory extended cholecystectomy (AEC)—the GB is removed with a small wedge of liver and subjected to frozen section histopathological examination (Fig. 13.11) (Kapoor et al. 2016).

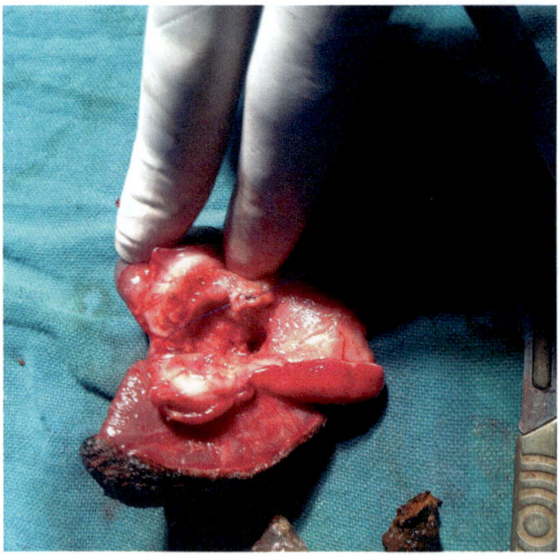

Fig. 13.11 Specimen of anticipatory extended cholecystectomy (AEC)—removal of the gall bladder (GB) with a small wedge of liver—we have described AEC in patients with thick-walled GB with a low preoperative suspicion of gall bladder cancer (in patients a high preoperative suspicion of gall bladder cancer, extended cholecystectomy should be done)

ALL GBs removed for a preoperative diagnosis of benign (stone) disease MUST be opened in the operation room itself (before the laparoscopic ports are removed or the abdomen is closed), washed in running water, and carefully examined (may be with a magnifying glass) by the operating surgeon for any suspicious lesion, e.g., ulcer, nodule, polyp, induration, wall thickening, etc. Any suspected area should be marked with a suture and the GB sent for frozen section histopathological examination. In expert hands, frozen section should have >90% sensitivity and 100% specificity (i.e. no false positive); accuracy for the depth of invasion, however, may not be very high. If the frozen section diagnosis is positive for malignancy, EC should be performed. Imprint cytology of the GB mucosa has also been described to confirm grossly evident carcinoma and to detect macroscopically inapparent (incidental) carcinoma (Otero et al. 2008).

13.2 Incidental GBC

13.2.1 Incidence

Incidence of incidental GBC is about 1–3% of all cholecystectomies; 9/1663 (0.54%) laparoscopic cholecystectomies performed at Nagoya (1991–2003) turned out to be incidental GBC (Yamamoto et al. 2005). In Korea, 1 in 150 (0.7%) cholecystectomy turned out to be an incidental GBC (Choi et al. 2015). Seventy-three (1.6%) incidental GBCs were diagnosed in 4629 cholecystectomies performed at Asan Medical Center Seoul South Korea (1998–2014) (Ahn et al. 2016). Incidental GBC was found in 155 (0.8%) of 20,584 cholecystectomies performed in Tunisia between 2003 and 2016 (Charfi et al. 2018). Swedish Register for gall stone surgery included 36,255 cases (2007–2014)—215 (0.6%) were found to have incidental GBC (Muszynska et al. 2017). In Turkey, incidental (called unsuspected by the authors) GBC was found in 5 (0.4%) of 1294 cholecystectomy specimens (Dincel et al. 2018). In the United States, 26 (0.45%) of 5796 cholecystectomies revealed incidental GBC (Goussous et al. 2018). More and more incidental GBCs are being diagnosed as more and more cholecystectomies are being performed because of universal application of US as the first investigation for any abdominal symptom and because threshold for offering and accepting cholecystectomy is becoming lower with laparoscopic cholecystectomy (LC). The proportion of incidental GBC in all cases of GBC varies from region to region. In Chile, 368 (39%) of 1366 cases of GBC seen between 1987 and 2005 were incidental (Roa et al. 2014). Only 20% of all 46 GBCs diagnosed at Yokohama Japan vs more than 60% of those diagnosed in Chile and at MSKCC New York USA were incidental GBCs (Butte et al. 2011b). In the United States, about half (47%) of all cases of GBC are incidental GBC (Shih et al. 2007; Duffy et al. 2008). Out of 445 GBC patients who underwent resection at a consortium of ten institutions in the United States from 2000 to 2015, as many as 266 (60%) were incidental GBC (Ethun et al. 2017a). The rates of incidental GBC may be higher in patients who are old, present with acute cholecystitis or empyema, have elevated levels of serum alkaline phosphatase (ALP), those with choledocholithiasis, those who have porcelain GB, Mirizzi syndrome, or GB polyp (Muszynska et al. 2017; Goussous et al. 2018). Incidental GBC was found in 6.5% of patients undergoing emergency versus 0.4% of patients undergoing elective cholecystectomy (n = 6329) between 2011 and 2017 in Brazil (Figueiredo et al. 2020). Muszynska et al. (2020) analyzed the data of 28,915 patients (derivation cohort) and 7851 patients (validation cohort) registered in the nationwide Swedish Registry for Gallstone Surgery (GallRiks) and developed a risk score model to predict incidental GBC in patients undergoing cholecystectomy.

13.2.2 Issues

The key issues in the management of incidental GBC are

1. Is a reoperation required or is follow-up alone sufficient (after the index simple cholecystectomy)?
2. Which patients should undergo reoperation?
3. What investigative workup is required before reoperation?
4. When should the reoperation be performed?
5. What should be the extent of reoperation?

13.2.3 Which Patients Should Undergo Reoperation?

This depends on the probability of finding residual disease in the GB bed or the lymph nodes at reoperation which in turn depends largely on the T stage. In patients with a tumor at the GB neck, residual disease may be present in the cystic duct remnant also.

Residual disease was found at reoperation in 46% of 115 patients (most of these had T2 or more disease) managed at six hepatobiliary centers in the United States; 0%, 10%, and 36% in liver and 13%, 31%, and 46% in the lymph nodes (LNs) in T1, T2, and T3 disease, respectively; overall 38% in T1, 57% in T2, and 77% in T3 (Pawlik et al. 2007). Residual disease was found in 100 (74%) of 146 patients with incidental GBC who were reoperated. The incidence of residual disease found at reoperation increased with increasing T stage viz. T1 (50%), T2 (66%), T3 (85%), T4 (100%) (Duffy et al. 2008). Four hundred and forty-nine GBC patients were operated at ten institutions in USA (2000–2015)—262 (58%) were incidental GBC who underwent reoperation. T stage, grade, lymphovascular invasion (LVI), and perineural invasion (PNI) were associated with increased risk of locoregional disease and distant disease at reoperation. Each of these characteristics was assigned a numerical value (Tis = 0, T1 = 1, T2 = 2, T3/T4 = 3; well differentiated = 1, moderately differentiated = 2, poorly differentiated = 3; LVI negative = 1, LVI positive = 2; PNI negative = 1, PNI positive = 2)—these values added to a GBC predictive risk score (GBRS) of 3–10. The scores were classified as 3–4 (low risk), 5–7 (intermediate risk), and 8–10 (high risk) (Ethun 2016). This score to predict residual disease was later validated in 56 patients with incidental GBC by Mochizuki et al. (2018). Two hundred and fifty-four incidental GBCs were managed at the Memorial Sloan Kettering Cancer Center (MSKCC) New York USA between 1992 and 2015—188 (74%) were reoperated—locoregional residual disease was found in 82 (32%), and distant residual disease in 69 (27%) patients; residual disease in the GB bed and lymph nodes increases with T stage and degree of differentiation. The chances of finding residual disease at reoperation were more in patients with T3 disease and in patients whose tumor had poor differentiation. The chances of finding residual disease at reoperation were T3—87%, T1b/T2 + poor differentiation—67%, T1b/T2 + well/moderate differentiation 35% (Creasy et al. 2017). Vinuela et al. (2017) reviewed 187 patients with incidental GBC who underwent oncologic extended resection (OER) in Chile and the United States. Residual cancer was found in 73 (39%) patients. T3 status, LVI, and PNI were associated with residual cancer. In a report from Chile and Argentina, residual disease was found in 58 (35%) of 168 patients with incidental GBC who underwent reresection; the incidence of residual disease was 20% in T1b, 24% in T2, and 72% in T3 disease (Gil et al. 2019).

One of the tenets of safety, in order to avoid a bile duct injury, during LC is to remain to the right of the cystic lymph node (LN). This would mean that the GB specimen will not include the cystic LN—nodal status, therefore, will be NX (not known). Even if the cystic LN is included in the GB specimen and is negative for metastasis, it does not necessarily mean N0 status because the cystic LN is not a sentinel LN i.e. other LNs can be positive even if the cystic LN is negative. Positivity of LNs increases with the T stage—T1a < 5%, T1b 10–20%, T2 40–60%, and T3, T4 > 75%. At reoperation in 248 patients with incidental GBC, LNs were positive in 33% patients in T2, 58% in T3, and 69% in T4 (Fong et al. 2000).

The International Study Group of HPB Cancer in Brazil has recently developed an evidence-based consensus for the management of patients with incidental GBC (Grupo Internacional de Estudos de Câncer Hepatopancreatobiliar - ISG-HPB-Cancer et al. 2020).

13.2.4 Investigations

The aim of workup of a patient with incidental GBC is the same as in any other patient with GBC, i.e., to find out an oncological reason to not operate upon the patient because if such a reason is present and it is either missed, neglected, or ignored, the reoperation will be futile. All patients with incidental GBC should have a detailed clinical examination to look for any distant metastasis (liver nodule, ascites, pelvic deposits, left supraclavicular LN, umbilical nodule, port/scar nodule), more so if there has been a delay after the index cholecystectomy. All patients with inciden-

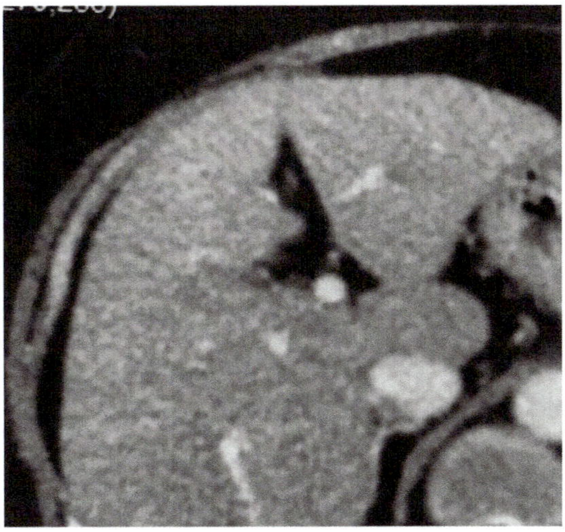

Fig. 13.12 CT, in a patient with incidental gall bladder cancer, shows a hypodense lesion in the gall bladder fossa—suggestive of residual/recurrent disease

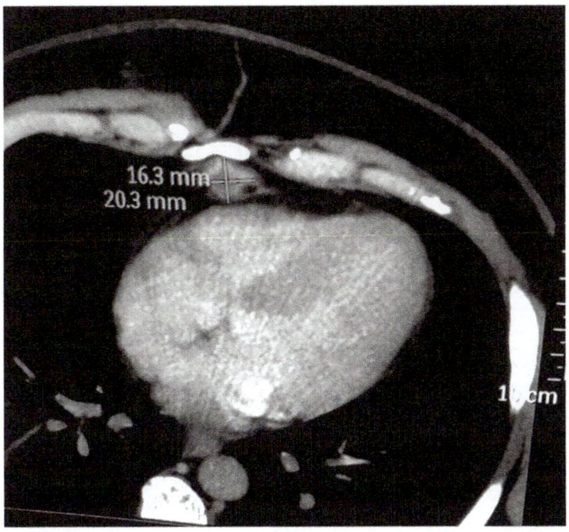

Fig. 13.13 CT chest, in a patient with incidental gall bladder cancer, shows an anterior mediastinal nodule (distant metastasis)

tal GBC should have an abdominal US and contrast-enhanced CT (abdomen Fig. 13.12, pelvis, and chest Fig. 13.13) or MRI, again to detect any metastasis and to find out any residual disease in the GB bed or in the LNs. CT, however, cannot detect very small lesions and may not differentiate between postoperative changes and residual disease in the GB bed.

FDG PET has a sensitivity of 78% and specificity of 80% for detecting residual disease

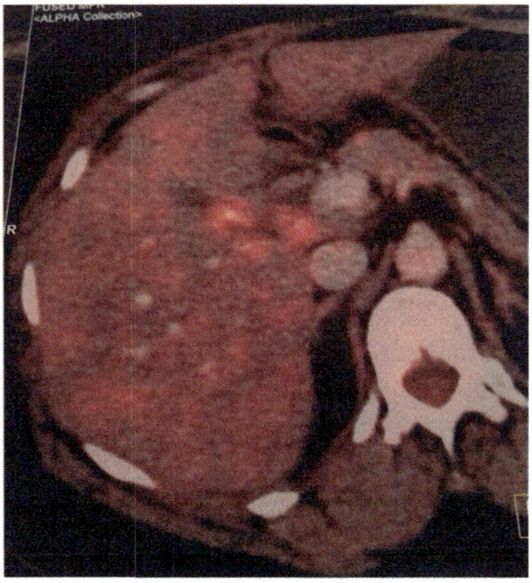

Fig. 13.14 PET scan, in a patient with incidental gall bladder cancer, shows FDG activity in the gall bladder fossa and adjacent lymph nodes

(Fig. 13.14) in incidental GBC (Anderson et al. 2004). It detected metastatic disease in a significant number of patients and is recommended to detect metastases (Corvera et al. 2008). Shukla et al. (2008) performed PET in 80 patients with incidental GBC—as many as 55 (70%) had disseminated disease and 24 had potentially resectable disease—21 out of these 24 could be resected and 7 out of 21 were found to have residual disease. Butte et al. (2009) observed that PET reduced the number of nontherapeutic reoperations in incidental GBC. PET detected disseminated disease in 10 (31%) of 32 patients; it changed the management in 8 (25%). PET caused a change in management in only 13% of 63 patients with incidental GBC (cf. 31% with non-incidental GBC) (Leung et al. 2014). Tata Memorial Hospital (TMH) Mumbai India group used PET-CT to detect residual disease before revision surgery in 108 patients with incidental GBC. PET was negative in 64 (59%) patients. Chances of finding residual disease at reoperation were less (23% vs. 52%) in PET negative patients. pT1b patients with no uptake on PET were not found to have any residual disease at reoperation. Based on this observation, the authors recommended observation rather than reoperation for PET negative pT1b patients (Goel et al. 2016).

PET should definitely be done if there has been a delay in reoperation and in advanced i.e. T3 or node-positive disease, or aggressive biology, i.e., poor differentiation, LVI, PNI, tumors. PET, however, may be false-positive in the immediate postoperative period—it becomes more specific when performed 4–6 weeks after the index cholecystectomy.

At MSKCC New York USA, 136 patients with incidental GBC were reoperated—19 had dissemination. Staging laparoscopy (SL) was performed in 46—it could detect dissemination in only 2/10 that had dissemination. Staging laparoscopy was not found to be as useful in incidental GBC as in preoperatively diagnosed GBC. Yield of SL was likely to be higher in patients with advanced (T2, T3) lesion, poor differentiation, late presentation for reoperation, and history of bile spill during the index cholecystectomy (Butte et al. 2011a). The Author (VKK), however, recommends that every patient with GBC (including incidental GBC) MUST have the benefit of SL before a laparotomy is performed as the detection of a metastasis is an absolute contraindication for any surgery in GBC.

13.2.5 Timing of Reoperation

Earlier, it was believed that reoperation for CEC for incidental GBC should be performed as early as possible after the index cholecystectomy because delay in reoperation increases the risk of dissemination and reduces the benefit in terms of survival.

Ausania et al. (2013) proposed an intentional delay of 3 months before reoperation—this approach selected out aggressive tumors which would not have in any case benefited from the reoperation. Median survival in 24 patients who underwent resection was 54.8 months versus 9.7 months in other 24 who had unresectable disease. Two hundred and seven (46%) of 449 GBC patients with incidental GBC underwent reoperation at ten US academic institutions (2004–2014) at <4 weeks (n = 25, 12%), 4–8 weeks (n = 91, 44%) or >8 weeks (n = 91, 44%). Longest median survival was seen in those operated at 4–8 weeks (40 months) versus those operated early (17 months) or late (22 months). T stage, reoperation at <4 weeks or >8 weeks, presence of residual disease, R2 resection, and LN involvement were predictors of poor survival (Ethun et al. 2017c). A contrary view has, however, been expressed in a Chinese report of 80 incidental GBCs—patients who were reoperated within 2 weeks (n = 37) had better (median 86 months) survival than those who were operated between 2 weeks and 1 month (n = 26, median 26 months) and those who were operated after 1 month (n = 17, median 27 months) (Du et al. 2018). Another approach is to use neoadjuvant (before reoperation) chemotherapy to select out cases which develop progression of the disease, especially distant metastases, and resect only good biology tumors (Cherkassky and D'Angelica 2019; Cherkassky and Jarnagin 2019). Neoadjuvant chemotherapy, however, is not the standard of care in GBC and should not be offered to potentially resectable cases. Laparoscopic re-resection (n = 65) for incidental GBC has been shown to be oncologically non-inferior to open re-resection (n = 190) in a retrospective multicenter analysis (Vega et al. 2020).

13.2.6 Extent of Reoperation

Early GBC is defined as T1a/T1b and N0 disease. Whether T2 can also be considered as early is a matter of debate; T2 (perimuscular/subserosal) GBC can be stage II (T2N0), III (T2N1), or even IVB (T2N2) disease and should be considered advanced GBC. Early GBC is rarely diagnosed preoperatively (most cases are detected incidentally on histopathological examination of the gall bladder removed for a presumed preoperative diagnosis of stone disease). A polypoidal (papillary) GBC, in the absence of GS, in a well-distended normal wall GB may be detected on US in early stages. Most patients with incidental GBC have pT2 (about half) or pT1 (about one-third) tumors (Søreide et al. 2019). In Chile, 33% of 368 incidental GBCs were advanced (beyond muscularis propria) (Roa et al. 2014). In Tis (carcinoma in situ) and T1a (involving lamina propria only) tumor, LN metastases are present in <5% of cases, recurrence rates are low and survival rates are high (5 year >95%) after simple cholecystectomy only; reoperation is, therefore, not required. National Cancer Database (NCDB) USA analysis of 4015 patients operated between 2004 and 2014 included 246 T1a tumors—positive LN was seen in as many as 13% T1a lesions but, surprisingly, there was no survival benefit of LN resection (Köhn et al. 2018). T1a stage should be reconfirmed by preparing more sections if the formalin-fixed specimen and/or paraffin-embedded blocks are available and/or review of the slides by an experienced pathologist. Intraepithelial extension of the tumor into the RAS may indicate reoperation even in T1a disease. If bile spill had occurred during the index cholecystectomy, chemotherapy should be advised.

T1b (muscularis propria) tumors can have lymphatic and venous invasion; incidence of LN metastases is significant (10–20%). Controversy still persists about the need for reoperation in T1b disease. This is because some groups have reported good long-term survival after simple cholecystectomy alone—10-year survival of 87% in 13 patients (Wakai et al. 2001) and 5-year survival of 100% in 39 cases (Shirai et al. 1992) and 88% in 49 cases (de Aretxabala et al. 2009). In a retrospective analysis of 47 T1b patients, 18 of whom underwent radical resection with regional LN dissection but 29 underwent simple cholecystectomy only, survival after simple cholecystectomy was same as that after radical resection; additional radical resection was not recommended by the authors for T1b disease (Yuza et al. 2020). Earlier reports suggested that simple cholecystectomy alone is enough for T1b lesion and reoperation (for CEC) is not required but many recent reports have reported high rates of recurrence after simple cholecystectomy for T1b lesions—only 50% 1-year survival after simple cholecystectomy in T1b (Principe et al. 2006). In an analysis of 464 patients with T1b GBC from the NCDB, overall 5-year survival after SC was only 48% (Vo et al. 2019). Moreover, some reports where EC was performed for T1b lesion found significant (14% Kumar et al. 2019, 15% Vo et al. 2019) rates of LN metastasis in T1b lesion thus emphasizing the need for EC in T1b lesion.

Lee et al. (2011) performed pooled systematic analysis of 29 publications (up to 2008) including 1266 patients with T1 GBC—706 (56%) T1a and 560 (44%) T1b. In T1a patients, simple cholecystectomy was performed in 590 (84%) (open in 321, 54% and lap in 269, 46%) while EC was performed in 110 (16%) (15% performed as reoperation). In T1b patients, simple cholecystectomy was performed in 375 (67%) (open in 76% and lap in 24%), while EC was performed in 168 (30%) (26% performed as reoperation). LN metastases were found in 1.8% cases in T1a and 11% in T1b. In T1a, simple cholecystectomy resulted in 100% 5-year survival. Recurrence was seen in 1.1% cases in T1a and 9.3% in T1b. The authors concluded that there was no definite evidence that EC is advantageous over SC for T1b—but at the same time mentioned that because LN metastasis is considerable, regional lymphadenectomy should be performed. An analysis of 237 patients with T1b GBC who underwent surgical resection (SC 116, EC 121) at 14 centers in South Korea, Japan, Chile, and the United States showed similar survival outcome (5-year OS 93.7% vs. 95.5%) after SC or EC and concluded that SC is adequate and EC is not required for T1b (Kim et al. 2018). In a meta-analysis of 22 articles with 2578 patients with T1 GBC, SC and EC showed comparable survival patterns in both T1a and T1b (Lee et al. 2018a). A retrospective analysis of 2112 T1 and T2 GBCs operated from 2004 to 2014 identified in the SEER database revealed that LN excision did not offer survival benefit in T1a and T1b cases (benefit was seen only in T2 patients) (Steffen et al. 2019).

The Author (VKK), however, disagrees with these recommendations and advocates reoperation for CEC for T1b incidental GBC. This is the Indian "Buddhist" Middle Path described by the author (Kapoor 2007), i.e., an aggressive approach toward early (and incidental) GBC so that no opportunity for cure is missed. In the German Registry experience of 883 cases of incidental GBC, reresection improved survival in T1b from 34% to 75% and reresection was recommended (Goetze and Paolucci 2014a, c). A recent review (Søreide et al. 2019) on the topic also recommends reresection for T1b incidental GBC.

Clinical data from 277 patients with T1b GBC who received curative surgical treatment between 2004 and 2015 were collected from the SEER database. Only 127 of these 277 patients underwent lymphadenectomy—23 of 127 had tumor <1 cm in diameter and none of these had LN metastases; 104 of these 127 had tumor >1 cm in diameter and 15 (14%) of these had LN metastases. In patients with tumor <1 cm, there was no difference in survival between SC and EC. EC provided survival benefit over SC in patients with tumor >1 cm (Wang et al. 2019).

During simple cholecystectomy, the plane of dissection is subserosal, i.e., between the GB wall (muscle) and the cystic plate. This means that the tumor plane is likely to be breached and there will be a high chance of residual disease in the GB bed in T2 (perimuscular/subserosal) disease. Rate of LN metastasis is high (40–60%), and residual disease will be found at reoperation in about 50% of cases. Recurrence rates are high after SC and 5-year survival after simple cholecystectomy is only 20–40% (19% Fong et al. 2000, 20% de Aretxabala et al. 2009, 25% Goetze and Paolucci 2008 and 40% Shirai et al. 1992); reoperation for CEC provides better 5-year survival (41% Goetze and Paolucci 2008, 59% Fong et al. 2000, 62% Fuks et al. 2011, 70% de Aretxabala et al. 2009, 90% Shirai et al. 1992). A large experience with 410 patients with T2 GBC operated in 14 university hospitals in South Korea recommended EC (including wedge resection of GB bed for T2 tumors). Since systemic recurrences were common, adjuvant chemotherapy was also recommended (Lee et al. 2018b).

Four hundred and thirty-seven patients with incidental GBC who underwent reoperation for T2 GBC were classified as peritoneal side and hepatic side. Higher rates of vascular invasion (51% vs. 19%), neural invasion (33% vs. 8%), and LN metastases (40% vs. 17%) were seen in hepatic side versus peritoneal side tumors. Five-year survival was less (43% vs. 65%) in hepatic side versus peritoneal side disease (Shindoh et al. 2015). Lee et al. (2015) also classified T2 disease as hepatic or peritoneal. The 8th edition of AJCC TNM staging has subclassified T2 into T2a (peritoneal side) and T2b (hepatic side). Worse 5-year survival (72% vs. 96%) has been reported in pT2b (n = 56) than pT2a (n = 25) (Toge et al. 2019).

Peritoneal side (n = 99) disease had better (85% vs. 72%) 5-year survival than hepatic side (n = 93) disease in a six center review from South Korea. In peritoneal side T2 tumor, RC with liver resection provided similar (71% vs. 55%) survival as RC without liver resection. In hepatic side T2, RC with liver resection resulted in better (80% vs. 30%) survival than RC without liver resection. The authors recommend RC with lymphadenectomy alone without liver resection in peritoneal side disease (Lee et al. 2017). Park et al. (2018) reviewed 78 patients with T2 GBC and recommended hepatic resection for tumors located on hepatic side only and not for those on the peritoneal side. Eighty-one patients with T2 GBC treated in South Korea between 1999 and 2017 were retrospectively analyzed—36 of these 81 had peritoneal side (T2a) and 45 had hepatic side (T2b) tumors; hepatic resection was performed in 44 (T2a = 20 and T2b = 24) patients, while 37 (T2a = 16 and T2b = 21) did not have hepatic resection. Recurrence rates were higher (44% vs. 8%) in T2b than in T2a. Three-year OS was better (97% vs. 76%) in T2a than in T2b tumors. Hepatic resection did not improve survival in either T2a (94% vs. 100%) or T2b (71% vs. 100%). The Authors recommend that hepatic resection is not essential in curative treatment of T2 GBC (Cho et al. 2019). Another recent report of 84 T2 incidental GBCs showed that hepatectomy (n = 36) did not improve survival (66% vs. 60%)—the authors recommended lymphadenectomy only (Li et al. 2019). But the Author (VKK) does not agree with these recommendations and advocates a proper CEC, including both liver wedge resection and lymphadenectomy, in ALL patients with T2 disease, irrespective of whether it is peritoneal side or hepatic side. This is the Indian "Buddhist" Middle Path described by the author (Kapoor 2009), i.e., an aggressive approach toward early (and incidental) GBC so that no opportunity for cure is missed. In an analysis of 1251 patients in the National Cancer Database (NCDB) (2009–2012), liver resection improved the survival regardless of the tumor location in pT2 disease (Lafaro et al. 2020). Kohya et al. (2010) classified T2 GBC into three groups based on the extent of subserosal invasion—minimal, medium, and massive. They recommended partial hepatectomy and extrahepatic bile duct resection (EHBDR) in patients with medium and massive subserosal invasion. The German Registry experience with 624 cases of incidental GBC, in fact, recommends segments IVB + V liver resection (rather than just liver wedge) for T2 incidental GBC (Goetze and Paolucci 2010). Toge et al. (2019) recommended that the extent of lymphadenectomy should not be changed in pT2a (vs. pT2b) tumors.

Kawahara et al. (2017) classified T2 tumors as

1. P-type—tumor in the GB fundus (Gf) or body (Gb) and on the free peritoneal side—full-thickness cholecystectomy (FTC) and regional LN dissection.
2. H-type—tumor in the GB fundus (Gf) or body (Gb) and in contact with the liver in the GB bed—GB bed resection and regional LN dissection.
3. N-type—tumor located in the GB neck (Gn)—GB bed resection, bile duct resection, and regional LN dissection.

Ideally speaking, T3 disease should have been diagnosed preoperatively but most series of incidental GBC have a significant proportion of patients with T3 tumor—14/51 incidental GBC were T3 (de Aretxabala et al. 2018); 81/266 incidental GBCs were T3 and 11 were even T4 (Ethun et al. 2017b). No patient with T3 survived for 5 years after SC (Shirai et al. 1992; Fuks et al. 2011), 5-year survival in T3 after SC was only 8% (Goetze and Paolucci 2008). No survival benefit was seen after reoperation in 32 (out of total 85 incidental GBC) patients with T3 disease—5-year survival in T3 even after reoperation was 17% (Goetze and Paolucci 2008). Other reports showed better survival after reoperation in T3 disease 19% versus 0% (Fuks et al. 2011) and 21% (Fong et al. 2000). Even German Registry has recently reported better results in T3 incidental GBC after radical resections done in 75/282 patients (Goetze and Paolucci 2014a). Reresection improved survival in even pT3 disease (23 vs. 10 months) (Lundgren et al. 2019). Though the benefit of reoperation in T3 incidental GBC is debated, the patient should be given the benefit of doubt and advised reoperation, albeit with a questionable benefit in terms of survival. Surprisingly, even in 81 consecutive T3 unexpected (incidental) GBC, there was no difference in OS between anatomic hepatectomy (IVB + V) and wedge hepatectomy (Yu et al. 2019).

Simple cholecystectomy in T4 disease results in R2 resection which is associated with poor survival; there is no advantage of reoperation for CEC.

The maximum benefit, in terms of increase in survival, of reoperation accrues to patients with T2 incidental GBC. By and large, most patients with incidental GBC (except those with a distant metastasis) should be offered the benefit of reoperation for CEC. However, for various reasons, many patients with incidental GBC are either not advised or are not willing to undergo reoperation; all these patients should then receive adjuvant chemotherapy (and radiotherapy) as the second-best option. Adjuvant therapy after SC is a potential alternative to reoperation for CEC for incidental GBC—SC + adjuvant therapy resulted in median survival of 16.4 versus 10.7 months after EC (Kasumova et al. 2017).

The diagnosis of incidental GBC comes as an unexpected, unpleasant, and unwelcome shock to the patient as well as the surgeon. The patient, however, needs to be assured that incidental GBC is usually early, resectable, and potentially curable stage of GBC, unlike a preoperative diagnosis of GBC where the disease is usually advanced, unresectable, and incurable. Median survival in incidental GBC was 16 months cf. 5 months in GBC which was diagnosed preoperatively (Duffy et al. 2008). In most instances, simple cholecystectomy alone (which has been performed) is an incomplete operation/treatment for the incidental GBC and the patient requires an expert opinion for further management. Patients with incidental GBC should be referred to a high-volume center for liver resections because such centers are more

(61% vs. 41%) likely to perform reoperation for liver resection when it is indicated, especially for T1b and T2–T3 GBC (Goetze and Paolucci 2014b). CEC for incidental GBC can be open, laparoscopic (Gumbs and Hoffman 2010), or robotic (Araujo et al. 2019).

Ideally, the surgeon who performed the index cholecystectomy should record (but this will have to be done for all cholecystectomies as the surgeon does not know at the time of cholecystectomy as to which GB will turn out to have an incidental GBC) whether GB perforation occurred causing bile spill, whether a bag was used for GB extraction and which port was used for GB extraction. The surgeon/oncologist who is managing an incidental GBC should retrospectively review the preoperative investigations to see whether there was any suspicion of GBC in the history or on imaging which was missed, (s)he must contact/speak to the surgeon who performed the index cholecystectomy to review the operative findings and the details of the operative procedure viz. whether GB perforation occurred causing bile spill, whether a bag was used for GB extraction and which port was used for GB extraction, and the pathologist who examined the GB to review the details of the histopathology viz. T stage, site (i.e. fundus, body or neck; hepatic or peritoneal) of the tumor, cystic duct margin status, cystic LN (if included in the specimen) status, grade, lymphovascular invasion (LVI), perineural invasion (PNI) and pericapsular invasion (PCI) in the lymph node. In real-life clinical practice, these details are invariably not available as the index cholecystectomy was done at one hospital and the patient is referred to another hospital for definitive management of incidental GBC.

At reoperation for CEC, the cystic duct stump (Fig. 13.15) should be identified and, if possible, excised—the excised cystic duct stump should be sent for frozen section histopathological examination which, if positive, mandates CBD excision (Shukla et al. 2008). CBD excision at CEC, however, increased the morbidity from 23% to 60% and did not improve survival (Fuks et al. 2011). In a two center (United States and China) retrospective analysis of 179 patients with incidental GBC who underwent subsequent oncological extended resection (OER), 33 (17%) were found to have a positive cystic duct margin. CBD excision was performed in 42 (23%) patients. Positivity of the cystic duct margin reduced the 5-year OS from 57% to 34% (Vega et al. 2019).

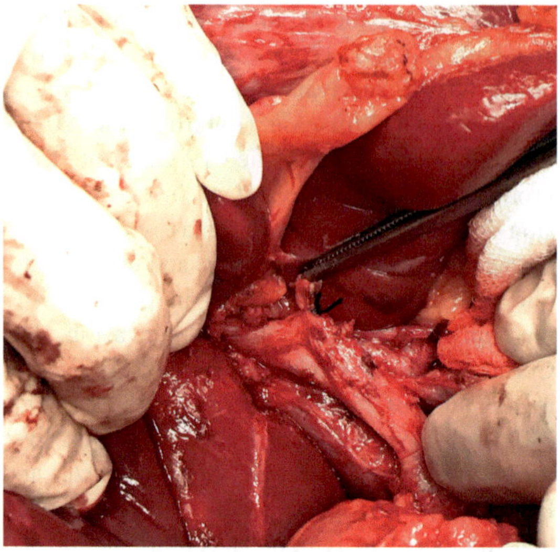

Fig. 13.15 During the reoperation for incidental gall bladder cancer, the cystic duct stump should be looked for, biopsied, and sent for frozen section histopathological examination; if it is positive, common bile duct excision is indicated

13.2.7 Port-Site Excision

Routine port-site excision (PSE) (Fig. 13.16a, b) during the reoperation for incidental GBC remains controversial. Whether all ports or only the port of GB extraction (if known) or the epigastric and umbilical ports (as one of them is likely to be the port of GB extraction) should be excised is also a matter of debate. Many surgeons are of the opinion that port-site metastases (PSM) indicates distant disease; port-site excision during CEC is more a staging (and not a therapeutic) procedure—for deciding adjuvant therapy and predicting prognosis. Hundred and thirteen patients with incidental GBC were managed at the MSKCC New York USA over 17 years—port-site metastasis was found in 13 (19%) of 69 patients in whom PSE was performed it was seen in only T2 or T3 tumors.

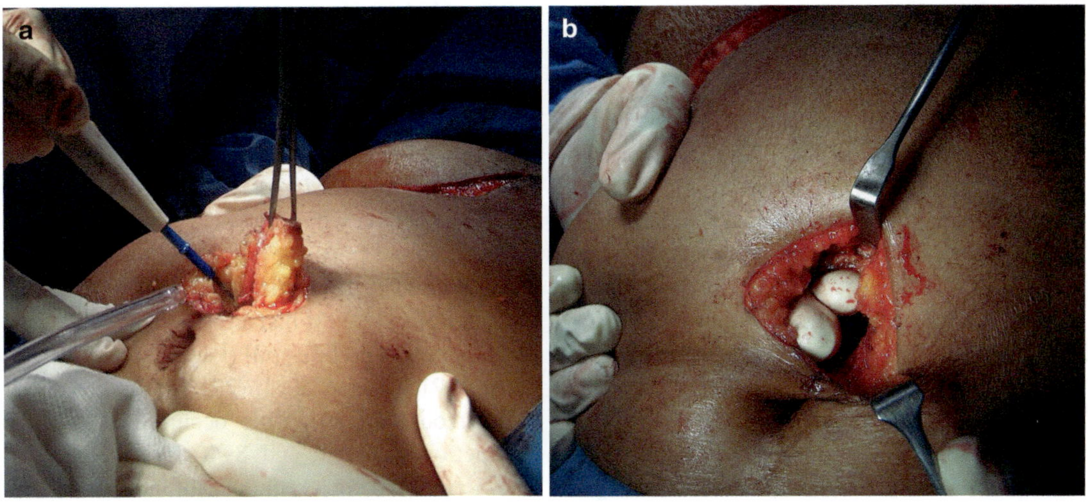

Fig. 13.16 (**a** and **b**) Port-site excision during reoperation (completion extended cholecystectomy) for incidental gall bladder cancer

Median survival in patients who developed PSM was 17 months cf. 42 months in those who did not have PSM. In patients who had R0 resection, PSE in 69 patients (vs. no PSE in 44 patients) did not affect overall or disease-free survival (Maker et al. 2012). PSE in 54 out of 148 patients who underwent reresection did not improve survival (1-, 3-, and 5-year survival 77%, 58%, and 21% with PSE vs. 78%, 55%, and 33% without PSE) in the French Registry experience (1998–2008) with 218 incidental GBCs; 8% of patients who had PSE developed an incisional hernia (Fig. 13.17) (Fuks et al. 2013). Fifty-seven (70%) of 81 patients with PSM died of cancer at a median of 13 (1–36) months; 49 out of 53 (92%) died within 2 years of LC (Berger-Richardson et al. 2017). Four hundred and forty-nine GBCs were resected in ten institutions in USA between 2000 and 2015—reoperation for incidental GBC was performed in 266—193 of 266 patients with incidental GBC underwent reresection—47 (24%) had PSE during the reresection. Three-year survival in patients who underwent PSE was 65% versus 43% in those who did not have PSE; median survival was 89 versus 30 months (p=0.06)—PSE, however, was not recommended by the authors (Ethun et al. 2017d). PSE is not recommended in the AHPBA consensus statement (Aloia et al. 2015), the NCCN guidelines (Benson et al. 2019a), and in the Brazilian consensus (Grupo Internacional de Estudos de Câncer Hepatopancreatobiliar—ISG-HPB-Cancer et al. 2020).

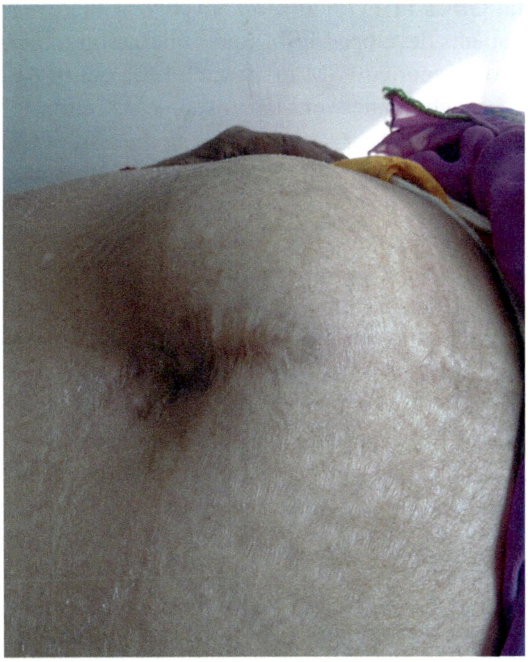

Fig. 13.17 Incisional hernia at the site of excision of the umbilical port

13.2.8 Port-Site Metastases

Recurrence at the access port wound following laparoscopic management of cancer is called port-site metastasis (PSM). The incidence of PSM in patients with colon cancer who undergo laparoscopic colonic resection is <1%. But unlike colon cancer, GBC has high propensity for peritoneal seeding/metastasis. Scar metastases are seen even after open cholecystectomy for GBC in about 7% of cases. Most cholecystectomies are now performed laparoscopically. LC has a higher risk of GB perforation and bile spill, which further increases the risk of PSM. In case of GBC, PSM occurs most frequently after LC for presumed GSD where the final histopathology reveals GBC, i.e., incidental GBC.

An international survey of surgeons in Austria, Germany, and Switzerland revealed 409 incidental GBCs in 117,840 LCs. Seventy of these 409 patients developed PSM (the same group of surgeons reported PSM in 19, i.e., 4.6% out of 412 cases who underwent laparoscopic resection for colorectal cancer)—it was seen at the port of GB extraction in 49 patients but was present at other ports in 37 patients. In as many as 52 out of 70 patients, the tumor was confined to the GB wall (T0 n = 13, T1 n = 13, and T2 n = 36) (Paolucci et al. 1999). Paollucci (2001) in a review of four international surveys and 75 case reports (1991–1999) found that 14–30% of patients with incidental GBC developed PSM. In a systematic review of 27 papers, quality-weighted incidence of PSM after laparoscopic resection of incidental GBC was 18.6% in seven papers in the historic era (1991–1999); it came down to 10.3% in the 20 papers in the modern era (2000–2014). PSM occurred as frequently (10%) in early GBC as in advanced GBC (13%) (Berger-Richardson et al. 2017). These rates of PSM are, however, underestimates as the true incidence may be even higher, if looked for.

Cancer cells are known to have predilection for healing wounds which are rich in growth factors. PSMs can occur due to direct (contact) contamination of the parietes during extraction of the GB at the extraction port site or they may be caused by the pneumoperitoneum, gas currents, and chimney effect causing contamination of all ports; GB perforation and bile spill, which occur very frequently during LC, also cause port-site seeding. That is why PSM occurs not only at the GB extraction port site but at the non-extraction port sites also. Fifty-nine of 70 (84%) patients who developed PSM had an intact unopened GB, i.e., there was no bile spill (Paolucci et al. 1999). Berger-Richardson et al. (2017) found that 101 (53%) out of 190 PSMs occurred at the GB extraction port site and 89 (47%) at the non-extraction port site (keeping in mind that there is only one GB extraction site and three non-extraction sites). The risk of PSM can be reduced by avoiding GB perforation and bile spill during the cholecystectomy and with the routine use of a specimen retrieval bag in all cases, but this will prevent PSM at the extraction port site only, not at the non-extraction port sites.

PSM may be considered as a local or distant deposit. PSM is usually an indicator of peritoneal dissemination and is associated with poor survival. Early (say within 6 months) PSM indicates aggressive biology disease; it suggests peritoneal dissemination and prognosticates poor outcome and poor survival. Rarely, PSM is an isolated deposit, i.e., it is a local port-site implantation due to contamination of the port site during extraction of the GB and there is no diffuse peritoneal dissemination or any other metastasis (on CT or PET scan Fig. 13.18a, b). Port-site excision (metastatectomy) with adjuvant chemotherapy may help in such a case, though with a high risk of recurrence. The excision has to be wide, i.e., at least 1 cm around the metastasis (one has to keep in mind the possibility of an oblique or zigzag port tract) and full thickness, i.e., from the skin to the peritoneum (Fig. 13.19a, b). Reconstruction may require use of flaps or mesh. There are anecdotal reports of long-term survival after excision of PSM, probably in such cases.

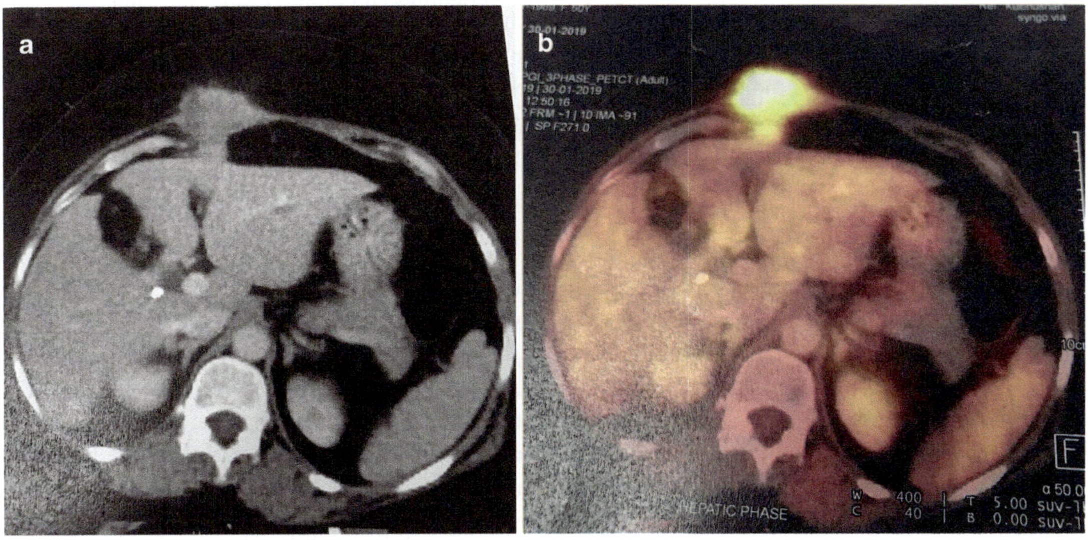

Fig. 13.18 Isolated port site metastasis on (**a**) CT and (**b**) PET

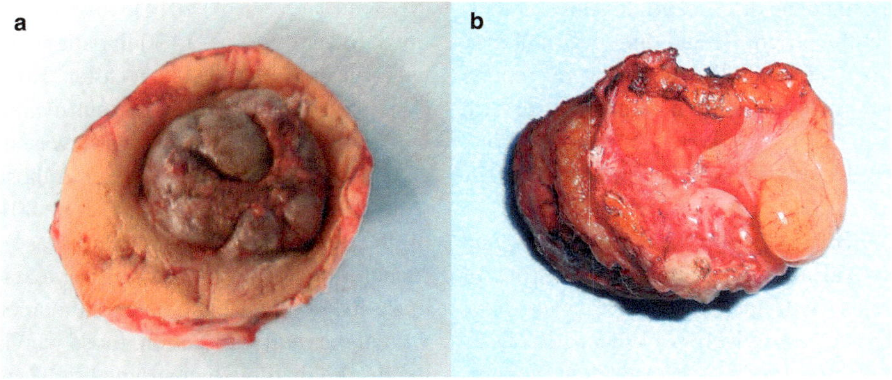

Fig. 13.19 Excision of port-site metastasis (**a**) wide (**b**) full thickness. (Image courtesy Dr. Ami Javed, GB Pant Hospital New Delhi)

13.3 Adjuvant Therapy

Indications for use of adjuvant therapy in incidental GBC are, by and large, the same as in any other patient with GBC, i.e., T2 or more, node positive, margin positive, poor histological features, i.e., poor differentiation, LVI, PNI, PCI. In addition, patients who had bile spill during the index cholecystectomy and those who had papillary tumor should also receive adjuvant chemotherapy, irrespective of the T or N status. Risk of recurrence is more (38% vs. 27%) in patients in whom GB perforation occurred versus those in whom GB perforation did not occur during the index cholecystectomy (Goetze and Paolucci 2009).

13.4 Survival

Incidental GBC is usually in the early stages, is more frequently resectable, and has better outcome than non-incidental (obvious or suspected) GBC. Incidental GBC may represent a distinct biology than non-incidental (obvious or suspected) GBC. Four hundred and forty-five resections were performed between 2000 and 2015 in ten institutions in the United States—266 of these were for incidental GBC. Incidental GBC had less high-grade tumor (31% vs. 50%), lymphovascular invasion (LVI) (54% vs. 64%), and node positivity (49% vs. 60%) and has better outcome than non-incidental GBC even in the same stage; median survival in patients with incidental GBC was 32 months (vs. 17 months in patients with non-incidental GBC) (Ethun et al. 2017a).

Some surgeons believe that reoperation for incidental GBC is mainly for staging and prognosis rather than to improve survival (Watson et al. 2017) because if no residual disease is found at reoperation, the reoperation was not required and if residual disease is found at reoperation the reoperation will not improve survival. The Author (VKK), however, strongly recommends reoperation for incidental GBC as it will correctly and completely stage the disease, guide adjuvant therapy, predict the prognosis and outcome, and may even improve survival. There are several reports which show that reoperation improved survival vs. no reoperation—26 versus 5 months (Fong et al. 2000), 18 versus 6 months (Shih et al. 2007). Reresection increased the survival in T2 and T3 incidental GBC (Fuks et al. 2011). One, 3-, and 5-year survival after reresection in 148 (out of 218) patients with incidental GBC was 76%, 54%, and 41%, respectively (Fuks et al. 2011).

Factors which predict survival after reoperation for incidental GBC are T, N, margin, residual disease, and resection status. Barreto et al. (2014) reported their results of reresection in 127 patients with incidental GBC—the most important predictor of recurrence was LN metastasis; delay in reoperation did not influence the survival. Nodal status at reoperation is an important predictor for survival—5-year survival was 73% without nodal involvement versus 27% with nodal involvement (Pawlik et al. 2007). In a French report of 50 patients with incidental GBC who underwent reoperation, T3 tumor and LN involvement were found to be risk factors for survival. Three-year survival was 85%, 31%, and 0%, and median survival 80, 22, and 13 months in patients with none, one, or two of these risk factors (Addeo et al. 2018). Whether the index cholecystectomy was open, laparoscopic, or laparoscopic converted to open does not affect the prognosis of patients with incidental GBC (Goetze and Paolucci 2013a). Residual disease is, probably, the most important predictor of outcome after reoperation in incidental GBC. In the French Surgical Association registry, a 10-year-experience of university and regional hospitals, 5-year survival in presence of residual disease was 17% vs. 68% in absence of residual disease (Fuks et al. 2011). At the MSKCC New York USA (1995–2005), 206/435 (47%) GBCs were incidental—136 (66%) of these 206 were reoperated—median survival in patients with no residual disease was 72 months vs. 19 months in those with residual disease even after R0 resection and 13 months after R1/R2 resection (Duffy et al. 2008). DFS in patients with residual disease was 11.2 vs. 93.4 months in those without residual disease (Butte et al. 2014). Five-year DFS was much lower (19% vs. 74%) in patients with residual cancer (73/187) even after R0 resection (Vinuela et al. 2017). Median survival in patients with residual disease (n = 58) was much less (20 months vs. 63 months) than in those without residual disease (n = 110) (Gil et al. 2019). None of the patients with residual disease found at reoperation survived beyond 3 years (Kumar et al. 2019). In pT2 patients with incidental GBC who underwent reresection, those who had residual disease had median survival of 32 months vs. median survival not reached in those without residual disease (Lundgren et al. 2019). Data of 463 patients with incidental GBC in the Netherlands Cancer Registry were analyzed—median OS in patients without residual disease was better than in those with residual disease (not reached vs. 23 months); pT3 and pN1 were predictive factors for residual disease (de Savornin Lohman et al. 2020). Intraoperative spillage (n = 12) was associated with decreased progression free survival (PFS) in 66 patients with incidental GBC (Blakely et al. 2019).

It was earlier believed that patients with GBC who first underwent simple cholecystectomy with a diagnosis of GSD and were found to have incidental GBC on histopathological examination of the GB and undergo reoperation for CEC have a poorer outcome as compared to those who undergo a one-stage EC with a preoperative diagnosis of GBC. But recent reports show that as long as R0 resection status can be achieved, outcomes are similar. Survival of 80 patients who underwent initial non-curative cholecystectomy followed by definitive resection in the second stage (at reoperation) was no different than 22 who had a one-stage definitive EC after a preoperative diagnosis of GBC (Fong et al. 2000). Vega et al. (2019), on the other hand, reported poorer (31% vs. 85%) 3-year survival in T2 GBC when reoperation, i.e., CEC, was performed after simple cholecystectomy showing incidental GBC than when it was diagnosed preoperatively and one-stage EC was performed. The last word on the optimum management of incidental GBC, is however, yet to be said!

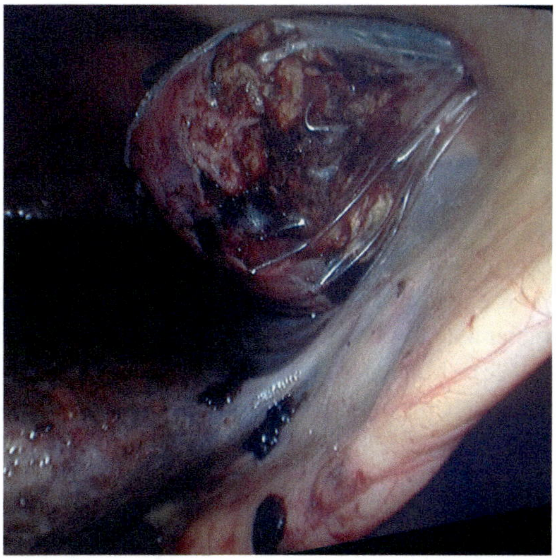

Fig. 13.20 Preferably, all gall bladders removed for gall stones should be extracted in a bag to avoid contamination of the port wound in order to avoid port site metastasis, in case it turns out to be incidental gall bladder cancer

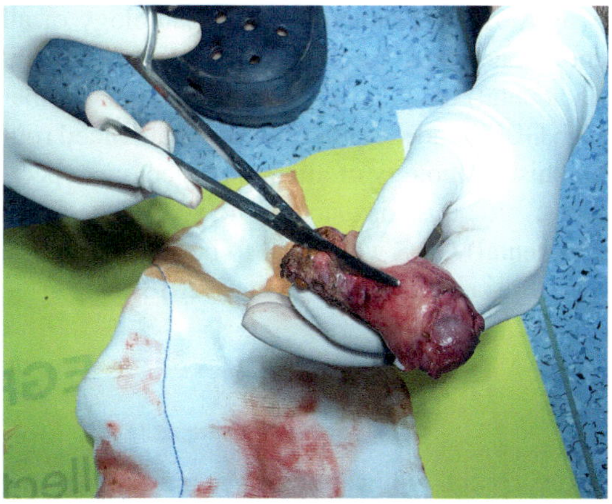

Fig. 13.21 It must be a routine practice to open the gall bladder (GB) specimen and carefully examine the GB wall and mucosa for any abnormality such as thickening, nodule, ulcer, or polyp; if such a finding is present, frozen section histopathological examination should be done

13.5 Prevention

Every effort must be made to avoid GB perforation and bile spill during LC. German Registry experience of 592 cases of incidental GBC showed that recurrence rate was as high as 38% in 73 cases in whom GB perforation occurred during the index laparoscopic cholecystectomy (Goetze and Paolucci 2009). In an analysis of 82 incidental GBCs, bile spill was reported in 55 (67%) cases during the index cholecystectomy. Peritoneal dissemination was more (24% vs. 4%) frequent in patients who had bile spill (Horkoff et al. 2019). In another report of 66 incidental GBCs, bile spill (and drain placement) was associated with poorer PFS and OS (Blakely et al. 2019). If bile spill occurs, irrigation with copious amounts of saline should be performed (Tumer et al. 2005). The Author (VKK) suggests distilled water instead of saline as it will cause, autolysis of spilled cancer cells, if any. GB should be extracted in a bag (Fig. 13.20) to avoid contamination of the port wound in order to prevent port-site metastasis. Once GB perforation has occurred, use of a specimen retrieval bag does not reduce the risk of recurrence (Goetze and Paolucci 2009).

It must be a routine practice to open the GB specimen (Fig. 13.21) and carefully examine the GB wall and mucosa for any abnormality such as thickening, nodule, ulcer, or polyp. If such an abnormality is found, it should be marked by a suture and the GB should be subjected to frozen section histopathological examination. If malignancy is found, an extended cholecystectomy should be performed at that time only by adding liver wedge resection and lymphadenectomy.

Some reports suggest that based on macroscopic examination of the GB specimen, the surgeon should be able to select out those GBs which need a microscopic examination by the pathologist, and this can reduce routine histopathological examination by about 80% (Corten et al. 2019a). The 2016 Dutch national guidelines on handling of a removed gallbladder for cholelithiasis propose a selective histopathologic policy (Sel-HP) rather than routine policy (Rout-HP) (Corten et al. 2019b). Macroscopic examination of the GB specimen by the surgeon followed by selective histopathological examination has been suggested by others also to reduce costs (Firat et al. 2019). The Author (VKK), however, strongly disagrees with this approach and is of the opinion that all GBs, even if they look grossly normal, MUST be subjected to histopathological examination. This is the only way that a true incidental GBC which is usually in early stages and has a potential for cure by reoperation can be detected. Agarwal et al. (2012) recommended histopathology of all cholecystectomy specimens to detect inapparent (incidental) GBC. A report from Pakistan, another high GBC incidence area, also recommended routine histopathology of all cholecystectomy specimens; if this is not followed subclinical (incidental) GBC would fail to be identified with disastrous results (Siddiqui et al. 2013).

13.6 Missed GBC

Some recent publications have questioned the routine practice of histopathological examination of every GB after cholecystectomy because of the low yield of finding an incidental GBC in a macroscopically grossly normal-looking GB; they recommend selective histopathological examination of only those GBs which have a macroscopic (gross) abnormality (Corten et al. 2019a; Firat et al. 2019). This is to reduce the workload of the pathologists and to reduce the costs of management. It is also argued that if at all any incidental GBC is present in a macroscopically grossly normal-looking GB, it is likely to be early (Tis or T1a) for which simple cholecystectomy alone (which has already been done) is enough and nothing else is required. However, almost half of the incidental GBCs are likely to be T1b, T2, or T3 where simple cholecystectomy alone is not enough, and reoperation for CEC will be required. A grossly abnormal GB, according to the Author (Kapoor 2006) is, however, unsuspected GBC which merits a frozen section histopathological examination followed by an immediate completion EC, if positive. The true incidental GBC is one which is detected only on histopathological examination in a grossly normal-looking GB.

In many instances, after cholecystectomy for a presumed preoperative diagnosis of GSD, if and when the GB looks apparently (grossly) normal to the surgeon, it is not sent for histopathological examination. Some of these patients present during the follow-up, usually after a few months, with symptoms suggestive of recurrence of GBC viz. pain, jaundice, vomiting, anorexia, and weight loss; examination may reveal a "GB" lump and evidence of distant spread including a palpable nodule at one of the port sites. Imaging (US and CT) shows a GB fossa mass (Fig. 13.22a, b) or liver metastases. This is because an early GBC, which was not grossly apparent, was missed because the GB was not sent for histopathological examination. Almost all of these missed recurrent GBCs, except an occasional localized port-site metastasis, are invariably unresectable. Agarwal et al. (2012) reported 77 cases which did not have histopathology of the GB after cholecystectomy and presented after a median of 152 days with recurrence—38 were operated but resectability was only 8% and median survival was only 10 months. Some of these patients with "missed" recurrent GBC who present with obstructive jaundice are misdiagnosed as post-cholecystectomy "benign" biliary stricture and referred for repair in the form of Roux-en-Y hepaticojejunostomy (Fig. 13.23) (Sharma et al. 2008). If the GB were subjected to histopathological examination, the incidental GBC would have been detected; it would have been an early GBC which could be resected at reoperation (CEC) and would have resulted in long-term survival, may be even cure. But missing the GBC means inevitable death in what was a potentially curable disease.

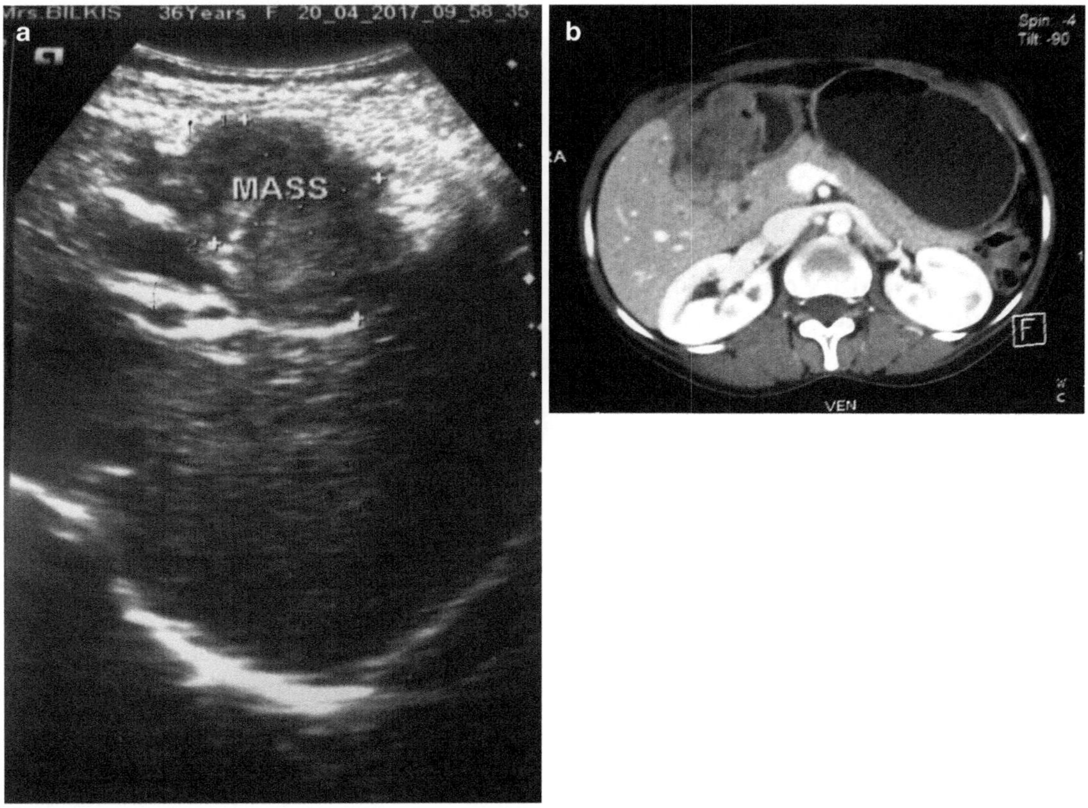

Fig. 13.22 "Missed" gall bladder cancer (**a**) US (**b**) CT shows a soft tissue mass in the gall bladder fossa infiltrating the prepyloric antrum

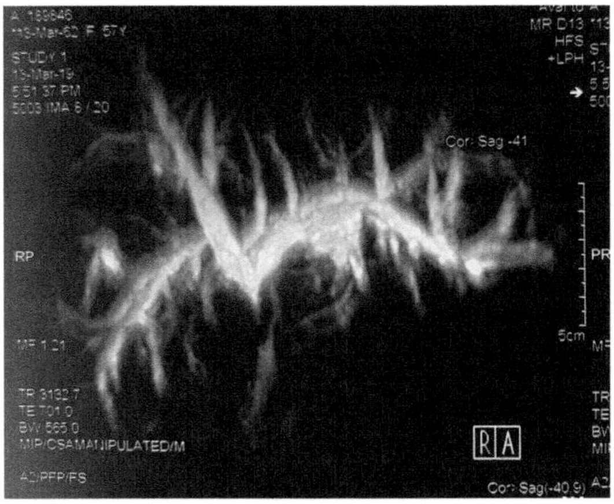

Fig. 13.23 MRC shows high (hilar) biliary block in a patient with post-cholecystectomy jaundice who was referred to us as benign biliary stricture (for repair with Roux-en-Y hepaticojejunostomy)—further investigations revealed it to be "missed" gall bladder cancer

The Author (VKK) strongly recommends that all GBs removed for a preoperative diagnosis of GSD should be opened, preferably by the surgeon himself, before the ports are removed (or the abdomen is closed), washed in running tap water to remove all bile and the mucosa carefully examined (preferably with a magnifying glass) to look for any suspicious area such as GB wall thickening, nodule, ulcer, or polyp. If such a lesion is present, the GB should be subjected to frozen section histopathological examination. If frozen section histopathological examination of the GB reveals malignancy, an EC is completed at that time only by removing a 2 cm wedge of liver and adding lymphadenectomy. Even if the GB looks grossly normal, it should ALWAYS be subjected to routine histopathological examination to detect an incidental GBC.

A few hundred US Dollars (or Japanese Yens, Korean Wons, or Indian Rupees) and a few minutes of the pathologist's time are worth an expense to save the life of a patient.

Incidental GBC is mostly curable but is usually mismanaged.

Invited Commentary on Incidental Gall Bladder Cancer

Thorsten Oliver Goetze

The preferred definition of incidental gall bladder cancer (GBC), according to the Author's (VKK) opinion (Kapoor 2001b), is GBC detected for the first time on histopathological examination of the removed GB (by open or laparoscopic simple cholecystectomy). In the German Registry (GR) of Incidental Gallbladder Carcinoma (IGBC) more than 1000 cases have been collected so far and the definition for registering a patient in the GR (Goetze and Paolucci 2013a) is nearly the same, i.e., the diagnosis of GBC was first made by the pathologist after cholecystectomy for benign reasons and is, therefore, consistent with the majority of literature. A gallbladder carcinoma is suspected preoperatively in only 30% of all patients (Varshney et al. 2002; Wullstein et al. 2002); the remaining 70% of all cases are incidentally discovered by the pathologist (so-called incidental or occult gallbladder carcinoma) (Box and Edge 1999; Copher et al. 1995). A gallbladder carcinoma is found in 0.2–2.9% of all cholecystectomies (Romano et al. 2001; Toyonaga et al. 2003). After a simple cholecystectomy, it is important to perform radical re-resection according to the NCCN, ESMO, and German-S3 Guidelines (Valle et al. 2016; Benson et al. 2019b; Gutt et al. 2018). The mentioned guidelines and the data of the GR support a radical completion surgery (stage-adjusted therapy) in cases of T1b and more advanced stages. T1b GBCs significantly benefit from radical surgery and are patients with a realistic potential to be cured. Hepatic resection should be performed to obtain clear margins. In IGBC, a radical re-resection usually consists of wedge resection in segments IVB and V or bisegmentectomy of segments IVB and V as the minimal volume required. Liver resections should always be combined with a standardized lymphadenectomy along the hepatoduodenal ligament for therapeutic and staging reasons. Especially in such early cases like T1b IGBC completion surgery should eradicate the micrometastatic disease, which is usually PET negative. Endo et al. (2004) showed that in T2 cancers most of micrometastatic lesions are within 1 cm of the gallbladder bed and very few were located 1–2 cm away from it. The indication of a PET directly after cholecystectomy in this situation seems debatable because of methodic reasons. Otherwise, if a PET shows residual disease away from the GB bed in liver, the curative claim of a second surgery seems to be debatable.

Gallbladder neoplasms show a high incidence of locoregional failure after surgical resection, with early spread to celiac, retropancreatic, and aortocaval nodes as well as occult liver spread (Endo et al. 2004). The rate of positive lymph nodes is 31.2% in T2 and 45.5% in T3 stage carcinomas (Endo et al. 2004; Bartlett et al. 1996). Lymphatic spread beyond the hepatoduodenal ligament generally represents distant metastatic disease, and a cure in such patients by a pure surgical concept does not seem to be achievable. Therefore, there is a need for a systemic therapy as early as possible in the course of treatment of IGBCs. The landmark trial, UK ABC-02 by Valle et al. (2010) compared gemcitabine/cisplatin with gemcitabine alone in locally advanced or metastatic (palliative situation) cholangio- and gallbladder carcinomas and showed clear superiority of the combination, with significant improvements for progression-free survival (PFS) (8 vs. 5 months, $p < 0.001$) and overall survival (OS) (11.7 vs. 8.1 months, $p < 0.001$). Basically, the study indicates the sensitivity of this disease toward chemotherapy and provides a rationale for the use of this chemotherapeutic doublet in neoadjuvant/perioperative settings also.

For improving disease control and cure rates of patients with immediate radical re-resection (IRR) in T2–3 IGBCs, it may be meaningful to implement early additional systemic therapy. The earliest moment to apply chemotherapy would be directly after simple cholecystectomy in IGBCs. The encouraging results of neoadjuvant/perioperative concepts in esophagogastric, stomach, rectal, and other malignancies provide an additional rationale to use this treatment in the early phase of IGBC management. However, due to the fact that two-third of GBCs are incidental findings after simple cholecystectomy, an earlier start of a systemic therapy in IGBC will not be realistic. Furthermore, preoperatively discovered GBCs are usually too advanced for neoadjuvant/perioperative concepts.

Recently the results of two randomized trials were presented which evaluated the role of either gemcitabine and oxaliplatin (PRODIGE 12) (Edeline et al. 2019) or capecitabine (BILCAP) (Primrose et al. 2019b) compared to observation alone in biliary tract including gallbladder cancer. The primary endpoint of PRODIGE 12 trial was relapse-free survival (RFS). The study showed no significant benefit according to relapse-free survival and overall survival. Therefore, the authors concluded that there was no benefit for GEMOX over surveillance in the adjuvant setting and GEMOX chemotherapy was not recommended in the adjuvant situation (Edeline et al. 2019). The most recent results of the BILCAP phase III trial (Primrose et al. 2019b) in 447 patients showed a significantly improved OS only in the PP (Per-Protocol)-population. In a sensitivity analysis, adjusting for further prognostic factors (gender, nodal status, and histological grade) there was a significant benefit for adjuvant chemotherapy. However, in the overall ITT (Intention-To-Treat)-population, the trial was negative. To conclude, there are trends for improvement in OS due to adjuvant therapy, but data demonstrating a significant improvement for adding adjuvant therapy after a curative resection are lacking. Nevertheless, adjuvant capecitabine was currently defined as the adjuvant standard of care (SoC) therapy.

Because of high rates of disease recurrence and poor survival rates in IGBC following surgical resection and the inadequacy of treatment modalities in the pure adjuvant therapy there is a need for an earlier intervention in the course of the disease. Due to the prognostic improvements of patients in other tumor entities (e.g., gastric, colorectal) (Cunningham et al. 2006; Al-Batran et al. 2019) treated with neoadjuvant or perioperative therapy there is a strong rationale to use these concepts in biliary and gallbladder cancers. In Germany, the GAIN trial with perioperative cisplatin + gemcitabine right after simple cholecystectomy and before IRR has just started recruitment. GAIN is a multicenter, randomized, controlled, open-label phase III study including patients with pT2–3N−ve or pT1–3N+ve IGBCs after simple cholecystectomy and patients with resectable/borderline resectable cholangiocarcinomas (ICC/ECC) scheduled to receive perioperative chemotherapy or surgery alone. GAIN was based on and initiated by the investigators of the German Registry for Incidental Gallbladder Carcinoma (GR).

All efforts must be made to cure the early stage IGBCs, including radical surgery and systemic therapy options. Compromise in the treatment of these patients with a realistic chance of cure will quickly lead to a non-curative palliative setting. On the other hand, it is necessary to avoid the so-called pseudo-curative surgery in patients with too advanced disease where a good systemic palliative chemotherapy is better than performing multivisceral resections with doubtful prognostic benefit.

Invited Commentary on Incidental Gall Bladder Cancer

Shishir K. Maithel

Professor VK Kapoor has written a very complete and elegant review of incidental gallbladder cancer (GBC). I offer my brief comments on a few select topics: diagnosis and frozen section analysis, staging and predicting residual disease, extent of operation, and adjuvant/neoadjuvant therapy.

The Author (VKK) mentions the use of intraoperative fine needle aspiration (FNA) in making a diagnosis of GBC. I need to emphasize caution with this approach. Intraoperatively, the FNA would most likely be performed via a peritoneal approach, as opposed to through the liver. Also, in this clinical situation, the intended mass or nodule is likely small and thus multiple passes may be necessary. FNA introduces the risk of peritoneal spillage of bile, which in the setting of GBC can be devastating for the patient as it has been associated with early development of peritoneal disease. Furthermore, re-resection after a diagnosis of incidental GBC has not been shown to be associated with reduced survival or worse outcomes compared to performing an extended or "radical" cholecystectomy at the index operation. Finally, obtaining an accurate tissue specimen from the FNA, namely one that can not only make the diagnosis but also correctly delineate the T-stage to guide operative therapy, can be difficult, and thus I am skeptical of the utility of intraoperative FNA. If the index of suspicion for cancer is high enough to warrant an extended cholecystectomy without tissue diagnosis, and it can be performed safely, then I am of the opinion that it is reasonable to perform after obtaining informed consent from the patient and/or family.

In a similar vein, most laparoscopic cholecystectomies that are performed worldwide are not performed by specialty-trained hepatobiliary surgeons or surgical oncologists; they are performed by general surgeons. Thus, the value of in-depth frozen section analysis as described by Professor Kapoor needs to be questioned. If, in the majority of cases, the surgical expertise is not available to do anything with the information gained from the frozen section analysis in the operating room, then why do it in the first place? Furthermore, re-resection at some interval of time after the index cholecystectomy is not associated with worse outcomes than performing the oncologic operation at the index operation, and in fact, as suggested by two studies, may actually be better.

Once the diagnosis is made, adequate staging and best determination of residual disease are paramount in guiding further therapy. Professor Kapoor has covered staging thoroughly; I only emphasize that a PET scan must be interpreted with caution, particularly in the early postoperative period when evaluating the operative field. It is extremely difficult to accurately differentiate residual disease or positive lymph nodes from merely reactive inflammation resulting from the index operation. Currently, the standard of care to estimate residual disease is to base it off the T-stage alone. As Professor Kapoor highlighted, Ethun et al. (2017a) developed a risk score that utilizes other adverse pathologic characteristics routinely available after the index operation, namely lymphovascular invasion (LVI), perineural invasion (PNI), and grade, to more accurately predict the incidence of residual disease. I would encourage clinicians to incorporate this risk score into their decision making, as it may help further personalize management of patients with T1b disease or of high-risk patients that are marginal operative candidates.

The extent of operation has nicely been covered by Professor Kapoor, and is also detailed in the consensus statement put forth by the American Hepato-Pancreato-Biliary Association (AHPBA)/ Society of Surgical Oncology (SSO)/Society for Surgery of the Alimentary Tract (SSAT) to which Professor Kapoor has already alluded. I would like to make a few comments on this topic. I whole heartedly agree with Professor Kapoor that we should be aggressive surgically for T1b disease, unless of course patient co-morbidity is a contraindication, and that the "side" of T2 disease (i.e., T2a vs. T2b) should not affect the decision to perform a re-resection. I would also add that while a complete portal lymphadenectomy should be routinely performed, removing distant lymph nodes (i.e., celiac axis or aortocaval) should not be considered standard of care as metastases to these lymph node basins is considered distant metastases and removal of them does not usually translate into prolonged survival. Finally, given the strong association of port-site involvement with the early development of peritoneal disease, routine port-site resection is not recommended, as Professor Kapoor has pointed out as well.

There remains the issue of other therapies besides resection for incidental GBC. The largest obstacle with determining the best course of other therapy for this disease is its scarcity and the fact that it is grouped together with all other biliary cancers (i.e., cholangiocarcinoma of all sites) in clinical trials. Despite it being well known that these biliary malignancies are all unique in their molecular signatures and biologic behavior, they have all been lumped together for the purpose of clinical trials in order to optimize the feasibility of completing the trial. Given that this is the best information that we have, despite its limitations, the BILCAP trial has defined the standard of care adjuvant therapy after re-resection of incidental GBC to be 6 months of capecitabine (Primrose et al. 2019b). This recommendation is regardless of margin status or lymph node status, and has been endorsed by the ASCO Adjuvant Guidelines Committee (Shroff et al. 2019). Interestingly, given the exceedingly low rate of margin positive resections for incidental GBC given the nature of the disease, it is my opinion that radiation has a limited, if any, role in the management of this disease.

Finally, as Professor Kapoor has highlighted, the survival of patients with incidental GBC has much left to be desired and has tremendous room for improvement. While prevention would be the ideal scenario, given its low incidence, the implementation of screening programs or performing prophylactic cholecystectomies outside the context of a very high-risk population is not a realistic option. In the same vein as pancreas cancer, we need to develop more effective systemic therapy for this disease and perhaps, administering neoadjuvant chemotherapy prior to re-resection would help eradicate micrometastatic disease and optimize patient selection for those who would most benefit from re-resection. This trial needs to be conducted in a disease-specific manner, focusing only on incidental GBC, and can only be accomplished with the cooperation and collaboration of the international community. Efforts to do exactly this are underway.

References

Chapter References

Addeo P, Centonze L, Locicero A, Faitot F, Jedidi H, Felli E, Fuchshuber P, Bachellier P. Incidental gallbladder carcinoma discovered after laparoscopic cholecystectomy: identifying patients who will benefit from reoperation. J Gastrointest Surg. 2018;22(4):606–14. https://doi.org/10.1007/s11605-017-3655-z. Epub 2017 Dec 22.

Agarwal AK, Kalayarasan R, Singh S, Javed A, Sakhuja P. All cholecystectomy specimens must be sent for histopathology to detect inapparent gallbladder cancer. HPB (Oxford). 2012;14(4):269–73. https://doi.org/10.1111/j.1477-2574.2012.00443.x. Epub 2012 Feb 26.

Ahn Y, Park CS, Hwang S, Jang HJ, Choi KM, Lee SG. Incidental gallbladder cancer after routine cholecystectomy: when should we suspect it preoperatively and what are predictors of patient survival? Ann Surg Treat Res. 2016;90(3):131–8. https://doi.org/10.4174/astr.2016.90.3.131. Epub 2016 Feb 26.

Aloia TA, Járufe N, Javle M, Maithel SK, Roa JC, Adsay V, Coimbra FJ, Jarnagin WR. Gallbladder cancer: expert consensus statement. HPB (Oxford). 2015;17(8):681–90. https://doi.org/10.1111/hpb.12444.

Anderson CD, Rice MH, Pinson CW, Chapman WC, Chari RS, Delbeke D. Fluorodeoxyglucose PET imaging in the evaluation of gallbladder carcinoma and cholangiocarcinoma. J Gastrointest Surg. 2004;8(1):90–7.

Araujo RLC, de Sanctis MA, Coelho TRV, Felippe FEC, Burgardt D, Wohnrath DR. Robotic surgery as an alternative approach for reoperation of incidental gallbladder cancer. J Gastrointest Cancer. 2019; https://doi.org/10.1007/s12029-019-00264-3.

Ausania F, Tsirlis T, White SA, French JJ, Jaques BC, Charnley RM, Manas DM. Incidental pT2-T3 gallbladder cancer after a cholecystectomy: outcome of staging at 3 months prior to a radical resection. HPB (Oxford). 2013;15(8):633–7. https://doi.org/10.1111/hpb.12032. Epub 2013 Jan 7

Barreto SG, Pawar S, Shah S, Talole S, Goel M, Shrikhande SV. Patterns of failure and determinants of outcomes following radical re-resection for incidental gallbladder cancer. World J Surg. 2014;38(2):484–9. https://doi.org/10.1007/s00268-013-2266-4.

Benson AB, D'Angelica MI, Abbott DE, Abrams TA, Alberts SR, Anaya DA, Anders R, Are C, Brown D, Chang DT, Cloyd J, Covey AM, Hawkins W, Iyer R, Jacob R, Karachristos A, Kelley RK, Kim R, Palta M, Park JO, Sahai V, Schefter T, Sicklick JK, Singh G, Sohal D, Stein S, Tian GG, Vauthey JN, Venook AP, Hammond LJ, Darlow SD. Guidelines insights: hepatobiliary cancers, Version 2.2019. J Natl Compr Cancer Netw. 2019a;17(4):302–10. https://doi.org/10.6004/jnccn.2019.0019.

Berger-Richardson D, Chesney TR, Englesakis M, Govindarajan A, Cleary SP, Swallow CJ. Trends in port-site metastasis after laparoscopic resection of incidental gallbladder cancer: a systematic review. Surgery. 2017;161(3):618–27. https://doi.org/10.1016/j.surg.2016.08.007. Epub 2016 Oct 13.

Blakely AM, Wong P, Chu P, Warner SG, Raoof M, Singh G, Fong Y, Melstrom LG. Intraoperative bile spillage is associated with worse survival in gallbladder adenocarcinoma. J Surg Oncol. 2019; https://doi.org/10.1002/jso.25617.

Butte JM, Redondo F, Waugh E, Meneses M, Pruzzo R, Parada H, Amaral H, De La Fuente HA. The role of PET-CT in patients with incidental gallbladder cancer. HPB (Oxford). 2009;11(7):585–91.

Butte JM, Gönen M, Allen PJ, D'Angelica MI, Kingham TP, Fong Y, Dematteo RP, Blumgart L, Jarnagin WR. The role of laparoscopic staging in patients with incidental gallbladder cancer. HPB (Oxford). 2011a;13(7):463–72. https://doi.org/10.1111/j.1477-2574.2011.00325.x. Epub 2011 Jun 7.

Butte JM, Matsuo K, Gönen M, D'Angelica MI, Waugh E, Allen PJ, Fong Y, DeMatteo RP, Blumgart L, Endo I, De La Fuente H, Jarnagin WR. Gallbladder cancer: differences in presentation, surgical treatment, and survival in patients treated at centers in three countries. J Am Coll Surg. 2011b;212(1):50–61. https://doi.org/10.1016/j.jamcollsurg.2010.09.009. Epub 2010 Nov 12.

Butte JM, Kingham TP, Gönen M, D'Angelica MI, Allen PJ, Fong Y, DeMatteo RP, Jarnagin WR. Residual disease predicts outcomes after definitive resection for incidental gallbladder cancer. J Am Coll Surg. 2014;219(3):416–29. https://doi.org/10.1016/j.jamcollsurg.2014.01.069. Epub 2014 May 16.

Charfi S, Gouiaa N, Mnif H, Chtourou L, Tahri N, Abid B, Mzali R, Boudawara TS. Histopathological findings in cholecystectomies specimens: a single institution study of 20,584 cases. Hepatobiliary Pancreat Dis Int. 2018;17(4):345–8. https://doi.org/10.1016/j.hbpd.2018.06.008. Epub 2018 Jun 26.

Chen C, Geng Z, Shen H, Song H, Zhao Y, Zhang G, Li W, Ma L, Wang L. Long-term outcomes and prognostic factors in advanced gallbladder cancer: focus on the advanced T stage. PLoS One. 2016;11(11):e0166361. https://doi.org/10.1371/journal.pone.0166361. eCollection 2016.

Cherkassky L, D'Angelica M. Gallbladder cancer: managing the incidental diagnosis. Surg Oncol Clin N Am. 2019;28(4):619–30. https://doi.org/10.1016/j.soc.2019.06.005. Review.

Cherkassky L, Jarnagin W. Selecting treatment sequence for patients with incidental gallbladder cancer: a neoadjuvant approach versus upfront surgery. Updat Surg. 2019;71(2):217–25. https://doi.org/10.1007/s13304-019-00670-z. Epub 2019 Jun 28.

Cho JK, Lee W, Jang JY, Kim HG, Kim JM, Kwag SJ, Park JH, Kim JY, Park T, Jeong SH, Ju YT, Jung EJ, Lee YJ, Hong SC, Jeong CY. Validation of the oncologic effect of hepatic resection for T2 gallbladder cancer: a retrospective study. World J Surg Oncol. 2019;17(1):8. https://doi.org/10.1186/s12957-018-1556-6.

Choi KS, Choi SB, Park P, Kim WB, Choi SY. Clinical characteristics of incidental or unsuspected gallbladder cancers diagnosed during or after cholecystectomy: a systematic review and meta-analysis. World J Gastroenterol. 2015;21(4):1315–23. https://doi.org/10.3748/wjg.v21.i4.1315.

Clemente G. Unexpected gallbladder cancer: surgical strategies and prognostic factors. World J Gastrointest Surg. 2016;8(8):541–4. https://doi.org/10.4240/wjgs.v8.i8.541.

Corten BJGA, Alexander S, van Zwam PH, Leclercq WKG, Roumen RMH, Slooter GD. Outcome of surgical inspection of the gallbladder in relation to final pathology. J Gastrointest Surg. 2019a;23(6):1130–4. https://doi.org/10.1007/s11605-018-3921-8. Epub 2018 Aug 21.

Corten BJGA, Leclercq WKG, Dejong CH, Roumen RMH, Slooter GD. Selective histological examination after cholecystectomy: an analysis of current daily practice in The Netherlands. World J Surg. 2019b; https://doi.org/10.1007/s00268-019-05077-w.

Corvera CU, Blumgart LH, Akhurst T, DeMatteo RP, D'Angelica M, Fong Y, Jarnagin WR. 18F-fluorodeoxyglucose positron emission tomography influences management decisions in patients with biliary cancer. J Am Coll Surg. 2008;206(1):57–65. Epub 2007 Oct 1

Creasy JM, Goldman DA, Gonen M, Dudeja V, Askan G, Basturk O, Balachandran VP, Allen PJ, DeMatteo RP, D'Angelica MI, Jarnagin WR, Peter Kingham T. Predicting residual disease in incidental gallbladder cancer: risk stratification for modified treatment strategies. J Gastrointest Surg. 2017;21(8):1254–61. https://doi.org/10.1007/s11605-017-3436-8. Epub 2017 May 8.

de Aretxabala X, Roa I, Hepp J, Maluenda F, Mordojovich G, Leon J, Roa JC. Early gallbladder cancer: is further treatment necessary? J Surg Oncol. 2009;100(7):589–93. https://doi.org/10.1002/jso.21389.

de Aretxabala X, Oppliger F, Solano N, Rencoret G, Vivanco M, Carvajal D, Hepp J, Roa I. Laparoscopic management of incidental gallbladder cancer. Surg Endosc. 2018;32(10):4251–5. https://doi.org/10.1007/s00464-018-6173-5. Epub 2018 Jun 20.

de Savornin Lohman EAJ, van der Geest LG, de Bitter TJJ, et al. Re-resection in incidental gallbladder cancer: survival and the incidence of residual disease. Ann Surg Oncol. 2020;27(4):1132–42. https://doi.org/10.1245/s10434-019-08074-4.

Dincel O, Goksu M, Hatipoglu HS. Importance of routine histopathological examination of a gallbladder surgical specimen: unexpected gallbladder cancer. J Cancer Res Ther. 2018;14(6):1325–9. https://doi.org/10.4103/0973-1482.187301.

Du J, Yang XW, Wen ZJ, Xue C, Wu YM, Wu MC, Zhang LL. Relationship between prognosis and time interval from cholecystectomy to reoperation in postoperative incidental gallbladder carcinoma. Chin Med J (Engl). 2018;131(20):2503–5. https://doi.org/10.4103/0366-6999.243565.

Duffy A, Capanu M, Abou-Alfa GK, Huitzil D, Jarnagin W, Fong Y, D'Angelica M, Dematteo RP, Blumgart LH, O'Reilly EM. Gallbladder cancer (GBC): 10-year experience at Memorial Sloan-Kettering Cancer Centre (MSKCC). J Surg Oncol. 2008;98(7):485–9. https://doi.org/10.1002/jso.21141.

Ethun CG, Le N, Lopez-Aguiar AG, Pawlik TM, Poultsides G, Tran T, Idrees K, Isom CA, Fields RC, Krasnick BA, Weber SM, Salem A, Martin RCG, Scoggins CR, Shen P, Mogal HD, Schmidt C, Beal E, Hatzaras I, Shenoy R, Russell MC, Maithel SK. Pathologic and prognostic implications of incidental versus nonincidental gallbladder cancer: a 10-institution study from the United States Extrahepatic Biliary Malignancy Consortium. Am Surg. 2017a;83(7):679–86.

Ethun CG, Postlewait LM, Le N, Pawlik TM, Buettner S, Poultsides G, Tran T, Idrees K, Isom CA, Fields RC, Jin LX, Weber SM, Salem A, Martin RC, Scoggins C, Shen P, Mogal HD, Schmidt C, Beal E, Hatzaras I, Shenoy R, Merchant N, Cardona K, Maithel SK. A novel pathology-based preoperative risk score to predict locoregional residual and distant disease and survival for incidental gallbladder cancer: a 10-institution study from the U.S. Extrahepatic Biliary Malignancy Consortium. Ann Surg Oncol. 2017b;24(5):1343–50. https://doi.org/10.1245/s10434-016-5637-x. Epub 2016 Nov 3

Ethun CG, Postlewait LM, Le N, Pawlik TM, Buettner S, Poultsides G, Tran T, Idrees K, Isom CA, Fields RC, Jin LX, Weber SM, Salem A, Martin RC, Scoggins C, Shen P, Mogal HD, Schmidt C, Beal E, Hatzaras I, Shenoy R, Kooby DA, Maithel SK. Association of optimal time interval to re-resection for incidental gallbladder cancer with overall survival: a multi-institution analysis from the US Extrahepatic Biliary Malignancy Consortium. JAMA Surg. 2017c;152(2):143–9. https://doi.org/10.1001/jamasurg.2016.3642. Erratum in: JAMA Surg. 2017;152(2):211.

Ethun CG, Postlewait LM, Le N, Pawlik TM, Poultsides G, Tran T, Idrees K, Isom CA, Fields RC, Krasnick BA, Weber SM, Salem A, Martin RCG, Scoggins CR, Shen P, Mogal HD, Schmidt C, Beal E, Hatzaras I, Shenoy R, Cardona K, Maithel SK. Routine port-site excision in incidentally discovered gallbladder cancer is not associated with improved survival: a multi-institution analysis from the US Extrahepatic Biliary Malignancy Consortium. J Surg Oncol. 2017d;115(7):805–11. https://doi.org/10.1002/jso.24591. Epub 2017 Feb 23.

Figueiredo WR, Santos RR, Paula MMDRC. Comparative incidence of incidental gallbladder cancer in emergency cholecystectomies versus in elective cholecystectomies. Incidência comparativa de câncer incidental de vesícula biliar em colecistectomias de urgência versus colecistectomias eletivas. Rev Col Bras Cir. 2020;46(6):e20192366. https://doi.org/10.1590/0100-6991e-20192366.

Firat YD, Idiz UO, Cakir C, Yardimci E, Yazici P, Bektasoglu H, Bozkurt E, Ucak R, Gucin Z, Uresin T, Hasbahceci M. Prospective multi-center study of surgeon's assessment of the gallbladder compared to histopathological examination to detect incidental malignancy. Langenbecks Arch Surg. 2019; https://doi.org/10.1007/s00423-019-01800-2.

Fong Y, Jarnagin W, Blumgart LH. Gallbladder cancer: comparison of patients presenting initially for definitive operation with those presenting after prior noncurative intervention. Ann Surg. 2000;232(4):557–69.

Fuks D, Regimbeau JM, Le Treut YP, Bachellier P, Raventos A, Pruvot FR, Chiche L, Farges O. Incidental gallbladder cancer by the AFC-GBC-2009 Study Group. World J Surg. 2011;35(8):1887–97. https://doi.org/10.1007/s00268-011-1134-3.

Fuks D, Regimbeau JM, Pessaux P, Bachellier P, Raventos A, Mantion G, Gigot JF, Chiche L, Pascal G, Azoulay D, Laurent A, Letoublon C, Boleslawski E, Rivoire M, Mabrut JY, Adham M, Le Treut YP, Delpero JR, Navarro F, Ayav A, Boudjema K, Nuzzo G, Scotte M, Farges O. Is port-site resection necessary in the surgical management of gallbladder cancer? J Visc Surg. 2013;150(4):277–84. https://doi.org/10.1016/j.jviscsurg.2013.03.006. Epub 2013 May 9.

Gil L, de Aretxabala X, Lendoire J, Duek F, Hepp J, Imventarza O. Incidental gallbladder cancer: how residual disease affects outcome in two referral HPB centers from South America. World J Surg. 2019;43(1):214–20. https://doi.org/10.1007/s00268-018-4762-z.

Goel M, Tamhankar A, Rangarajan V, Patkar S, Ramadwar M, Shrikhande SV. Role of PET CT scan in redefining treatment of incidental gall bladder carcinoma. J Surg Oncol. 2016;113(6):652–8. https://doi.org/10.1002/jso.24198. Epub 2016 Feb 5.

Goetze TO. Gallbladder carcinoma: prognostic factors and therapeutic options. World J Gastroenterol. 2015;21(43):12211–7. https://doi.org/10.3748/wjg.v21.i43.12211. Review.

Goetze TO, Paolucci V. Benefits of reoperation of T2 and more advanced incidental gallbladder carcinoma: analysis of the German registry. Ann Surg. 2008;247(1):104–8.

Goetze TO, Paolucci V. Use of retrieval bags in incidental gallbladder cancer cases. World J Surg. 2009;33(10):2161–5. https://doi.org/10.1007/s00268-009-0163-7.

Goetze TO, Paolucci V. Adequate extent in radical re-resection of incidental gallbladder carcinoma: analysis of the German Registry. Surg Endosc. 2010;24(9):2156–64. https://doi.org/10.1007/s00464-010-0914-4. Epub 2010 Feb 23.

Goetze TO, Paolucci V. Prognosis of incidental gallbladder carcinoma is not influenced by the primary access technique: analysis of 837 incidental gallbladder carcinomas in the German Registry. Surg Endosc. 2013a;27(8):2821–8. https://doi.org/10.1007/s00464-013-2819-5. Epub 2013 Feb 13.

Goetze TO, Paolucci V. [Incidental T1b-T3 gallbladder carcinoma. Extended cholecystectomy as an underestimated prognostic factor-results of the German registry]. Chirurg. 2014a;85(2):131–8. https://doi.org/10.1007/s00104-013-2587-8. German.

Goetze TO, Paolucci V. Influence of high- and low-volume liver surgery in gallbladder carcinoma. World J Gastroenterol. 2014b;20(48):18445–51. https://doi.org/10.3748/wjg.v20.i48.18445.

Goetze TO, Paolucci V. [Immediate radical re-resection of incidental T1b gallbladder cancer and the problem of an adequate extent of resection (results of the German Registry "Incidental Gallbladder Cancer")].

Zentralbl Chir. 2014c;139(Suppl 2):e43–8. https://doi.org/10.1055/s-0030-1262698. Epub 2011 Mar 1. German.

Goussous N, Maqsood H, Patel K, Ferdosi H, Muhammad N, Sill AM, Kowdley GC, Cunningham SC. Clues to predict incidental gallbladder cancer. Hepatobiliary Pancreat Dis Int. 2018;17(2):149–54. https://doi.org/10.1016/j.hbpd.2018.02.001. Epub 2018 Feb 19.

Grupo Internacional de Estudos de Câncer Hepatopancreatobiliar - ISG-HPB-Cancer, Coimbra FJF, Torres OJM, et al. Brazilian consensus on incidental gallbladder carcinoma. Arq Bras Cir Dig. 2020;33(1):e1496. https://doi.org/10.1590/0102-6720 20190001e1496.

Gumbs AA, Hoffman JP. Laparoscopic completion radical cholecystectomy for T2 gallbladder cancer. Surg Endosc. 2010;24(12):3221–3. Epub 2010 May 25

Horkoff MJ, Ahmed Z, Xu Y, Sutherland FR, Dixon E, Ball CG, Bathe OF. Adverse outcomes after bile spillage in incidental gallbladder cancers: a population-based study. Ann Surg. 2019; https://doi.org/10.1097/SLA.0000000000003325.

Kapoor VK. Incidental gallbladder cancer. Am J Gastroenterol. 2001a;96(3):627–9. Review.

Kapoor VK. Gallbladder cancer: a global perspective. J Surg Oncol. 2006;93(8):607–9.

Kapoor VK. Advanced gallbladder cancer: Indian "middle path". J Hepatobiliary Pancreat Surg. 2007;14(4):366–73. Epub 2007 Jul 30.

Kapoor VK, Behari A. Surgical procedures for gall bladder cancer. BAOJ Cancer Res Ther. 2017;3:037.

Kapoor VK, Singh R, Behari A, Sharma S, Kumar A, Prakash A, Singh RK, Kumar A, Saxena R. Anticipatory extended cholecystectomy: the 'Lucknow' approach for thick walled gall bladder with low suspicion of cancer. Chin Clin Oncol. 2016;5(1):8. https://doi.org/10.3978/j.issn.2304-3865.2016.02.07.

Kasumova GG, Tabatabaie O, Najarian RM, Callery MP, Ng SC, Bullock AJ, Fisher RA, Tseng JF. Surgical management of gallbladder cancer: simple versus extended cholecystectomy and the role of adjuvant therapy. Ann Surg. 2017;266(4):625–31. https://doi.org/10.1097/SLA.0000000000002385.

Kawahara R, Shirahama T, Arai S, Muroya D, Nomura Y, Fukutomi S, Shirahama N, Takagi K, Goto Y, Akashi M, Maruyama Y, Sakai H, Ishikawa H, Hisaka T, Yasunaga M, Horiuchi H, Okuda K, Akagi Y, Tanaka H. Evaluation of surgical procedures for T2 gallbladder cancer in terms of recurrence and prognosis. Kurume Med J. 2017;63(1.2):15–22. https://doi.org/10.2739/kurumemedj.MS65005. Epub 2017 Mar 22.

Kim HS, Park JW, Kim H, Han Y, Kwon W, Kim SW, Hwang YJ, Kim SG, Kwon HJ, Vinuela E, Járufe N, Roa JC, Han IW, Heo JS, Choi SH, Choi DW, Ahn KS, Kang KJ, Lee W, Jeong CY, Hong SC, Troncoso A, Losada H, Han SS, Park SJ, Yanagimoto H, Endo I, Kubota K, Wakai T, Ajiki T, Adsay NV, Jang JY. Optimal surgical treatment in patients with T1b gallbladder cancer: an international multicenter study. J Hepatobiliary Pancreat Sci. 2018;25(12):533–43. https://doi.org/10.1002/jhbp.593.

Köhn N, Maubach J, Warschkow R, Tsai C, Nussbaum DP, Candinas D, Gloor B, Schmied BM, Blazer DG III, Worni M. High rate of positive lymph nodes in T1a gallbladder cancer does not translate to decreased survival: a population-based, propensity score adjusted analysis. HPB (Oxford). 2018;20(11):1073–81. https://doi.org/10.1016/j.hpb.2018.05.007. Epub 2018 Jun 8.

Kohya N, Kitahara K, Miyazaki K. Rational therapeutic strategy for T2 gallbladder carcinoma based on tumor spread. World J Gastroenterol. 2010;16(28):3567–72.

Kumar S, Bhoriwal S, Muduly D, Kar M, Sharma A, Pathy S, Shukla NK, Deo SVS. Multimodality management of incidentally detected gall bladder cancer: long term results from a tertiary care cancer centre. J Gastrointest Oncol. 2019;10(1):128–33. https://doi.org/10.21037/jgo.2018.09.10.

Lafaro K, Blakely AM, Melstrom LG, et al. Prognostic impact of tumor location in resected gallbladder cancer: a national cohort analysis. J Surg Oncol. 2020; https://doi.org/10.1002/jso.26107.

Lee SE, Jang JY, Lim CS, Kang MJ, Kim SW. Systematic review on the surgical treatment for T1 gallbladder cancer. World J Gastroenterol. 2011;17(2):174–80. https://doi.org/10.3748/wjg.v17.i2.174. Review.

Lee H, Choi DW, Park JY, Youn S, Kwon W, Heo JS, Choi SH, Jang KT. Surgical strategy for T2 gallbladder cancer according to tumor location. Ann Surg Oncol. 2015;22(8):2779–86. https://doi.org/10.1245/s10434-014-4300-7. Epub 2014 Dec 18.

Lee W, Jeong CY, Jang JY, Kim YH, Roh YH, Kim KW, Kang SH, Yoon MH, Seo HI, Yun SP, et al. Do hepatic-sided tumors require more extensive resection than peritoneal-sided tumors in patients with T2 gallbladder cancer? Results of a retrospective multicenter study. Surgery. 2017;162(3):515–24. https://doi.org/10.1016/j.surg.2017.05.004.

Lee H, Kwon W, Han Y, Kim JR, Kim SW, Jang JY. Optimal extent of surgery for early gallbladder cancer with regard to long-term survival: a meta-analysis. J Hepatobiliary Pancreat Sci. 2018a;25(2):131–41. https://doi.org/10.1002/jhbp.521. Epub 2017 Dec 14. Review.

Lee SE, Kim SW, Han HS, Lee WJ, Yoon DS, Cho BH, Choi IS, Kim HJ, Hong SC, Lee SM, Choi DW, Park SJ, Kim HJ, Jang JY, Korean Pancreas Surgery Club. Surgical strategy for T2 gallbladder cancer: nationwide multicenter survey in Korea. J Korean Med Sci. 2018b;33(28):e186. https://doi.org/10.3346/jkms.2018.33.e186. eCollection 2018 Jul 9.

Leung U, Pandit-Taskar N, Corvera CU, D'Angelica MI, Allen PJ, Kingham TP, DeMatteo RP, Jarnagin WR, Fong Y. Impact of pre-operative positron emission tomography in gallbladder cancer. HPB (Oxford). 2014;16(11):1023–30. https://doi.org/10.1111/hpb.12282. Epub 2014 Jun 4

Li G, Kim JH, Jung W, Hwang JC, Yang MJ, Kim JH, Yoo BM, Kim WH. Significance of hepatectomy in patients diagnosed with T2 gallbladder cancer. Surg Laparosc Endosc Percutan Tech. 2019; https://doi.org/10.1097/SLE.0000000000000703.

Lundgren L, Muszynska C, Ros A, Persson G, Gimm O, Andersson B, Sandström P. Management of incidental gallbladder cancer in a national cohort. Br J Surg. 2019;106(9):1216–27. https://doi.org/10.1002/bjs.11205. Epub 2019 Jul 1.

Maker AV, Butte JM, Oxenberg J, Kuk D, Gonen M, Fong Y, Dematteo RP, D'Angelica MI, Allen PJ, Jarnagin WR. Is port site resection necessary in the surgical management of gallbladder cancer? Ann Surg Oncol. 2012;19(2):409–17.

Mochizuki T, Abe T, Amano H, Hanada K, Hattori M, Kobayashi T, Nakahara M, Ohdan H, Noriyuki T. Efficacy of the gallbladder cancer predictive risk score based on pathological findings: a propensity score-matched analysis. Ann Surg Oncol. 2018;25(6):1699–708. https://doi.org/10.1245/s10434-018-6444-3. Epub 2018 Apr 6.

Muszynska C, Lundgren L, Lindell G, Andersson R, Nilsson J, Sandström P, Andersson B. Predictors of incidental gallbladder cancer in patients undergoing cholecystectomy for benign gallbladder disease: Results from a population-based gallstone surgery registry. Surgery. 2017;162(2):256–63. https://doi.org/10.1016/j.surg.2017.02.009. Epub 2017 Apr 8.

Muszynska C, Nilsson J, Lundgren L, et al. A risk score model to predict incidental gallbladder cancer in patients scheduled for cholecystectomy. Am J Surg. 2020; https://doi.org/10.1016/j.amjsurg.2020.01.039.

Otero JC, Proske A, Vallilengua C, Luján M, Poletto L, Otero JR, Pezzotto SM, Celoria G. Gallbladder carcinoma: intraoperative imprint cytology, a helpful and valuable screening procedure. J Hepatobiliary Pancreat Surg. 2008;15(2):157–60. https://doi.org/10.1007/s00534-007-1253-2. Epub 2008 Apr 6.

Paolucci V, Schaeff B, Schneider M, Gutt C. Tumor seeding following laparoscopy: international survey. World J Surg. 1999;23(10):989–95; discussion 996–7.

Park TJ, Ahn KS, Kim YH, Kim TS, Hong JH, Kang KJ. The optimal surgical resection approach for T2 gallbladder carcinoma: evaluating the role of surgical extent according to the tumor location. Ann Surg Treat Res. 2018;94(3):135–41. https://doi.org/10.4174/astr.2018.94.3.135. Epub 2018 Feb 28.

Pawlik TM, Gleisner AL, Vigano L, Kooby DA, Bauer TW, Frilling A, Adams RB, Staley CA, Trindade EN, Schulick RD, Choti MA, Capussotti L. Incidence of finding residual disease for incidental gallbladder carcinoma: implications for re-resection. J Gastrointest Surg. 2007;11(11):1478–86; discussion 1486–7.

Principe A, Del Gaudio M, Ercolani G, Golfieri R, Cucchetti A, Pinna AD. Radical surgery for gallbladder carcinoma: possibilities of survival. Hepatogastroenterology. 2006;53(71):660–4.

Qadan M, Kingham TP. Technical aspects of gallbladder cancer surgery. Surg Clin North Am. 2016;96(2):229–45. https://doi.org/10.1016/j.suc.2015.12.007.

Roa I, Ibacache G, Muñoz S, de Aretxabala X. Gallbladder cancer in Chile: pathologic characteristics of survival and prognostic factors: analysis of 1,366 cases. Am J Clin Pathol. 2014;141(5):675–82. https://doi.org/10.1309/AJCPQT3ELN2BBCKA.

Sharma A, Behari A, Sikora SS, Kumar A, Saxena R, Kapoor VK. Post-cholecystectomy biliary strictures: not always benign. J Gastroenterol Hepatol. 2008;23(7 Pt 2):e63–6. Epub 2007 Jul 20.

Shih SP, Schulick RD, Cameron JL, Lillemoe KD, Pitt HA, Choti MA, Campbell KA, Yeo CJ, Talamini MA. Gallbladder cancer: the role of laparoscopy and radical resection. Ann Surg. 2007;245(6):893–901.

Shindoh J, de Aretxabala X, Aloia TA, Roa JC, Roa I, Zimmitti G, Javle M, Conrad C, Maru DM, Aoki T, et al. Tumor location is a strong predictor of tumor progression and survival in T2 gallbladder cancer: an international multicenter study. Ann Surg. 2015;261(4):733–9. https://doi.org/10.1097/SLA.0000000000000728.

Shirai Y, Yoshida K, Tsukada K, Muto T. Inapparent carcinoma of the gallbladder. An appraisal of a radical second operation after simple cholecystectomy. Ann Surg. 1992;215(4):326–31.

Shukla PJ, Barreto G, Neve R, Mohandas KM, Shrikhande SV. Can we do better than 'incidental' gallbladder cancer? Hepatogastroenterology. 2007;54(80):2184–5.

Shukla PJ, Barreto G, Kakade A, Shrikhande SV. Revision surgery for incidental gallbladder cancer: factors influencing operability and further evidence for T1b tumours. HPB (Oxford). 2008;10(1):43–7. https://doi.org/10.1080/13651820701867794.

Siddiqui FG, Memon AA, Abro AH, Sasoli NA, Ahmad L. Routine histopathology of gallbladder after elective cholecystectomy for gallstones: waste of resources or a justified act? BMC Surg. 2013;13:26. https://doi.org/10.1186/1471-2482-13-26.

Søreide K, Guest RV, Harrison EM, Kendall TJ, Garden OJ, Wigmore SJ. Systematic review of management of incidental gallbladder cancer after cholecystectomy. Br J Surg. 2019;106(1):32–45. https://doi.org/10.1002/bjs.11035.

Steffen T, Ebinger SM, Tarantino I, Widmann B. Prognostic impact of lymph node excision in T1 and T2 gallbladder cancer: a population-based and propensity score-matched SEER analysis. J Gastrointest Surg. 2019; https://doi.org/10.1007/s11605-019-04175-3.

Toge K, Sakata J, Hirose Y, Yuza K, Ando T, Soma D, Katada T, Miura K, Takizawa K, Kobayashi T, Wakai T. Lymphatic spread of T2 gallbladder carcinoma: regional lymphadenectomy is required independent of tumor location. Eur J Surg Oncol. 2019; https://doi.org/10.1016/j.ejso.2019.03.038.

Tumer AR, Yüksek YN, Yasti AC, Gözalan U, Kama NA. Dropped gallstones during laparoscopic cholecystectomy: the consequences. World J Surg. 2005;29(4):437–40.

Vega EA, Vinuela E, Sanhueza M, Mege R, Caracci M, Diaz C, Diaz A, Okuno M, Joechle K, Goumard C, Chun YS, Tzeng CD, Lee JE, Vauthey JN, Conrad C. Positive cystic duct margin at index cholecystectomy in incidental gallbladder cancer is an important negative prognosticator. Eur J Surg Oncol. 2019;45(6):1061–8. https://doi.org/10.1016/j.ejso.2019.01.013. Epub 2019 Jan 24.

Vega EA, De Aretxabala X, Qiao W, et al. Comparison of oncological outcomes after open and laparoscopic re-resection of incidental gallbladder cancer. Br J Surg. 2020;107(3):289–300. https://doi.org/10.1002/bjs.11379.

Vinuela E, Vega EA, Yamashita S, Sanhueza M, Mege R, Cavada G, Aloia TA, Chun YS, Lee JE, Vauthey JN, Conrad C. Incidental gallbladder cancer: residual cancer discovered at oncologic extended resection determines outcome: a report from high- and low-incidence countries. Ann Surg Oncol. 2017;24(8):2334–43. https://doi.org/10.1245/s10434-017-5859-6. Epub 2017 Apr 17.

Vo E, Curley SA, Chai CY, Massarweh NN, Tran Cao HS. National failure of surgical staging for T1b gallbladder cancer. Ann Surg Oncol. 2019;26(2):604–10. https://doi.org/10.1245/s10434-018-7064-7. Epub 2018 Nov 29.

Wakai T, Shirai Y, Yokoyama N, Nagakura S, Watanabe H, Hatakeyama K. Early gallbladder carcinoma does not warrant radical resection. Br J Surg. 2001;88(5):675–8.

Wang Z, Li Y, Jiang W, Yan J, Dai J, Jiao B, Yin Z, Zhang Y. Simple cholecystectomy is adequate for patients with T1b gallbladder adenocarcinoma < 1 cm in diameter. Front Oncol. 2019;9:409. https://doi.org/10.3389/fonc.2019.00409. eCollection 2019.

Watson H, Dasari B, Wyatt J, Hidalgo E, Prasad R, Lodge P, Toogood G. Does a second resection provide a survival benefit in patients diagnosed with incidental T1b/T2 gallbladder cancer following cholecystectomy? HPB (Oxford). 2017;19(2):104–7. https://doi.org/10.1016/j.hpb.2016.11.006. Epub 2016 Dec 13.

Yamaguchi K, Tsuneyoshi M. Subclinical gallbladder carcinoma. Am J Surg. 1992;163(4):382–6.

Yamamoto H, Hayakawa N, Kitagawa Y, Katohno Y, Sasaya T, Takara D, Nagino M, Nimura Y. Unsuspected gallbladder carcinoma after laparoscopic cholecystectomy. J Hepatobiliary Pancreat Surg. 2005;12(5):391–8.

Yu LH, Yuan B, Fu XH, Yu WL, Liu J, Zhang YJ. Does anatomic resection get more benefits than wedge hepatectomy on the prognosis for pT3 unsuspected gallbladder cancer? J Laparoendosc Adv Surg Tech A. 2019; https://doi.org/10.1089/lap.2018.0690.

Yuza K, Sakata J, Prasoon P, et al. Long-term outcomes of surgical resection for T1b gallbladder cancer: an institutional evaluation. BMC Cancer. 2020;20(1):20. https://doi.org/10.1186/s12885-019-6507-2.

Zhong H, Hao TT, Chen Y, Luo F. Unexpected gallbladder cancer during or after laparoscopic cholecystectomy: risk factors and experience of diagnosis and treatment of 22 cases. Am Surg. 2019;85(6):671–5.

References for Commentary Notes by Thorsten Oliver Goetze

Al-Batran SE, Homann N, Pauligk C, Goetze TO, et al. Perioperative chemotherapy with fluorouracil plus leucovorin, oxaliplatin, and docetaxel versus fluorouracil or capecitabine plus cisplatin and epirubicin for locally advanced, resectable gastric or gastro-oesophageal junction adenocarcinoma (FLOT4): a randomised, phase 2/3 trial. Lancet. 2019;393(10184):1948–57.

Bartlett DL, Fong Y, Fortner JG, Brennan MF, Blumgart LH. Long-term results after resection for gallbladder cancer. Implications for staging and management. Ann Surg. 1996;224(5):639–46.

Benson AB, D'Angelica MI, Abbott DE, et al. Guidelines insights: hepatobiliary cancers, Version 2.2019. J Natl Compr Cancer Netw. 2019b;17(4):302–10.

Box JC, Edge SB. Laparoscopic cholecystectomy and unsuspected gallbladder carcinoma. Semin Surg Oncol. 1999;16:327–31.

Copher JC, Rogers JJ, Dalton ML. Trocar-site metastasis following laparoscopic cholecystectomy for unsuspected carcinoma of the gallbladder. Surg Endosc. 1995;9:348–50.

Cunningham D, Allum WH, Stenning SP, Thompson JN, Van de Velde CJ, Nicolson M, et al. Perioperative chemotherapy versus surgery alone for resectable gastroesophageal cancer. N Engl J Med. 2006;355(1):11–20.

Edeline J, Bonnetain F, Phelip JM, Watelet J, Hammel P, Joly J-P, et al. Gemox versus surveillance following surgery of localized biliary tract cancer: results of the PRODIGE 12-ACCORD 18 (UNICANCER GI) phase III trial. J Clin Oncol. 2019;37(8):658–67. https://doi.org/10.1200/JCO.18.00050. Epub 2019 Feb 1

Endo I, Shimada H, Takimoto A, et al. Microscopic liver metastasis: prognostic factor for patients with pT2 gallbladder carcinoma. World J Surg. 2004;28(7):692–6.

Gutt C, Jenssen C, Barreiros AP, Götze TO, Stokes CS, Jansen PL, Neubrand M, Lammert F; [Updated S3-Guideline for Prophylaxis, Diagnosis and Treatment of Gallstones. German Society for Digestive and Metabolic Diseases (DGVS) and German Society for Surgery of the Alimentary Tract (DGAV) - AWMF Registry 021/008]. Z Gastroenterol. 2018;56(8):912–966. https://doi:10.1055/a-0644-2972. Epub 2018 Aug 1.

Kapoor VK. Incidental gallbladder cancer. Am J Gastroenterol. 2001b;96(3):627–9.

Romano F, Franciosi C, Caprotti R, et al. Laparoscopic cholecystectomy and unsuspected gallbladder cancer. Eur J Surg Oncol. 2001;27:225–8.

Toyonaga T, Chijiiwa K, Nakano K, et al. Completion radical surgery after cholecystectomy for accidentally

undiagnosed gallbladder carcinoma. World J Surg. 2003;27:266–71.
Valle J, Wasan H, Palmer DH, Cunningham D, Anthoney A, Maraveyas A, et al. Cisplatin plus gemcitabine versus gemcitabine for biliary tract cancer. N Engl J Med. 2010;362(14):1273–81.
Valle JW, Borbath I, Khan SA, Huguet F, Gruenberger T, Arnold D. Biliary cancer: ESMO Clinical Practice Guidelines for diagnosis, treatment and follow-up. Ann Oncol. 2016;27(Suppl 5):v28–37.
Varshney S, Buttirini G, Gupta R. Incidental carcinoma of the gallbladder. Eur J Surg Oncol. 2002;28:4–10.
Wullstein C, Woeste G, Barkhausen S, et al. Do complications related to laparoscopic cholecystectomy influence the prognosis of gallbladder cancer? Surg Endosc. 2002;16:828–32.

References for Commentary Notes by Shishir K. Maithel

Primrose JN, Fox RP, Palmer DH, Malik HZ, Prasad R, Mirza D, Anthony A, Corrie P, Falk S, Finch-Jones M, Wasan H, Ross P, Wall L, Wadsley J, Evans JTR, Stocken D, Praseedom R, Ma YT, Davidson B, Neoptolemos JP, Iveson T, Raftery J, Zhu S, Cunningham D, Garden OJ, Stubbs C, Valle JW, Bridgewater J, BILCAP Study Group. Capecitabine compared with observation in resected biliary tract cancer (BILCAP): a randomised, controlled, multicentre, phase 3 study. Lancet Oncol. 2019b;20(5):663–73. https://doi.org/10.1016/S1470-2045(18)30915-X. Epub 2019 Mar 25
Shroff RT, Kennedy EB, Bachini M, Bekaii-Saab T, Crane C, Edeline J, El-Khoueiry A, Feng M, Katz MHG, Primrose J, Soares HP, Valle J, Maithel SK. Adjuvant therapy for resected biliary tract cancer: ASCO clinical practice guideline. J Clin Oncol. 2019;37(12):1015–27. https://doi.org/10.1200/JCO.18.02178. Epub 2019 Mar 11

Adjuvant Therapy in Gall Bladder Cancera

14

Vinay K. Kapoor

Surgical resection (Fig. 14.1) is the mainstay of management of potentially resectable gall bladder cancer (GBC) and is the only option which offers a chance of cure. Adjuvant therapy further improves recurrence free as well as overall survival. Patients with possibly resectable disease should be offered upfront surgery with an aim for intent-to-cure (R0) resection but nonsurgical (chemo/radio) therapy plays an important role in a large majority of patients even after resection as well as in those who have unresectable disease. Most reports on adjuvant therapy include all biliary tract cancers (BTC), i.e., GBC and cholangiocarcinoma; very little evidence is available for GBC alone. Most of the available studies are retrospective single-institution analyses of small number of cases using empiric heterogeneous therapies, generating low-level evidence for adjuvant therapy. There is, thus, a dearth of good and strong data to make any recommendations about adjuvant therapy in GBC. The role and place of adjuvant therapy in GBC are not so well established as in esophagogastric, pancreatic and colorectal cancers (CRC), and hepatocellular carcinoma (HCC).

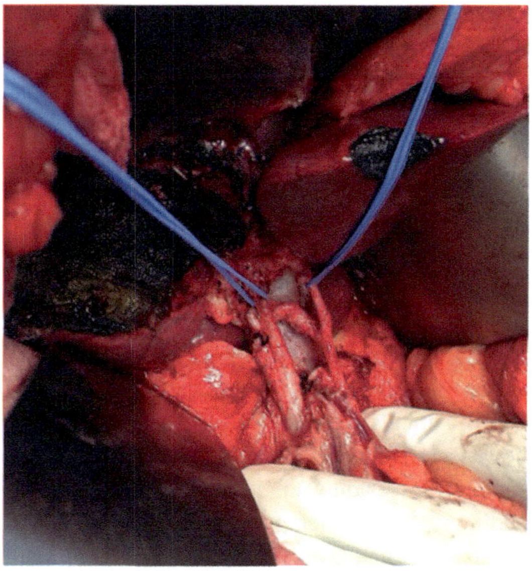

Fig. 14.1 Operative picture of extended cholecystectomy; liver wedge and skeletonized common bile duct (in left blue sling) and hepatic artery (in right blue sling) and portal vein (posterior) are seen—surgical resection (extended cholecystectomy showed here) is the mainstay of management of gall bladder cancer

14.1 Adjuvant Therapy

Majority of patients with GBC develop recurrence—locoregional and/or metastatic—even after an apparent R0 surgical resection; there is, therefore, a role of adjuvant (chemo and/or radio) therapy which should preferably be started within

Please also see an Invited Commentary on Adjuvant Therapy in Gall Bladder Cancer by Milind Javle (pp **_**)

V. K. Kapoor (✉)
Department of Surgical Gastroenterology, Sanjay Gandhi Post-Graduate Institute of Medical Sciences (SGPGIMS), Lucknow, Uttar Pradesh, India
e-mail: vkkapoor.india@gmail.com

V. K. Kapoor (ed.), *A Pictorial Treatise on Gall Bladder Cancer*,
https://doi.org/10.1007/978-981-15-5289-2_14

8–12 weeks of surgery. The duration of adjuvant therapy is usually 6 months. Need and decision for adjuvant treatment after surgical resection require knowledge of recurrence pattern whether locoregional, i.e., GB bed in the liver or lymph nodes or distant (liver, peritoneal, and extra-abdominal) after an intent-to-cure potentially curative R0 resection. After an R0 resection, most recurrences are metastatic thus suggesting that adjuvant chemotherapy will be a more rational strategy. Ninety-seven patients with GBC underwent resection (90% of the resections were margin negative) at the Memorial Sloan Kettering Cancer Center (MSKCC) New York USA. Follow-up was short (median 24 months) but still 53/80 (66%) patients in whom information was available had recurrence. Median time to recurrence was 11.5 months. Locoregional recurrence alone occurred in only 15% of cases; initial recurrence was at a distant site, with or without associated locoregional recurrence, in 85% of cases suggesting that chemotherapy should always be used (Jarnagin et al. 2003). In a report from South Korea, recurrences after surgical resection in T2 GBC were more often systemic (78%) than local (22%)—adjuvant chemotherapy is, therefore, recommended (Lee et al. 2018). Patients who undergo R2 or R1 resection, however, have a high risk of local recurrence and should receive adjuvant radiotherapy (RT) also, in addition to chemotherapy.

In a National Cancer Database (NCDB) analysis of 6825 patients with GBC (2004–2014), 2168 (32%) received adjuvant therapy—adjuvant therapy improved survival (Kasumova et al. 2017). In another NCDB (2004–2012) analysis of 1335 T1–T3, N1, M0 GBC, median survival with adjuvant therapy after surgery was better (19.6 vs. 13.3 months) versus surgery alone (Tran Cao et al. 2018).

14.2 Indications for Adjuvant Therapy

Patients with good performance status (ECOG 0/1) and normal/near normal (<2 times normal) renal and liver functions can be offered adjuvant therapy.

There are no predictive markers for selection of patients likely to respond to adjuvant therapy. Duffy et al. (2008) stated that no institutional standard exists with regard to the decision to administer adjuvant therapy or the type of adjuvant therapy in GBC. In a meta-analysis of 6712 patients with BTC (of who 1797 received adjuvant therapy), benefit of adjuvant therapy was seen in patients with node-positive disease (HR 0.49) and also those who underwent margin positive resection (HR 0.36) (Horgan et al. 2012). A meta-analysis of ten retrospective studies evaluating the role of adjuvant therapy after resection showed advantage of adjuvant therapy in stage II and III, node-positive patients and after R1 resection (Ma et al. 2015). Benefit of adjuvant chemotherapy has been observed in T2 or more GBC (Bergquist et al. 2018). Adjuvant chemotherapy was given to 30 out of 88 in completely resected T2N0 GBC patients—it reduced distant failure rates but did not improve OS (Kattepur et al. 2019).

T2 (Fig. 14.2) or beyond, node-positive (Fig. 14.3), margin positive (R1 resection status), gross residual disease (R2 resection status), e.g., non-curative simple cholecystectomy, poor histological features, e.g., poor differentiation (Fig. 14.4), lymphovascular invasion (LVI) (Fig. 14.5), perineural invasion (PNI) (Fig. 14.6), pericapsular invasion (PCI) in the metastatic LN are indications for adjuvant therapy.

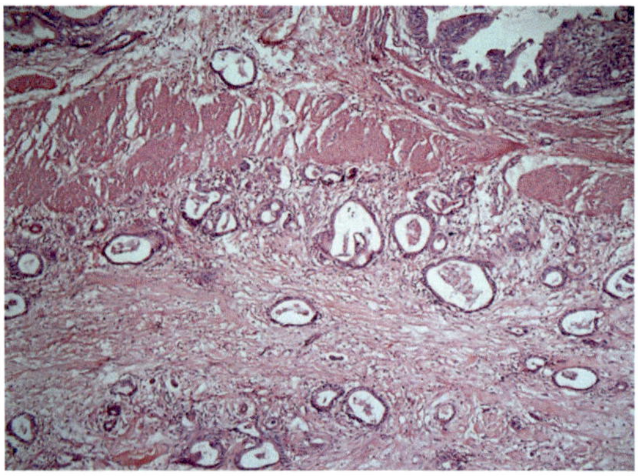

Fig. 14.2 Microphotograph shows adenocarcinoma infiltrating the perimuscular connective tissue (T2)—T2 or more disease is an indication for adjuvant therapy in gall bladder cancer

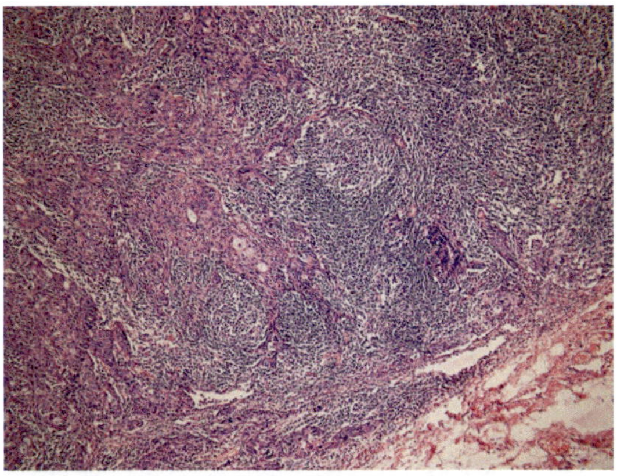

Fig. 14.3 Microphotograph shows tumor deposits in a lymph node—positive lymph node status is an indication for adjuvant therapy in gall bladder cancer, irrespective of the T stage

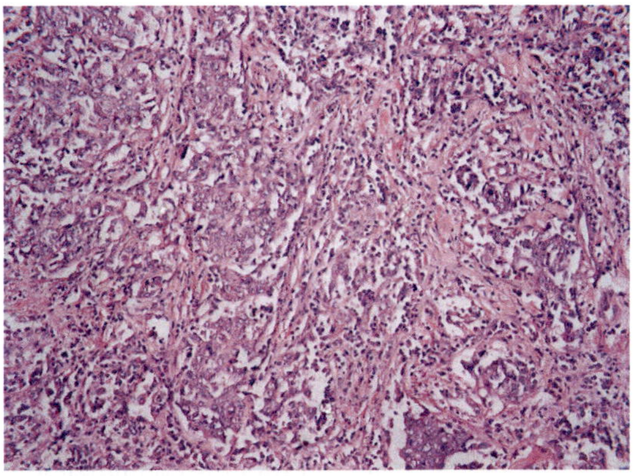

Fig. 14.4 Microphotograph shows poorly differentiated adenocarcinoma—poor differentiation of the tumor is an indication for adjuvant therapy in gall bladder cancer, irrespective of the T and N stage

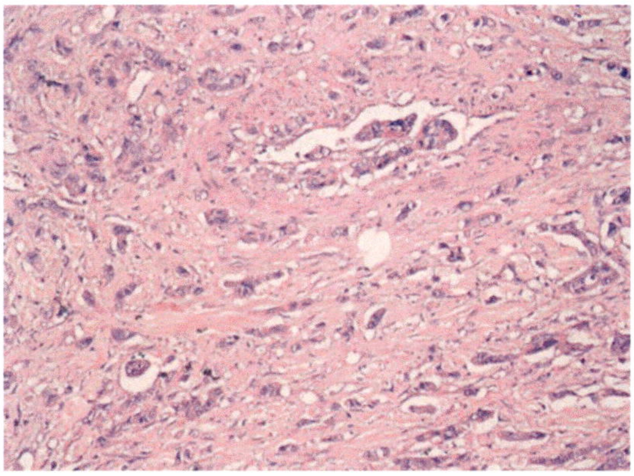

Fig. 14.5 Microphotograph shows tumor deposits in a lymphatic vessel—presence of lympho-vascular invasion (LVI) in the primary tumor is an indication for adjuvant therapy in gall bladder cancer, irrespective of the T and N stage

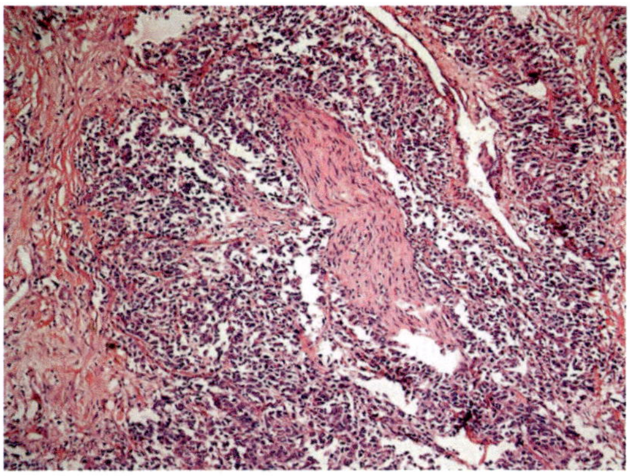

Fig. 14.6 Microphotograph shows tumor deposits around a nerve trunk—presence of perineural invasion (PNI) in the primary tumor is an indication for adjuvant therapy in gall bladder cancer, irrespective of the T and N stage

On the other hand, there are several reports which show conflicting results with no benefit of adjuvant therapy. A Japanese review of 3000 patients did not show any benefit of adjuvant therapy (Kayahara and Nagakawa 2007). Glazer et al. (2012) observed that neither neoadjuvant nor adjuvant therapy improved survival in patients with BTC who were resected with wide (1 cm negative) margins. Fluoro-pyramidine-based chemotherapy ($n = 84$) was compared with surveillance only ($n = 279$) following R0 resection in stage I–III GBC—after propensity score matching (PSM), no difference in 5-year recurrence-free survival (RFS) (51% vs. 65%) and overall survival (OS) (66% vs. 70%) was observed (Go et al. 2016). Four thousand seven hundred and seventy-five T2–T3 node-positive patients who underwent resection with grossly negative margins (R0 or R1) were reported to the NCDB between 2004 and 2011—adjuvant chemotherapy was administered to 29% patients and chemoradiation to 14%. T3 or node-positive tumors had a modest survival advantage with adjuvant chemoradiotherapy but the survival curves converged after 5 years of follow-up. The authors questioned the curative potential of adjuvant therapy justifying placebo-controlled trials of chemotherapy (Mantripragada et al. 2016).

The National Comprehensive Cancer Network (NCCN) guidelines recommend adjuvant fluoropyramidine/gemcitabine-based chemotherapy/chemoradiation for all except T1N0 tumors. European Society of Medical Oncology (ESMO) recommends postoperative adjuvant chemoradiotherapy in high-risk cases. American Society of Clinical Oncology (ASCO) recommends adjuvant chemotherapy with capecitabine for 6 months in patients who have undergone resection; chemoradiotherapy is recommended after R1 resection (Shroff et al. 2019).

14.3 Chemotherapy

Fluoro-pyrimidine, i.e., 5 fluorouracil (5 FU) (425 mg/m^2 as IV bolus on days 1–5 every 28 days) was the first drug used for chemotherapy in GBC; it was later combined with leucovorin (20 mg/m^2). Infusional 5 FU is better than IV bolus. In a multicenter prospective randomized phase III trial of pancreatobiliary tumors, including 140 GBC patients, who underwent non-curative resection, two courses of infusional 5 FU started on postoperative week 1 + mitomycin C on the day of surgery followed by prolonged administration of oral 5 FU until disease recurrence were used—5-year disease-free survival (DFS) was 20% versus 12%, and overall survival (OS) was 26% versus 14% as compared to observation only. There was no benefit of adjuvant chemotherapy after R0 resection; benefit was seen in node-positive patients (Takada et al. 2002); but this regime is not usually followed now. Oral prodrug of 5 FU, i.e., capecitabine (Fig. 14.7) (2000 mg/m^2 daily or 1000 mg/m^2 twice daily for 14 of every 21 days) has also been used; it has been combined with oxaliplatin (cap-ox) also. In Bilcap, a randomized controlled multicenter (44 HPB centers in the UK) phase III study (2006–2014) including 447 patients with BTC (GBC $n = 79$), oral capecitabine 1250 mg/m^2 twice daily (commencing within 16 weeks of surgery) on days 1–14 of 21 day cycle × 8 cycles showed benefit (overall survival OS 51 vs. 36 months, median recurrence-free survival RFS 24 vs. 18 months) over observation alone after macroscopically complete resection (Primrose et al. 2019a). S-1, an oral fluoro-pyramidine that includes three agents—florafur (tegafur), gimeracil, and oteracil is used in Japan.

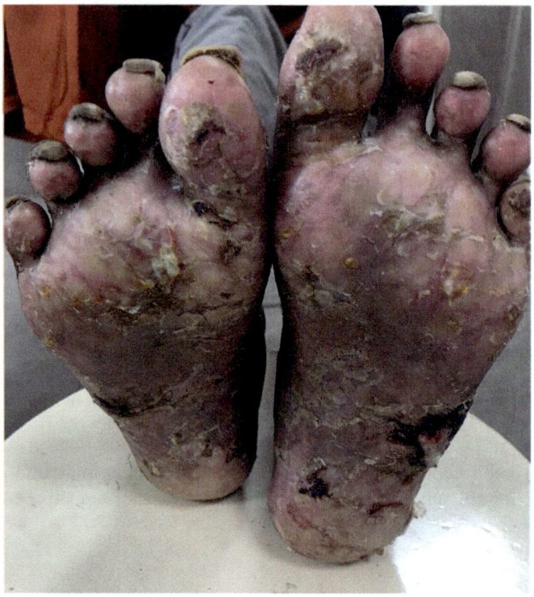

Fig. 14.7 Picture shows soles of a patient with capecitabine-related hand and foot syndrome—capecitabine plays an important role in adjuvant therapy in gall bladder cancer

Gemcitabine (1000 mg/m^2 weekly for 3 out of every 4 weeks for 6 months) is the preferred chemotherapeutic agent now, either alone or with platinum-based drugs (cisplatin or oxaliplatin). Superiority of gemcitabine + cisplatin (gem-cis or cis-gem) over gemcitabine alone was proved in a Japanese multicenter study (Okusaka et al. 2010). Gemcitabine on day 1 plus oxaliplatin on day 2 every 2 weeks has the same outcome as gemcitabine + cisplatin but with less toxicity. In French Prodige 12-ACCORD 18-UNICANCER GI multicenter (33 centers), open-label, randomized phase III trial (2009–2014) including 196 localized BTCs, adjuvant gemcitabine 1000 mg/m^2 on day 1 + oxaliplatin 85 mg/m^2 on day 2 of every 14 days (gem-ox) started within

3 months × 12 cycles versus surveillance following R0 or R1 resection surgery showed that it was feasible but provided no improvement in recurrence-free survival (RFS) (median 30 vs. 19 months; 4 years 39% vs. 33%) and overall survival (OS) (76 vs. 51 months). Adverse events were more (grade 3: 62% vs. 18%; grade 4: 11% vs. 3%) in the chemotherapy group (Edeline et al. 2019a). ACTICCA is a randomized multinational phase III trial of adjuvant gemcitabine (1000 mg/m^2 and cisplatin 25 mg/m^2 on days 1 and 8 every 21 days × 6 cycles) versus capecitabine (1250 mg/m^2 BID days 1–14 of 21 days × 8 cycles) versus observation alone after curative-intent resection in BTC (Stein et al. 2015). A recent report from Japan showed the feasibility and potential efficacy of gemcitabine, S-1, and leucovorin (GSL) in 12 patients with GBC (Takahara et al. 2019).

There is no established second-line chemotherapy for GBC if the patient does not respond to the first-line drugs, i.e., gemcitabine and cisplatin but FOLFOX has been suggested (Javle et al. 2019).

Cytoreductive surgery (CRS) with hyperthermic intraperitoneal chemotherapy (HIPEC) has been used in patients with peritoneal metastases in some cancers. It was used in 5 GBC patients (out of a total of 1069 CRS + HIPEC procedures in various cancers treated between 1991 and 2013)—organs resected included omentum, liver, colon, ovary, and diaphragm—3 year and median survival were 30% and 22 months, respectively (Randle et al. 2014).

Intra-arterial adjuvant chemotherapy through a catheter placed in the common hepatic artery (CHA) or proper hepatic artery (PHA) to reduce the risk of hepatic metastasis after resection has been reported (Chen et al. 2018).

14.4 Radiotherapy

Many recurrences after an apparent intent-to-cure (R0) resection are local (GB bed in liver) and regional (LNs) thus emphasizing the role of RT as adjuvant therapy. Role of postoperative adjuvant RT alone after surgical resection, however, is not well established. Adjuvant RT resulted in better local control (59% vs. 36%) and 5-year survival (8.9% vs. 2.9%) after resections in 85 patients with stage IV GBC—RT was most useful after R1 resection (cf. R0 or R2 resection) (Todoroki et al. 1999). At the Mayo Clinic, Rochester MN USA 21 patients who received adjuvant external beam RT (EBRT) and 5 FU after curative resection had 64% 5-year survival versus 33% in a historical cohort after R0 resection alone (Kresl et al. 2002). In a SEER database (1992–2002) of more than 3000 patients, median survival was better (14 months) with adjuvant RT than after surgery alone (8 months); the advantage was even more (16 vs. 5 months) in LN-positive cases (Mojica et al. 2007). In SEER data (1988–2003) of 4180 patients with GBC who underwent resection, 760 received adjuvant RT—patients with T2 or more and node-positive disease benefited from adjuvant RT (Wang et al. 2011). In a survival analysis of 279 operated patients, radiotherapy improved OS in patients with positive resection margin cases (Lim et al. 2013). Wang et al. (2008) derived a risk model for estimation of potential survival benefit by addition of post resection RT and generated a comparative nomogram and online risk prediction tool.

A systematic review and meta-analysis of 14 studies including 9364 patients showed the benefit of adjuvant RT in patients with node-positive disease and after R1 resection (Kim et al. 2018).

Postoperative adjuvant EBRT includes 40–50 Gy to the lymph node areas and 55–60 Gy to the tumor bed; it may be combined with 5 FU as radiosensitizer. The main issue in using RT for GBC is radiation-induced liver disease (RILD) which manifests as hepatomegaly, ascites, and deranged liver function tests (LFT) any time after 2 weeks; it may even progress to liver failure and cause death. Post-RT gastroduodenal bleeding in the short term (Lee et al. 2017) and stricture (Fig. 14.8) in the long term are complications of EBRT. CT simulation allows better delineation of the target structures as well as the adjacent organs at risk (OAR). Gross tumor volume (radiographically evident) and clinical target volume (CTV) including potential microscopic disease are calculated. A margin is added to the CTV to obtain the planning target volume (PTV). 3D conformal RT and intensity-modulated RT (IMRT) allow dose escalation with less damage to the

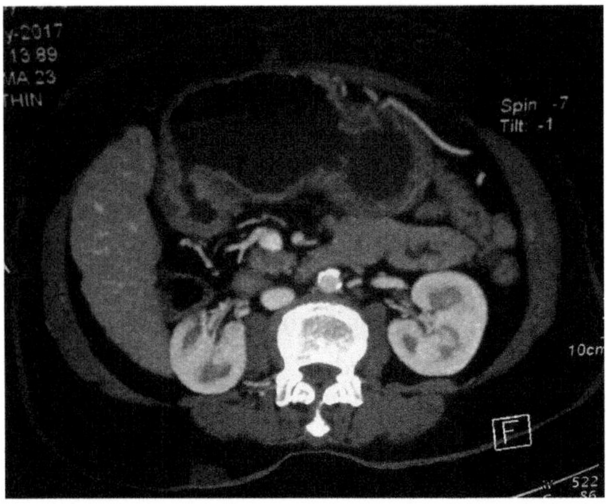

Fig. 14.8 CT shows pyloric thickening as a result of radiotherapy; repeated upper gastrointestinal endoscopic biopsies were negative for recurrent disease—radiotherapy plays an important role in adjuvant therapy in gall bladder cancer

OAR. Image-guided RT (IGRT) and stereotactic body RT (SBRT), i.e., limited number of high-dose fractions delivered conformally to the target, are also useful. Intraoperative RT (IORT) has the advantage of delivering a large dose (10–20 Gy) of RT in a single fraction to the tumor while sparing or minimizing exposure of the adjacent normal structures. This is followed by postoperative adjuvant EBRT in the usual doses. Todoroki et al. (1991) reported single dose (20–30 Gy) IORT in 10/27 stage IV (T4 N0-1) GBC patients who underwent resection—3-year survival in 10 patients who received IORT was 10% versus 0% in 17 patients who did not receive IORT. IORT, however, has the problem of availability and logistics. Advanced techniques of RT, e.g., proton beam therapy offer newer avenues in ablative RT (Verma and Crane 2019).

Patients who have jaundice are very frequently unresectable; palliation is provided by placing biliary stents. Endoscopic stents are preferred but patients with high (hilar) obstruction often require percutaneous transhepatic biliary intervention. These stents are likely to get blocked due to tumor ingrowth. Intraluminal brachytherapy (ILBT) has been used to increase the patency of the biliary stents (Wang et al. 2011). If brachytherapy is to be used, external access is required which means that biliary drainage should be external or internal–external and a large diameter (8–14 Fr) catheter is required. Brachytherapy can be high-dose rate (HDR) where the catheter is connected to the machine or low-dose rate (LDR) where the iridium source is introduced into the percutaneous transhepatic biliary drainage (PTBD) tube. In a systematic review and meta-analysis of 12 studies including 641 patients (out of which 340 received ILBT) with malignant obstructive jaundice in whom stent was placed, ILBT reduced the risk of stent occlusion and improved survival (Xu et al. 2018).

14.5 Chemoradiotherapy (CRT)

Chemoradiotherapy (CRT) may be better than RT or chemo alone.

Gemcitabine 1000 mg/m^2 IV on days 1 and 8 + capecitabine 650 mg/m^2 or 1000 mg/m^2 twice daily or 1500 mg/m^2 per day on days 1–14 of every 21 days × 4 cycles followed by chemoradiotherapy (CRT) (capecitabine + RT 40–50 Gy to LNs and 55–60 Gy to the tumor bed) has also been used. In a SEER (1995–2005) analysis of 1137 patients with GBC who underwent resection, 126 received chemotherapy, and 126 received CRT—CRT was better than chemo alone (Wang et al. 2011). Southwest Oncology Group Phase II single-arm trial of adjuvant gemcitabine + capecitabine followed by concurrent capecitabine and RT in 79 patients (GBC + intrahepatic cholangiocarcinoma) showed good tolerance with 2-year OS of 65% and median survival of 35 months (Ben-Josef et al. 2015a). In an NCDB analysis (1998–2006) of 6690 cases, 15% received adjuvant chemotherapy and RT—it was associated with improved survival (HR 0.77, 0.66–0.90), more so in node-positive patients (HR 0.64, 0.53–0.78) (Hoehn et al. 2015). Hundred and twelve patients who underwent extended surgery for GBC at six National Cancer Institute (NCI) designated cancer centers in USA (1985–2008)—61% received adjuvant RT (93% of these received concurrent chemotherapy also). Patients who received adjuvant RT had more (57% vs. 16%) advanced T stage, LN involvement (63% vs. 18%), and positive margins (37%

vs. 9%), but 5-year overall survival OS was equal (49% vs. 52.5%) suggesting an advantage of CRT over chemotherapy alone (Wang et al. 2015). In a multi-institutional consortium database (2000–2015), 61 (21%) patients received chemotherapy and 44 (15%) received CRT after 291 curative-intent resections—adjuvant therapy improved survival but only in high-risk cases, i.e., T3/T4, LN metastasis, and R1 resection status (Kim et al. 2016). Addition of RT further improved the survival benefit of adjuvant chemotherapy—it was 27 months for extended cholecystectomy + chemotherapy + RT versus 15.9 for extended cholecystectomy + chemotherapy (no RT) (Kasumova et al. 2017). In the NCDB (2004–2012) analysis of 1335 node-positive GBC patients, 5-year survival was better with adjuvant chemoradiotherapy (24.7 vs. 14.3 months) versus adjuvant chemotherapy alone after surgery. Adjuvant CRT following surgery was associated with lower risk of death than after surgery alone whether margin negative (HR 0.66) or margin positive (HR 0.54) (Tran Cao et al. 2018). Concurrent chemoradiotherapy (cCRT) followed by adjuvant chemotherapy is better; cCRT improved survival from 13 to 27 months (Gu et al. 2018). Verma and Crane (2019) recommended consideration of CRT for node-positive or margin-positive disease; Gamboa and Maithel (2020) suggested consideration of CRT after R1 resection.

A systemic review of 27 articles (3 systemic reviews and 24 observational studies) concluded that existing evidence for adjuvant therapy is not robust; evidence was moderate, poor, and very poor for adjuvant chemotherapy, CRT and RT, respectively. Adjuvant therapy may improve overall survival in patients with advanced stages of the disease, positive LNs, and positive surgical margins (Manterola et al. 2019).

14.6 Neoadjuvant Therapy

The term adjuvant therapy was coined for the use of chemotherapy even after an intent-to-cure (R0) resection for early breast cancer, presumably to decrease the risk of recurrence (especially distant metastases) by taking care of the micrometastases, based on the concept that cancer, even to begin with, is a systemic disease. The same concept, when applied before operation in patients with resectable disease, has been called neoadjuvant therapy (NAT). The term neoadjuvant therapy is now being used loosely even for locally advanced borderline resectable or even unresectable disease, though the purists, including the Author (VKK), believe that this should be called downsizing/downstaging therapy. NAT has an established role in esophagus, stomach, rectum, and pancreas cancer. Response to NAT is assessed by imaging, i.e., CT/PET-CT (Fig. 14.9a, b) using RECIST/PERCIST criteria—complete response (CR), partial response (PR), stable disease (SD), and progressive disease (PD). Response rate (RR) is CR + PR while clinical benefit rate (CBR) is CR + PR + SD. Patients who received NAT before surgery should receive postoperative adjuvant chemotherapy after resection to complete six cycles of perioperative therapy.

Another major advantage of the use of NAT is assessment of the biology and aggressiveness of the tumor and selection of less aggressive tumors with good biology for resection. Patients with biologically aggressive disease declare themselves as progressive disease (locoregional or metastases) and are excluded from surgical resection as they will not benefit from resection thus improving the overall survival of the cohort.

A large number of patients with GBC have locoregionally advanced but nonmetastatic possibly unresectable or difficult to resect (borderline resectable) disease; NAT is a theoretical option. Definitions of unresectable or borderline resectable GBC are, however, not well defined as the resectability of GBC depends on the aggressiveness of the surgical approach. There is, however, very little evidence on the role of NAT in GBC and NAT is not a standard of care. Pre NAT biliary drainage (endoscopic or percutaneous) is performed in patients with jaundice to bring the serum bilirubin down to normal.

de Aretxabala et al. (2004) used continuous infusion of 5 FU for 5 days plus RT 45 Gy in 23 patients—14 (60%) were operated—5 were alive at follow-up of 44 months. Kato et al. (2015) reported 22 patients with unresectable BTC

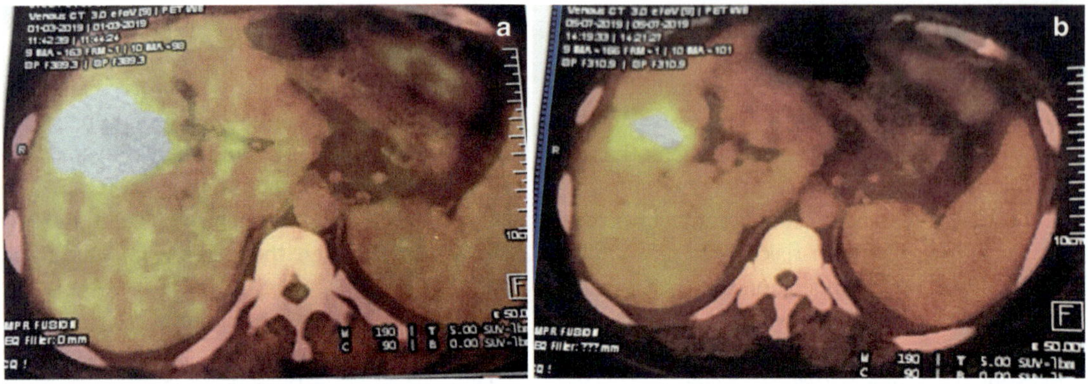

Fig. 14.9 (**a**) Pre neoadjuvant therapy (NAT) PET showing large tumor. (**b**) Post NAT PET showing significant regression in the size of the tumor—NAT is being studied in locally advanced possibly unresectable gall bladder cancer; response is evaluated with CT and/or PET

(GBC $n = 7$) who received gemcitabine (1000 mg/m^2 IV once a week for 3 weeks every 4 weeks)—8 patients in whom obvious downsizing and even disappearance of vascular invasion was observed could be resected (R0 resection $n = 4$, R1 resection $n = 4$); 6 patients had recurrence but 2 were alive at 13 and 42 months without recurrence. Sirohi et al. (2015) in a retrospective analysis of 37 patients treated between 2009 and 2013 showed the advantage of neoadjuvant chemotherapy (NACT) (gemcitabine + cisplatin) in locally advanced GBC—response rate was 68%—17 patients could undergo R0 resection; patients who were operated had median OS of 26 months. Agrawal et al. (2016) used neoadjuvant chemoradiotherapy (45 Gy external RT along with weekly concurrent cisplatin 35 mg/m^2 and 5 FU 500 mg) in locally advanced GBC—resection could be performed in 6/40 cases. Neoadjuvant concurrent chemoradiation (gemcitabine 300 mg/m^2/week × 5 weeks) and helical tomotherapy (57 Gy over 25 fractions to the tumor and 45 Gy over 25 fractions to the LNs) was used in 28 patients with locally advanced (T3–T4 with large porta nodes) GBC—PET was used to rule out metastases. Chemoradiation could be completed in 25 patients—20 had complete or partial response, 18 were operated and R0 resection was achieved in 14 patients. Five-year OS in patients with R0 resection was 47% (Engineer et al. 2016). At the MSKCC New York USA (1992–2015), 74 patients with GBC received neoadjuvant chemotherapy (gemcitabine alone or gemcitabine + cisplatin)—17 (23%) had progressive disease, 38 (5%) stable disease, and 19 (26%) showed partial response—22 (30%) were operated—10 (14%) could be resected. Median OS in ten patients who underwent resection after NACT was 51 months cf. 14 months for the entire cohort and 11 months for unresectable patients (Creasy et al. 2017). Chaudhari et al. (2018) reported 160 patients (140 had T3/T4 disease and 105 were node positive) with GBC who received NACT from 2010 to 2016. They used gemcitabine 1000 mg/m^2 as a 30 min infusion and cisplatin 25 mg/m^2 on days 1 and 8 of a 21-day cycle or gemcitabine 1000 mg/m^2 on day 1 as a 100-min infusion and oxaliplatin 100 mg/m^2 over 2 h on day 2 of every 14 days. Response rate was 53% and clinical benefit rate (CBR) was 70%. Curative intent resection could be performed in 66 (41%) patients. OS and DFS in patients who underwent curative-intent resection were 49 and 25 months, respectively.

A systematic review of six studies including 474 patients of which 398 (84%) received NACT and 76 (16%) received neoadjuvant chemoradiotherapy (NACRT), however, observed that there is insufficient data to support the routine use of NACT or NACRT in advanced GBC (Hakeem et al. 2019).

Role of NAT (after the index cholecystectomy and before reoperation for completion of extended cholecystectomy CEC) in patients with incidental GBC is even less defined. de Aretxabala

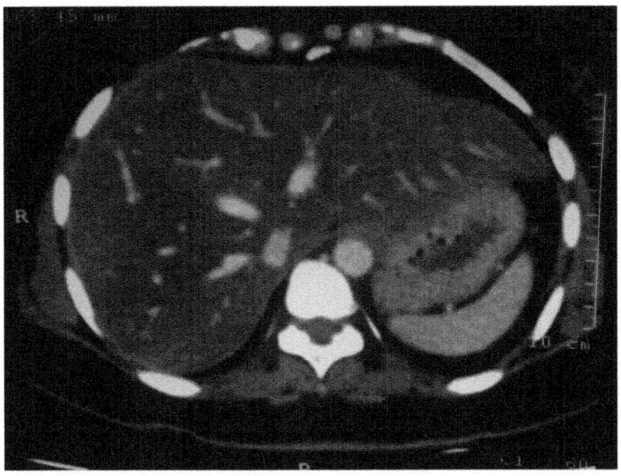

Fig. 14.10 CT shows a fatty liver (density less than that of the spleen)—chemotherapy can cause chemotherapy-associated steatohepatitis (CASH) which can make the subsequent liver resection technically difficult

et al. (1999) were the first to report use of preoperative CRT (continuous infusion of 5 FU 350 mg/m^2 on days 1–5 and 21–25 + 180 cGy/fraction 5 days/week total 4500 cGy) in 18 out of 27 patients who were found to have GBC after cholecystectomy—15 were reoperated and resection was performed in 13; 7 were alive at 24 months. Kasumova et al. (2017) also reported adjuvant/neoadjuvant chemotherapy followed by reoperation for CEC after simple cholecystectomy and detection of incidental GBC on histopathological examination of the GB.

Chemotherapy may cause chemotherapy-associated steato-hepatitis (CASH) (Fig. 14.10), which decreases the hypertrophic response of the liver to portal vein embolization (PVE) and makes the liver parenchymal transection technically difficult. Patients who receive NAT, especially radiation, have higher morbidity—bile leak was seen in 6/26 (43%) patients 2 of whom required reoperation (Engineer et al. 2016).

14.7 Targeted Therapy

For many cancers, mutated proteins represent targets for novel therapeutic agents which are more specific, more efficacious, and less toxic than conventional chemotherapy. Molecular biology of GBC has not been well studied and is ill understood (see Chap. 4). There are no known targets and no established biological therapy for GBC. Actionable mutations of molecules such as EGFR, VEGF, VEGFR, mTOR, HER2/neu, PDL-1, PD-1, MET, PIK3CA, cadherin, MEK1, MEK2, etc. which can be actionable targets for potential therapy are being studied in GBC (Javle et al. 2019; Mishra et al. 2019). Various intracellular signaling pathways, e.g., angiogenesis, ErbB, Hedgehog, AKT/MAPK/ERK, Notch, PI3K/AKD/mTOR, etc. have been identified for GBC. They can be potential targets for biological therapy (Bizama et al. 2015; Valle et al. 2017).

Erlotinib (oral tyrosine kinase inhibitor TKI), sorafenib (TKI against vascular endothelial growth factor receptor VEGFR and platelet-derived growth factor receptor PDGFR), cetuximab (anti-EGFR), trastuzumab (anti HER2), bevacizumab (a monoclonal antibody MCA targeting vascular endothelial growth factor VEGF), have been used in GBC. Celecoxib—a selective inhibitor of cyclo-oxygenase (COX) was found to have an inhibitory effect on proliferation of GBC cells (Deng et al. 2017); this may have a therapeutic implication as cox-2 overexpression was seen by us in 57/64 GBCs (Ghosh et al. 2000). EGFR overexpression was seen on IHC in 44/50 patients with GBC (weak in 10, moderate in 26, and strong in 8). MSI as a sign of mismatch repair deficiency is a predictor of response to anti-PD-1 therapy (Le et al. 2015). Li et al. (2019) demonstrated therapeutic activity of PD-L1 monoclonal antibody (sapitinib and atezolizumab) in GBC cells.

14.8 Definitive (Palliative) Therapy

Majority of patients with GBC have metastatic or unresectable locally advanced disease and are candidates for palliative therapy only. In addition to nonsurgical (endoscopic or percutaneous) interventions, chemotherapy, and/or radiotherapy may play a role as palliative/definitive therapy. Response rate of various chemotherapy regimens is about 10–30%.

ABC-02 is a multicenter phase III study of BTC (including 149 GBC)—six cycles of gemcitabine 1000 mg/m^2 on days 1 and 8 + cisplatin 25 mg/m^2 on days 1 and 8 of every 21 days resulted in better mOS (11.7 vs. 8.1 months) and PFS (8 vs. 5 months) than gemcitabine alone 1000 mg/m^2 on days 1, 8, and 15 of every 28 days but with higher rates (25% vs. 17%) of grade 3 or 4 neutropenia (Valle et al. 2010). A randomized trial of gemcitabine + oxaliplatin (gem-ox) versus 5 FU + leucovorin versus best supportive care (BSC) in unresectable GBC (n = 81) reported RR of 32%, 14%, and 0% and mOS of 9.5, 4.6, and 4.5 months, respectively (Sharma et al. 2010). In an NCDB USA (2004–2012) analysis of 1335 node-positive patients, surgery was performed in 1123 patients while 212 had no surgery. Median OS was 19.6 months after surgery plus adjuvant therapy (adjuvant chemoradiotherapy 24.7 months vs. adjuvant chemotherapy 14.3 months), 13.3 months after surgery alone, 11.6 months after nonsurgical therapy, and 8.3 months after no treatment (Tran Cao et al. 2018). In 173 patients with unresectable stage IVB GBC, cisplatin 25 mg/m^2 + gemcitabine 1000 mg/m^2 IV on days 1 and 8 of 21 days cycle achieved disease control (complete response (CR), partial response (PR) + stable disease (SD)) in 60%; OS was 8.1 months (You et al. 2019).

An experimental study showed that photodynamic therapy (PDT) had an antitumor effect on NOZ (a GBC cell line) tumor cells treated with indo-cynanine green (ICG)-lactosomes thus suggesting the possibility of near-infrared fluorescence (NIRF) imaging to guide PDT (Hishikawa et al. 2019).

Adjuvant, as well as neoadjuvant, therapy in GBC needs much more evidence before it can become the standard of care.

Invited Commentary on Adjuvant Therapy in Gall Bladder Cancer

Milind Javle

Introduction

Gallbladder cancer (GBC) is an important health care problem in Asia and Latin America, while gradually declining in incidence in the Western world. An estimated 5000 cases are diagnosed annually in the United States annually and this disease disproportionately affects certain minorities, including Alaskan Natives and American Indians. Between the years 2007 and 2011, GBC incidence rates declined across all racial and ethnic groups in the United States, with the exception of non-Hispanic Blacks wherein an increase in incidence of 2.2% per year was noted (Henley et al. 2015). Unfortunately, most patients are diagnosed at an advanced disease stage: 40% with regional spread or lymph nodal involvement and 40% with distant metastases. Thus, patients with localized, resectable disease that are candidates for adjuvant therapy represent a minority of the population. Furthermore, most patients in the United States are diagnosed with GBC incidentally after cholecystectomy for presumed gallstone cholecystitis. GBC is detected at a frequency of 0.2–3% of all cholecystectomies in the United States (Kanlioz et al. 2019; Cherkassky and D'Angelica 2019).

Although surgery is potentially curative, recurrence occurs in over a third patients undergoing resection and the median time to recurrence is less than 1 year. Depth of tumor invasion (T3), lymphovascular invasion (LVI), and residual disease are associated with a higher recurrence risk (Aloia et al. 2015).

In patients with T2 disease, patients with tumors on the hepatic side had higher rates of vascular invasion, neural invasion, nodal metastasis, and consequently poorer survival than patients with tumors on the peritoneal side (Shindoh et al. 2015). The primary sites of recurrence include distant sites such as the peritoneum (65%), locoregional (15%), and both locoregional and distant (20%) (Margonis et al. 2016). These factors need to be accounted for while considering adjuvant therapy.

Adjuvant Therapy Trials

Until recently, there were no prospective, randomized clinical trials of adjuvant therapy versus observation for biliary tract cancer (BTC) and to date, there has not been a trial exclusively for GBC Investigators from Princess Margaret Cancer Center, Toronto ON Canada performed a literature-based meta-analysis of 20 studies that included 6712 patients with BTC and had received either adjuvant therapy or surveillance. There was a nonsignificant improvement in overall survival with any adjuvant therapy compared with surgery alone ($p = 0.06$) in their analysis and no difference was noted between GBC and bile duct tumors ($p = 0.68$). The greatest benefit of adjuvant therapy occurred in patients with node-positive disease and R1 resection margins (Horgan and Knox 2018).

Beyond this analysis, adjuvant therapy for biliary cancer has been guided by the following three prospective clinical trials:

1. The SWOG 0809 was an intergroup phase II clinical trial of adjuvant gemcitabine and capecitabine for four cycles followed by chemoradiotherapy for patients with extrahepatic cholangiocarcinoma and GBC. A total of 79 patients were enrolled; a 2-year survival of 65% with a median survival of 35 months met the preplanned clinical endpoints of the study (Ben-Josef et al. 2015b). Interestingly, there was a nonsignificant survival difference between R0 and R1 patients. This trial has established the adjuvant therapy standard for patients undergoing resection, especially those with R1 margins.
2. The PRODIGE–ACCORD study randomized 200 resected BTC patients, which included 20% with GBC, to gemcitabine + oxaliplatin (GEMOX) versus observation. This study was powered to detect an improvement in relapse-free survival from 18 to 30 months (HR of 0.60) (Edeline et al. 2019b). The study did demonstrate a numerical superiority with GEMOX, but was underpowered to detect a significant difference. GEMOX may represent a viable alternative for patients that are unable to tolerate other agents, such as capecitabine or cisplatin.
3. The BILCAP study from the UK randomized 447 patients with BTC to adjuvant capecitabine versus observation (Primrose et al. 2019b). The median survival was 51 months in the capecitabine arm versus 36 months with observation. This difference was not significant in an intention to treat analysis. However, in a protocol-specified analysis, this difference did meet the statistical bar and also indicated an improved relapse-free survival with capecitabine. Notably, 20% patients enrolled in BILCAP had GBC and although the trial was not powered to detect survival differences in various BTC types, subset analysis did not detect an improved survival with capecitabine for GBC patients (HR = 0.84, $p = 0.596$).

Based on the above data, however, adjuvant capecitabine after resection and radiotherapy for R1 margins represent the current standards in North America.

Future Approaches to Adjuvant Therapy

Further refinement of chemotherapy is expected from the ongoing ACTICCA-1 trial from Europe, which compares adjuvant gemcitabine and cisplatin with capecitabine after surgical resection. Recent developments in next-generation sequencing (NGS) for BTC have highlighted actionable mutations, such as in the *FGFR*, *EGFR*, *IDH1*, *Her2/neu*, and *BRAF* genes (Javle et al. 2016). A fraction of GBC is enriched with *Her2/neu* and *EGFR* amplification and targeted approaches in the adjuvant setting are worthy of consideration (Javle et al. 2014).

In summary, while several recent trials have created new adjuvant therapy choices for patients with resected BTC, these therapies are still suboptimal for GBC and a dedicated study for this population is needed.

References

Chapter References

Agrawal S, Mohan L, Mourya C, Neyaz Z, Saxena R. Radiological downstaging with neoadjuvant therapy in unresectable gall bladder cancer cases. Asian Pac J Cancer Prev. 2016;17(4):2137–40.

Ben-Josef E, Guthrie KA, El-Khoueiry AB, Corless CL, Zalupski MM, Lowy AM, Thomas CR Jr, Alberts SR, Dawson LA, Micetich KC, Thomas MB, Siegel AB, Blanke CD. SWOG S0809: a phase II intergroup trial of adjuvant capecitabine and gemcitabine followed by radiotherapy and concurrent capecitabine in extrahepatic cholangiocarcinoma and gallbladder carcinoma. J Clin Oncol. 2015a;33(24):2617–22. https://doi.org/10.1200/JCO.2014.60.2219. Epub 2015 May 11

Bergquist JR, Shah HN, Habermann EB, Hernandez MC, Ivanics T, Kendrick ML, Smoot RL, Nagorney DM, Borad MJ, McWilliams RR, Truty MJ. Adjuvant systemic therapy after resection of node positive gallbladder cancer: time for a well-designed trial? (Results of a US-national retrospective cohort study). Int J Surg. 2018;52:171–9. https://doi.org/10.1016/j.ijsu.2018.02.052. Epub 2018 Feb 26

Bizama C, Garcia P, Espinoza JA, Weber H, Leal P, Nervi B, et al. Targeting specific molecular pathways holds promise for advanced gallbladder cancer therapy. Cancer Treat Rev. 2015;41(3):222–34. https://doi.org/10.1016/j.ctrv.2015.01.003.

Chaudhari VA, Ostwal V, Patkar S, Sahu A, Toshniwal A, Ramaswamy A, Shetty NS, Shrikhande SV, Goel M. Outcome of neoadjuvant chemotherapy in "locally advanced/borderline resectable" gallbladder cancer: the need to define indications. HPB (Oxford). 2018;20(9):841–7. https://doi.org/10.1016/j.hpb.2018.03.008. Epub 2018 Apr 26

Chen C, Feng W, Zheng Y, Bao Y, Feng M. Intra-arterial chemotherapy improved survival of stage 2–3 gallbladder cancer after curative resection. Onco Targets Ther. 2018;11:2975–9. https://doi.org/10.2147/OTT.S166246. eCollection 2018.

Creasy JM, Goldman DA, Dudeja V, Lowery MA, Cercek A, Balachandran VP, Allen PJ, DeMatteo RP, Kingham TP, D'Angelica MI, Jarnagin WR. Systemic chemotherapy combined with resection for locally advanced gallbladder carcinoma: surgical and survival outcomes. J Am Coll Surg. 2017;224(5):906–16. https://doi.org/10.1016/j.jamcollsurg.2016.12.058. Epub 2017 Feb 13

de Aretxabala X, Roa I, Burgos L, Cartes R, Silva J, Yañez E, Araya JC, Villaseca M, Quijada I, Vittini C. Preoperative chemoradiotherapy in the treatment of gallbladder cancer. Am Surg. 1999;65(3):241–6.

de Aretxabala X, Losada H, Mora J, Roa I, Burgos L, Yáñez E, Quijada I, Roa JC. [Neoadjuvant chemoradiotherapy in gallbladder cancer]. Rev Med Chil. 2004;132(1):51-57. Spanish.

Deng M, Qin Y, Chen X, Li D, Wang Q, Zheng H, et al. Combination of celecoxib and PD184161 exerts synergistic inhibitory effects on gallbladder cancer cell proliferation. Oncol Lett. 2017;13(5):3850–8. https://doi.org/10.3892/ol.2017.5914.

Duffy A, Capanu M, Abou-Alfa GK, Huitzil D, Jarnagin W, Fong Y, D'Angelica M, Dematteo RP, Blumgart LH, O'Reilly EM. Gallbladder cancer (GBC): 10-year experience at Memorial Sloan-Kettering Cancer Centre (MSKCC). J Surg Oncol. 2008;98(7):485–9. https://doi.org/10.1002/jso.21141.

Edeline J, Benabdelghani M, Bertaut A, Watelet J, Hammel P, Joly JP, Boudjema K, Fartoux L, Bouhier-Leporrier K, Jouve JL, Faroux R, Guerin-Meyer V, Kurtz JE, Assénat E, Seitz JF, Baumgaertner I, Tougeron D, de la Fouchardière C, Lombard-Bohas C, Boucher E, Stanbury T, Louvet C, Malka D, Phelip JM. Gemcitabine and oxaliplatin chemotherapy or surveillance in resected biliary tract cancer (PRODIGE 12-ACCORD 18-UNICANCER GI): a randomized phase III study. J Clin Oncol. 2019a;37(8):658–67. https://doi.org/10.1200/JCO.18.00050. Epub 2019 Feb 1.

Engineer R, Goel M, Chopra S, Patil P, Purandare N, Rangarajan V, Ph R, Bal M, Shrikhande S, Shrivastava SK, Mehta S. Neoadjuvant chemoradiation followed by surgery for locally advanced gallbladder cancers: a new paradigm. Ann Surg Oncol. 2016;23(9):3009–15. https://doi.org/10.1245/s10434-016-5197-0. Epub 2016 Apr 13

Gamboa AC, Maithel SK. The landmark series: gallbladder cancer. Ann Surg Oncol. 2020;27(8):2846–58. https://doi.org/10.1245/s10434-020-08654-9.

Ghosh M, Kawamoto T, Koike N, Fukao K, Yoshida S, Kashiwagi H, Kapoor VK, Agarwal S, Krishnani N, Uchida K, Miwa M, Todoroki T. Cyclooxygenase expression in the gallbladder. Int J Mol Med. 2000;6(5):527–32.

Glazer ES, Liu P, Abdalla EK, Vauthey JN, Curley SA. Neither neoadjuvant nor adjuvant therapy increases survival after biliary tract cancer resection with wide negative margins. J Gastrointest Surg. 2012;16(9):1666–71. https://doi.org/10.1007/s11605-012-1935-1. Epub 2012 Jul 10

Go SI, Kim YS, Hwang IG, Kim EY, Oh SY, Ji JH, Song HN, Park SH, Park JO, Kang JH. Is there a role for adjuvant therapy in R0 resected gallbladder cancer?: a propensity score-matched analysis. Cancer Res Treat. 2016;48(4):1274–85. Epub 2016 Feb 12

Gu B, Qian L, Yu H, Hu J, Wang Q, Shan J, Shi L, Liu H, Yang Q, Liang X, Cai X, Sun X. Concurrent chemoradiotherapy in curatively resected gallbladder carcinoma: a propensity score-matched analysis. Int J Radiat Oncol Biol Phys. 2018;100(1):138–45. https://doi.org/10.1016/j.ijrobp.2017.09.029. Epub 2017 Sep 20

Hakeem AR, Papoulas M, Menon KV. The role of neoadjuvant chemotherapy or chemoradiotherapy for advanced gallbladder cancer - a systematic review. Eur J Surg Oncol. 2019;45(2):83–91. https://doi.org/10.1016/j.ejso.2018.08.020. Epub 2018 Sep 7

Hishikawa H, Kaibori M, Tsuda T, et al. Near-infrared fluorescence imaging and photodynamic therapy with indocyanine green lactosomes has antineoplastic effects for gallbladder cancer. Oncotarget. 2019;10(54):5622–31. https://doi.org/10.18632/oncotarget.27193.

Hoehn RS, Wima K, Ertel AE, Meier A, Ahmad SA, Shah SA, Abbott DE. Adjuvant therapy for gallbladder cancer: an analysis of the national cancer data base. J

Gastrointest Surg. 2015;19(10):1794–801. https://doi.org/10.1007/s11605-015-2922-0. Epub 2015 Aug 21

Horgan AM, Amir E, Walter T, Knox JJ. Adjuvant therapy in the treatment of biliary tract cancer: a systematic review and meta-analysis. J Clin Oncol. 2012;30(16):1934–40. https://doi.org/10.1200/JCO.2011.40.5381. Epub 2012 Apr 23. Review

Jarnagin WR, Ruo L, Little SA, Klimstra D, D'Angelica M, DeMatteo RP, Wagman R, Blumgart LH, Fong Y. Patterns of initial disease recurrence after resection of gallbladder carcinoma and hilar cholangiocarcinoma: implications for adjuvant therapeutic strategies. Cancer. 2003;98(8):1689–700.

Javle M, Zhao H, Abou-Alfa GK. Systemic therapy for gallbladder cancer. Chin Clin Oncol. 2019;8(4):44. https://doi.org/10.21037/cco.2019.08.14.

Kasumova GG, Tabatabaie O, Najarian RM, Callery MP, Ng SC, Bullock AJ, Fisher RA, Tseng JF. Surgical management of gallbladder cancer: simple versus extended cholecystectomy and the role of adjuvant therapy. Ann Surg. 2017;266(4):625–31. https://doi.org/10.1097/SLA.0000000000002385.

Kato A, Shimizu H, Ohtsuka M, Yoshitomi H, Furukawa K, Takayashiki T, Nakadai E, Kishimoto T, Nakatani Y, Yoshidome H, Miyazaki M. Downsizing chemotherapy for initially unresectable locally advanced biliary tract cancer patients treated with gemcitabine plus cisplatin combination therapy followed by radical surgery. Ann Surg Oncol. 2015;22(Suppl 3):S1093–9. https://doi.org/10.1245/s10434-015-4768-9. Epub 2015 Aug 4

Kattepur AK, Patkar S, Goel M, Ramaswamy A, Ostwal V. Role of adjuvant chemotherapy in resected T2N0 gall bladder cancer. J Gastrointest Surg. 2019;23(11):2232–8. https://doi.org/10.1007/s11605-019-04104-4.

Kayahara M, Nagakawa T. Recent trends of gallbladder cancer in Japan: an analysis of 4,770 patients. Cancer. 2007;110(3):572–80.

Kim Y, Amini N, Wilson A, Margonis GA, Ethun CG, Poultsides G, Tran T, Idrees K, Isom CA, Fields RC, Krasnick B, Weber SM, Salem A, Martin RC, Scoggins C, Shen P, Mogal HD, Schmidt C, Beal E, Hatzaras I, Shenoy R, Cardona K, Maithel SK, Pawlik TM. Impact of chemotherapy and external-beam radiation therapy on outcomes among patients with resected gallbladder cancer: a multi-institutional analysis. Ann Surg Oncol. 2016;23(9):2998–3008. https://doi.org/10.1245/s10434-016-5262-8. Epub 2016 May 11

Kim BH, Kwon J, Chie EK, Kim K, Kim YH, Seo DW, Narang AK, Herman JM. Adjuvant chemoradiotherapy is associated with improved survival for patients with resected gallbladder carcinoma: a systematic review and meta-analysis. Ann Surg Oncol. 2018;25(1):255–64. https://doi.org/10.1245/s10434-017-6139-1. Epub 2017 Oct 27

Kresl JJ, Schild SE, Henning GT, Gunderson LL, Donohue J, Pitot H, Haddock MG, Nagorney D. Adjuvant external beam radiation therapy with concurrent chemotherapy in the management of gallbladder carcinoma. Int J Radiat Oncol Biol Phys. 2002;52(1):167–75.

Le DT, Uram JN, Wang H, Bartlett BR, Kemberling H, Eyring AD, Skora AD, Luber BS, Azad NS, Laheru D, Biedrzycki B, Donehower RC, Zaheer A, Fisher GA, Crocenzi TS, Lee JJ, Duffy SM, Goldberg RM, de la Chapelle A, Koshiji M, Bhaijee F, Huebner T, Hruban RH, Wood LD, Cuka N, Pardoll DM, Papadopoulos N, Kinzler KW, Zhou S, Cornish TC, Taube JM, Anders RA, Eshleman JR, Vogelstein B, Diaz LA Jr. PD-1 blockade in tumors with mismatch-repair deficiency. N Engl J Med. 2015;372(26):2509–20. https://doi.org/10.1056/NEJMoa1500596. Epub 2015 May 30

Lee J, Lim DH, Park HC, Yu JI, Choi DW, Choi SH, Heo JS. Predictive factors of gastroduodenal bleeding after postoperative radiotherapy in biliary tract cancer. Jpn J Clin Oncol. 2017;47(4):328–33. https://doi.org/10.1093/jjco/hyw205.

Lee SE, Kim SW, Han HS, Lee WJ, Yoon DS, Cho BH, Choi IS, Kim HJ, Hong SC, Lee SM, Choi DW, Park SJ, Kim HJ, Jang JY, Korean Pancreas Surgery Club. Surgical strategy for T2 gallbladder cancer: nationwide multicenter survey in Korea. J Korean Med Sci. 2018;33(28):e186. https://doi.org/10.3346/jkms.2018.33.e186. eCollection 2018 Jul 9

Li M, Liu F, Zhang F, Zhou W, Jiang X, Yang Y, Qu K, Wang Y, Ma Q, Wang T, Bai L, Wang Z, Song X, Zhu Y, Yuan R, Gao Y, Liu Y, Jin Y, Li H, Xiang S, Ye Y, Zhang Y, Jiang L, Hu Y, Hao Y, Lu W, Chen S, Gu J, Zhou J, Gong W, Zhang Y, Wang X, Liu X, Liu C, Liu H, Liu Y, Liu Y. Genomic *ERBB2*/*ERBB3* mutations promote PD-L1-mediated immune escape in gallbladder cancer: a whole-exome sequencing analysis. Gut. 2019;68(6):1024–33. https://doi.org/10.1136/gutjnl-2018-316039. Epub 2018 Jun 28

Lim H, Seo DW, Park DH, Lee SS, Lee SK, Kim MH, Hwang S. Prognostic factors in patients with gallbladder cancer after surgical resection: analysis of 279 operated patients. J Clin Gastroenterol. 2013;47(5):443–8. https://doi.org/10.1097/MCG.0b013e3182703409. PMID: 23188077.

Ma N, Cheng H, Qin B, Zhong R, Wang B. Adjuvant therapy in the treatment of gallbladder cancer: a meta-analysis. BMC Cancer. 2015;15:615. https://doi.org/10.1186/s12885-015-1617-y.

Manterola C, Duque G, Grande L, de Aretxabala X, Conejeros R, Otzen T, García N. A systematic review of the effectiveness of adjuvant therapy for patients with gallbladder cancer. HPB (Oxford). 2019; https://doi.org/10.1016/j.hpb.2019.02.019.

Mantripragada KC, Hamid F, Shafqat H, Olszewski AJ. Adjuvant therapy for resected gallbladder cancer: analysis of the national cancer data base. J Natl Cancer Inst. 2016;109(2). pii: djw202.

Mishra SK, Kumari N, Krishnani N. Molecular pathogenesis of gallbladder cancer: an update. Mutat Res. 2019;816–818:111674. https://doi.org/10.1016/j.mrfmmm.2019.111674.

Mojica P, Smith D, Ellenhorn J. Adjuvant radiation therapy is associated with improved survival for gallbladder carcinoma with regional metastatic disease. J Surg Oncol. 2007;96(1):8–13.

Okusaka T, Nakachi K, Fukutomi A, Mizuno N, Ohkawa S, Funakoshi A, Nagino M, Kondo S, Nagaoka S, Funai J, Koshiji M, Nambu Y, Furuse J, Miyazaki M, Nimura Y. Gemcitabine alone or in combination with cisplatin in patients with biliary tract cancer: a comparative multicentre study in Japan. Br J Cancer. 2010;103(4):469–74. https://doi.org/10.1038/sj.bjc.6605779. Epub 2010 Jul 13

Primrose JN, Fox RP, Palmer DH, Malik HZ, Prasad R, Mirza D, Anthony A, Corrie P, Falk S, Finch-Jones M, Wasan H, Ross P, Wall L, Wadsley J, Evans JTR, Stocken D, Praseedom R, Ma YT, Davidson B, Neoptolemos JP, Iveson T, Raftery J, Zhu S, Cunningham D, Garden OJ, Stubbs C, Valle JW, Bridgewater J, BILCAP Study Group. Capecitabine compared with observation in resected biliary tract cancer (BILCAP): a randomised, controlled, multicentre, phase 3 study. Lancet Oncol. 2019a;20(5):663–73. https://doi.org/10.1016/S1470-2045(18)30915-X. Epub 2019 Mar 25. Erratum in: Lancet Oncol. 2019 Apr 2.

Randle RW, Levine EA, Clark CJ, Stewart JH, Shen P, Votanopoulos KI. Cytoreductive surgery with hyperthermic intraperitoneal chemotherapy for gallbladder cancer: a retrospective review. Am Surg. 2014;80(7):710–3.

Sharma A, Dwary AD, Mohanti BK, Deo SV, Pal S, Sreenivas V, Raina V, Shukla NK, Thulkar S, Garg P, Chaudhary SP. Best supportive care compared with chemotherapy for unresectable gall bladder cancer: a randomized controlled study. J Clin Oncol. 2010;28(30):4581–6. https://doi.org/10.1200/JCO.2010.29.3605. Epub 2010 Sep 20

Shroff RT, Kennedy EB, Bachini M, Bekaii-Saab T, Crane C, Edeline J, El-Khoueiry A, Feng M, Katz MHG, Primrose J, Soares HP, Valle J, Maithel SK. Adjuvant therapy for resected biliary tract cancer: ASCO clinical practice guideline. J Clin Oncol. 2019;37(12):1015–27. https://doi.org/10.1200/JCO.18.02178. Epub 2019 Mar 11

Sirohi B, Mitra A, Jagannath P, Singh A, Ramadvar M, Kulkarni S, Goel M, Shrikhande SV. Neoadjuvant chemotherapy in patients with locally advanced gallbladder cancer. Future Oncol. 2015;11(10):1501–9. https://doi.org/10.2217/fon.14.308.

Stein A, Arnold D, Bridgewater J, Goldstein D, Jensen LH, Klümpen HJ, Lohse AW, Nashan B, Primrose J, Schrum S, Shannon J, Vettorazzi E, Wege H. Adjuvant chemotherapy with gemcitabine and cisplatin compared to observation after curative intent resection of cholangiocarcinoma and muscle invasive gallbladder carcinoma (ACTICCA-1 trial) - a randomized, multidisciplinary, multinational phase III trial. BMC Cancer. 2015;15:564. https://doi.org/10.1186/s12885-015-1498-0.

Takada T, Amano H, Yasuda H, Nimura Y, Matsushiro T, Kato H, Nagakawa T, Nakayama T. Is postoperative adjuvant chemotherapy useful for gallbladder carcinoma? A phase III multicenter prospective randomized controlled trial in patients with resected pancreaticobiliary carcinoma. Study Group of Surgical Adjuvant Therapy for Carcinomas of the Pancreas and Biliary Tract. Cancer. 2002;95(8):1685–95.

Takahara N, Isayama H, Nakai Y, Sasaki T, Saito K, Sato T, Hakuta R, Ishigaki K, Saito T, Hamada T, Mizuno S, Kogure H, Tada M, Koike K. A feasibility study of gemcitabine, S-1 and leucovorin combination therapy (GSL) for advanced biliary tract cancer. J Chemother. 2019;8:1–6. https://doi.org/10.1080/1120009X.2019.1626088.

Todoroki T, Iwasaki Y, Orii K, Otsuka M, Ohara K, Kawamoto T, Nakamura K. Resection combined with intraoperative radiation therapy (IORT) for stage IV (TNM) gallbladder carcinoma. World J Surg. 1991;15(3):357–66.

Todoroki T, Kawamoto T, Otsuka M, Koike N, Yoshida S, Takada Y, Adachi S, Kashiwagi H, Fukao K, Ohara K. Benefits of combining radiotherapy with aggressive resection for stage IV gallbladder cancer. Hepatogastroenterology. 1999;46(27):1585–91.

Tran Cao HS, Zhang Q, Sada YH, Chai C, Curley SA, Massarweh NN. The role of surgery and adjuvant therapy in lymph node-positive cancers of the gallbladder and intrahepatic bile ducts. Cancer. 2018;124(1):74–83. https://doi.org/10.1002/cncr.30968. Epub 2017 Aug 25

Valle J, Wasan H, Palmer DH, Cunningham D, Anthoney A, Maraveyas A, Madhusudan S, Iveson T, Hughes S, Pereira SP, Roughton M, Bridgewater J, ABC-02 Trial Investigators. Cisplatin plus gemcitabine versus gemcitabine for biliary tract cancer. N Engl J Med. 2010;362(14):1273–81. https://doi.org/10.1056/NEJMoa0908721.

Valle JW, Lamarca A, Goyal L, Barriuso J, Zhu AX. New horizons for precision medicine in biliary tract cancers. Cancer Discov. 2017;7(9):943–62. https://doi.org/10.1158/2159-8290.CD-17-0245.

Verma V, Crane CH. Contemporary perspectives on the use of radiation therapy for locally advanced gallbladder cancer. Chin Clin Oncol. 2019;8(4):41. https://doi.org/10.21037/cco.2019.08.12.

Wang SJ, Fuller CD, Kim JS, Sittig DF, Thomas CR Jr, Ravdin PM. Prediction model for estimating the survival benefit of adjuvant radiotherapy for gallbladder cancer. J Clin Oncol. 2008;26(13):2112–7. https://doi.org/10.1200/JCO.2007.14.7934. Epub 2008 Mar 31

Wang SJ, Lemieux A, Kalpathy-Cramer J, Ord CB, Walker GV, Fuller CD, Kim JS, Thomas CR Jr. Nomogram for predicting the benefit of adjuvant chemoradiotherapy for resected gallbladder cancer. J Clin Oncol. 2011;29(35):4627–32. https://doi.org/10.1200/JCO.2010.33.8020. Epub 2011 Nov 7

Wang J, Narang AK, Sugar EA, Luber B, Rosati LM, Hsu CC, Fuller CD, Pawlik TM, Miller RC, Czito BG, Tuli R, Crane CH, Ben-Josef E, Thomas CR Jr, Herman JM. Evaluation of adjuvant radiation therapy for resected gallbladder carcinoma: a multi-institutional experience. Ann Surg Oncol. 2015;22(Suppl 3):S1100–6. https://doi.org/10.1245/s10434-015-4685-y. Epub 2015 Jul 30

Xu X, Li J, Wu J, Zhu R, Ji W. A Systematic Review and Meta-analysis of Intraluminal Brachytherapy Versus Stent Alone in the Treatment of Malignant Obstructive Jaundice. Cardiovasc Intervent Radiol. 2018;41(2):206–217. https://doi.org/10.1007/s00270-017-1827-6. Epub 2017 Oct 26. PMID: 29075881.

You MS, Ryu JK, Choi YH, Choi JH, Huh G, Paik WH, Lee SH, Kim YT. Therapeutic outcomes and prognostic factors in unresectable gallbladder cancer treated with gemcitabine plus cisplatin. BMC Cancer. 2019;19(1):10. https://doi.org/10.1186/s12885-018-5211-y.

References for Commentary Notes

Aloia TA, Jarufe N, Javle M, et al. Gallbladder cancer: expert consensus statement. HPB (Oxford). 2015;17:681–90.

Cherkassky L, D'Angelica M. Gallbladder cancer: managing the incidental diagnosis. Surg Oncol Clin N Am. 2019;28:619–30.

Henley SJ, Weir HK, Jim MA, et al. Gallbladder cancer incidence and mortality, United States 1999–2011. Cancer Epidemiol Biomark Prev. 2015;24:1319–26.

Horgan AM, Knox JJ. Adjuvant therapy for biliary tract cancers. J Oncol Pract. 2018;14:701–8.

Javle M, Rashid A, Churi C, et al. Molecular characterization of gallbladder cancer using somatic mutation profiling. Hum Pathol. 2014;45:701–8.

Javle M, Bekaii-Saab T, Jain A, et al. Biliary cancer: Utility of next-generation sequencing for clinical management. Cancer. 2016;122:3838–47.

Kanlioz M, Ekici U, Ayva Y. Analysis of incidental gallbladder cancer in cholecystectomies. Cureus. 2019;11:e5710.

Margonis GA, Gani F, Buettner S, et al. Rates and patterns of recurrence after curative intent resection for gallbladder cancer: a multi-institution analysis from the US Extra-hepatic Biliary Malignancy Consortium. HPB (Oxford). 2016;18:872–8.

Shindoh J, de Aretxabala X, Aloia TA, et al. Tumor location is a strong predictor of tumor progression and survival in T2 gallbladder cancer: an international multicenter study. Ann Surg. 2015;261:733–9.

Prognosis and Survival in Gall Bladder Cancer

15

Vinay K. Kapoor

The 5-year survival of a patient with gall bladder cancer constitutes a medical curiosity. (Fortner and Pack 1958)

In gall bladder cancer (GBC), recurrences are fairly common even after an R0 (margin negative) resection. Recurrences are classified as locoregional (GB bed or hepatic resection margin and porta hepatis, hepatoduodenal ligament, and retroperitoneal lymph nodes LNs) or distant; common sites of distant recurrence are liver, peritoneum, and lung.

15.1 Follow-Up

Patients who undergo surgical resection with a curative intent should be followed up every 3 months for 1 year, every 6 months for another year, and then annually. Follow-up includes clinical evaluation (history of pain, jaundice, vomiting, anorexia, and weight loss; palpable lump, nodular hepatomegaly, and ascites on examination), liver function tests (LFT), tumor markers (CEA and CA 19.9), ultrasonography (US) (Fig. 15.1) and, may be, computed tomography (CT) (Fig. 15.2); positron emission tomography (PET) may be performed if a recurrence is suspected on the above evaluation. Recurrence is documented either by biopsy (image-guided fine needle aspiration cytology FNAC) confirmation or progressive disease on serial imaging.

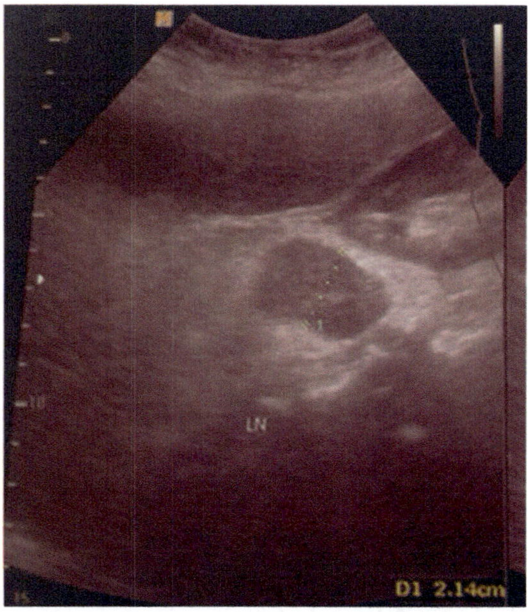

Fig. 15.1 US during the follow-up after surgical resection for gall bladder cancer shows recurrence in the form of a large lymph node

Please also see an Invited Commentary on Prognosis and Survival in Gall Bladder Cancer by Ryota Higuchi and Masakazu Yamamoto (pp **–**)

V. K. Kapoor (✉)
Department of Surgical Gastroenterology, Sanjay Gandhi Post-Graduate Institute of Medical Sciences (SGPGIMS), Lucknow, Uttar Pradesh, India
e-mail: vkkapoor.india@gmail.com

V. K. Kapoor (ed.), *A Pictorial Treatise on Gall Bladder Cancer*,
https://doi.org/10.1007/978-981-15-5289-2_15

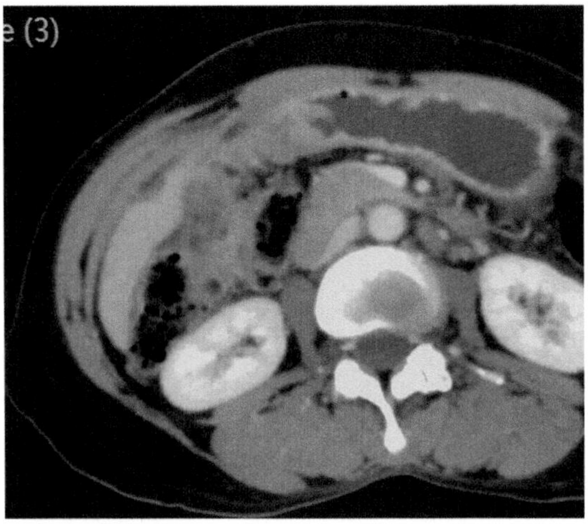

Fig. 15.2 CT during the follow-up after surgical resection for gall bladder cancer shows recurrence in the form of a soft tissue mass in the GB fossa

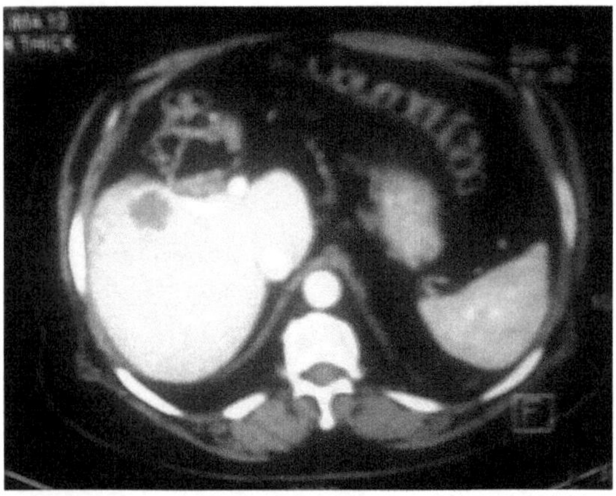

Fig. 15.3 CT during the follow-up after surgical resection for gall bladder cancer shows recurrence in the form of a liver metastasis

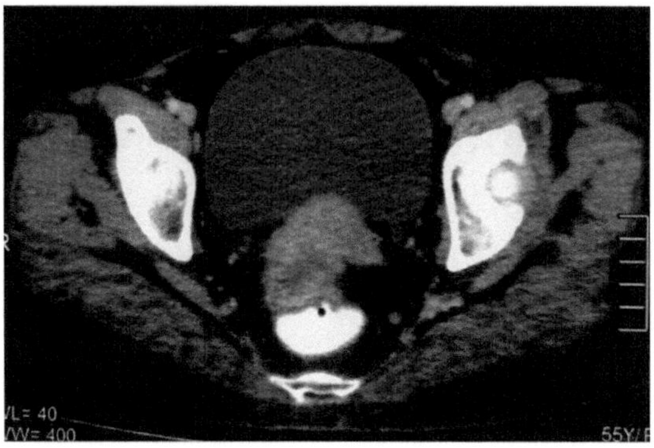

Fig. 15.4 CT during the follow-up after surgical resection for gall bladder cancer shows recurrence in the form of a pelvic deposit between the uterus anteriorly and the rectum posteriorly; it could be palpated on per rectal or per vaginal examination

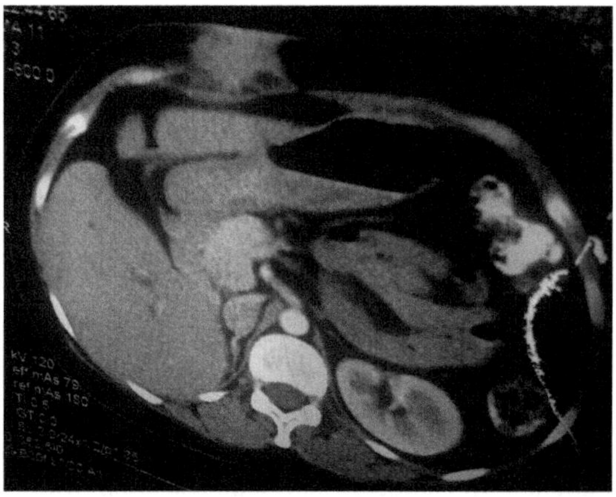

Fig. 15.5 CT during the follow-up after surgical resection for gall bladder cancer shows recurrence in the form of a deposit in the scar of the open operation

Recurrences in GBC occur early and are usually distant, e.g., liver (Fig. 15.3), peritoneal (Fig. 15.4), parietal (laparotomy scar Fig. 15.5 or laparoscopic port site Fig. 15.6). Ninety-seven patients with GBC underwent curative-intent resection at the Memorial Sloan Kettering Cancer Center (MSKCC) New York USA (1990–2001)—53/80 (66%) patients in whom follow-up was available had recurrence; median time to recurrence was 11.5 months, with 66% having recurrence within 24 months. As many as 85% of the recurrences were distant as well as locoregional and only 15% of the recurrences were isolated locoregional (i.e., no distant metastases) (Jarnagin et al. 2003). In a multi-institutional cohort of 217 GBC patients who underwent curative-intent surgery at ten institutions in the United States (2000–2014), 76 (35%) patients had recurrence (distant only in 66%, locoregional + distant in 18% and locoregional only in 16%) during a median follow-up of 30 months; median time to recurrence was 10 months and two-thirds of all recurrences occurred within 12 months. T3 disease (T4 disease was excluded from the analysis) and lymphovascular invasion (LVI) increased the risk of recurrence. Median overall survival among all patients was 16 months; 1-, 3-, and 5-year survival estimates

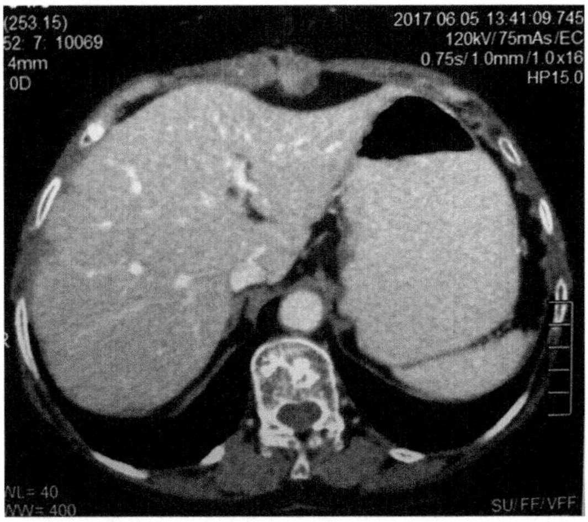

Fig. 15.6 CT during the follow-up after surgical resection for gall bladder cancer shows recurrence in the form of a port-site metastasis in the scar of the laparoscopic operation

for all patients were 80%, 54%, and 44%. Survival of patients who had recurrence was poorer than those without recurrence (1-, 3-, and 5-year survival 69% vs. 91%, 29% vs. 79%, and 16% vs. 76%). When interpreting these results, it needs to be, however, emphasized that patients with the highest risk of recurrence, i.e., those with T4 and N2 disease and those who had R2 resection, were excluded from the study (Margonis et al. 2016).

In several cancers, recurrences (including even distant metastases) can be resected for cure, but prognosis of recurrent GBC is invariably ominous because resection of recurrence is almost never an option. A review reported only three published reports of reresection for recurrence in GBC (Miyazaki et al. 2017). Reresection was performed in only 20 out of 135 cases with recurrence at the Nagoya University Japan (1991–2010); 5-year survival, however, was only 5%—survival was better if the initial disease-free interval was >2 years (Takahashi et al. 2015). In another report, reresection was performed between 2000 and 2014 in only nine GBC patients with recurrence—5-year survival of 24%, however, was achieved in this highly select group (Noji et al. 2015). Amemiya et al. (2008) reported anecdotal 13-year survival in a patient with GBC with extensive local nodal and metastatic disease who underwent central hepatic bisegmentectomy and para-aortic lymphadenectomy followed 2 months later by percutaneous ethanol injection (PEI) and transcatheter arterial embolization (TAE) for hepatic metastases followed 12 months later by retroperitoneal and iliac lymph node dissection with resection and reconstruction (with graft) of the external iliac artery followed 2 months later by radiotherapy for a paraesophageal lymph node. Kawamoto et al. (2018) reported anecdotal long-term (9 year and 6 months) survival in a patient with GBC who developed liver and peritoneal recurrences after an extended cholecystectomy, which were treated with a combination of microwave coagulo-necrotic therapy, chemotherapy, and radiotherapy.

15.2 Prognosis

GBC is a bad cancer per se (Kapoor 2015). It is one of the most lethal cancers with an abysmal prognosis and has one of the poorest outcomes of all cancers. As compared to 5-year survival of 70–75% for breast, 38–74% for colorectal, and 9–20% for stomach, 5-year survival for stage III GBC is a mere 7–8% (ACS n.d.). In most cancers, the survival curve plateaus after 5 years but in GBC recurrences and deaths continue to occur even after 5 years. Out of 166 patients with stage IV GBC who underwent major resections at the Nagoya University Japan, 25 survived for 3 years but only 15 survived for 5 years and only 7 for 10 years (Nishio et al. 2007). In another report of 165 T3, T4 GBC patients, 25 survived at 5 years but only 11 survived at 10 years (Igami et al. 2014).

Prognosis and outcome, to a great extent, are decided by the stage and the biology of the disease which in turn are determined by

1. T stage—Most reports mention T stage as one of the most important predictors of outcome but Sung et al. (2020), in analysis of 348 resected cases, surprisingly found no significant difference in survival between T1s-T1a, T1a-T1b, and T2a-T2b tumors. T2 has been subdivided into T2a (peritoneal side) and T2b (hepatic side) in the recent (8th) edition of AJCC-TNM but an analysis of 1251 patients

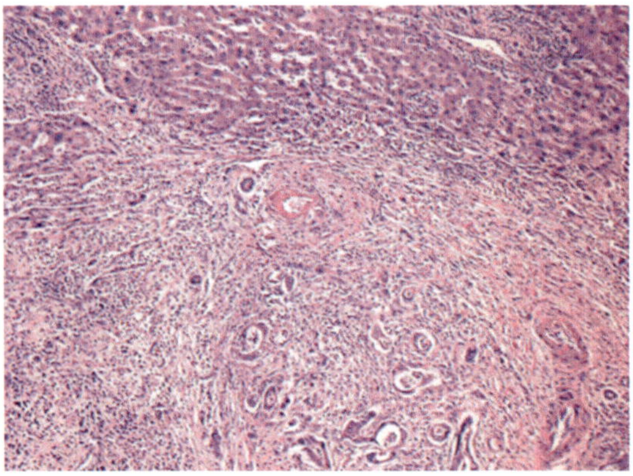

Fig. 15.7 Microphotograph shows adenocarcinoma of the gall bladder infiltrating the liver (T3)—risk of recurrence is higher and prognosis is poorer in patients with T3 or T4 tumor

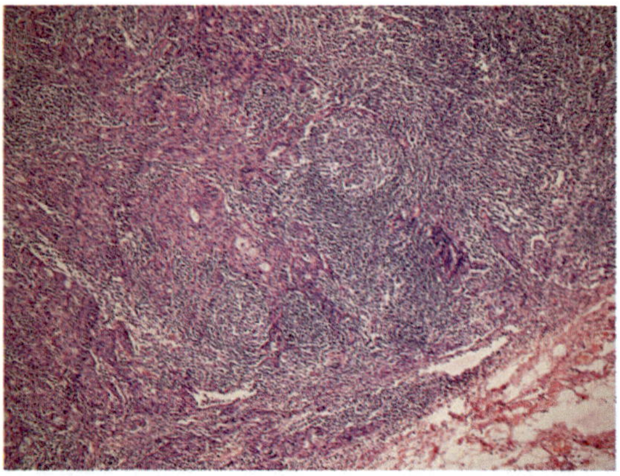

Fig. 15.8 Microphotograph shows tumor deposits in a lymph node—risk of recurrence is higher and prognosis is poorer in patients with node-positive disease

in the National Cancer Database (2009–2012) found no difference in survival between peritoneal and hepatic side T2 (Lafaro et al. 2020). T3 and T4 disease (Fig. 15.7) have worse outcome. Moreover, in these patients, those with jaundice have much worse outcome than those without (see Chap. 11).

2. N status—negative or positive (Fig. 15.8), site of lymph nodes, i.e., whether beyond the hepatoduodenal ligament, number (removed, positive, and negative).

   NOTE Some earlier reports (Bartlett et al. 1996; Benoist et al. 1998) reported no long-term survival in node-positive patients and questioned the role of operation in such cases but that does not hold true today and most series report 5-year survival in even node-positive patients. Shirai et al. (2012) reported 43% 5-year survival (22 actual 5-year survivors) in node-positive patients.

   In a large (n = 4534) survival analysis from Japan, 5-year (51% in N0 vs. 29% in N1 vs. 11% in N2) and median (65 months in N0 vs. 25 months in N1 and 13 months in N2) survival were much better in node-negative than in node-positive patients (Ishihara et al. 2016). In a large report from India, median survival in node-negative patients was much higher (62 vs. 14 months) than in node-positive patients (Mishra et al. 2017). Greater LN dissection has been shown to be associated with better survival (Tran and Nissen 2015). Lymph node ratio (LNR), i.e., number of metastatic LNs/number of retrieved LNs >0.5 is a poor prognostic marker (Negi et al. 2011). LNR is an important predictor of prognosis—5-year survival was 33% if LNR was <0.15 versus 10% if LNR >0.15 (Birnbaum et al. 2015). Analysis of 214 patients, who underwent curative resection in a multi-institutional database in USA (2000–2015), revealed that LNR provided better prognostic discrimination (Amini et al. 2016). The number of positive LNs also determines survival. Five-year survival in T2M0 with 1–2 positive LNs was 83% versus 50% in T2 M0 with 3 or more positive LNs. Similarly, 5-year survival in T3M0 with 1–2 positive LNs was 46% versus 0% in T3M0 with 3 or more positive LNs (Sakata et al. 2017). The number of negative LNs (NLN) is also an important predictor of better survival—patients with 2 or more NLN had better 5-year survival than those with 0 or 1 NLN in all stages (Lin et al. 2018). Positive LNs (PLN), LNR, and log odds of positive LNs (LODDS) were found to be the best prognostic discriminants for recurrence and survival (Lee et al. 2019).

3. Histological features, e.g., grade (poor differentiation) (Fig. 15.9), lymphovascular invasion (LVI) (Fig. 15.10), perineural invasion

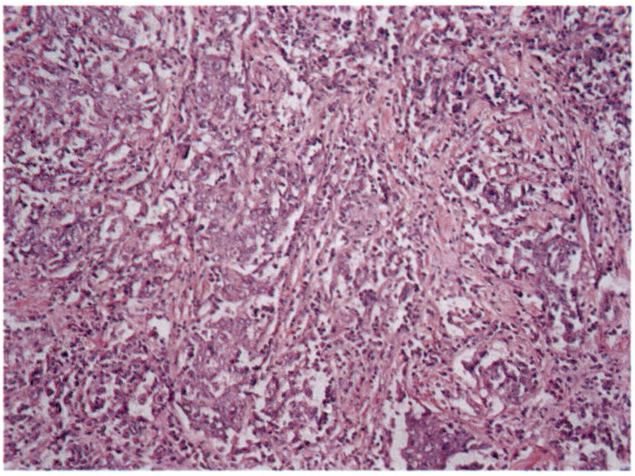

Fig. 15.9 Microphotograph shows poorly differentiated adenocarcinoma—risk of recurrence is higher and prognosis is poorer in patients showing poor differentiation in the primary tumor

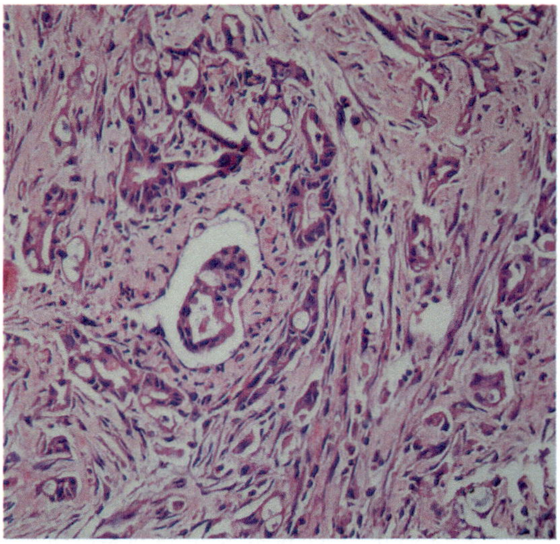

Fig. 15.10 Microphotograph shows tumor deposits in a lymphatic vessel—risk of recurrence is higher and prognosis is poorer in patients showing lymphovascular invasion (LVI) in the primary tumor

(PNI) (Fig. 15.11), and pericapsular invasion (PCI) in the LNs.

4. R (resection status) viz. R0 versus R1 or R2. Five-year disease specific survival (DSS) was mere 8% after R1 or R2 resection ($n = 104$) vs. 52% after R0 resection ($n = 168$) (Higuchi et al. 2014). In 338 patients with advanced GBC who were treated in Xian China from 2008 to 2012—curative resection provided much better survival than non-curative resection (1-, 3-, and 5-year survival was 59%, 47%, and 44% vs. 13%, 9%, and 8%); median survival was also longer (22 vs. 3 months) after curative resection. In the curative resection group, positive margin, LN metastasis, and poor differentiation were risk factors for poor outcome (Chen et al. 2016).

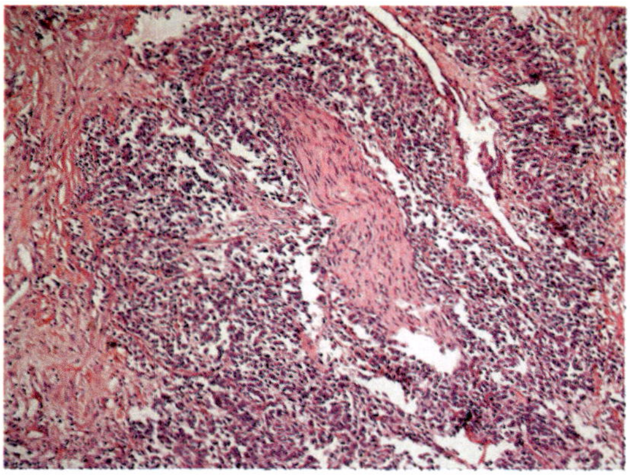

Fig. 15.11 Microphotograph shows tumor deposits around a nerve trunk—risk of recurrence is higher and prognosis is poorer in patients showing perineural invasion (PNI) in the primary tumor

Todoroki et al. (1999a) reported better survival in females. Higuchi et al. (2014) also reported better (42% vs. 29%) 5-year DSS in women as compared to men. In an analysis of 9041 cases from the SEER database (1988–2013), 5-year survival was lowest (13.9%) in widowed versus divorced/separated (18.7%); those who were never married had lower survival (20.2%) versus best married (21.1%) (Bai et al. 2017).

Presence of preoperative inflammation, i.e., acute cholecystitis or cholangitis within 2 weeks of operation in 23 out of 88 patients was associated with lower 3-year survival (33% vs. 73%); even after R0 resection (Han et al. 2011). Inflammatory markers have been found to affect the prognosis in various cancers. Elevated neutrophil to lymphocyte ratio (NLR) in GBC makes a bad cancer even worse (Beal et al. 2016). High (>4.33) neutrophil to lymphocyte ratio (NLR) was associated with worse outcome in the form of 1-, 3-, and 5-year overall survival (63%, 12%, and 8% vs. 76%, 43%, and 34%) (Liu et al. 2019a). High (>0.24) monocyte to lymphocyte ratio (MLR) (Choi et al. 2019) and high (>143.7) platelet to lymphocyte ratio (PLR) (Zhu et al. 2019) are also markers of poor prognosis.

Preoperative fasting hyperglycemia is an independent indicator of poor prognosis after surgery in GBC (Zheng et al. 2019). Fibrinogen plays an important regulatory role in inflammation which controls angiogenesis, proliferation, and migration of tumor. Serum albumin reflects the nutritional status of the patient. Elevated fibrinogen albumin ratio correlated with unfavorable overall survival in GBC (Wu et al. 2018). Radiographic sarcopenia, determined by skeletal muscle mass index using computed tomography (CT), predicted survival—1-, 3-, and 5-year survival in patients with radiological sarcopenia ($n = 88$) was 64%, 42%, and 36% versus 84%, 63%, and 54% in those without radiographic sarcopenia ($n = 70$); on multivariate analysis, radiographic sarcopenia, as also stage, radicality, intraoperative blood loss, and adjuvant therapy, was a significant (HR 1.7) prognostic factor for survival (Lee et al. 2020). Total metabolic tumor volume (MTV) on ^{16}F-FDG PET was a significant factor for predicting overall survival (OS) (Chun et al. 2019).

Red cell distribution width (RDW) has been shown to be associated with tumor stage in many cancers—higher levels of RDW indicate advanced stage in GBC (Gupta et al. 2019). Actual neutrophil count, lymphocyte monocyte ratio, albumin, and neutrophil–lymphocyte ratio (ALAN) score has been described to predict median overall survival (OS) in advanced biliary cancer—5 months in high risk, 12 months in intermediate risk, and 22 months in low risk (Salati et al. 2019). Overall survival was less in patients with low high-density lipoprotein—cholesterol (HDL-C) levels ($n = 42$) as compared to those with normal HDL-C levels ($n = 57$) (Yuan et al. 2019).

CA 19.9 is a prognostic marker to predict survival (Mochizuki et al. 2018; Liu et al. 2019b). In GBC patients with jaundice, patients with CA 19.9 <50 UI/mL had longer (40 vs. 12 months) survival than those with CA 19.9 >50 UI/mL (Tran et al. 2017). After laparoscopic resection in 47 patients with tumor confined to the GB wall, 5-year survival was better (85% vs. 69%) in patients with normal CA 19.9 level (Zhang et al. 2018). Therapeutic index based on 3-year OS was better in patients with CA 19.9 <200 UI/mL than in those with CA 19.9 >200 UI/mL (Sahara et al. 2020).

Five-year DSS was less with operating time >360 min (24% vs. 50%) and bleeding >2000 mL (13% vs. 52%) (Higuchi et al. 2014). In 61 (23%) out of 262 patients who underwent curative-intent resection for GBC at a ten-institution consortium in USA (2000–2015)—survival after surgical resection was poorer (median 20 vs. 32 months) in patients who received perioperative blood transfusion (Lopez-Aguiar et al. 2018). Postoperative complications also predicted poor survival (Mochizuki et al. 2018).

A nomogram including age, sex, T stage, histology, and number of LNs derived from the data on 789 patients in the SEER database better predicted survival than AJCC 7th edition TNM stage (Chen et al. 2019). Another nomogram, including age, ECOG performance status, hemoglobin, alkaline phosphatase, tumor size, and metastases, was found to be superior to TNM staging in predicting OS in 528 patients (Yadav et al. 2020). Like in some other cancers, patients with GBC treated at an Academic Medical Center (AMC) had lower 30-day and 90-day mortality and better OS than those treated at a Community Cancer Center (CCC) (Melillo et al. 2020).

15.3 Survival

GBC has one of the poorest outcomes of all cancers with a high mortality to incidence ratio. Five-year survival for stage III GBC is 7–8% cf. 70–75% for same stage breast cancer, 38–74%, for colorectal cancer, and 9–20% for stomach cancer (ACS). Cure still eludes and outcome is dismal with poor survival in most patients with GBC since majority of them have advanced (metastatic/locoregional) disease at the time of diagnosis and are inoperable, unresectable, and incurable. There is lack of effective adjuvant therapy in resected cases. Majority of patients who undergo even an apparently curative (R0) resection develop recurrence because of the aggressive biology of the disease and recurrences are invariably unresectable.

Overall median survival in GBC is 6–12 months and 5-year survival is still in single digit in the range of 5–10%. Metastatic disease has a median survival of 6 months (Duffy et al.

2008). Median survival without treatment is 3 months. Long-term survival and potential cure are possible only in early (T1T2, N0; stage I, II) GBC. Anecdotal long-term survival has been reported in few patients with advanced (T3 or N+, stage III) GBC. Long-term survival is very unlikely in T4 disease even after major resection. Patients who are unresectable or have metastatic disease rarely live beyond 1–2 years. This is more a reflection of the aggressive biology of the disease rather than failure of treatment.

Most reports on GBC mention median and 5-year actuarial survival; very few reports mention long-term (10 year) survival and actual long-term survivors. The Niigata University group reported 20-year survival in 47 patients with T1b GBC operated between 1982 and 2018 (Yuza et al. 2020).

Survival rates of GBC reported from the United States are very low, even in early stages of the disease—5-year survival in more than 10,000 patients treated between 1989 and 1996 was mere 50% in Stage I and 28% in Stage II (ACS). Five-year survival in 2330 patients in the SEER database in the United States was 12% (Carriaga and Henson 1995). At the MSKCC New York USA, 5-year survival rates were 54% for AJCC stage II, 28% for stage III, and 25% for stage IV (Fong et al. 2000). In a later report from the MSKCC, 435 GBCs (37% of which were stage IV) were seen—136 were operated—123 underwent curative resection—median overall survival was 10 months (stage I–III 13 months, stage IV 6 months, incidental GBC 16 months) (Duffy et al. 2008). Long-term (median follow-up 58 months) outcome was available in 104 patients managed at the MSKCC New York USA—actuarial 5-year disease-specific survival (DSS) was 42%; 5-year survival in 63 patients with T3/T4 GBC who underwent resection was 25%; nearly all long-term survivors had N0 disease (D'Angelica et al. 2009). Some older series (Bartlett et al. 1996; Benoist et al. 1998) had also reported no long-term survival in node-positive patients. In a National Cancer Database (NCDB) USA (2004–2012) analysis, surgery was performed in 1123 patients while 212 had no surgery. Median OS was 19.6 months after surgery plus adjuvant therapy, 13.3 months after surgery alone, 11.6 months after nonsurgical therapy, and 8.3 months after no treatment (Tran Cao et al. 2018).

Much better survival has been reported from Japan. Five-year survival in an early (1976–1998) Japanese series of 135 patients who underwent resection was 36% (100% for stage I, 78% for stage II, 69% for stage III, and 11% for stage IV); there were 22 actual 5-year survivors but only 3 of these 22 had stage IV disease (Todoroki et al. 1999b). In a review of 4424 cases from Japan, 5-year survival was 83% for AJCC 5th edition stage I, 70% for stage II, 45% for stage III, 23% for stage IVA, and 9% for stage IVB (Kayahara et al. 2008). The Japanese Biliary Tract Cancer Statistics Registry enrolled 2067 patients with GBC between 1998 and 2004—resection rate was 69%; overall 5-year survival was 42%—88% for Japan Society of Biliary Surgery (JSBS) stage I, 69% for stage II, 42% for stage III, 23% for stage IVA, and 6% for stage IVB (Miyakawa et al. 2009). Overall 5-year survival in 4534 GBC cases in Japan (2008–2013) was 40% (91% in stage I, 71% in stage II, and 30% in stage III) (Ishihara et al. 2016). At the Tokyo Women's Medical University, resection was performed in 382 patients between 1969 and 2012—5-year survival was 99% in AJCC stage I (n = 87), 85% in stage II (n = 32), 40% in stage IIIA (n = 35), 53% in stage IIIB (n = 56), and 0% in stage IVA (n = 30) and 18% in stage IVB (n = 141) (Higuchi and Yamamoto 2014). The Nagoya University Japan group has reported its results in advanced GBC—59 patients with stage IV GBC underwent radical resection (1979–1994); only six survived for more than 5 years—these were patients without celiac, superior mesenteric, or para-aortic lymph node involvement (Kondo et al. 2001). The Nagoya University Japan group again reported 72 patients with stage IV GBC—mortality was 14 (19%) and only 11 patients survived <3 years; 5-year survival was not mentioned (Kondo et al. 2003). Recently, the Nagoya University Japan group reported 166 patients with stage IV GBC who underwent resection—mortality was 14% and 5-year survival was 12%; 15 patients survived for 5 years

(Nishio et al. 2007). Three-, 5-, and 10-year survival was 34%, 25%, and 16%, and median survival was 1.5 years in 165 patients with advanced (T3, T4) GBC resected at Nagoya between 1979 and 2011 (Igami et al. 2014). The Tokyo Women's Medical University Japan reported its results in 274 patients with advanced (beyond muscularis propria) GBC who were operated between 1969 and 2012; overall 5-year disease-specific survival (DSS) was 37%—85%, 67%, 28%, and 11% for JSBS stage II ($n = 33$), III ($n = 50$), IVa ($n = 46$), and IVb ($n = 141$), respectively; median survival was 22 months and there were 56 five-year survivors, but the number of actual 10-year survivors was not mentioned (Higuchi et al. 2014).

In a large report of 1366 cases (1987–2005) from Chile, all patients with disease beyond the GB wall died before 50 months (Roa et al. 2014).

Two hundred and seventy-nine patients with GBC were operated in South Korea (1992–2009), R0 resection was achieved in 164 (35 SC, 129 EC)—median overall survival was 26 months; 5-year survival was 95% in stage I, 76% in stage II, 45% in stage IIIA, 22% in stage IIIB, and <5% in stage IV (Lim et al. 2013). Six hundred and ninety-two patients with GBC were operated at the Seoul National University South Korea between 1987 and 2014—curative resection could be performed in 59% and 5-year survival after curative resection was 67% (Chang et al. 2016).

There are very few reports on GBC from Europe. Cumulative experience of the French Surgical Association (FSA) with 724 patients, 85% of which had T3/T4 disease, showed median survival of 3 months and 1 year and 5-year survival of 14% and 5%, respectively (Cubertafond et al. 1994). Sweden Regional Cancer Center West identified 546 GBCs (2000–2014)—median survival was 4.7 months (2000–2004), 4.8 months (2000–2009), and 6.1 months (2010–2014) (Lindnér et al. 2018).

Mishra et al. (2017) reported only 11 actual 5-year survivors (stage I = 3, II = 5 and III = 3; 9 node negative and 2 node positive; only 3 with adjacent organs involvement) out of 437 patients with GBC at a tertiary care hospital in India.

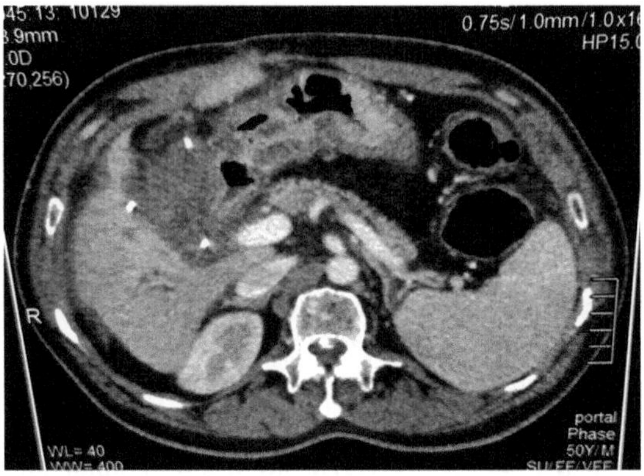

Fig. 15.12 CT shows early (within a few months) recurrence in the gall bladder fossa infiltrating the duodenum (surgical clips can also be seen) in a patient with node-positive disease with lymphovascular invasion (LVI) and perineural invasion (PNI) in the primary tumor

15.4 Incidental GBC

Overall survival in incidental GBC was more (32 vs. 17 months) than non-incidental GBC (Ethun et al. 2017). Presence or absence of residual disease at reoperation is the most important predictor of survival in incidental GBC (see Chap. 13).

GBC is uncommon in the West and has, therefore, not received much attention. Early GBC is difficult to diagnose. Clinically obvious GBC is usually advanced and needs major resections. These surgical procedures are associated with significant morbidity and mortality. Recurrences are common (Fig. 15.12) and survival poor, even after R0 resection. Role of adjuvant therapy is not well established.

> *With all the factors pitched against it, GBC is a bad cancer per se* (Kapoor 2015).

Invited Commentary on Prognosis and Survival in Gall Bladder Cancer

Ryota Higuchi and Masakazu Yamamoto

Professor VK Kapoor has reviewed the follow-up, recurrence, prognosis, prognostic factors, and surgical outcomes after gallbladder cancer (GBC) surgery. For patients with GBC, the only treatment that can be expected to result in a cure is surgical resection; however, recurrence rates are high, even with radical resection, as noted by Professor VK Kapoor. Therefore, the development of effective adjuvant therapies to improve treatment results is expected.

Primrose et al. recently reported a randomized controlled multicenter phase 3 study (Capecitabine compared with observation in resected biliary tract cancer [BILCAP] trial (Primrose et al. 2019)) that evaluated the effectiveness of capecitabine as a postoperative adjuvant chemotherapy for biliary tract cancers, with the exception of duodenal papilla cancer. In their intention to treat analysis of 447 participants, the median overall survival in the surgery-only group was 36.4 months compared to 51.1 months in the surgery with capecitabine group (hazard ratio [HR] 0.81, 95% confident interval [CI]; 0.63–1.04, $p = 0.097$). Though prognostic prolongation was observed no superiority was shown. In per-protocol analysis of 430 patients, the median overall survival for the surgery alone group was 36.1 months compared to 52.7 months for the surgery plus capecitabine group (HR 0.75, 95% CI; 0.58–0.97, $p = 0.028$). A significant effect in terms of improving prognosis with capecitabine was suggested by per-protocol analysis. A prognostic effect of 15 months was observed; therefore, it may be possible that capecitabine will be accepted as a standard postoperative adjuvant treatment overseas.

Manterola et al. (2019) conducted a systematic review of the treatment after GBC surgery. Twenty-seven reports of treatments met the selection criteria (3 systematic reviews and 24 observational studies). The evidence for chemotherapy, chemoradiotherapy, and radiotherapy was reported as moderate, poor, and very poor, respectively. Although the available evidence is inconclusive, Manterola et al. (2019) noted that adjuvant therapy may improve overall survival in patients with positive lymph node metastases, positive surgical resection margins, or advanced-stage cancer.

Currently, the Adjuvant S-1 for Cholangiocarcinoma Trial (ASCOT) (Nakachi et al. 2018) is being conducted to verify the efficacy of the tegafur, gimeracil, and oteracil potassium combination drug (S-1), and the Adjuvant Chemotherapy With Gemcitabine and Cisplatin Compared to Standard of Care After Curative Intent Resection of Biliary Tract Cancer (ACTICCA-1) trial (Stein et al. 2015) are being conducted to verify the efficacy of gemcitabine plus cisplatin. The results of these trials are expected to improve the outcomes after surgery for GBC.

The biliary tract cancer clinical practice guidelines (Yoshitomi et al. 2015) state that there is no clear consensus on factors indicating unresectability due to local progression in GBC. In addition, it is said that "cases with distant metastasis are treated as unresectable because they have little significance for resection regardless of the occupied site and are more harmful than good." However, case reports have mentioned that there are cases of long-term survival by multidisciplinary treatment, including surgery and chemotherapy, even when initial distant metastasis is observed. In recent years, even patients who could not undergo resection at the first visit have been reported to be able to undergo conversion surgery. Downsizing chemotherapy for initially unresectable locally advanced GBC has also been reported (Kato et al. 2015). Further advances in chemotherapy and chemoradiotherapy may be expected to change the respectability status and improve surgical outcomes by therapeutic interventions.

References

Chapter References

ACS. www.cancer.org.

Amemiya T, Yokoyama Y, Oda K, Nishio H, Ebata T, Abe T, Igami T, Nagino M, Nimura Y. A patient with gallbladder cancer with paraaortic lymph node and hepatic metastases who has survived for more than 13 years after the primary extended radical operation. J Hepatobiliary Pancreat Surg. 2008;15(6):648–51. https://doi.org/10.1007/s00534-007-1316-4. Epub 2008 Nov 7.

Amini N, Kim Y, Wilson A, Margonis GA, Ethun CG, Poultsides G, Tran T, Idrees K, Isom CA, Fields RC, Krasnick B, Weber SM, Salem A, Martin RC, Scoggins C, Shen P, Mogal HD, Schmidt C, Beal E, Hatzaras I,

Shenoy R, Maithel SK, Pawlik TM. Prognostic implications of lymph node status for patients with gallbladder cancer: a multi-institutional study. Ann Surg Oncol. 2016;23(9):3016–23. https://doi.org/10.1245/s10434-016-5243-y. Epub 2016 May 5

Bai DS, Chen P, Qian JJ, Jin SJ, Jiang GQ. Effect of marital status on the survival of patients with gallbladder cancer treated with surgical resection: a population-based study. Oncotarget. 2017;8(16):26404–13. https://doi.org/10.18632/oncotarget.15476.

Bartlett DL, Fong Y, Fortner JG, Brennan MF, Blumgart LH. Long-term results after resection for gallbladder cancer. Implications for staging and management. Ann Surg. 1996;224(5):639–46. https://doi.org/10.1097/00000658-199611000-00008.

Beal EW, Wei L, Ethun CG, Black SM, Dillhoff M, Salem A, Weber SM, Tran T, Poultsides G, Son AY, Hatzaras I, Jin L, Fields RC, Buettner S, Pawlik TM, Scoggins C, Martin RC, Isom CA, Idrees K, Mogal HD, Shen P, Maithel SK, Schmidt CR. Elevated NLR in gallbladder cancer and cholangiocarcinoma - making bad cancers even worse: results from the US Extrahepatic Biliary Malignancy Consortium. HPB (Oxford). 2016;18(11):950–7. https://doi.org/10.1016/j.hpb.2016.08.006. Epub 2016 Sep 24

Benoist S, Panis Y, Fagniez PL. Long-term results after curative resection for carcinoma of the gallbladder. French University Association for Surgical Research. Am J Surg. 1998;175(2):118–22. https://doi.org/10.1016/s0002-9610(97)00269-9.

Birnbaum DJ, Viganò L, Russolillo N, Langella S, Ferrero A, Capussotti L. Lymph node metastases in patients undergoing surgery for a gallbladder cancer. Extension of the lymph node dissection and prognostic value of the lymph node ratio. Ann Surg Oncol. 2015;22(3):811–8. https://doi.org/10.1245/s10434-014-4044-4. Epub 2014 Sep 9

Carriaga MT, Henson DE. Liver, gallbladder, extrahepatic bile ducts, and pancreas. Cancer. 1995;75(1 Suppl):171–90. https://doi.org/10.1002/1097-0142(19950101)75:1+<171::aid-cncr2820751306>3.0.co;2-2.

Chang J, Jang JY, Lee KB, Kang MJ, Jung W, Shin YC, Kim SW. Improvement of clinical outcomes in the patients with gallbladder cancer: lessons from periodic comparison in a tertiary referral center. J Hepatobiliary Pancreat Sci. 2016;23(4):234–41. https://doi.org/10.1002/jhbp.330. Epub 2016 Mar 1

Chen C, Geng Z, Shen H, Song H, Zhao Y, Zhang G, Li W, Ma L, Wang L. Long-term outcomes and prognostic factors in advanced gallbladder cancer: focus on the advanced T stage. PLoS One. 2016;11(11):e0166361. https://doi.org/10.1371/journal.pone.0166361. eCollection 2016.

Chen M, Cao J, Zhang B, Pan L, Cai X. A nomogram for prediction of overall survival in patients with node-negative gallbladder cancer. J Cancer. 2019;10(14):3246–52. https://doi.org/10.7150/jca.30046.

Choi YH, Lee JW, Lee SH, Choi JH, Kang J, Lee BS, Paik WH, Ryu JK, Kim YT. A high monocyte-to-lymphocyte ratio predicts poor prognosis in patients with advanced gallbladder cancer receiving chemotherapy. Cancer Epidemiol Biomark Prev 2019;28(6):1045-1051. doi: https://doi.org/10.1158/1055-9965. EPI-18-1066. Epub 2019 Mar 6.

Chun YJ, Jeung HC, Park HS, Park JS, Rha SY, Choi HJ, Lee JH, Jeon TJ. Significance of metabolic tumor volume and total lesion glycolysis measured using ^{18}F-FDG PET/CT in locally advanced and metastatic gallbladder carcinoma. Yonsei Med J. 2019;60(7):604–10. https://doi.org/10.3349/ymj.2019.60.7.604.

Cubertafond P, Gainant A, Cucchiaro G. Surgical treatment of 724 carcinomas of the gallbladder carcinoma: long term results. Ann Surg. 1994;219:275–80. https://doi.org/10.1097/00000658-199403000-00007.

D'Angelica M, Dalal KM, DeMatteo RP, Fong Y, Blumgart LH, Jarnagin WR. Analysis of the extent of resection for adenocarcinoma of the gallbladder. Ann Surg Oncol. 2009;16(4):806–16. https://doi.org/10.1245/s10434-008-0189-3.

Duffy A, Capanu M, Abou-Alfa GK, Huitzil D, Jarnagin W, Fong Y, D'Angelica M, Dematteo RP, Blumgart LH, O'Reilly EM. Gallbladder cancer (GBC): 10-year experience at Memorial Sloan-Kettering Cancer Centre (MSKCC). J Surg Oncol. 2008;98(7):485–9. https://doi.org/10.1002/jso.21141.

Ethun CG, Le N, Lopez-Aguiar AG, Pawlik TM, Poultsides G, Tran T, Idrees K, Isom CA, Fields RC, Krasnick BA, Weber SM, Salem A, Martin RCG, Scoggins CR, Shen P, Mogal HD, Schmidt C, Beal E, Hatzaras I, Shenoy R, Russell MC, Maithel SK. Pathologic and prognostic implications of incidental versus nonincidental gallbladder cancer: a 10-institution study from the United States Extrahepatic Biliary Malignancy Consortium. Am Surg. 2017;83(7):679–86.

Fong Y, Jarnagin W, Blumgart LH. Gallbladder cancer: comparison of patients presenting initially for definitive operation with those presenting after prior noncurative intervention. Ann Surg. 2000;232(4):557–69. https://doi.org/10.1097/00000658-200010000-00011.

Fortner JG, Pack GT. Clinical aspects of primary carcinoma of the gallbladder. AMA Arch Surg. 1958;77(5):742–50. https://doi.org/10.1001/archsurg.1958.01290040090011.

Gupta A, Gupta S, Gupta A, Gupta A, Goyal B, Agrawal S, Joshua LM, Kumar U, Ravi B, Kant R. Red cell distribution width: a surrogate biomarker to predict tumor burden in carcinoma gallbladder. Niger J Surg. 2019;25(2):198–202. https://doi.org/10.4103/njs.NJS_22_19.

Han HS, Cho JY, Yoon YS, Ahn KS, Kim H. Preoperative inflammation is a prognostic factor for gallbladder carcinoma. Br J Surg. 2011;98(1):111–6. https://doi.org/10.1002/bjs.7265. Epub 2010 Oct 29

Higuchi R, Yamamoto M. Aggressive surgical management and treatment outcomes of gallbladder cancer.

In: Agarwal A, Fong Y, editors. Carcinoma of the gall bladder. New Delhi: Elsevier; 2014. p. 175–83.

Higuchi R, Ota T, Araida T, Kajiyama H, Yazawa T, Furukawa T, Yoshikawa T, Takasaki K, Yamamoto M. Surgical approaches to advanced gallbladder cancer: a 40-year single-institution study of prognostic factors and resectability. Ann Surg Oncol. 2014;21(13):4308–16. https://doi.org/10.1245/s10434-014-3885-1. Epub 2014 Jul 15

Igami T, Ebata T, Yokoyama Y, Sugawara G, Nagino M. Advanced resectable gallbladder cancer: diagnosis and surgical approach. In: Agarwal A, Fong Y, editors. Carcinoma of the gall bladder. New Delhi: Elsevier; 2014. p. 89–105.

Ishihara S, Horiguchi A, Miyakawa S, Endo I, Miyazaki M, Takada T. Biliary tract cancer registry in Japan from 2008 to 2013. J Hepatobiliary Pancreat Sci. 2016;23(3):149–57. https://doi.org/10.1002/jhbp.314. Epub 2016 Jan 26

Jarnagin WR, Ruo L, Little SA, Klimstra D, D'Angelica M, DeMatteo RP, Wagman R, Blumgart LH, Fong Y. Patterns of initial disease recurrence after resection of gallbladder carcinoma and hilar cholangiocarcinoma: implications for adjuvant therapeutic strategies. Cancer. 2003;98(8):1689–700. https://doi.org/10.1002/cncr.11699.

Kapoor VK. Is gall bladder cancer a bad cancer per se? World J Gastrointest Surg. 2015;7:107–9. https://doi.org/10.4240/wjgs.v7.i7.107.

Kawamoto M, Wada Y, Koya N, Takami Y, Saitsu H, Ishizaki N, Tabata M, Onishi H, Nakamura M, Morisaki T. Long-term survival of a patient with recurrent gallbladder carcinoma, treated with chemotherapy, immunotherapy, and surgery: a case report. Surg Case Rep. 2018;4(1):115. https://doi.org/10.1186/s40792-018-0512-6.

Kayahara M, Nagakawa T, Nakagawara H, Kitagawa H, Ohta T. Prognostic factors for gallbladder cancer in Japan. Ann Surg. 2008;248(5):807–14. https://doi.org/10.1097/SLA.0b013e31818a1561.

Kondo S, Nimura Y, Kamiya J, Nagino M, Kanai M, Uesaka K, Yuasa N, Sano T, Hayakawa N. Five-year survivors after aggressive surgery for stage IV gallbladder cancer. J Hepatobiliary Pancreat Surg. 2001;8(6):511–7. https://doi.org/10.1007/s005340100018.

Kondo S, Nimura Y, Kamiya J, Nagino M, Kanai M, Uesaka K, Yuasa N, Sano T, Hayakawa N. Factors influencing postoperative hospital mortality and long-term survival after radical resection for stage IV gallbladder carcinoma. World J Surg. 2003;27(3):272–7. . Epub 2003 Feb 27. https://doi.org/10.1007/s00268-002-6654-4.

Lafaro K, Blakely AM, Melstrom LG, et al. Prognostic impact of tumor location in resected gallbladder cancer: a national cohort analysis. J Surg Oncol. 2020; https://doi.org/10.1002/jso.26107.

Lee W, Jeong CY, Kim YH, et al. Validation of the prognostic performance in various nodal staging systems for gallbladder cancer: results of a multicenter study. Langenbecks Arch Surg. 2019;404(5):581–8. https://doi.org/10.1007/s00423-019-01807-9.

Lee EC, Park SJ, Lee SD, Han SS, Kim SH. Effects of sarcopenia on prognosis after resection of gallbladder cancer. J Gastrointest Surg. 2020;24(5):1082–91. https://doi.org/10.1007/s11605-019-04198-w.

Lim H, Seo DW, Park DH, Lee SS, Lee SK, Kim MH, Hwang S. Prognostic factors in patients with gallbladder cancer after surgical resection: analysis of 279 operated patients. J Clin Gastroenterol. 2013;47(5):443–8. https://doi.org/10.1097/MCG.0b013e3182703409.

Lin JY, Bai DS, Zhou BH, Chen P, Qian JJ, Jin SJ, Jiang GQ. Positive relationship between number of negative lymph nodes and duration of gallbladder cancer cause-specific survival after surgery. Cancer Manag Res. 2018;10:6961–9. https://doi.org/10.2147/CMAR.S187857. eCollection 2018

Lindnér P, Holmberg E, Hafström L. Gallbladder cancer - no improvement in survival over time in a Swedish population. Acta Oncol. 2018;57(11):1482–9. https://doi.org/10.1080/0284186X.2018.1478124. Epub 2018 Jun 22

Liu F, Hu HJ, Ma WJ, Yang Q, Wang JK, Li FY. Prognostic significance of neutrophil-lymphocyte ratio and carbohydrate antigen 19-9 in patients with gallbladder carcinoma. Medicine (Baltimore). 2019a;98(8):e14550. https://doi.org/10.1097/MD.0000000000014550. PMID: 30813165; PMCID: PMC6407978.

Liu F, Wang JK, Ma WJ, Yang Q, Hu HJ, Li FY. Clinical value of preoperative CA19-9 levels in evaluating resectability of gallbladder carcinoma. ANZ J Surg. 2019b;89(3):E76–80. https://doi.org/10.1111/ans.14893. Epub 2018 Oct 10

Lopez-Aguiar AG, Ethun CG, McInnis MR, Pawlik TM, Poultsides G, Tran T, Idrees K, Isom CA, Fields RC, Krasnick BA, Weber SM, Salem A, Martin RCG, Scoggins CR, Shen P, Mogal HD, Schmidt C, Beal EW, Hatzaras I, Shenoy R, Cardona K, Maithel SK. Association of perioperative transfusion with survival and recurrence after resection of gallbladder cancer: a 10-institution study from the US Extrahepatic Biliary Malignancy Consortium. J Surg Oncol. 2018;117(8):1638–47. https://doi.org/10.1002/jso.25086. Epub 2018 May 14

Margonis GA, Gani F, Buettner S, et al. Rates and patterns of recurrence after curative intent resection for gallbladder cancer: a multi-institution analysis from the US extra-hepatic biliary malignancy consortium. HPB (Oxford). 2016;18:872–8. https://doi.org/10.1016/j.hpb.2016.05.016. Epub 2016 Aug 13

Melillo A, Linden K, Spitz F, Atabek U, Gaughan J, Hong YK. Disparities in treatment for gallbladder carcinoma: does treatment site matter? J Gastrointest Surg. 2020;24(5):1071–6. https://doi.org/10.1007/s11605-019-04389-5.

Mishra PK, Saluja SS, Prithiviraj N, Varshney V, Goel N, Patil N. Predictors of curative resection and long term survival of gallbladder cancer - a retrospective analysis. Am J Surg. 2017;214(2):278–86. https://doi.org/10.1016/j.amjsurg.2017.02.006. Epub 2017 Feb 9

Miyakawa S, Ishihara S, Horiguchi A, Takada T, Miyazaki M, Nagakawa T. Biliary tract cancer treatment: 5,584 results from the Biliary Tract Cancer Statistics Registry from 1998 to 2004 in Japan. J Hepatobiliary Pancreat Surg. 2009;16(1):1–7. https://doi.org/10.1007/s00534-008-0015-0. Epub 2008 Dec 26

Miyazaki M, Shimizu H, Yoshitomi H, Kato A, Furukawa K, Takayashiki T, Kuboki S, Takano S, Ohtsuka M. Clinical implication of surgical resection for recurrent biliary tract cancer: does it work or not? Ann Gastroenterol Surg. 2017;1(3):164–70. https://doi.org/10.1002/ags3.12036. eCollection 2017 Sep. Review

Mochizuki T, Abe T, Amano H, Hanada K, Hattori M, Kobayashi T, Nakahara M, Ohdan H, Noriyuki T. Efficacy of the gallbladder cancer predictive risk score based on pathological findings: a propensity score-matched analysis. Ann Surg Oncol. 2018;25(6):1699–708. https://doi.org/10.1245/s10434-018-6444-3. Epub 2018 Apr 6

Negi SS, Singh A, Chaudhary A. Lymph nodal involvement as prognostic factor in gallbladder cancer: location, count or ratio? J Gastrointest Surg. 2011;15(6):1017–25. https://doi.org/10.1007/s11605-011-1528-4. Epub 2011 Apr 13.

Nishio H, Nagino M, Ebata T, Yokoyama Y, Igami T, Nimura Y. Aggressive surgery for stage IV gallbladder carcinoma; what are the contraindications? J Hepatobiliary Pancreat Surg. 2007;14(4):351–7. Epub 2007 Jul 30. https://doi.org/10.1007/s00534-006-1187-0.

Noji T, Tsuchikawa T, Mizota T, Okamura K, Nakamura T, Tamoto E, Shichinohe T, Hirano S. Surgery for recurrent biliary carcinoma: results for 27 recurrent cases. World J Surg Oncol. 2015;13:82. https://doi.org/10.1186/s12957-015-0507-8.

Roa I, Ibacache G, Muñoz S, de Aretxabala X. Gallbladder cancer in Chile: pathologic characteristics of survival and prognostic factors: analysis of 1,366 cases. Am J Clin Pathol. 2014;141(5):675–82. https://doi.org/10.1309/AJCPQT3ELN2BBCKA.

Sahara K, Tsilimigras DI, Maithel SK, et al. Survival benefit of lymphadenectomy for gallbladder cancer based on the therapeutic index: an analysis of the US Extrahepatic Biliary Malignancy Consortium. J Surg Oncol. 2020;121(3):503–10. https://doi.org/10.1002/jso.25825.

Sakata J, Kobayashi T, Ohashi T, Hirose Y, Takano K, Takizawa K, Miura K, Ishikawa H, Toge K, Yuza K, Soma D, Ando T, Wakai T. Prognostic heterogeneity of the seventh edition of UICC Stage III gallbladder carcinoma: which patients benefit from surgical resection? Eur J Surg Oncol. 2017;43(4):780–7. https://doi.org/10.1016/j.ejso.2017.01.001. Epub 2017 Jan 19

Salati M, Caputo F, Cunningham D, Marcheselli L, Spallanzani A, Rimini M, Gelsomino F, Reggiani-Bonetti L, Andrikou K, Rovinelli F, Smyth E, Baratelli C, Kouvelakis K, Kalaitzaki R, Gillbanks A, Michalarea V, Cascinu S, Braconi C. The A.L.A.N. score identifies prognostic classes in advanced biliary cancer patients receiving first-line chemotherapy. Eur J Cancer. 2019;117:84–90. https://doi.org/10.1016/j.ejca.2019.05.030. Epub 2019 Jul 2

Shirai Y, Sakata J, Wakai T, Ohashi T, Ajioka Y, Hatakeyama K. Assessment of lymph node status in gallbladder cancer: location, number, or ratio of positive nodes. World J Surg Oncol. 2012;10:87. https://doi.org/10.1186/1477-7819-10-87.

Sung YN, Song M, Lee JH, et al. Validation of the 8th Edition of the American Joint Committee on Cancer Staging System for Gallbladder Cancer and implications for the follow-up of patients without node dissection. Cancer Res Treat. 2020;52(2):455–68. https://doi.org/10.4143/crt.2019.271.

Takahashi Y, Ebata T, Yokoyama Y, Igami T, Sugawara G, Mizuno T, Nimura Y, Nagino M. Surgery for recurrent biliary tract cancer: a single-center experience with 74 consecutive resections. Ann Surg. 2015;262(1):121–9. https://doi.org/10.1097/SLA.0000000000000827.

Todoroki T, Kawamoto T, Otsuka M, Koike N, Yoshida S, Takada Y, Adachi S, Kashiwagi H, Fukao K, Ohara K. Benefits of combining radiotherapy with aggressive resection for stage IV gallbladder cancer. Hepatogastroenterology. 1999a;46(27):1585–91.

Todoroki T, Kawamoto T, Takahashi H, Takada Y, Koike N, Otsuka M, Fukao K. Treatment of gallbladder cancer by radical resection. Br J Surg. 1999b;86(5):622–7. https://doi.org/10.1046/j.1365-2168.1999.01085.x.

Tran Cao HS, Zhang Q, Sada YH, Chai C, Curley SA, Massarweh NN. The role of surgery and adjuvant therapy in lymph node-positive cancers of the gallbladder and intrahepatic bile ducts. Cancer. 2018;124(1):74–83. https://doi.org/10.1002/cncr.30968. Epub 2017 Aug 25

Tran TB, Nissen NN. Surgery for gallbladder cancer in the US: a need for greater lymph node clearance. J Gastrointest Oncol. 2015;6(5):452–8. https://doi.org/10.3978/j.issn.2078-6891.2015.062.

Tran TB, Norton JA, Ethun CG, Pawlik TM, Buettner S, Schmidt C, Beal EW, Hawkins WG, Fields RC, Krasnick BA, Weber SM, Salem A, Martin RCG, Scoggins CR, Shen P, Mogal HD, Idrees K, Isom CA, Hatzaras I, Shenoy R, Maithel SK, Poultsides GA. Gallbladder cancer presenting with jaundice: uniformly fatal or still potentially curable? J Gastrointest Surg. 2017;21(8):1245–53. https://doi.org/10.1007/s11605-017-3440-z. Epub 2017 May 11

Wu WY, Zhang HH, Xiong JP, Yang XB, Bai Y, Lin JZ, Long JY, Zheng YC, Zhao HT, Sang XT. Prognostic significance of the fibrinogen-to-albumin ratio in gallbladder cancer patients. World J Gastroenterol. 2018;24(29):3281–92. https://doi.org/10.3748/wjg.v24.i29.3281.

Yadav S, Tella SH, Kommalapati A, et al. A novel clinically based staging system for gallbladder cancer. J Natl Compr Cancer Netw. 2020;18(2):151–9. https://doi.org/10.6004/jnccn.2019.7357.

Yuan B, Fu J, Yu WL, Fu XH, Qiu YH, Yin L, Zhu B, Zhang YJ. Prognostic value of serum high-density lipoprotein cholesterol in patients with gallbladder cancer. Rev Esp Enferm Dig. 2019;111(11):839–84. https://doi.org/10.17235/reed.2019.6201/2019.

Yuza K, Sakata J, Prasoon P, et al. Long-term outcomes of surgical resection for T1b gallbladder cancer: an institutional evaluation. BMC Cancer. 2020;20(1):20. https://doi.org/10.1186/s12885-019-6507-2.

Zhang L, Hou C, Xu Z, Wang L, Ling X, Xiu D. Laparoscopic treatment for suspected gallbladder cancer confined to the wall: a 10-year study from a single institution. Chin J Cancer Res. 2018;30(1):84–92. https://doi.org/10.21147/j.issn.1000-9604.2018.01.09.

Zheng P, Wang X, Hong Z, Shen F, Zhang Q. Preoperative fasting hyperglycemia is an independent prognostic factor for postoperative survival after gallbladder carcinoma radical surgery. Cancer Manag Res. 2019;11:1425–32. https://doi.org/10.2147/CMAR.S192273. eCollection 2019.

Zhu S, Yang J, Cui X, Zhao Y, Tao Z, Xia F, Chen L, Huang J, Ma X. Preoperative platelet-to-lymphocyte ratio and neutrophil-to-lymphocyte ratio as predictors of clinical outcome in patients with gallbladder cancer. Sci Rep. 2019;9(1):1823. https://doi.org/10.1038/s41598-018-38396-4.

References for Commentary Notes

Kato A, Shimizu H, Ohtsuka M, et al. Downsizing chemotherapy for initially unresectable locally advanced biliary tract cancer patients treated with gemcitabine plus cisplatin combination therapy followed by radical surgery. Ann Surg Oncol. 2015;22(Suppl 3):S1093–9.

Manterola C, Duque G, Grande L, et al. A systematic review of the effectiveness of adjuvant therapy for patients with gallbladder cancer. HPB (Oxford). 2019;21(11):1427–35.

Nakachi K, Konishi M, Ikeda M, et al. A randomized Phase III trial of adjuvant S-1 therapy vs. observation alone in resected biliary tract cancer: Japan Clinical Oncology Group Study (JCOG1202, ASCOT). Jpn J Clin Oncol. 2018;48:392–5.

Primrose JN, Fox RP, Palmer DH, et al. Capecitabine compared with observation in resected biliary tract cancer (BILCAP): a randomised, controlled, multicentre, phase 3 study. Lancet Oncol. 2019;20:663–73.

Stein A, Arnold D, Bridgewater J, et al. Adjuvant chemotherapy with gemcitabine and cisplatin compared to observation after curative intent resection of cholangiocarcinoma and muscle invasive gallbladder carcinoma (ACTICCA-1 trial) - a randomized, multidisciplinary, multinational phase III trial. BMC Cancer. 2015;15:564.

Yoshitomi H, Miyakawa S, Nagino M, et al. Updated clinical practice guidelines for the management of biliary tract cancers: revision concepts and major revised points. J Hepatobiliary Pancreat Sci. 2015;22:274–8.

16 Prevention of Gall Bladder Cancer

Vinay K. Kapoor

Most patients with gall bladder cancer (GBC) present with advanced unresectable disease as early GBC is elusive (Kapoor et al. 1996). Overall outcome is poor and survival is short. GBC is more common in certain geographical areas and some ethnic groups. Prevention, therefore, becomes important, especially in high incidence areas and populations. Primary prevention is not an option as the etiology of GBC cf. tobacco for lung cancer, viral hepatitis B and C for hepatocellular carcinoma (HCC), is not known. The next best option is secondary prevention, i.e., preventive cholecystectomy for asymptomatic GS.

16.1 Asymptomatic GS

Innocent GS is a myth (William Mayo et al. 1911).

The symptom of gall stones (GS) is biliary colic—dull steady continuous constant (not colicky) pain in the right hypochondrium or epigastrium lasting for more than 1 h, which is sometimes provoked by a heavy or fatty meal and which may radiate to the right shoulder. Asymptomatic GS are detected incidentally on US (Fig. 16.1) (or any other imaging) done for a non-GI, e.g., gynecological or urological indication or in presence of vague atypical non-biliary abdominal symptoms, e.g., dyspepsia (but no biliary colic), indigestion, bloating, etc. or during pregnancy or as a part of a routine health checkup. Asymptomatic GS are very common; in a review of 9332 postmortems, only 14% of those with GS had had a cholecystectomy, indicating that the remaining 86% were probably asymptomatic (Khan 2004). Cholecystectomy may be performed for asymptomatic GS for two rea-

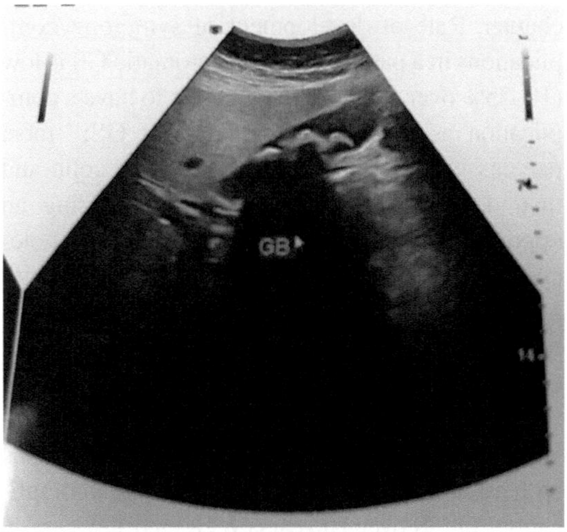

Fig. 16.1 US shows multiple gall stones (GS) in a distended gall bladder—GS are the most important risk factor for gall bladder cancer; more and more asymptomatic GS are being detected with the increasing use of US

Please also see an Invited Commentary on Prevention of Gall Bladder Cancer by Nicolas Jarufe (pp **–**)

V. K. Kapoor (✉)
Department of Surgical Gastroenterology, Sanjay Gandhi Post-Graduate Institute of Medical Sciences (SGPGIMS), Lucknow, Uttar Pradesh, India
e-mail: vkkapoor.india@gmail.com

V. K. Kapoor (ed.), *A Pictorial Treatise on Gall Bladder Cancer*,
https://doi.org/10.1007/978-981-15-5289-2_16

sons—one to avoid future symptoms and complications of GS, e.g., acute cholecystitis, common bile duct (CBD) stone, acute cholangitis, acute pancreatitis, and second to prevent GBC in the future. We Behari and Kapoor 2012 introduced the terms "prophylactic" for cholecystectomy done for asymptomatic GS to avoid future symptoms/complications and "preventive" for cholecystectomy done for asymptomatic GS to prevent GBC in the future. Concomitant (incidental) cholecystectomy is cholecystectomy done for asymptomatic GS during laparotomy/laparoscopy for some other indication. Asymptomatic GS were present in 284 patients with CRC who were operated in Korea (2004–2011), 143 underwent cholecystectomy—bile duct injury (BDI) occurred in 1 (0.7%); remaining 139 were followed for 33 months—8 required cholecystectomy for biliary complications during the follow up (Lee et al. 2015).

16.2 Prophylactic Cholecystectomy

"Prophylactic" cholecystectomy is cholecystectomy done for asymptomatic GS to avoid future symptoms/complications. "Prophylactic" cholecystectomy is not the topic for discussion in this chapter. Rate of development of symptoms/complications in a patient with asymptomatic GS is low (10–25% over 5–15 years). It is rare to have a complication as the first presentation of GS; most patients will present first with a biliary colic and then develop a complication thus providing an opportunity for an elective intervention (i.e., cholecystectomy) for the GS. Only 18% of persons with asymptomatic GS developed biliary pain over a period of 20 years (Lowenfels et al. 1985). Annual complication rate in presence of asymptomatic GS was 0.3–1.2% (GREPCO 1984). Theoretical calculations revealed that only 15 out of 10,000 persons with asymptomatic GS will die because of complications of GS over 10 years (WGO n.d.).

Some of the indications for prophylactic cholecystectomy in a person with asymptomatic GS are

1. Patients undergoing solid organ transplantation—GS are likely to become symptomatic in organ transplant recipients within 2 years of the transplant; complications of GS are more difficult to diagnose in these patients because of immunosuppression.
2. Chronic hemolytic syndromes, e.g., sickle cell disease (SCD)—symptoms of GS may be difficult to differentiate from those of a vaso-occlusive crisis.
3. Diabetes—elderly diabetics are at a higher risk to die from complications of GS.

16.3 Preventive Cholecystectomy

"Preventive" cholecystectomy is cholecystectomy done for asymptomatic GS to prevent GBC in the future. Cholecystectomy for asymptomatic GS will prevent GBC in 100% of cases as the target organ itself is removed. An inverse relationship between cholecystectomy rates and incidence of GBC has been observed. Risk of development of GBC in persons with asymptomatic GS is, however, low. Europe has high prevalence (10% of all adults) of GS (2–3 times more in women versus men; more with increasing age; about 30% in women above 65 years), but incidence rates of GBC are low. Risk of development of cancer was low—0.3% over 30 years, 0.25% for women, and 0.12% for men. Only 1 GBC was seen in 118 persons with asymptomatic GS followed for 10 years in the Group for Epidemiology and Prevention of Cholelithiasis (GREPCO 1984). Only five GBCs were seen in 2583 persons with asymptomatic GS over a follow-up for 13.3 years (Maringhini et al. 1987). When 1000 persons with asymptomatic GS were followed up for 7000 patient-years, none developed GBC (Ransohoff and Gracie 1993). No GBC occurred in 580 persons with asymptomatic GS over 9 years (Festi et al. 2010).

The duration of follow-up in these studies is not very long; these results cannot, therefore, be applied to young patients with asymptomatic GS. These data are from low GBC incidence areas/populations. Risk of GBC in asymptomatic GS in high GBC incidence areas is not known. There is a need to study the natural history (vis-à-vis the risk of GBC) of asymptomatic GS in high GBC incidence areas, such as north India. Risk of GBC in patients with asymptomatic GS varies from one population to other—in a case control study of 139 GBC and 2399 patients with GS, 20-year cumulative risk of GBC was 1.5% in American Indian women versus only 0.1% in Black women (Lowenfels et al. 1985).Cholecystectomy was performed in 150 patients with asymptomatic GS in eastern India, histopathology revealed adenocarcinoma in 1, carcinoma in situ in 1, and metaplasia in 24 (Ibrarullah et al. 2018). Similar findings have been reported from Chile (Csendes et al. 1998).

Secondary prevention of GBC, in the form of preventive cholecystectomy is, however, an invasive, expensive, and risky option. One has to weigh the risks of operation which increases with increasing age and comorbidities versus the benefits in terms of prevention of GBC. Death from the complications of the operation is real and immediate versus the risk of GBC which is hypothetical and occurs later (after several years). Laparoscopic cholecystectomy carries a small but definite risk of BDI which is around 0.5% (1 in 200). Other complications of cholecystectomy include post-cholecystectomy duodenogastric reflux, bile-induced diarrhea, and incisional hernia. In the long term, there is a slightly increased risk of right colon cancer after cholecystectomy. Incidence rate ratio of colorectal cancer (CRC) in 55,960 persons who underwent cholecystectomy was 1.3 (1.2–1.5) as compared to 574,668 who did not have a cholecystectomy (Shao and Yang 2005). Hazard ratio (HR) of CRC in 5850 persons who underwent cholecystectomy versus 62,180 without GS was 1.6 (Chen et al. 2014).

According to a Cochrane Database Systemic Review, there is no evidence to either recommend or refuse surgery for asymptomatic GS (Gurusamy and Samraj 2007). Preventive cholecystectomy is not recommended as a routine for anyone and everyone with asymptomatic GS. Those who are at the highest risk to develop GBC need to be identified and "preemptive" cholecystectomy offered to them. But unlike in other cancers, e.g., alfa-fetoprotein (AFP) for cirrhotics to detect early HCC or endoscopy to detect early colorectal cancer (CRC) in inflammatory bowel disease (IBD), there are no surveillance options to detect early GBC in patients with asymptomatic GS. In the absence of strong data and good quality evidence, it has to be a highly subjective decision of the patient and the physician together, based on the evaluation and assessment of the anticipated risks, expected benefits, and personal choices. Selective preventive cholecystectomy *MAY* be considered in a young patient with a large stone (Fig. 16.2) or a GB packed with stones (Fig. 16.3) (Kapoor 2006),

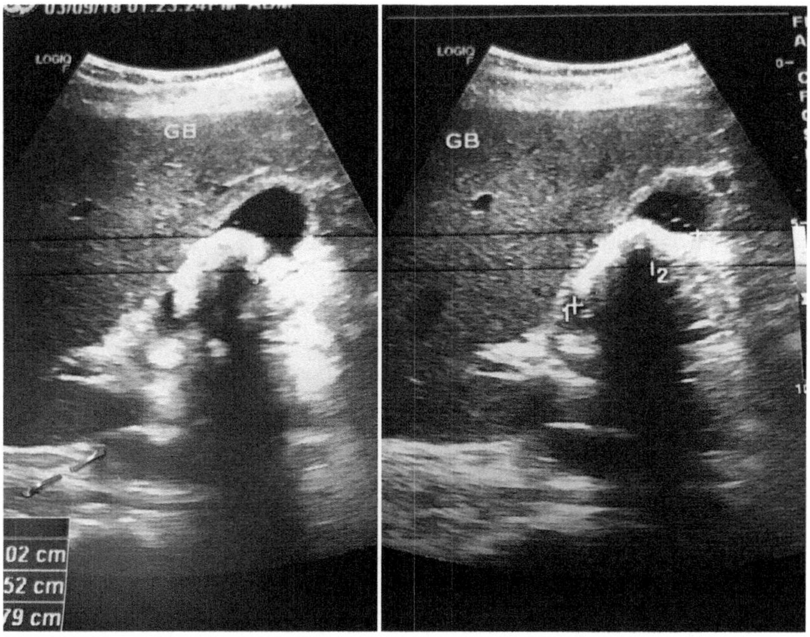

Fig. 16.2 US shows a large (4 cm) gall stone (GS); large (>3 cm) gall stones carry a higher risk of gall bladder cancer

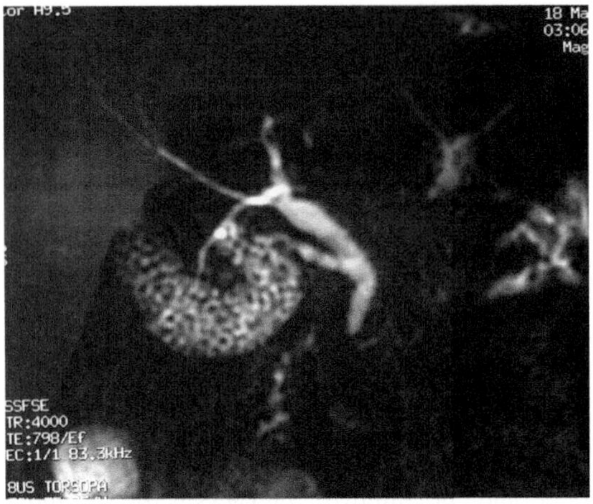

Fig. 16.3 MRC shows a gall bladder (GB) packed with gall stones (GS)—high GS/GB volume ratio carries a higher risk of gall bladder cancer

more so in a nonfunctioning GB (Dutta et al. 2005) in a high incidence geographical area or ethnic group. WGO Practice Guidelines recommend preventive cholecystectomy in patients with asymptomatic GS living in high-risk areas such as Chile and Bolivia. Lowenfels et al. (1985) calculated that while 769 cholecystectomies will be required to prevent one GBC in low-risk population, only 67 cholecystectomies will prevent one GBC in high-risk population. In Chile, under the public health care system program of explicit health guarantee (EHG) started in 2006 (minsal.cl/portal), universal ultrasound (US) screening is advised for all women in the age group of 40–49 years—prophylactic (preventive) cholecystectomy is then recommended in patients with even asymptomatic GS (Roa and de Aretxabala 2015). This program has been extended to men and women in the age group of 35–49 years with at least one risk factor, e.g., Mapuche surname, obesity, low socioeconomic status (SES), multiparity, etc. The cost-effectiveness of this program is, however, questionable (Salazar et al. 2019). There is a need to identify a biomarker which can identify those amongst asymptomatic GS having the highest risk of developing GBC so that "preemptive" cholecystectomy can be offered to them (Kapoor 2006).

In some situations, patients with even asymptomatic GS should be operated because of an increased risk of GBC. Thick-walled GB (Fig. 16.4) on US is usually benign, i.e., chronic cholecystitis (CC) or xantho-granulomatous cholecystitis (XGC) but is more likely to harbor an incidental GBC than a normal thickness GB; cholecystectomy should be advised for all thick-walled GBs. We have described anticipatory extended cholecystectomy (AEC) for diffuse TWGBs with a low suspicion of cancer - the GB is removed with a small wedge of liver and subjected to frozen section histopathological examination (Kapoor et al. 2016) (see Chap. 13). Porcelain GB (Fig. 16.5) also carries a higher risk of GBC. Machado (2016) after reviewing the published literature on porcelain GB, recommended selective preventive cholecystectomy and warned that nonoperative approach may

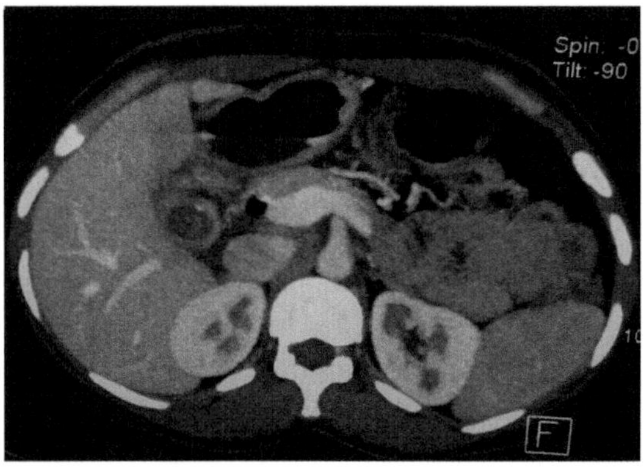

Fig. 16.4 CT shows a diffuse thick walled gall bladder (TWGB)—a TWGB is more likely to have a gall bladder cancer; all TWGBs should be operated

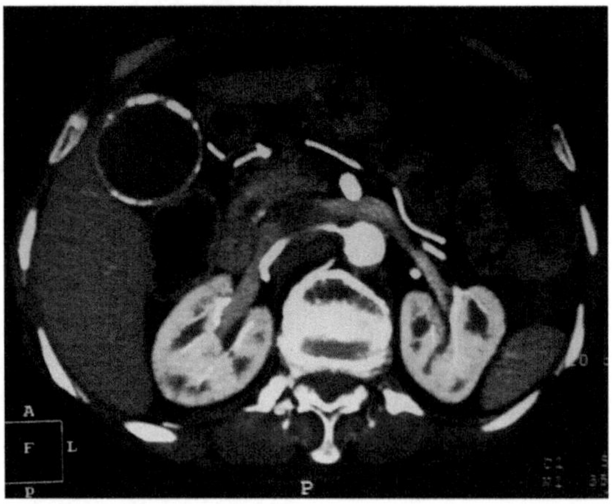

Fig. 16.5 CT shows calcified gall bladder (GB) wall (porcelain GB)—porcelain GB carries a higher risk of gall bladder cancer; all porcelain GBs should be operated

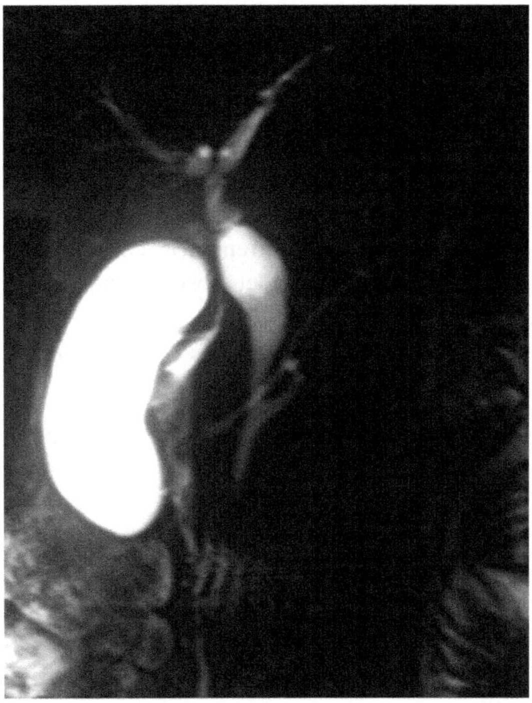

Fig. 16.6 MRCP shows a long common channel of the common bile duct and the pancreatic duct, i.e., anomalous pancreaticobiliary ductal union (APBDU)—APBDU is associated with a higher risk of biliary tract cancer, including gall bladder cancer; APBDU is an indication for a preventive cholecystectomy

require prolonged (even lifelong) follow-up. Anomalous pancreaticobiliary ductal union (APBDU) (Fig. 16.6) without cystic dilatation of the CBD and single large sessile polyp (Fig. 16.7), especially in a high-risk person, are other indications for preventive cholecystectomy.

16.4 Tertiary Prevention

Tertiary prevention is in the form of early diagnosis of GBC. There is no serum-based marker, e.g., PSA for prostate, which can be used for screening of the population, at least in high incidence areas. US is a universally available, easy, noninvasive, not too expensive screening tool but the yield (in terms of no. detected/no. screened) is very low and whatever cancers are detected on US are not early but advanced (T2 or beyond). Three out of four GBCs detected on annual US screening of population in Niigata, Japan were in advanced stages (Ogoshi et al. 1999). GB is not easily amenable to endoscopic inspection cf. esophagus, stomach, and colorectum, where endoscopic screening of high-risk population may help in early diagnosis.

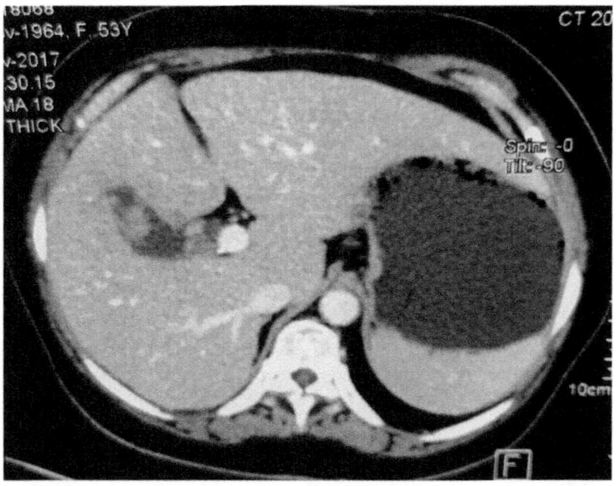

Fig. 16.7 CT shows a gall bladder (GB) polyp—GB polyps may be neoplastic; all GB polyps detected on US need further evaluation with Doppler, EUS, CT, MRI, etc.

16.5 Quaternary Prevention

Quaternary prevention is detection of GBC in a GB removed with a presumed preoperative diagnosis of symptomatic GS. All GBs removed with a presumed diagnosis of GS should be opened (Fig. 16.8) by the surgeon in the operation room (OR) itself, washed with running tap water (Fig. 16.9), and examined for a suspicious area, e.g., wall thickening, nodule, plaque, or ulcer which should be marked with an identifying suture and subjected to frozen section histopathological examination. There are several reports (Corten et al. 2019b) which recommend that a macroscopically normal-looking GB may not be subjected to histopathological examination to reduce the workload of the pathologists and to save costs but most of these reports are from low GBC incidence areas. We have sounded a strong note of caution in accepting these recommendations, especially in high GBC incidence areas, as this (i.e. routine histopathological examination of ALL GB specimens) is the only way to diagnose early GBC. Most early GBCs are detected as an incidental finding on histopathological examina-

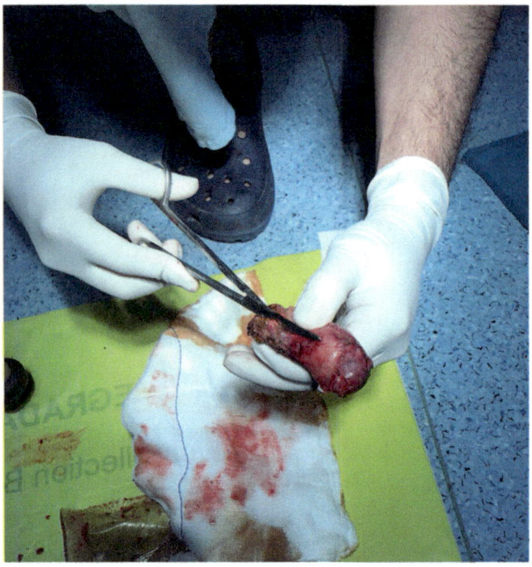

Fig. 16.8 All gall bladders removed for gall stones should be opened by the surgeon in the operation room itself and examined carefully for any suspicious lesion which if found should be subjected to frozen section histopathological examination

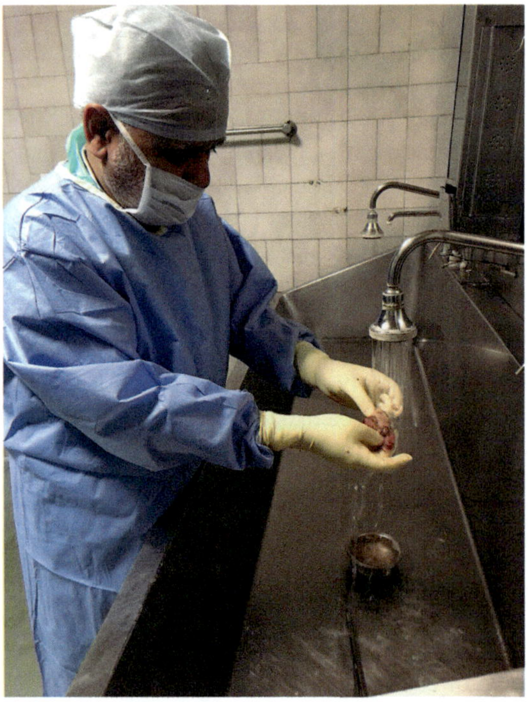

Fig. 16.9 The Author (VKK) washing an opened gall bladder removed for gall stones—the mucosal surface of all gall bladders removed for gall stones should be washed in running water and examined carefully for any suspicious lesion which if found should be subjected to frozen section histopathological examination

tion of the GB removed with a presumed diagnosis of GS (Behari and Kapoor 2012). They need reoperation for completion extended cholecystectomy (CEC) which carries a high possibility for cure. If all GBs are not subjected to histopathological examination as a routine, an early GBC may be missed and the patient may present a few months later with a recurrent GBC causing jaundice and/or gastric outlet obstruction—missed GBC (Sharma et al. 2008).

An early GBC missed is a life lost (that too in a few months' time)!

In the vast desert of gallstone disease, prevention of GBC remains elusive like a mirage!

Invited Commentary on Prevention of Gallbladder Cancer

Nicolas Jarufe

This chapter deals with the prevention of gallbladder cancer (GBC) in a very detailed way by delivering arguments based on the literature that support the ideas raised. The emphasis is on preventive cholecystectomy for asymptomatic gallbladder stones (GS) to avoid cancer formation.

Multiple risk factors have been associated with GBC; cholelithiasis, age, obesity, multiparity, female sex, postmenopausal status and estrogen use, gallbladder wall calcification (porcelain gallbladder), adenomatous polyps, genetic factors (race/ethnic group), diets rich in fats and carbohydrates, tobacco, low socioeconomic status, exposure to carcinogens and chronic inflammation of the biliary system, either by chronic infection (*Opisthorchis viverrini*, *Salmonella typhi*, and *paratyphi*), by drugs (isoniazid, methyldopa) or congenital anomalies (choledochal cysts, congenital bile duct dilation, anomalous pancreatobiliary junction or primary sclerosing cholangitis) among others. However, cholelithiasis corresponds to the main associated factor, giving a risk four to seven times greater. More than 95% of patients with GBC in Chile have associated cholelithiasis, representing the most important risk factor for this disease. In Chile, for example, 98% of those with GBC have cholelithiasis, generally associated with a single and large calculus. The female sex has a 3:1 ratio increasing with age with a maximum incidence between the sixth and seventh decade of life. The vast majority of gallbladder polyps correspond to cholesterol, inflammatory or hyperplastic pseudopolyps, with no malignant potential. However, adenomatous polyps, mainly those greater than 1 cm (risk of 45–67% in 10–15 mm polyps), solitary and sessile, risk that increases if other have a risk of progressing to cancer, a risk factors are present.

In order to reduce the death rate from GBC in Chile, a public health program was created where gallbladder surgery is guaranteed to all people with stones between the ages of 35 and 49 since 2006 (described in the Kapoor chapter). Some papers have been published where changes in incidence and mortality have been demonstrated, especially in women. Mortality rates in women in 2006 were 25 per 100,000 population decreasing to 20/100,000 in 2012. In both sexes, it dropped from 10 to 8/100,000 in the same period. Therefore, in high incidence countries such as Chile, there is no such discussion, and GS are always operated independently of the symptoms or their size.

With regard to early diagnosis (tertiary prevention), as described by Kapoor, there is no blood marker with reliable sensitivity for GBC. Abdominal ultrasound is a very good method to discover gallstones, however, for cancer it is of low sensitivity apart from advanced cases.

Only 25% of the GBC are diagnosed before or during surgery, the remaining 75% is detected during the pathological analysis of the cholecystectomy specimen. In the macroscopic analysis done by the pathologist, 33.1% of advanced cancers and 70% of incipient cancers are not apparent, due to the predominance of flat lesions and many times also masked by exacerbated chronic inflammatory processes that may be present in up to 41% of surgical specimens with GBC. This fact raises the need for the appropriate systematic sampling of routine cholecystectomy specimens in order to rule out an invisible (incidental) GBC. In our experience, the macroscopic analysis after fixation in buffered formalin extended on a paraffin plate for a period of at least 12 h, sampling a randomized central entire longitudinal section that includes all segments viz. fundus, body and neck of the GB allows the detection of 100% of preneoplastic and neoplastic lesions. Once a preneoplastic or neoplastic lesion is diagnosed, the total mapping of the gallbladder should be carried out in order to ensure that the maximum infiltration of the wall is correctly recorded. In this process, the correct identification of the cystic duct edge (margin), and serous (peritoneal) and hepatic side of the gallbladder are paramount since it has been established that when subserous tumors (pT2) totally or partially compromise the hepatic side of the GB (without compromising the surgical edge), they have a worse prognosis than when it is confined to the serous (peritoneal) side of the GB (Shindoh et al. 2014).

The muscular tunic is irregular and discontinuous, not acting as a real containment barrier for tumor infiltration into deeper layers, facilitating pseudodiverticular mucosal evagination through these areas of least resistance that can reach even the subserosa, these are produced due to increased intracavitary pressure related to the presence of GS and they are known as Rokistanky–Aschoff sinuses (RAS), with similar characteristics to what occurs in diverticulosis of the large intestine secondary to constipation. The intraepithelial extension of the neoplastic surface lesion in the RAS, which can be found in up to 17.8% of cases with incipient (pT1a and pT1b) carcinomas, without showing clear infiltration beyond the glandular epithelial basement membrane, is not considered by the TNM classification to define a higher T. Despite this, recent publications have shown that patients with incipient (pT1a and pT1b) tumors (pT1a and pT1b) with extension of the epithelial lesion in the RAS have a significantly lower survival. The incipient carcinoma is a disease of good prognosis even with simple cholecystectomy, with actuarial survival of 92.3% and 90.4% at 5 and 10 years, respectively. Patients with pT1a and pT1b with lesions that extend to the RAS behave like subserous tumors (pT2) with a survival of close to 60% and 50%, respectively. When the cases with extension to the RAS are eliminated from the analysis, the 10-year survival rises to 100% in intramucosal

(T1a) cancers and 93% to intramuscular (T1b) cancers (Roa et al. 2013). These figures raise the need to evaluate a second surgery in patients with intramucosal tumors (pT1a) that present extension of the lesions in the RAS. Given the current evidence, it is reasonable to recommend the directed study of the RAS involvement when reassessing an incidental GBC, particularly in those patients with T1a lesions.

As a final comment, like Kapoor describes in the chapter, given the poor prognosis of GBC, prevention plays an important role. This should be oriented to the investigation of cholelithiasis, especially in people at risk as described in the text. Preventive cholecystectomy is of low morbidity and should be indicated in all patients with cholelithiasis even if it is asymptomatic since the vast majority of GBC are associated with GS. Once the gallbladder is removed, a detailed pathological examination that includes the involvement of RAS is essential in order to take the best therapeutic option.

References

Chapter References

Behari A, Kapoor VK. Asymptomatic gallstones (AsGS) - to treat or not to? Indian J Surg. 2012;74(1):4–12. https://doi.org/10.1007/s12262-011-0376-5. Epub 2011 Dec 3.

Chen YK, Yeh JH, Lin CL, Peng CL, Sung FC, Hwang IM, Kao CH. Cancer risk in patients with cholelithiasis and after cholecystectomy: a nationwide cohort study. J Gastroenterol. 2014;49(5):923–31. https://doi.org/10.1007/s00535-013-0846-6. Epub 2013 Jun 28

Corten BJGA, Leclercq WKG, Dejong CH, Roumen RMH, Slooter GD. Selective histological examination after cholecystectomy: an analysis of current daily practice in The Netherlands. World J Surg. 2019b; https://doi.org/10.1007/s00268-019-05077-w.

Csendes A, Smok G, Burdiles P, Díaz JC, Maluenda F, Korn O. Histological findings of gallbladder mucosa in 95 control subjects and 80 patients with asymptomatic gallstones. Dig Dis Sci. 1998;43(5):931–4.

Dutta U, Nagi B, Garg PK, Sinha SK, Singh K, Tandon RK. Patients with gallstones develop gallbladder cancer at an earlier age. Eur J Cancer Prev. 2005;14(4):381–5.

Festi D, Reggiani ML, Attili AF, Loria P, Pazzi P, Scaioli E, Capodicasa S, Romano F, Roda E, Colecchia A. Natural history of gallstone disease: expectant management or active treatment? Results from a population-based cohort study. J Gastroenterol Hepatol. 2010;25(4):719–24. https://doi.org/10.1111/j.1440-1746.2009.06146.x.

GREPCO. Prevalence of gallstone disease in an Italian adult female population. Rome Group for the Epidemiology and Prevention of Cholelithiasis (GREPCO). Am J Epidemiol. 1984;119(5):796–805.

Gurusamy KS, Samraj K. Cholecystectomy versus no cholecystectomy in patients with silent gallstones. Cochrane Database Syst Rev 2007;(1):CD006230. Review.

Ibrarullah M, Baisakh MR, Dash AP, Mohapatra A, Sahoo SK, Agarwal A. Cholecystectomy for asymptomatic gallstones: clinicopathological study. Trop Gastroenterol. 2018;39(2):62–7.

Kapoor VK. Cholecystectomy in patients with asymptomatic gallstones to prevent gall bladder cancer—the case against. Indian J Gastroenterol. 2006;25(3):152–4.

Kapoor VK, Pradeep R, Haribhakti SP, Sikora SS, Kaushik SP. Early carcinoma of the gallbladder: an elusive disease. J Surg Oncol. 1996;62(4):284–7.

Kapoor VK, Singh R, Behari A, Sharma S, Kumar A, Prakash A, Singh RK, Kumar A, Saxena R. Anticipatory extended cholecystectomy: the 'Lucknow' approach for thick walled gall bladder with low suspicion of cancer. Chin Clin Oncol. 2016;5(1):8. https://doi.org/10.3978/j.issn.2304-3865.2016.02.07.

Khan HN. Re: Asymptomatic gallstones in the laparoscopic era. JR Coll Surg Edin 2002; 14: 742–748. Surgeon. 2004;2(2):115; author reply 116.

Lee SY, Jang JH, Kim DW, Park J, Oh HK, Ihn MH, Han HS, Oh JH, Park SJ, Kang SB. Incidental cholecystectomy in patients with asymptomatic gallstones undergoing surgery for colorectal cancer. Dig Surg. 2015;32(3):183–9. https://doi.org/10.1159/000380961. Epub 2015 Mar 28

Lowenfels AB, Lindström CG, Conway MJ, Hastings PR. Gallstones and risk of gallbladder cancer. J Natl Cancer Inst. 1985;75(1):77–80.

Machado NO. Porcelain gallbladder: decoding the malignant truth. Sultan Qaboos Univ Med J. 2016;16(4):e416–21. https://doi.org/10.18295/squmj.2016.16.04.003. Epub 2016 Nov 30. Review

Maringhini A, Moreau JA, Melton LJ III, Hench SV, Zinsmeister AR, DiMagno EP. Gallstones, gallbladder cancer, and other gastrointestinal malignancies. Ann Intern Med. 1987;107:30–5.

Mayo WJ. "Innocent" gall-stones a myth. JAMA. 1911;LVI(14):1021–24. https://doi.org/10.1001/jama.1911.02560140007005.

minsal.cl/portal.

Ogoshi K, Kato T, Saitou Y. Present status of ultrasonic mass screening for gallbladder cancer. In: Yamamoto M, Serra I, Endoh K, Ogoshi K, editors. Epidemiology of gallbladder and bile duct cancers. Niigata: Nishimura; 1999. p. 102–7.

Ransohoff DF, Gracie WA. Treatment of gallstones. Ann Intern Med. 1993;119(7 Pt 1):606–19.

Roa I, de Aretxabala X. Gallbladder cancer in Chile: what have we learned? Curr Opin Gastroenterol.

2015;31(3):269–75. https://doi.org/10.1097/MOG.0000000000000164. Review.

Salazar M, Ituarte C, Abriata MG, Santoro F, Arroyo G. Gallbladder cancer in South America: epidemiology and prevention. Chin Clin Oncol. 2019;8(4):32. https://doi.org/10.21037/cco.2019.07.12. Epub 2019 Aug 12

Shao T, Yang YX. Cholecystectomy and the risk of colorectal cancer. Am J Gastroenterol. 2005;100(8):1813–20.

Sharma A, Behari A, Sikora SS, Kumar A, Saxena R, Kapoor VK. Post-cholecystectomy biliary strictures: not always benign. J Gastroenterol Hepatol. 2008;23(7 Pt 2):e63–6. Epub 2007 Jul 20

World Gastroenterology Organization. https://www.worldgastroenterology.org/guidelines/global-guidelines/asymptomatic-gallstone-disease.

References for Commentary Notes

Roa JC, Tapia O, Manterola C, Villaseca M, Guzman P, Araya JC, et al. Early gallbladder carcinoma has a favorable outcome but Rokitansky-Aschoff sinus involvement is an adverse prognostic factor. Virchows Arch. 2013;463(5):651–61.

Shindoh J, de Aretxabala X, Aloia TA, Roa JC, Roa I, Zimmitti G, et al. Tumor location is a strong predictor of tumor progression and survival in T2 gallbladder cancer: an international multicenter study. Ann Surg. 2014;261(4):733–9.

17 Gall Bladder Cancer Memoirs

Vinay K. Kapoor

Gall bladder cancer (GBC), a "non-western" cancer, has a peculiar geographical prevalence being more common in central and south America (Bolivia, Chile, Colombia, and Ecuador), eastern and central Europe (Czech Republic, Germany, Hungary, Poland, and Slovakia), south Asia (India, Pakistan, Nepal, and Bangladesh), and east Asia (Japan, Korea, and China) and less common in the Western-developed world including North America (United States and Canada), UK and western Europe, and the Pacific (Australia and New Zealand).

Surgeons and scientists in two countries, Chile and Japan, had made significant contributions to "chole-cysto-oncology" much before the rest of the world, including myself, got interested in the disease. My treatise on GBC will be incomplete without my memoirs of my introduction to and interaction with colleagues in these two countries.

Dedication: I would like to dedicate this chapter to (Late) Dr. Takeshi Todoroki (Fig. 17.1) of the University of Tsukuba Japan, who had made significant contributions to the surgical management of gallbladder cancer (GBC) and who introduced me to Japan.

V. K. Kapoor (✉)
Department of Surgical Gastroenterology, Sanjay Gandhi Post-Graduate Institute of Medical Sciences (SGPGIMS), Lucknow, Uttar Pradesh, India
e-mail: vkkapoor.india@gmail.com

17.1 UK

A one-year Commonwealth Fellowship to the UK in 1996-97, at the invitation of Irving S Benjamin of the King's College Hospital London, allowed me to spend some time with Anthony J McMichael at the London School of Hygiene and Tropical Medicine and learn the ABC of epidemiology. It was here and then that I found out that GBC is common not only in North Indians but in the Native American Indians also.

17.2 USA

The 4-month Fulbright Visiting Lecturer Fellowship, at the invitation of John G Hunter of the Oregon Health & Science University (OHSU), Portland OR, enabled me to visit institutions in 14 states across USA including attending, at the invitation of Judith Kaur, the Native Circle meeting of scientists working with Native American people.

17.3 Eastern Europe

GBC is statistically 'common' in eastern and central Europe also but because of the small denominator (i.e. the population) and non-use of English in these countries, they do not figure in

V. K. Kapoor (ed.), *A Pictorial Treatise on Gall Bladder Cancer*,
https://doi.org/10.1007/978-981-15-5289-2_17

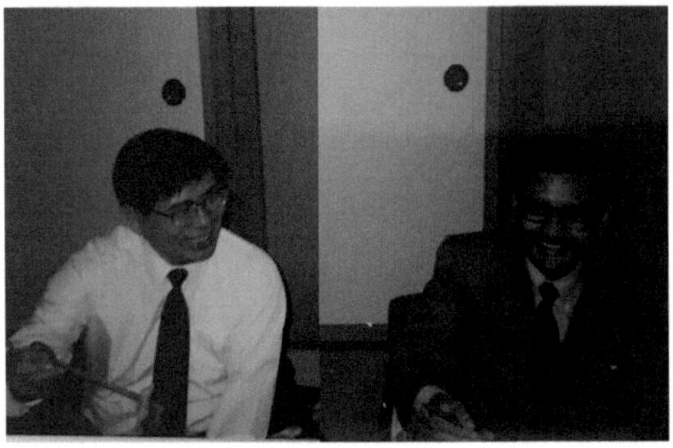

Fig. 17.1 The Author (VKK) with (Late) Dr. Takeshi Todoroki (Left) of Japan in 1998

the global GBC list. I did not, however, want to miss the opportunity to visit this relatively smaller GBC 'temple' also and a visit to Poland (Figs. 17.1 and 17.2), at the invitation of Zbigniew Biejat, materialized, courtesy a travel grant form Irving S Benjamin of the King's College Hospital London, during my one year stay in the UK on a Commonwealth Fellowship.

17.4 Chile: My Surgical "Pilgrimage"

Chile (with one of the highest incidence rates of GBC in the world), for chole-cysto-oncologists, i.e., those working with GBC, is what Vatican is to the Christians, Mecca to the Muslims and Sarnath Varanasi to the Buddhists. Ever since my involvement with GBC started way back in 1988 when I was at the All India Institute of Medical Sciences (AIIMS), New Delhi India we have been reading, discussing, and following articles written by Xabier (pronounced as Khavier) de Aretxabala (pronounced as Arexabala) (Fig. 17.3) and Ivan Roa, surgeon and pathologist, respectively from the University of Temuco in Chile (incidentally, their interest with GBC also started around the same time as ours (de Aretxabala et al. 1990)).

The national society meetings of the surgeons in Chile and South America are conducted in Spanish and no international surgical congress has been held in Chile. So, I grabbed the opportunity to go to Chile when I saw the flyer for a World Congress, though of Internal Medicine, to be held at Santiago in Chile. The view of the snow-capped peaks of the Andes as I looked out of the window on the Miami to Santiago flight which was flying parallel to the mountain range on its western (Chilean) side was breathtaking. At 6 a.m., the golden glow of the sunrise behind the peaks on their eastern (Argentinean) side virtually put the snow on fire. Incidentally, the border between the two countries in the high mountains is decided by the direction of the flow of water in a river—if the river flows eastwards the hill belongs to Argentina, if westwards it is Chile! The "residency" habit of catching a sleep whenever and wherever possible helped me to avoid a jet lag even after a 4 leg (Lucknow–Delhi–London–Miami–Santiago), 48 h, 20,000-km journey across four continents and I was awake and fresh enough to go with Dr. Aretxabala and his wife Isabel for a drive to the top of the Serra (Hill) San Cristobel (Fig. 17.4) followed by a Peruvian dinner on the very evening of my arrival in Santiago.

Chile, more than 4000 km long and less than 120 km wide at its narrowest part, is probably the "slimmest" country in the world. It shares its borders with Peru and Bolivia to its north and Argentina to its east. Chile is a geographical wonder where the ocean (Pacific) and high mountain ranges (Andes) are within visible distances from each other. The mountain ranges of the Andes and the coastal mountains come within 40 m of each other at one place. It is a goldmine (or may be "coppermine!" Chile is the largest producer and exporter of copper in the world—no wonder the lawns of the La Moneda presidential palace in the heart of the city are decorated with copper flowers (Fig. 17.5) and the front of the majestic Marriott Hotel in the newer western quarters of the city is copper and not the usual glass) of natural beauty—Lapis Lazuli is another Chilean exclusivity (the only other place where it is still found is Afghanistan).

The top of the Serra (Hill) San Cristobel in the northern part of the city with a pristine white statue of Virgin Mary at its top (Isabel informed me that the statue was built in France in the same factory where the Eiffel Tower was assembled)

Fig. 17.2 Outline of a continuing medical education (CME) program at

Oddział Warszawski Towarzystwa Chirurgów Polskich
III Klinika Chirurgii II Wydziału Lekarskiego AM
Szpital Czerniakowski, ul.Stępińska 19/25
00-739 Warszawa, tel/fax (0-22) 41 04 93

XIII Międzynarodowe Targi "Medica, Laboratorium '97"

DZIEŃ CHIRURGII

22 października 1997, Pałac Kultury i Nauki
Sala Rudniewa, godzina 15.30-17.30

Uprzejmie zapraszamy na posiedzenie naukowe Oddziału Warszawskiego Towarzystwa Chirurgów Polskich w czasie trwania targów.

Program:

A.Borkowski
Endoskopowe leczenie nowotworów górnych dróg moczowych

P.Nyckowski
Diagnostyka i leczenie przerzutów do wątroby

P.Andziak, W.Noszczyk
Udrożnienie tętnicy szyjnej wewnętrznej u chorych z krytycznym zwężeniem lub niedrożnością po stronie przeciwnej

J.M.Krusiewicz, T.Szczęsny
Współczesne możliwości torakoskopii

W.Rowiński
Postępy w chirurgii transplantacyjnej

V.Kapoor
Gallbladder cancer

Po posiedzeniu zapraszamy na kawę w imieniu firmy ***Pharmacia&Upjohn***

Sekretarz O.W. T.Ch.P — Prezes O.W.T.Ch.P.

dr med. Zbigniew Biejat — Prof.dr hab.med. Jerzy A.Pola_ski

offers the best view of the sprawling city of Santiago (Fig. 17.6) and is a very popular picnic spot for the families many of which could be seen walking and even cycling to the 800 m top of the hill. Mote Con Huesillo (Fig. 17.7), a refreshing drink of peach and cereal (though it was a bit too sweet even for a person like me with a sweet tooth—a tinge of salt and lime could have probably made it taste even better), was very welcome. A small Basque church and tree—most Chileans have a Basque (in northern Spain) background (Dr. Aretxabala informed me that his grandfather also came from Spain to Chile). A small (I thought it was an open drain until I was told it was a river) but turbulent Mapocho (crazy) river runs through the city—it is so named because once in about a decade it overflows and floods parts of the city.

GBC is the commonest cause of death in women in Chile, yet Chile (like India) still does

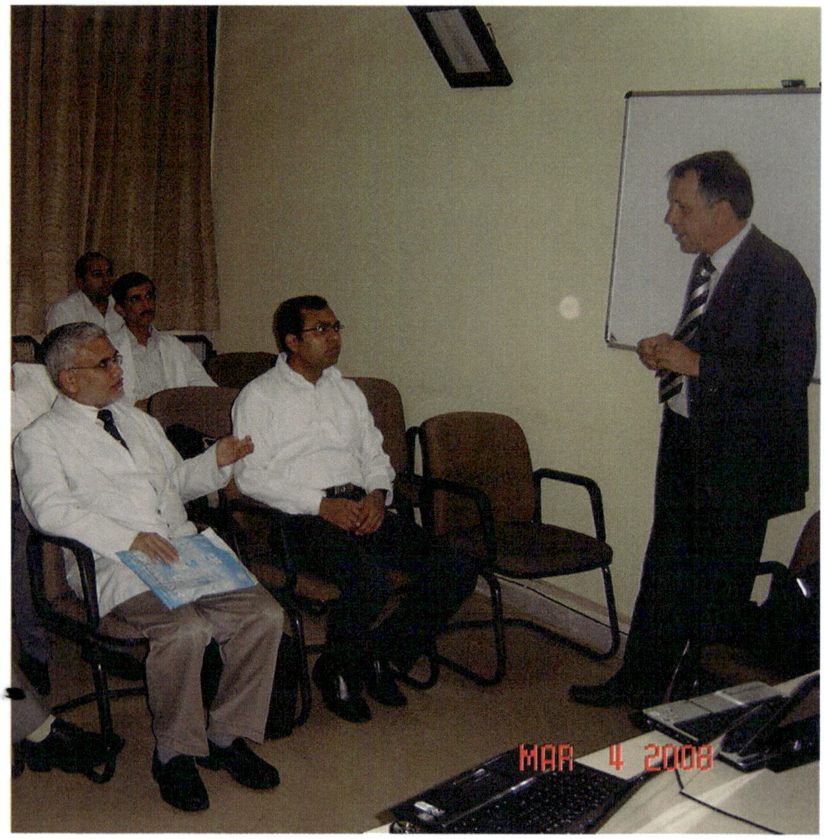

Fig. 17.3 Xabier de Aretxabala during his visit to the Sanjay Gandhi Post-Graduate Institute of Medical Sciences (SGPGIMS), Lucknow India in 2008

not have a national GBC registry. Other than GBC, there is very little Indian in Chile—I could see a few Indian cars on the roads and the Phillips bulb in the small but cozy room of my Tulip Inn was a Made in India and the bath towels were also Fabricado en India. Empanada, a popular Chilean snack, is very much like the Indian "*samosa*" but filled with meat (instead of vegetables). Some Chilean women, with their facial features, wheatish skin color, and black hair could easily pass of as Indian. Healthcare in Chile is similar to that in India—public (government) hospitals where the treatment is virtually free to anyone and everyone are busy, crowded, and always full but those who can afford and who have a private insurance go to one of the 5-star hotel-like private hospitals such as Clinica Alemana (German), which has two buildings on either side of a busy city road with an underground tunnel connecting the two, which gives one a feeling of walking through an airport terminal.

The similarities, however, end there. Chile is a developed and disciplined democracy now after having seen military rule for 18 long years from 1973 to 1990 (surprisingly as many as 46% of Chilean people had voted for the continuation of the Military rule as it brought discipline and order to the country and boosted its economy—now one of the strongest in South America). My criteria for including a country in the "developed" list are parameters such as whether you feel safe to travel in public transport even after it is dark, you can drive between cities at a speed of 100–120 km without having to stop at a traffic signal, and you can drink water straight from the tap. Unlike in India, where the language changes from one state to another and sometimes even within the state, Spanish is spoken not only in all parts of Chile but almost over the entire South American continent. It is mandatory for every family in Chile to send the children to school and receive education up to secondary level (12th)—a

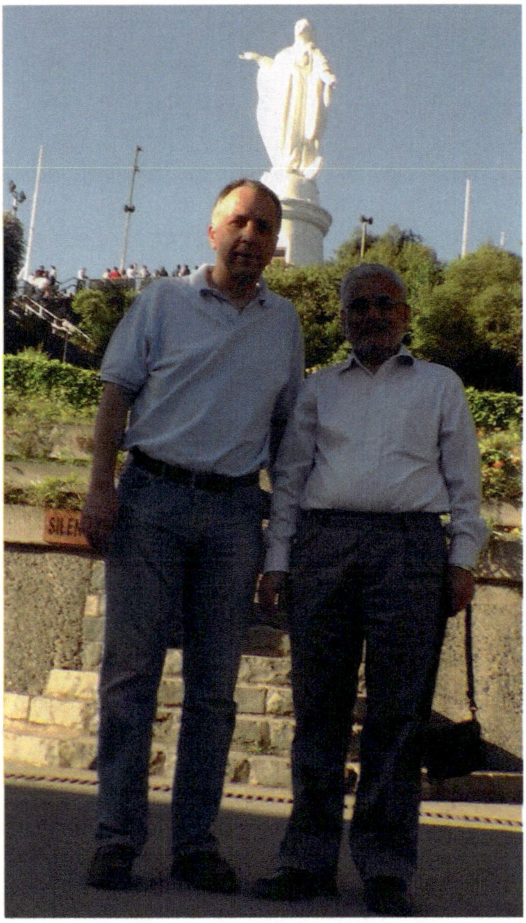

Fig. 17.4 The Author (VKK) with Xabier de Aretxabala (Left) at the Serra San Cristobel, Temuco Chile

large number of youth thus want to enter a college/university but there are not enough seats in the public institutions resulting in a large number of private universities (including medical); the private Alemana Clinic is also attached to a private university. We, in India, also differ with Dr. Aretxabala in the philosophy of management of T1b (muscularis propria) GBC—while he reported 88% 5-year survival in 49 patients with T1b GBC after simple cholecystectomy only (de Aretxabala et al. 2009), we recommend extended cholecystectomy for T1b disease (Wagholikar et al. 2002).

I also had a good chance to enjoy a cup of tea at the French Le Fornis Cafe in the Alemana Clinic and share experiences and views on GBC with Prof Ivan Roa whose work I have always admired but I admired him even more now considering that even in a private hospital he has established excellent molecular biology facilities. Dr. Roa regretted that in Chile, most surgeons do not fix and send the GB to the pathologist in a proper manner, i.e., opened and stretched on a wax plate (to prevent its crumpling) and most pathologists do not take proper (i.e., along the length of the GB) and adequate (number) of sections (so as not to miss an incidental GBC); I did not have the courage to tell him that in India, not all GBs are even sent by the surgeons to the pathologists. Most (almost all) GBCs in Chile have gall stones (GS)—they very rarely see GBC without GS. Like in north India, most (80%) of their GS are multiple, mixed; about 15% are cholesterol solitaire and <5% are pigment GS. The native Mapuches in the South have higher prevalence of GS and are at a higher risk to develop GBC in the presence of GS. Based primarily on Dr. Roa's work, Chile now has a national program under which women between the ages of 40 and 60 are recommended to have ultrasonography (US) and if found to have GS are advised to undergo cholecystectomy. However, it is a bit too early to assess its impact on the incidence rates of GBC as the program started only a few years ago.

Dr. Carlos Benavides, the current president of the Chilean Surgical Society, works in the public San Borja (pronounced as Borha) Hospital but also goes to the private Alemana Clinic as the latter provides most of the money that he (and his family) can spend and enjoy, as salary from the public hospital is too small. A young pretty looking chief resident Patricia Rebolledo Caro took pictures after my lecture and emailed them to me even before I could open my email at the internet counter in the conference. After my lecture in his department, Dr. Carlos showed me around his hospital (especially the better areas built with the help of a Japanese grant) and was kind enough to drive me to Vespuchio Rieseco, my conference venue on the northern side of the city in his Audi.

I thought courtesy and hospitality are traits of the Eastern culture only. Chile, though geographically West, is culturally East. Where else but in

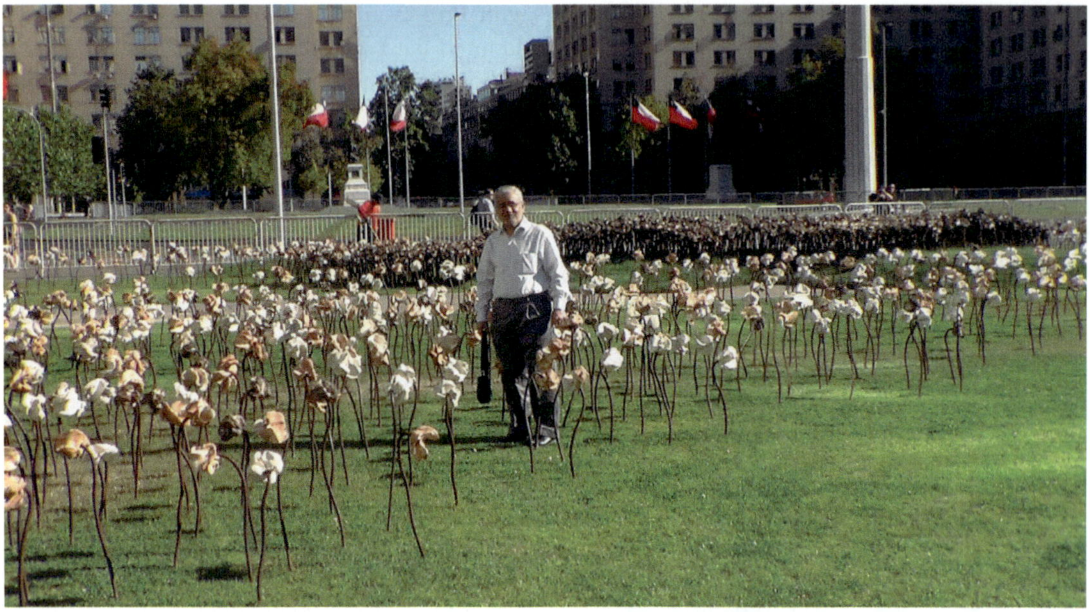

Fig. 17.5 Copper 'flowers' in the lawns of the La Moneda presidential palace in Santiago Chile

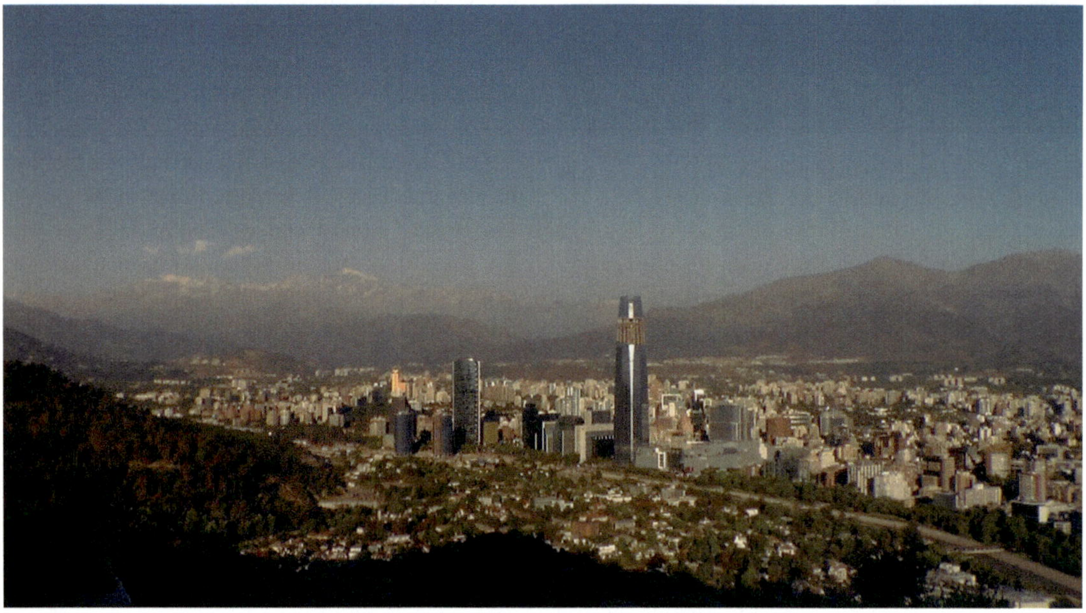

Fig. 17.6 Panoramic view of the city of Santiago Chile (with snow-capped peaks of Andes in the background)from the top of Serra San Cristobel

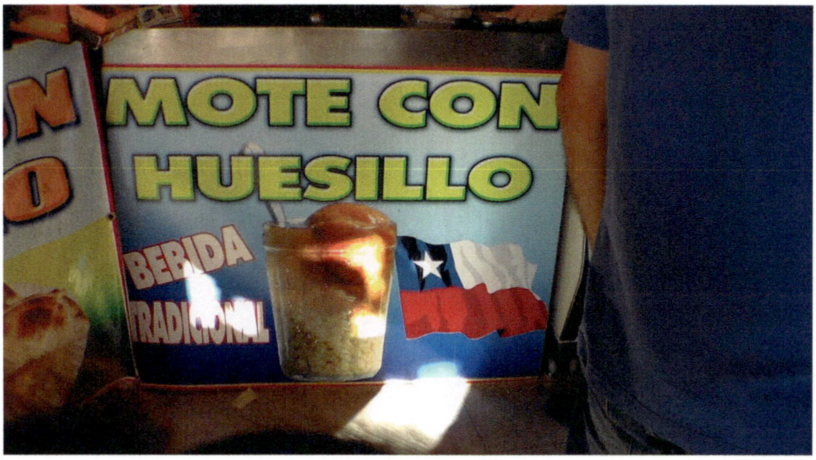

Fig. 17.7 Mote Con Huesillo – the refreshing peach and cereal drink

Chile the entire family of your host (in fact Dr. Aretxabala was not even my host, I had gone there on my own and "forced" my hospitality on him) will get involved to look after you—Dr. Aretxabala coming to the airport on a Sunday morning to receive me and then drop me to my hotel, carrying my bigger and heavier bag himself thus leaving only the lighter carry-on for me, leaving an envelope with some local currency for me at the hotel reception as banks would be closed on Sunday, his wife Isabel picking me up from my hotel to take me to his mother's house for a pure Spanish (not Chilean, not even Hispanic) dinner of *palla* (pronounced as pallya; similar to the Indian *biryani*) and she in advance checking with one of the few Indians in Santiago about the dietary preferences of Indian Hindus and then reconfirming it on the internet and preparing a vegetarian *palla* specially for me and finally, his son dropping me off to the airport, Dr. Carlos translating the salient points of the presentations made by his residents in Spanish for me, Dr. Nicolas Devaud dropping me to my hotel after my presentation, Dr. Ivan Roa taking the trouble to draw a map of the Plaza de Armas (Fig. 17.8) on a piece of paper with all the details such as the church, the man-on-the-horse statue, exit of metro, etc. to guide me to reach a shopping gallery where I could buy a replica of the Moai statue as a souvenir to take home.

Dr. Aretxabala took a full day off on a working day and took me on a long scenic drive on the 4–6 lane highway from Santiago through a tunnel beneath the Serra San Cristobel to the north through the mountains and some more tunnels to Casablanca (white house) valley with breathtaking landscapes and vineyards with tall propellers (which are put into use to move air during the extreme cold winters so as to avoid damage to the fragile fruit) lined by roses. Isabel-a fruit—a fruit expert herself—informed me that the roses pick up the disease before grapes thus giving time for appropriate measures to be taken (agriculture scientists and horticulturists have done better than what we physicians and surgeons have done to do something before gall stones turn malignant—wine is more precious and valued than human life!)). The drive took us to the garden city of Vina Del Mar with brightly colored multistoried houses on sloping hills (with many ascensors—wheeled cable cars to go to the top of each hill) on the coast of the Pacific Ocean. Most of the buildings seemed to be empty obviously so because they are second houses of people living in Santiago and are occupied only during the weekends and the summer (February) holidays. Farther and smaller towns of Reneca and Con Con were even more picturesque. We broke our journey for a fresh seafood lunch at the Yacht Club on the Ocean and a photo shoot with a Moai

Fig. 17.8 Map of Plaza de Armas hand-drawn by Ivan Roa

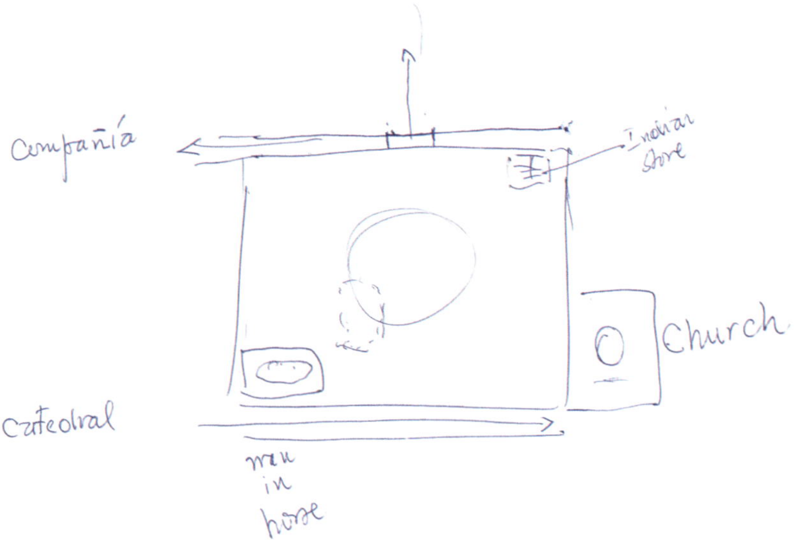

statue on the Pacific Coast donated by the people of the Eastern Island to the city of Vina Del Mar on its 400th anniversary. Picture postcard perfect port of Valparaiso—established in 1536 by the Spanish conquistadors used to be a very busy stopover earlier as ships going from Asia, Africa, and Europe to the West coast of the United States will have to stop there but lost its importance after the Panama Canal was built in 1914.

I always end my lecture on GBC abroad with a picture of Taj Mahal saying "not all stones are harmful, some are beautiful too." Had I known that the Easter Island (a 25 × 12 km island in the Pacific with a little more than 5000 inhabitants) is a part of Chile, I would have changed the picture to that of a Moai statue (Fig. 17.9) and said "some are mystical too."

PS: My bags were full of Indian food that I was carrying for my son Abhimanyu who is working in Ft Lauderdale, FL, USA. On my way back from Santiago to Miami, I did honestly declare to the customs about it and my bags were obviously opened for inspection. As the customs officer was opening all the packets and sniffing all the Indian snacks never seen by her before, flew out a moth from the bag and created a virtual hell with all the officers panicking around and looking for it. Good that GBC is not a vector-borne disease or else I could have been charged with a serious crime of importing an Indo-Chilean disease to the United States.

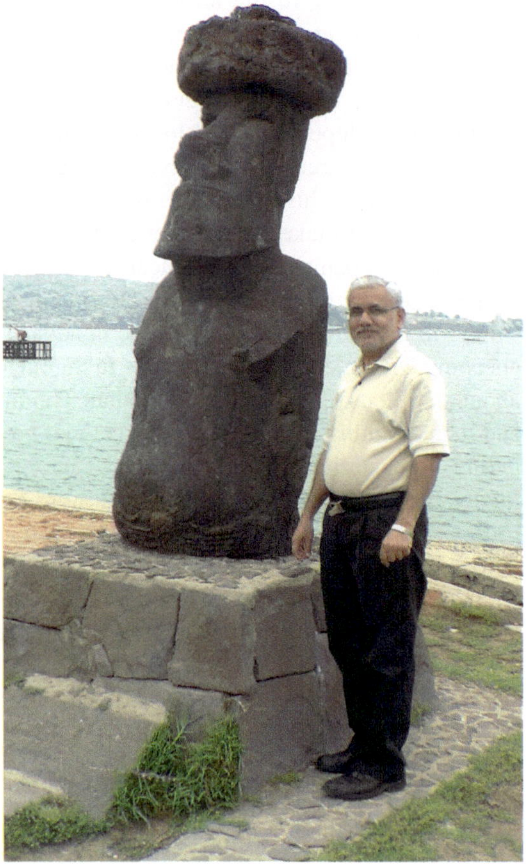

Fig. 17.9 The Author (VKK) with a Moai statue on the Pacific Coast of the city of Vina Del Mar in Chile

17.5 Japan

My *karmabhoomi* (the place of work) the Sanjay Gandhi Post-Graduate Institute of Medical Sciences (SGPGIMS), Lucknow India had a collaborative exchange program with the Nagoya University School of Medicine (NUSM), Nagoya Japan under the auspices of the Japan International Cooperation Agency (JICA). My first visit to Japan was in 1995 to attend the Annual Congress of the Japan Surgery Society (JSS) at the invitation of the colleagues from the NUSM (Fig. 17.10), followed by another visit the very next year to attend the JSS Congress at Chiba hosted by Masaru Miyazaki. New contacts led to more than 10 further visits to Japan to attend and contribute to the meetings of Eastern & Western Association of Liver Tumors (EWALT), International Association of Surgeons Gastroenterologists and Oncologists (IASGO), International Society for Digestive Surgery (ISDS), Japanese Society of Gastroenterological Surgery (JSGS), Japanese Society of Hepato-Biliary-Pancreatic Surgery (JSHBPS) and JSS (held every year during the cherry blossom season Fig. 17.11) at the invitations of several renowned Japanese surgeons including Norihiro Kokudo (Fig. 17.12), Masato Nagino, Akimasa Nakao (Fig. 17.13), Toshiaki Nonami, Mitsuo Shimada, Kyoichi Takaori, Kazuhiro Tsukada, Michiaki Unno, Toshifumi Wakai and Masakazu Yamamoto, and feast my eyes on rich Japanese heritage (Fig. 17.14) and enjoy the very warm Japanese hospitality (Fig. 17.15). During one of these visits, (Late) Takeshi Todoroki invited me to Tsukuba where my first research collaboration started with Masanao Miwa (Fig 17.16). In another visit, I was invited by Toshifumi Wakai to visit Niigata, a high GBC incidence area in Japan, where he introduced me to Yasuo Tsuchiya (Fig. 17.17) which blossomed into another research collaboration.

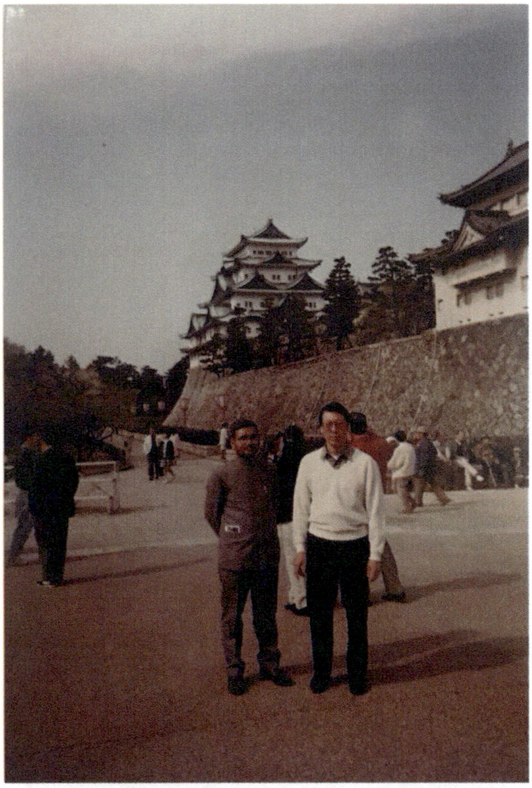

Fig. 17.10 The Author (VKK) with Toshiaki Nonami (Right) at Nagoya Castle 1995

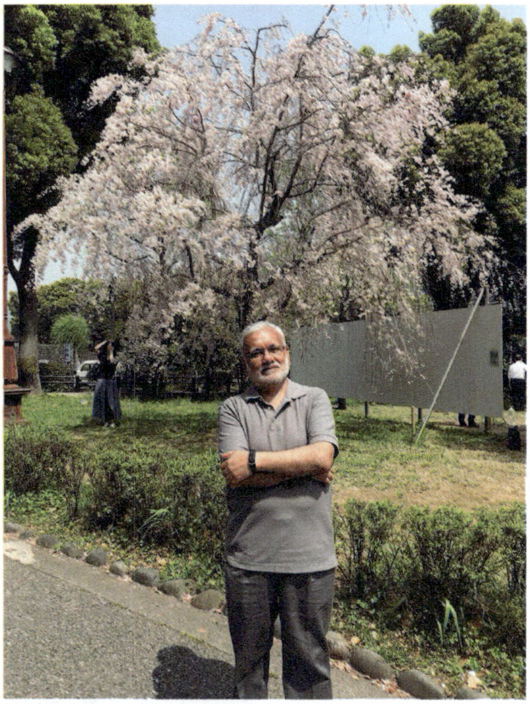

Fig. 17.11 The Annual Congresses of the Japan Surgery Society (JSS) are held every year during the cherry blossom season – the Author (VKK) during JSS 2018

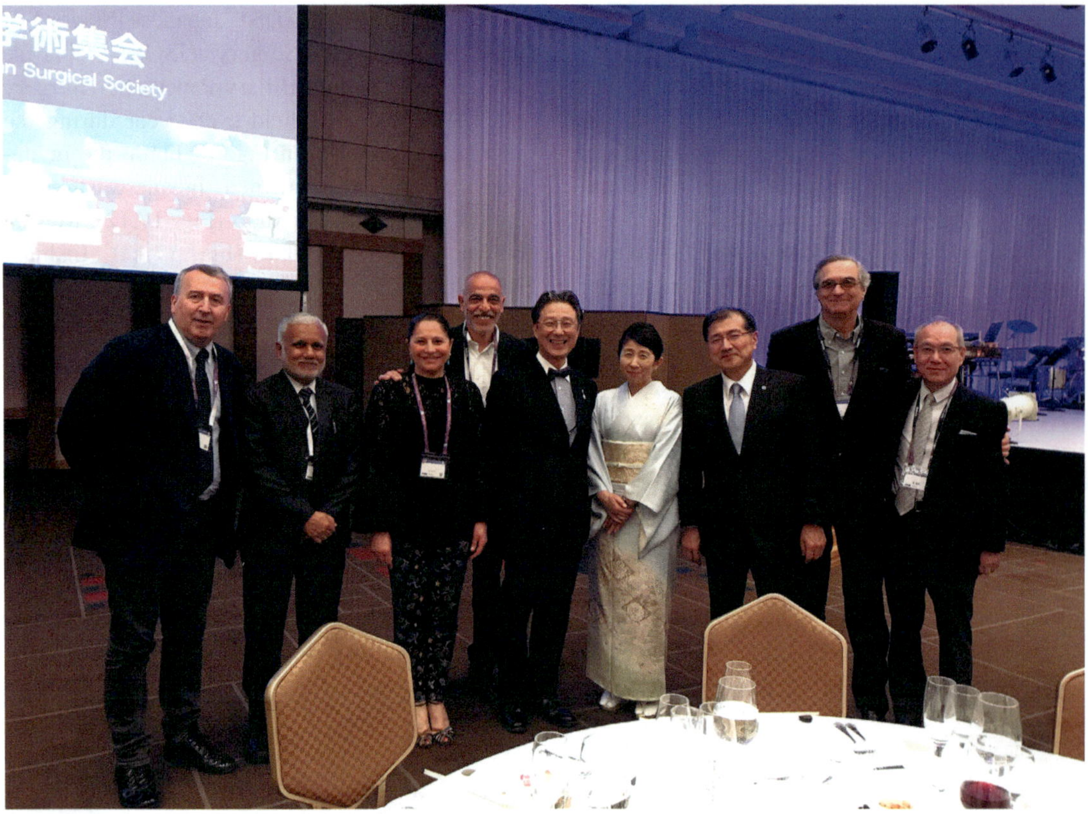

Fig. 17.12 The Author (VKK) (2nd from Left) with other international speakers at the Annual Congresses of the Japan Surgery Society (JSS) Tokyo 2018 at the invitation of Norihiro Kokudo (3rd from Right)

Fig. 17.13 The Author (VKK) with Akimasa Nakao (Left) during one of his visits to Japan

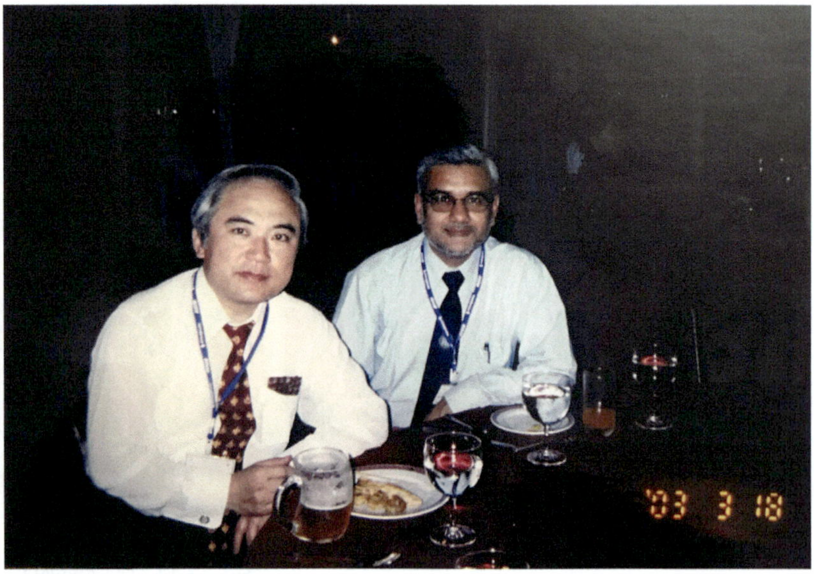

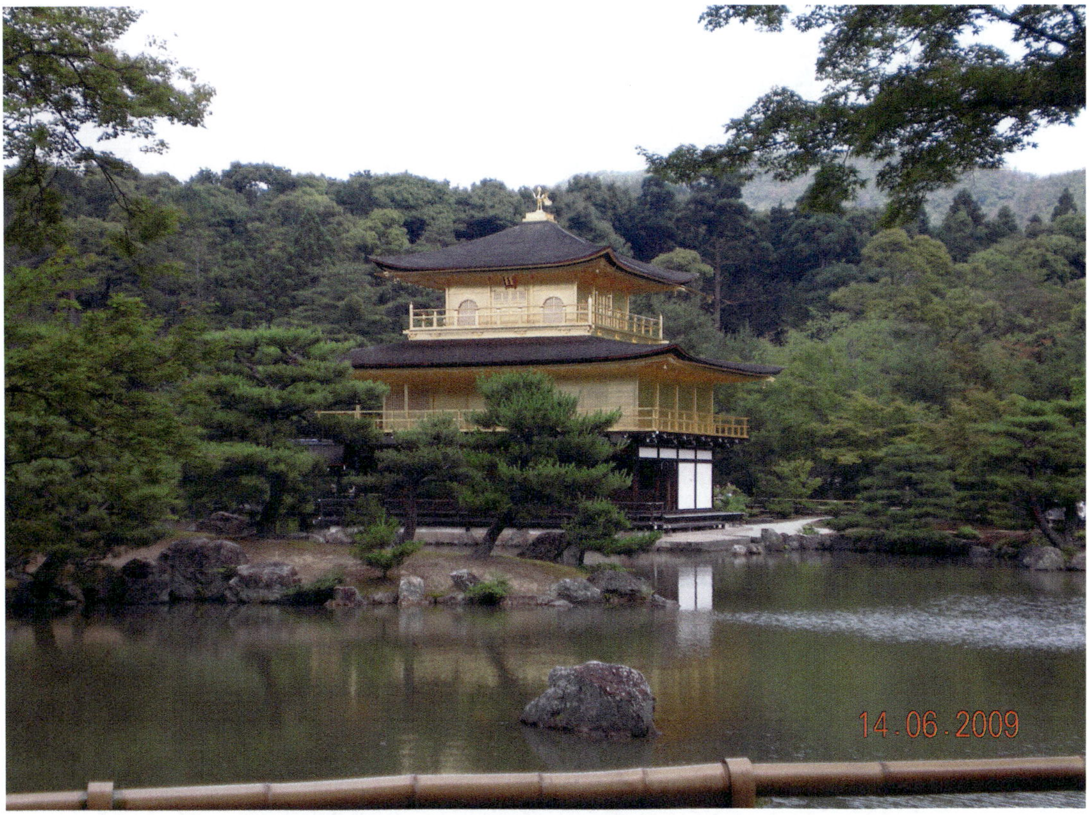

Fig. 17.14 Kinkaku-ji/ Rokuon-ji (Golden Pavilion) temple in Kyoto

Fig. 17.15 The Author (VKK) enjoying a Geisha dinner during one of the meetings in Japan

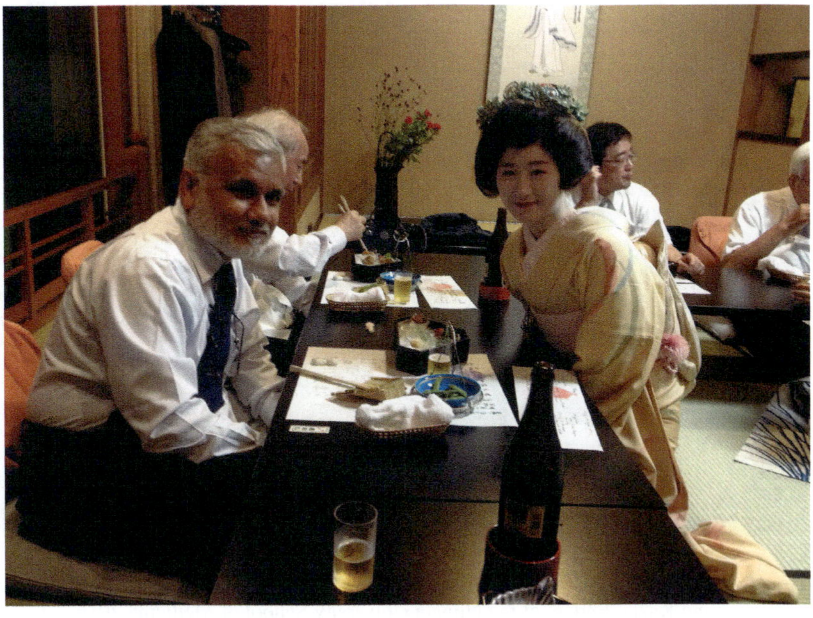

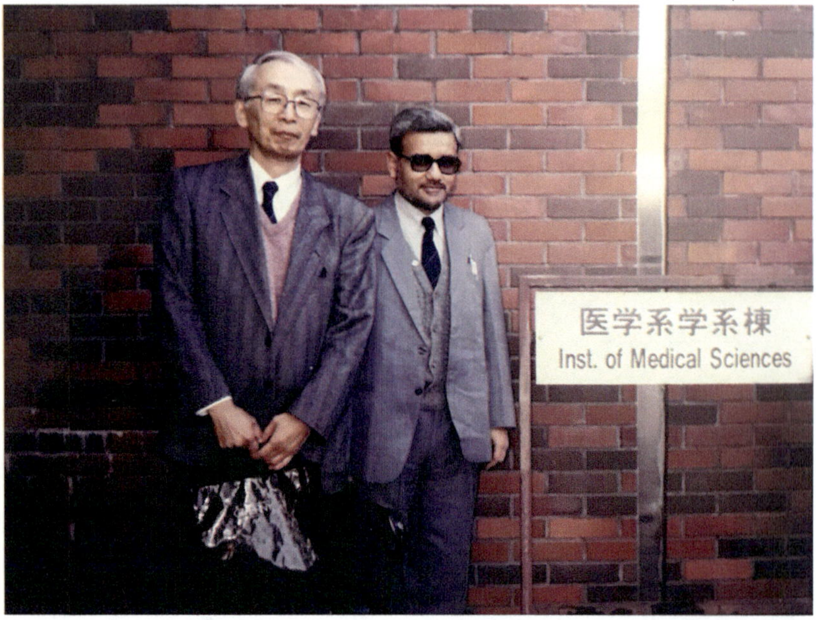

Fig. 17.16 The Author (VKK) with Masanao Miwa at the University of Tsukuba 1998

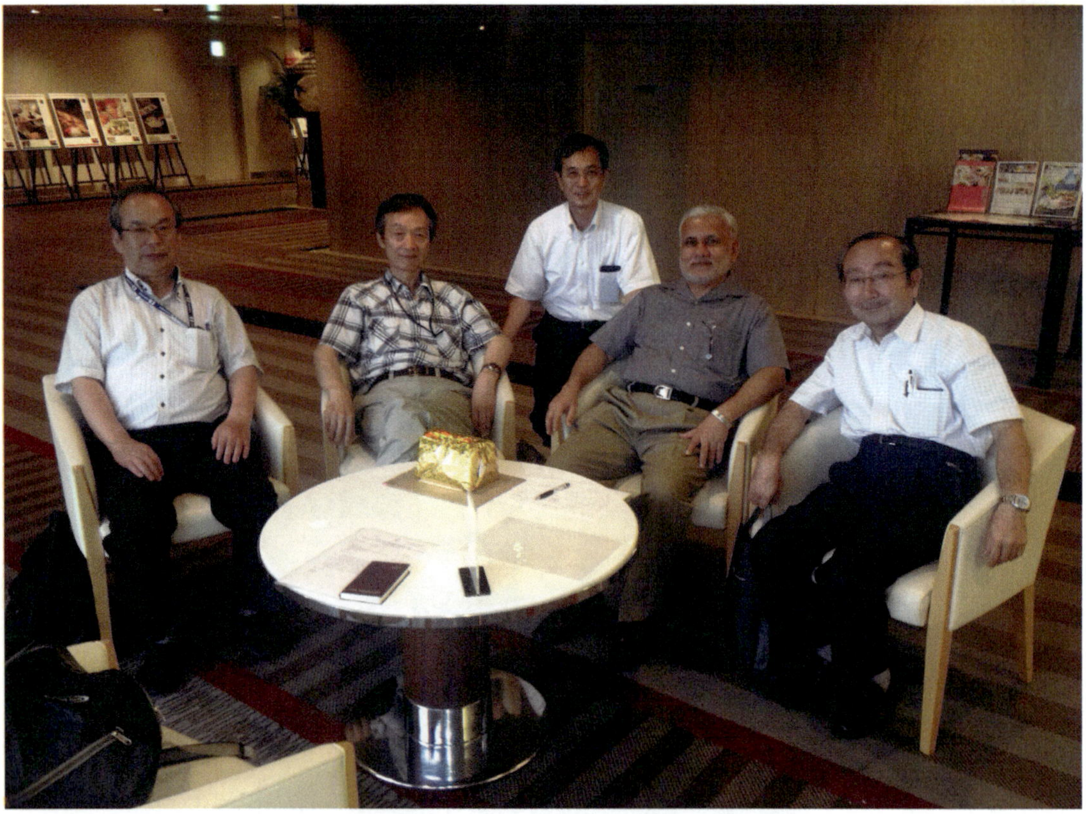

Fig. 17.17 The Author (VKK) (2nd from Right) with (from Left to Right) Toshikazu Ikoma, Tadashi Yamamoto, Yasuo Tsuchiya, and Kazuo Endoh, of the Niigata University School of Medicine 2016

17.5.1 How and Why Japanese Surgeons Are What They Are?

'He' was already performing percutaneous transhepatic cholangioscopy (PTCS) (Nimura and Shionoya 1986) for diagnosis of biliary tract cancers in 1986, a decade before I published my first article on gallbladder cancer (Kapoor et al. 1996). I have met him only a few times but every time we meet he would recognize me (or at least make me feel that he did), rise from his seat and greet me (with a bow, at the mid-body—not once but several times, in the usual Japanese way) even before I could wish him.

It was July 2014 when I went to Japan to attend the Annual Meeting of the Japanese Society of Gastroenterological Surgery (JSGS) at Koriyama in Fukushima prefecture where I had been nominated by the Indian Association of Surgical Gastroenterology (IASG) to represent it in a session on gallbladder cancer. Prof Toshifumi Wakai of Niigata University School of Medicine invited him and me to Niigata after the JSGS for a collaborative research group meeting. The three of us (Fig. 17.4) traveled from Koriyama to Niigata by train—each of one us pulled our bags (Prof Wakai had a small briefcase and a laptop bag, he had a briefcase and a backpack—from one of the IHPBA meetings and I had two heavy—Indian style—bags). While we were waiting for our train at Koriyama station, for the first time I noticed that one of his ear lobules had a "cauliflower" appearance; it was later that I came to know the reason when Prof Wakai in his introduction mentioned that in addition to being a leading hepatobiliary surgeon he is a black belt judoka also (obviously, even cancer cells cannot survive his aggressive moves). As we had a few minutes before the train arrived, I did not want to lose the golden opportunity—I requested a young man standing in the line behind us to take our picture (along with our bags). I positioned myself in such a way that he would be between Prof Wakai and me, but he gestured and said something in Japanese to the "photographer" who immediately moved his finger away from the shooting button of my Nikon Coolpix camera. I felt a bit embarrassed; is it that he is annoyed that I did not ask for his permission to have a picture with him. I was about to say sorry, when he put his firm, yet gentle, hand on my shoulder and said "You are our guest" and positioned himself to my side so that I would be in the center and then asked the gentleman to shoot (Fig. 17.18).

As soon as we exited the ticket gates at Niigata train station, two of Prof Wakai's residents were there to receive us—one for him and the other for me. They offered a hand to carry our bags—in my typical Indian senior consultant style I handed over one of my bags—obviously the heavier one—to the resident. A few seconds later as I looked behind, I was ashamed to see that not only Prof Wakai who is younger than me but also he—who is at least 15 years older than me—was pulling his bag himself with his backpack in his other hand.

My return flight from Narita to Delhi was at 6.30 PM and I wanted to reach the airport well in time (not wanting to repeat my last experience of a missed flight on an international trip). Prof Wakai had booked the two of us for 1212-1420 Niigata to Tokyo and 1433-1527 Tokyo to Narita trains. "Ten minutes (my calculation was based on the usual Indian rounding off of time to the nearest 10–15 minutes) at the busy Tokyo station is too little to change the train" I said. "Oh no, we have 13 minutes" he said, emphasizing on 13 as if there was a statistically significant difference between 10/15 and 13 minutes. I was still apprehensive and requested Prof Wakai to put me on an earlier Niigata to Tokyo train but the tickets had already been booked, and more importantly, they were more than certain that I will be able to make it. "Don't worry, I will guide you at Tokyo station" said he, who has guided surgeons not only in Japan but all over the world on how to do hepatectomies.

Guidance, I thought, will be in the form of he instructing me as to how to go from where we will alight at Tokyo station to the NarEx (Narita Express) platform. But it was not to be so; he virtually ran (once again with his bag and backpack) across the platform through milling crowds of people at Tokyo station and down the escalators,

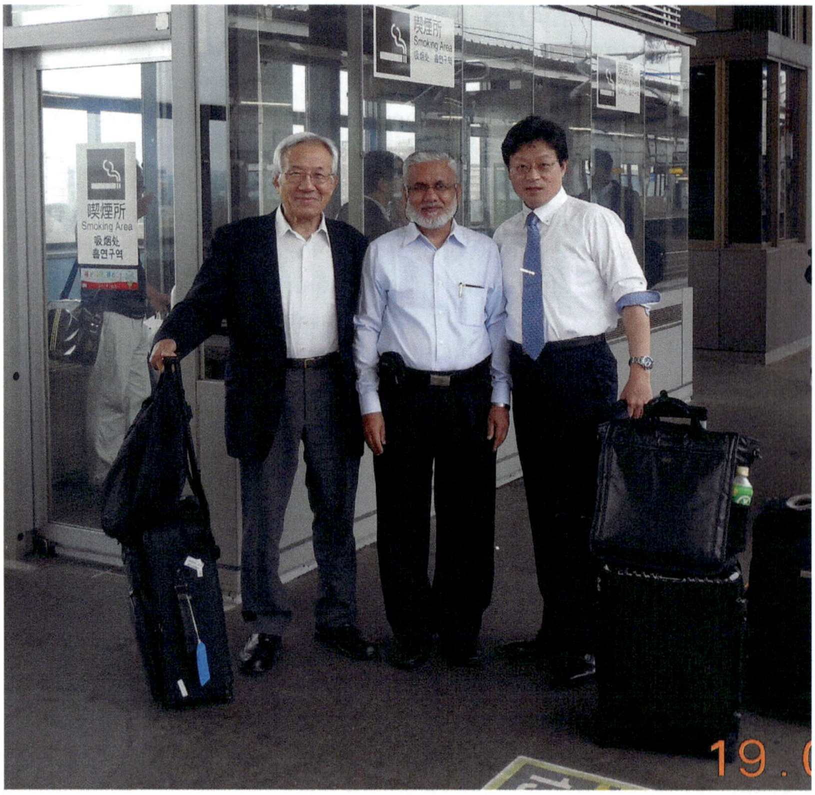

Fig. 17.18 The Author (VKK) with Yuji Nimura (Left) and Toshifumi Wakai (Right) in Japan

with me trailing him, till we reached the NarEx platform on basement 5 (B5) level. "Show me your ticket" he said and pointed toward one end of the train which was already there. He then went into the compartment and ushered me toward my reserved seat. It was after great persuasion that I could request him to leave the platform and move on with his onward journey to Nagoya before my train took off.

Results (in terms of mortality and survival) of surgery for most cancers are better in Japanese hands than in those of anybody else. Surgeons, especially in Europe and United States, sometimes attribute this to a different biology of the disease in Japan, but after observing surgeons all over the globe, I have no doubt in my mind at least that the Japanese (so also the Korean, Chinese, and Taiwanese) surgeons have the ultimate finesse and the best surgical skills in the world.

Just as he guided me at Tokyo train station, I am sure, is how senior surgeons of the kind of Yuji Nimura guide their trainees to perform surgery also and that is how and why Japanese surgeons are what they are.

To be great, you need not only might but also kindness. (Anpanman (the hero) to Ringo Bouya (his fan, a child) in a Japanese animation created by Takashi Yanese (1919–2013))

Acknowledgments Acknowledgments are due to the Indian Association of Surgical Gastroenterology (IASG) for the nomination and to the Japanese Society of Gastroenterological Surgery (JSGS) for the hospitality.

Section 17.5.1 has been reproduced with permission from Suture (May 2016; pp. 9–10) the Newsletter of the College of Surgeons of Sri Lanka.

References

de Aretxabala X, Roa I, Araya JC, Burgos L, Flores P, Huenchullan I, Miyazaki I. Operative findings in patients with early forms of gallbladder cancer. Br J Surg. 1990;77(3):291–3.

de Aretxabala X, Roa I, Hepp J, Maluenda F, Mordojovich G, Leon J, Roa JC. Early gallbladder cancer: is further treatment necessary? J Surg Oncol. 2009;100(7):589–93.

Kapoor VK, Pradeep R, Haribhakti SP, Sikora SS, Kaushik SP. Early carcinoma of the gall bladder - an elusive disease. J Surg Oncol. 1996;62:284–7.

Kapoor VK, McMichael AJ. Gall bladder cancer – an 'Indian' disease. National Medical Journal of India 2003;16:209–213. is available at http://archive.nmji.in/archives/volume%2016-4July%20August%202003/16-4%20final%20pdf/Review%20Article/RA.pdf.

Kapoor VK. An Indian meets the American Indians. National Medical Journal of India 2009;22:204–5. is available at http://archive.nmji.in/archives/Volume-22/Issue-4/PDF-volume-22-issue-4/Volume-22-issue-4-Spk-For-Myself.pdf.

Nimura Y, Shionoya S. [Diagnosis of bile duct and gallbladder carcinoma by percutaneous transhepatic cholangioscopy]. [Article in Japanese]. Gan No Rinsho. 1986;32(10):1246–8.

Wagholikar GD, Behari A, Krishnani NK, Kumar A, Sikora SS, Saxena R, Kapoor VK. Early gallbladder cancer. J Am Coll Surg. 2002;194:137–41.

Institutional Experiences in Gall Bladder Cancer

18

Vinay K. Kapoor

18.1 Databases

18.1.1 Global

https://gco.iarc.fr/

Global Cancer Observatory of the International Agency for Research against Cancer (IARC) is an interactive web-based platform presenting global cancer statistics using data from GLOBOCAN and Cancer Incidence in Five Continents (CI5) Vol XI.

http://ci5.iarc.fr

18.1.2 National Cancer Date Base (NCDB)

https://www.facs.org/quality-programs/cancer/ncdb

National Cancer Date Base (NCDB) USA, a joint venture of the Commission on Cancer (CoC) of the American College of Surgeons (ACS) and the American Cancer Society (ACS), is a prospective hospital based cancer registry that collects and reports data on more than 70% of all newly diagnosed cancers in more than 1500 CoC hospitals across the United States—20,142 cases of GBC were registered in the NCDB between 2004 and 2012.

18.1.3 Survey of Epidemiology and End Results (SEER)

https://seer.cancer.gov/

Survey of Epidemiology and End Results (SEER) database of National Cancer Institutes (NCI) in the United States is the largest publicly available cancer database in USA—12,180 GBCs enrolled between 2004 and 2015.

18.1.4 US-EBMC

United States Extrahepatic Biliary Malignancy Consortium (US—EBMC) of ten high volume academic medical centers in USA

- Johns Hopkins Hospital, Baltimore, MD
- New York University, New York, NY
- Ohio State University Wexner Medical Center and the James Cancer Hospital and Solove Research Institute, Columbus, OH
- Stanford University Medical Center, Stanford
- University of Louisville, Louisville, KY
- University of Wisconsin School of Medicine and Public Health, Madison, WI

V. K. Kapoor (✉)
Department of Surgical Gastroenterology, Sanjay Gandhi Post-Graduate Institute of Medical Sciences (SGPGIMS), Lucknow, Uttar Pradesh, India
e-mail: vkkapoor.india@gmail.com

V. K. Kapoor (ed.), *A Pictorial Treatise on Gall Bladder Cancer*,
https://doi.org/10.1007/978-981-15-5289-2_18

- Vanderbilt University Medical Center, Nashville, TN
- Wake Forest University, Winston–Salem, NC
- Washington University School of Medicine, St Louis, MO
- Winship Cancer Institute, Emory University, Atlanta, GA

18.2 Publications

18.2.1 Guidelines

- Aloia TA, Járufe N, Javle M, Maithel SK, Roa JC, Adsay V, Coimbra FJ, Jarnagin WR. Gallbladder cancer: expert consensus statement. HPB (Oxford). 2015;17(8):681–90. https://doi.org/10.1111/hpb.12444.

Expert consensus statement of Americas Hepato-Pancreato-Biliary Association (AHPBA)

- Benson AB, D'Angelica MI, Abbott DE, Abrams TA, Alberts SR, Anaya DA, Anders R, Are C, Brown D, Chang DT, Cloyd J, Covey AM, Hawkins W, Iyer R, Jacob R, Karachristos A, Kelley RK, Kim R, Palta M, Park JO, Sahai V, Schefter T, Sicklick JK, Singh G, Sohal D, Stein S, Tian GG, Vauthey JN, Venook AP, Hammond LJ, Darlow SD. Guidelines insights: hepatobiliary cancers, Version 2.2019. J Natl Compr Cancer Netw. 2019;17(4):302–10. https://doi.org/10.6004/jnccn.2019.0019.

National Comprehensive Cancer Network (NCCN) Guidelines

- Han HS, Yoon YS, Agarwal AK, Belli G, Itano O, Gumbs AA, Yoon DS, Kang CM, Lee SE, Wakai T, Troisi RI. Laparoscopic surgery for gallbladder cancer: an expert consensus statement. Dig Surg. 2019;36(1):1–6. https://doi.org/10.1159/000486207. Epub 2018 Jan 16.

Consensus statement for laparoscopic management of gallbladder cancer

- Lee SE, Kim KS, Kim WB, Kim IG, Nah YW, Ryu DH, Park JS, Yoon MH, Cho JY, Hong TH, et al. Practical guidelines for the surgical treatment of gallbladder cancer. J Korean Med Sci. 2014;29(10):1333–40. https://doi.org/10.3346/jkms.2014.29.10.1333.

Korean Association of Hepato-Biliary and Pancreas Surgery Guidelines

- Miyazaki M, Yoshitomi H, Miyakawa S, Uesaka K, Unno M, Endo I, Ota T, Ohtsuka M, Kinoshita H, Shimada K, Shimizu H, Tabata M, Chijiiwa K, Nagino M, Hirano S, Wakai T, Wada K, Isayama H, Okusaka T, Tsuyuguchi T, Fujita N, Furuse J, Yamao K, Murakami K, Yamazaki H, Kijima H, Nakanuma Y, Yoshida M, Takayashiki T, Takada T. Clinical practice guidelines for the management of biliary tract cancers 2015: the 2nd English edition. J Hepatobiliary Pancreat Sci. 2015;22(4):249–73. https://doi.org/10.1002/jhbp.233. Epub 2015 Mar 18.

Japanese Society of Hepato-Biliary-Pancreatic Surgery Guidelines

- Shukla HS, Sirohi B, Behari A, Sharma A, Majumdar J, Ganguly M, Tewari M, Kumar S, Saini S, Sahni P, Singh T, Kapoor VK, Sucharita V, Kaur T, Shukla DK, Rath GK. Indian Council of Medical Research consensus document for the management of gall bladder cancer. Indian J Med Paediatr Oncol. 2015;36(2):79–84. https://doi.org/10.4103/0971-5851.158829.

Indian Council of Medical Research consensus statement

- Valle JW, Borbath I, Khan SA, Huguet F, Gruenberger T, Arnold D; ESMO Guidelines Committee. Biliary cancer: ESMO Clinical Practice Guidelines for diagnosis, treatment and follow-up. Ann Oncol. 2016;27(Suppl 5):v28–37.

European Society of Medical Oncology Guidelines

18.2.2 Books

- Pandey M, Shukla VK, editors. Gallbladder cancer. New Delhi: Jaypee; 2004. p. 1–292.
- Agarwal A, Fong Y, editors. Carcinoma of the gallbladder. The current scenario. New Delhi: Elsevier; 2014. p. 1–183.

18.2.3 Special Issues of Journals

- Kapoor VK, Guest editor. Special topic on 'Gall Bladder Cancer'. Hepato-Gastroenterology (International Gastro-Surgical Club). 1999;46:1527–94. Contributors from Chile, France, Japan, Netherlands, UK and USA
- Shukla HS, Guest editor. Gall bladder cancer. J Surg Oncol. 2006;93:597–708.
- Ghassan K. Abou-Alfa. Chin Clin Oncol. 2019;8(4) August 2019.

18.3 Chile

18.3.1 Hospital Temuco, Universidad de la Frontera, Temuco Chile

Xabier de Aretxabala and Ivan Roa

- de Aretxabala X, Roa I, Araya JC, Burgos L, Flores P, Huenchullan I, Miyazaki I. Operative findings in patients with early forms of gallbladder cancer. Br J Surg. 1990;77(3):291–3.
- de Aretxabala X, Roa I, Burgos L, Araya JC, Fonseca L, Wistuba I, Flores P. Gallbladder cancer in Chile. A report on 54 potentially resectable tumors. Cancer. 1992;69(1):60–5.
- de Aretxabala X, Roa I, Araya JC, Burgos L, Flores P, Wistuba I, Villaseca MA, Sotomayor F, Roa JC. Gallbladder cancer in patients less than 40 years old. Br J Surg. 1994;81(1):111.
- de Aretxabala X, Roa I, Burgos L, Araya JC, Silva J, Siegel S. Laparoscopic cholecystectomy and gallbladder cancer. Surgery. 1995;117(4):479–80.
- Roa I, Araya JC, Villaseca M, De Aretxabala X, Riedemann P, Endoh K, Roa J. Preneoplastic lesions and gallbladder cancer: an estimate of the period required for progression. Gastroenterology. 1996;111(1):232–6.
- de Aretxabala XA, Roa IS, Burgos LA, Araya JC, Villaseca MA, Silva JA. Curative resection in potentially resectable tumours of the gallbladder. Eur J Surg. 1997;163(6):419–26.
- de Aretxabala X, Roa I, Burgos L, Cartes R, Silva J, Yañez E, Araya JC, Villaseca M, Quijada I, Vittini C. Preoperative chemoradiotherapy in the treatment of gallbladder cancer. Am Surg. 1999;65(3):241–6.
- Roa I, Araya JC, Villaseca M, Roa J, de Aretxabala X, Ibacache G. Gallbladder cancer in a high risk area: morphological features and spread patterns. Hepatogastroenterology. 1999;46(27):1540–6.
- de Aretxabala X, Roa I, Burgos L. Gallbladder cancer, management of early tumors. Hepatogastroenterology. 1999;46(27):1547–51. Review.
- de Aretxabala XA, Roa IS, Mora JP, Orellana JJ, Riedeman JP, Burgos LA, Silva VP, Cuadra AJ, Wanebo HJ. Laparoscopic cholecystectomy: its effect on the prognosis of patients with gallbladder cancer. World J Surg. 2004;28(6):544–7.
- de Aretxabala X, Roa I, Burgos L, Losada H, Roa JC, Mora J, Hepp J, Leon J, Maluenda F. Gallbladder cancer: an analysis of a series of 139 patients with invasion restricted to the subserosal layer. J Gastrointest Surg. 2006;10(2):186–92.
- Roa I, de Aretxabala X, Araya JC, Roa J. Preneoplastic lesions in gallbladder cancer. J Surg Oncol. 2006;93(8):615–23. Review.
- Roa I, Ibacache G, Roa J, Araya J, de Aretxabala X, Muñoz S. Gallstones and gallbladder cancer-volume and weight of gallstones are associated with gallbladder cancer: a case-control study. J Surg Oncol. 2006;93(8):624–8.
- de Aretxabala X, Roa I, Hepp J, Maluenda F, Mordojovich G, Leon J, Roa JC. Early gallbladder cancer: is further treatment necessary? J Surg Oncol. 2009;100(7):589–93. https://doi.org/10.1002/jso.21389.
- de Aretxabala X, Leon J, Hepp J, Maluenda F, Roa I. Gallbladder cancer: role of laparoscopy

in the management of potentially resectable tumors. Surg Endosc. 2010;24(9):2192–6. https://doi.org/10.1007/s00464-010-0925-1. Epub 2010 Feb 23.
- Roa I, Ibacache G, Muñoz S, de Aretxabala X. Gallbladder cancer in Chile: pathologic characteristics of survival and prognostic factors: analysis of 1,366 cases. Am J Clin Pathol. 2014;141(5):675–82. https://doi.org/10.1309/AJCPQT3ELN2BBCKA.
- Roa I, de Aretxabala X. Gallbladder cancer in Chile: what have we learned? Curr Opin Gastroenterol. 2015;31(3):269–75. https://doi.org/10.1097/MOG.0000000000000164. Review.
- de Aretxabala X, Oppliger F, Solano N, Rencoret G, Vivanco M, Carvajal D, Hepp J, Roa I. Laparoscopic management of incidental gallbladder cancer. Surg Endosc. 2018;32(10):4251–55. https://doi.org/10.1007/s00464-018-6173-5. Epub 2018 Jun 20.
- Gil L, de Aretxabala X, Lendoire J, Duek F, Hepp J, Imventarza O. Incidental gallbladder cancer: how residual disease affects outcome in two referral HPB centers from South America. World J Surg. 2019;43(1):214–20. https://doi.org/10.1007/s00268-018-4762-z.
- Vega EA, De Aretxabala X, Qiao W, et al. Comparison of oncological outcomes after open and laparoscopic re-resection of incidental gallbladder cancer. Br J Surg. 2020;107(3):289–300. https://doi.org/10.1002/bjs.11379.

18.4 Germany

Thorsten O Goetze and Vittorio Paolucci

The Central Registry of Incidental GBC of the German Society of Surgery, founded in 1997, covering 883 cases from 167 centers, has produced a large number of high-quality publications which virtually form the guidelines for management of incidental GBC.

- Paolucci V. Port site recurrences after laparoscopic cholecystectomy. J Hepatobiliary Pancreat Surg. 2001;8(6):535–43. Review.
- Goetze TO, Paolucci V. Does laparoscopy worsen the prognosis for incidental gallbladder cancer? Surg Endosc. 2006;20(2):286–93. Epub 2005 Dec 9.
- Goetze TO, Paolucci V. Benefits of reoperation of T2 and more advanced incidental gallbladder carcinoma: analysis of the German registry. Ann Surg. 2008;247(1):104–8.
- Goetze TO, Paolucci V. Immediate re-resection of T1 incidental gallbladder carcinomas: a survival analysis of the German Registry. Surg Endosc. 2008;22(11):2462–5. https://doi.org/10.1007/s00464-008-9747-9. Epub 2008 Feb 5.
- Goetze TO, Paolucci V. Use of retrieval bags in incidental gallbladder cancer cases. World J Surg. 2009;33(10):2161–5. https://doi.org/10.1007/s00268-009-0163-7.
- Goetze TO, Paolucci V. Adequate extent in radical re-resection of incidental gallbladder carcinoma: analysis of the German Registry. Surg Endosc. 2010;24(9):2156–64. https://doi.org/10.1007/s00464-010-0914-4. Epub 2010 Feb 23.
- Goetze TO, Paolucci V. The prognostic impact of positive lymph nodes in stages T1 to T3 incidental gallbladder carcinoma: results of the German Registry. Surg Endosc. 2012;26(5):1382–9. https://doi.org/10.1007/s00464-011-2044-z. Epub 2011 Nov 17.
- Goetze TO, Paolucci V. Prognosis of incidental gallbladder carcinoma is not influenced by the primary access technique: analysis of 837 incidental gallbladder carcinomas in the German Registry. Surg Endosc. 2013;27(8):2821–8. https://doi.org/10.1007/s00464-013-2819-5. Epub 2013 Feb 13.
- Goetze TO, Paolucci V. [Incidental T1b–T3 gallbladder carcinoma. Extended cholecystectomy as an underestimated prognostic factor-results of the German registry]. Chirurg. 2014;85(2):131–8. https://doi.org/10.1007/s00104-013-2587-8. German.
- Goetze TO, Paolucci V. Influence of high- and low-volume liver surgery in gallbladder carcinoma. World J Gastroenterol. 2014;20(48):18445–51. https://doi.org/10.3748/wjg.v20.i48.18445.

- Goetze TO, Paolucci V. [Immediate radical re-resection of incidental T1b gallbladder cancer and the problem of an adequate extent of resection (results of the German Registry "Incidental Gallbladder Cancer")]. Zentralbl Chir. 2014;139 Suppl 2:e43–8. https://doi.org/10.1055/s-0030-1262698. Epub 2011 Mar 1. German.

18.5 Japan

18.5.1 Nagoya University School of Medicine (NUSM), Nagoya Japan

Yuji Nimura and Masato Nagino

- Nimura Y, Hayakawa N, Kamiya J, Maeda S, Kondo S, Yasui A, Shionoya S. Hepatopancreatoduodenectomy for advanced carcinoma of the biliary tract. Hepatogastroenterology. 1991;38(2):170–5.
- Kondo S, Nimura Y, Hayakawa N, Kamiya J, Nagino M, Uesaka K. Regional and para-aortic lymphadenectomy in radical surgery for advanced gallbladder carcinoma. Br J Surg. 2000;87(4):418–22.
- Kondo S, Nimura Y, Kamiya J, Nagino M, Kanai M, Uesaka K, Yuasa N, Sano T, Hayakawa N. Five-year survivors after aggressive surgery for stage IV gallbladder cancer. J Hepatobiliary Pancreat Surg. 2001;8(6):511–7.

Out of 59 patients with stage IV GBC who underwent radial resection between 1979 and 1994, 6 survived for more than 5 years.

- Kondo S, Nimura Y, Hayakawa N, Kamiya J, Nagino M, Uesaka K. Extensive surgery for carcinoma of the gallbladder. Br J Surg. 2002;89(2):179–84.

Between 1979 and 1944, 116 GBC patients were operated—radical resection was performed in 80. Sixty-eight of these 80 patients had stage III/IV disease—they underwent ERH (n = 40), PD (n = 23), and/or portal vein resection (n = 23). Hospital mortality was 18%. Three and 5-year survival were 44% and 33% for Stage III and 24% and 17% for M0 stage IV disease and 7% and 3% for M1 stage IV disease.

- Kondo S, Nimura Y, Kamiya J, Nagino M, Kanai M, Uesaka K, Hayakawa N. Mode of tumor spread and surgical strategy in gallbladder carcinoma. Langenbecks Arch Surg. 2002;387(5–6):222–8. Epub 2002 Oct 2.

Review of 112 patients (stage I = 9, II = 11, III = 154 and IV = 78) who underwent curative resection; identified six types of spread

1. Hepatic bed type—large mass in GB fundes/body infiltrating the liver
2. Hepatic hilum type—small tumor in GB neck infiltrating the hepatic hilum
3. Hepatic bed + hilum type
4. LN type
5. Cystic duct type—small tumor in cystic duct infiltrating the CBD
6. Localized to GB

- Yamaguchi R, Nagino M, Oda K, Kamiya J, Uesaka K, Nimura Y. Perineural invasion has a negative impact on survival of patients with gallbladder carcinoma. Br J Surg. 2002;89(9):1130–6.
- Kondo S, Nimura Y, Kamiya J, Nagino M, Kanai M, Uesaka K, Yuasa N, Sano T, Hayakawa N. Factors influencing postoperative hospital mortality and long-term survival after radical resection for stage IV gallbladder carcinoma. World J Surg. 2003;27(3):272–7. Epub 2003 Feb 27.

Seventy-two patients (48, 67% had jaundice) with stage IV GBC underwent major procedures with curative intent—hospital mortality was 14 (19%); 11 patients survived more than 3 years (no mention of 5-year survival).

- Nagino M, Kamiya J, Nishio H, Ebata T, Arai T, Nimura Y. Two hundred forty consecutive portal vein embolizations before extended hepatectomy for biliary cancer: surgical outcome and long-term follow-up. Ann Surg. 2006;243(3):364–72.

Portal vein embolization (PVE) in 240 cases (GBC $n = 90$)

- Nishio H, Nagino M, Ebata T, Yokoyama Y, Igami T, Nimura Y. Aggressive surgery for stage IV gallbladder carcinoma; what are the contraindications? J Hepatobiliary Pancreat Surg. 2007;14(4):351–7. Epub 2007 Jul 30.

Seventy-nine major hepatectomy and 38 hepato-pancreato-duodenectomy (HPD) performed between 1996 and 2016

- Ebata T, Nagino M, Nishio H, Arai T, Nimura Y. Right hepatopancreatoduodenectomy: improvements over 23 years to attain acceptability. J Hepatobiliary Pancreat Surg. 2007;14(2):131–5. Epub 2007 Mar 27.

Fifty-eight hepato-pancreato-duodenectomy (HPD) (GBC $n = 33$) between 1981 and 2004

- Nishio H, Nagino M, Ebata T, Yokoyama Y, Igami T, Nimura Y. Aggressive surgery for stage IV gallbladder carcinoma; what are the contraindications? J Hepatobiliary Pancreat Surg. 2007;14(4):351–7. Epub 2007 Jul 30.

(1977–2004) 229 GBCs operated (stage I = 10, II = 11, III = 17, IV = 166)—96 had jaundice. One hundred and sixty-six stage IV patients—major hepatectomy 101, extrahepatic bile duct resection (EHBDR) 141, portal vein resection (PVR) 45, hepato-pancreato-duodenectomy (HPD) 33. Twenty-five survived for 3 years, 15 survived for 5 years, and 7 survived for 10 years. Median survival was 0.8 years and 3, 5, and 10 years survival were 19%, 12%, and 10%.

- Yokoyama Y, Nishio H, Ebata T, Abe T, Igami T, Oda K, Nimura Y, Nagino M. New classification of cystic duct carcinoma. World J Surg. 2008;32(4):621–6. https://doi.org/10.1007/s00268-007-9324-8.
- Nishio H, Ebata T, Yokoyama Y, Igami T, Sugawara G, Nagino M. Gallbladder cancer involving the extrahepatic bile duct is worthy of resection. Ann Surg. 2011;253(5):953–60. https://doi.org/10.1097/SLA.0b013e318216f5f3.
- Ebata T, Yokoyama Y, Igami T, Sugawara G, Takahashi Y, Nagino M. Portal vein embolization before extended hepatectomy for biliary cancer: current technique and review of 494 consecutive embolizations. Dig Surg. 2012;29(1):23–9. https://doi.org/10.1159/000335718. Epub 2012 Mar 15.

Portal vein embolization (GBC $n = 141$)

- Ebata T, Yokoyama Y, Igami T, Sugawara G, Mizuno T, Nagino M. Review of hepatopancreatoduodenectomy for biliary cancer: an extended radical approach of Japanese origin. J Hepatobiliary Pancreat Sci. 2014;21(8):550–5. https://doi.org/10.1002/jhbp.80. Epub 2014 Jan 27. Review.
- Takahashi Y, Ebata T, Yokoyama Y, Igami T, Sugawara G, Mizuno T, Nimura Y, Nagino M. Surgery for recurrent biliary tract cancer: a single-center experience with 74 consecutive resections. Ann Surg. 2015;262(1):121–9. https://doi.org/10.1097/SLA.0000000000000827.
- Igami T, Ebata T, Yokoyama Y, Sugawara G, Nagino M. Advanced resectable gallbladder cancer: diagnosis and surgical approach. In: Agarwal A, Fong Y, editors. Carcinoma of the gall bladder. New Delhi: Elsevier; 2014. p. 89–105.

Four hundred and eighty-five patients with GBC were treated between 1979 and 2011—292 (64%) underwent surgical resections—out of 192 resected patients, 165 had T3, T4—152 underwent hepatectomy (GB bed 22, segments IVB + V 21, central 4, right hepatectomy 89, ERH 16)—EHBDR was performed in 149 (90%), CRAO in 88 (53%), including HPD $n = 53$, PVR in 59 (36%) R0 resection status was achieved in 135 (82%) patients. Mortality in advanced (T3, T4) GBC was 12% (20/165). Three-, 5-, and 10-year survival in advanced GBC ($n = 165$) was 34%, 25%, and 16% median survival was 18 months; 25 patients survived more than 5 years and 11 patients survived more than 10 years.

- Igami T, Ebata T, Yokoyama Y, Sugawara G, Mizuno T, Yamaguchi J, Shimoyama Y, Nagino M. Combined extrahepatic bile duct resection for locally advanced gallbladder carcinoma: does it work? World J Surg. 2015;39(7):1810–7. https://doi.org/10.1007/s00268-015-3011-y.
- Mizuno T, Ebata T, Yokoyama Y, Igami T, Yamaguchi J, Onoe S, Watanabe N, Ando M, Nagino M. Major hepatectomy with or without pancreatoduodenectomy for advanced gallbladder cancer. Br J Surg. 2019;106(5):626–35. https://doi.org/10.1002/bjs.11088. Epub 2019 Feb 14.

One hundred and seventeen patients with GBC underwent major hepatectomy between 1996 and 2016 (including 38 HPD)—mortality 11/117 (9%) (7/38 18% for HPD)

18.5.2 Niigata University, Niigata Japan

Yoshio Shirai and Toshifumi Wakai

More than 1000 resection for GBC 1982–2018

- Shirai Y, Yoshida K, Tsukada K, Muto T, Watanabe H. Radical surgery for gallbladder carcinoma: long-term results. Ann Surg. 1992;216:565–8.
- Shirai Y, Yoshida K, Tsukada K, Muto T. Inapparent carcinoma of the gallbladder: an appraisal of a radical second operation after simple cholecystectomy. Ann Surg. 1992;215:326–31.
- Shirai Y, Yoshida K, Tsukada K, Muto T. Identification of the regional lymphatic system of the gallbladder by vital staining. Br J Surg. 1992;79:659–62.
- Ootani T, Shirai Y, Tsukada K, Muto T. Relationship between gallbladder carcinoma and the segmental type of adenomyomatosis of the gallbladder. Cancer. 1992;69:2647–52.
- Shirai Y, Yoshida K, Tsukada K, Muto T, Watanabe H. Early carcinoma of the gallbladder. Eur J Surg. 1992;158:545–8.
- Ohtani T, Shirai Y, Tsukada K, Hatakeyama K, Muto T. Carcinoma of the gallbladder: CT evaluation of lymphatic spread. Radiology. 1993;189:875–80.
- Tsukada K, Yoshida K, Aono S, Koyama Y, Shirai Y, Uchida K, Muto T. Major hepatectomy and pancreaticoduodenectomy for advanced carcinoma of the biliary tract. Br J Surg. 1994;81:108–10.
- Shirai Y, Tsukada K, Ohtani T, Watanabe H, Hatakeyama K. Hepatic metastases from carcinoma of the gallbladder. Cancer. 1995;75:2063–8.
- Tsukada K, Hatakeyama K, Kurosaki I, Uchida K, Shirai Y, Muto T, Yoshida K. Outcome of radical surgery for carcinoma of the gallbladder according to the TNM stage. Surgery. 1996;120:816–22.
- Ohtani T, Shirai Y, Tsukada K, Muto T, Hatakeyama K. Spread of gallbladder carcinoma: CT evaluation with pathologic correlation. Abdom Imaging. 1996;21:195–201.
- Shirai Y, Ohtani T, Tsukada K, Hatakeyama K. Combined pancreaticoduodenectomy and hepatectomy for patients with locally advanced gallbladder carcinoma: long term results. Cancer. 1997;80:1904–9.
- Tsukada K, Kurosaki I, Uchida K, Shirai Y, Oohashi Y, Yokoyama N, Watanabe H, Hatakeyama K. Lymph node spread from carcinoma of the gallbladder. Cancer. 1997;80:661–7.
- Yokoyama N, Shirai Y, Hatakeyama K. Immunohistochemical detection of lymph node micrometastases from gallbladder carcinoma using monoclonal anticytokeratin antibody. Cancer. 1999;85:1465–9.

- Nagakura S, Shirai Y, Yokoyama N, Hatakeyama K. Clinical significance of lymph node micrometastasis in gallbladder carcinoma. Surgery. 2001;129:704–13.
- Wakai T, Shirai Y, Yokoyama N, Nagakura S, Watanabe H, Hatakeyama K. Early gallbladder carcinoma does not warrant radical resection. Br J Surg. 2001;88(5):675–8.
- Wakai T, Shirai Y, Hatakeyama K. Radical second resection provides survival benefit for patients with T2 gallbladder carcinoma first discovered after laparoscopic cholecystectomy. World J Surg. 2002;26(7):867–71. Epub 2002 Apr 18.
- Oohashi Y, Shirai Y, Wakai T, Nagakura S, Watanabe H, Hatakeyama K. Adenosquamous carcinoma of the gallbladder warrants resection only if curative resection is feasible. Cancer. 2002;94:3000–5.
- Wakai T, Shirai Y, Yokoyama N, Ajioka Y, Watanabe H, Hatakeyama K. Depth of subserosal invasion predicts long-term survival after resection in patients with T2 gallbladder carcinoma. Ann Surg Oncol. 2003;10(4):447–54.
- Shirai Y, Wakai T, Hatakeyama K. Radical lymph node dissection for gallbladder cancer: indication and limitation. Surg Oncol Clin N Am. 2007;16:221–32.
- Nagahashi M, Shirai Y, Wakai T, Sakata J, Ajioka Y, Hatakeyama K. Perimuscular connective tissue contains more and larger lymphatic vessels than the shallower layers in human gallbladders. World J Gastroenterol. 2007;13(33):4480–3.
- Nagahashi M, Ajioka Y, Lang I, Szentirmay Z, Kasler M, Nakadaira H, Yokoyama N, Watanabe G, Nishikura K, Wakai T, Shirai Y, Hatakeyama K, Yamamoto M. Genetic changes of p53, K-ras, and microsatellite instability in gallbladder carcinoma in high-incidence areas of Japan and Hungary. World J Gastroenterol. 2008;14:70–5.
- Wakai T, Shirai Y, Tsuchiya Y, Nomura T, Akazawa K, Hatakeyama K. Combined major hepatectomy and pancreaticoduodenectomy for locally advanced biliary carcinoma: long-term results. World J Surg. 2008;32(6):1067–74. https://doi.org/10.1007/s00268-007-9393-8.

HPD in 28 patients (GBC $n = 11$)—mortality 21%; 5-year survival 11% median survival 9 months

- Wakai T, Shirai Y, Sakata J, Nagahashi M, Ajioka Y, Hatakeyama K. Mode of hepatic spread from gallbladder carcinoma: an immunohistochemical analysis of 42 hepatectomized specimens. Am J Surg Pathol. 2010;34(1):65–74. https://doi.org/10.1097/PAS.0b013e3181c467d4.

Description of modes of hepatic spread of GBC

- Sakata J, Shirai Y, Wakai T, Ajioka Y, Hatakeyama K. Number of positive lymph nodes independently determines the prognosis after resection in patients with gallbladder carcinoma. Ann Surg Oncol. 2010;17(7):1831–40. Epub 2010 Jan 15.

Analysis of 116 patients with GBC who underwent R0 radical resection—number, not location, of positive LNs determined the prognosis

- Wakai T, Ajioka Y, Nagino N, Yamaguchi N, Shirai Y, Hatakeyama K. Morphological features of early gallbladder carcinoma. Hepatogastroenterology. 2012;59(116):1013–7. https://doi.org/10.5754/hge11923.

Two hundred and twenty-nine patients with early GBC identified from surgical pathology database from 1982 to 2010—107 were protruding and 192 were superficial

- Wakai T, Shirai Y, Sakata J, Tsuchiya Y, Nomura T, Hatakeyama K. Surgical outcomes of minor hepatectomy for locally advanced gallbladder carcinoma. Hepatogastroenterology. 2012;59(119):2083–8.

Wedge resection in 58 patients and S4bS5 resection in 12 patients—3-year survival was 74% and 60%, respectively

- Shirai Y, Sakata J, Wakai T, Hatakeyama K. Full-thickness cholecystectomy with limited lymphadenectomy for gallbladder cancer. Hepatogastroenterology. 2012;59(117):1338–40. https://doi.org/10.5754/hge12276.

Cholecystectomy with removal of the entire cystic plate and removal of the first echelon LNs only in 12 elderly patients with comorbidities who had tumor confined to GB wall—5-year survival was 100% and median survival was 229 months

- Shirai Y, Wakai T, Sakata J, Hatakeyama K. Regional lymphadenectomy for gallbladder cancer: rational extent, technical details, and patient outcomes. World J Gastroenterol. 2012;18(22):2775–83. https://doi.org/10.3748/wjg.v18.i22.2775.

One hundred and fifty-two patients with GBC underwent "extended" portal LN dissection including first and second echelon LNs

- Shirai Y, Sakata J, Wakai T, Ohashi T, Hatakeyama K. "Extended" radical cholecystectomy for gallbladder cancer: long-term outcomes, indications and limitations. World J Gastroenterol. 2012;18(34):4736–43.

One hundred and forty-five patients with GBC underwent radical resection between 1982 and 2006—52 (T1 $n = 3$, T2 $n = 36$, T3 $n = 12$ and T4 $n = 1$) had extended radical cholecystectomy including the extrahepatic bile duct. Overall survival after extended radical cholecystectomy was 65% at 5 years and 53% at 10 years.

- Shirai Y, Sakata J, Wakai T, Ohashi T, Ajioka Y, Hatakeyama K. Assessment of lymph node status in gallbladder cancer: location, number, or ratio of positive nodes. World J Surg Oncol. 2012;10:87. https://doi.org/10.1186/1477-7819-10-87.

One hundred and thirty-five patients with GBC underwent radical resection with regional lymphadenectomy—the number of positive LNs (0, 1 to 3, or >3) was better predictor of survival than the location of the LNs.

- Sakata J, Kobayashi T, Tajima Y, Ohashi T, Hirose Y, Takano K, Takizawa K, Miura K, Wakai T. Relevance of dissection of the posterior superior pancreatico-duodenal lymph nodes in gallbladder carcinoma. Ann Surg Oncol. 2017;24(9):2474–81. https://doi.org/10.1245/s10434-017-5939-7. Epub 2017 Jun 26.

In 148 patients with GBC who underwent radical resection, 5-year survival in patients with posterior superior pancreaticoduodenal LN involvement was 56% versus 15% in those with LNs involved beyond these LNs

- Sakata J, Kobayashi T, Ohashi T, Hirose Y, Takano K, Takizawa K, Miura K, Ishikawa H, Toge K, Yuza K, Soma D, Ando T, Wakai T. Prognostic heterogeneity of the seventh edition of UICC Stage III gallbladder carcinoma: which patients benefit from surgical resection? Eur J Surg Oncol. 2017;43(4):780–7. https://doi.org/10.1016/j.ejso.2017.01.001. Epub 2017 Jan 19.

In 175 patients with GBC who underwent radical resection, 5-year survival in AJCC—UICC stage IIIB was better than in stage IIIA. Patients with 1–2 positive LNs had better survival than those with >3 positive LNs.

- Toge K, Sakata J, Hirose Y, Yuza K, Ando T, Soma D, Katada T, Miura K, Takizawa K, Kobayashi T, Wakai T. Lymphatic spread of T2 gallbladder carcinoma: regional lymphadenectomy is required independent of tumor location. Eur J Surg Oncol. 2019 30. pii: S0748-7983(19)30383-X. https://doi.org/10.1016/j.ejso.2019.03.038. [Epub ahead of print].

In 81 patients with T2 GBC, incidence of regional LN metastasis was higher (46% vs.

20%) in T2b ($n = 56$) versus T2a ($n = 25$) tumors, but the authors recommended that the extent of lymphadenectomy should be same for both

- Yuza K, Sakata J, Prasoon P, et al. Long-term outcomes of surgical resection for T1b gallbladder cancer: an institutional evaluation. BMC Cancer. 2020;20(1):20. Published 2020 Jan 6. https://doi.org/10.1186/s12885-019-6507-2.

18.5.3 Tokyo Womens Medical University (TWMU), Tokyo Japan

Masakazu Yamamoto and Ryota Higuchi

- Yamamoto M, Onoyama H, Ajiki T, Yamada I, Fujita T, Saitoh Y. Surgical results of operations for carcinoma of the gallbladder. Hepatogastroenterology. 1999;46(27):1552–6.
- Higuchi R, Yamamoto M. Aggressive surgical management and treatment outcomes of gallbladder cancer. In: Agarwal A, Fong Y, editors. Carcinoma of the gall bladder. New Delhi: Elsevier; 2014. p. 175–83.

Three hundred and eighty-two resections between 1969 and 2012—5-year survival 98.5% for UICC stage I ($n = 28$), 85% for II ($n = 32$), 40% for IIIA ($n = 35$), 53% for IIIB ($n = 56$), 0% for IVA ($n = 30$), and 18% for IVB. Mortality reduced from 13% in 239 cases manage between 1969 and 1999 to 3% in 143 cases managed during 2000–2013

- Higuchi R, Ota T, Araida T, Kajiyama H, Yazawa T, Furukawa T, Yoshikawa T, Takasaki K, Yamamoto M. Surgical approaches to advanced gallbladder cancer: a 40-year single-institution study of prognostic factors and resectability. Ann Surg Oncol. 2014;21(13):4308–16. https://doi.org/10.1245/s10434-014-3885-1. Epub 2014 Jul 15.
- Higuchi R, Yazawa T, Uemura S, Izumo W, Chaudhary RJ, Furukawa T, Yamamoto M. ENBD is associated with decreased tumor dissemination compared to PTBD in perihilar cholangiocarcinoma. J Gastrointest Surg. 2017;21(9):1506–14. https://doi.org/10.1007/s11605-017-3492-0. Epub 2017 Jul 18.
- Ota T, Araida T, Yamamoto M, Takasaki K. Operative outcome and problems of right hepatic lobectomy with pancreatoduodenectomy for advanced carcinoma of the biliary tract. J Hepatobiliary Pancreat Surg. 2007;14(2):155–8. Epub 2007 Mar 27.
- Chaudhary RK, Higuchi R, Yazawa T, Uemura S, Izumo W, Furukawa T, Kiyohara K, Yamamoto M. Surgery in node-positive gallbladder cancer: the implication of an involved superior retro-pancreatic lymph node. Surgery. 2019;165(3):541–7. https://doi.org/10.1016/j.surg.2018.09.003. Epub 2018 Oct 19.

18.6 South Korea

18.6.1 Seoul National University Bundang Hospital (SNUBH), Seongnam-si, South Korea

Ho-Seong Han and Yoo-Seok Yoon

- Cho JY, Han HS, Yoon YS, Ahn KS, Kim YH, Lee KH. Laparoscopic approach for suspected early-stage gallbladder carcinoma. Arch Surg. 2010;145(2):128–33.
- Kim H, Song JY, Cho JY, Yoon YS, Han HS, Lee HS, Ryu HS, Choe G. Strong cytoplasmic expression of COX2 at the invasive fronts of gallbladder cancer is associated with a poor prognosis. J Clin Pathol. 2010;63(12):1048–53.
- Han HS, Cho JY, Yoon YS, Ahn KS, Kim H. Preoperative inflammation is a prognostic factor for gallbladder carcinoma. Br J Surg. 2011;98(1):111–6.
- Yoon YS, Han HS, Cho JY, Choi Y, Lee W, Jang JY, Choi H. Is laparoscopy contraindicated for gallbladder cancer? A 10-year prospective cohort study. J Am Coll Surg. 2015;221(4):847–53. https://doi.org.10.1016/j.jamcollsurg.2015.07.010. Epub 2015 Jul 20.
- Park JH, Kim YH, Kim H, Yoon YS, Choi YR, Cho JY, Lee YJ, Han HS. Determining the

extent of cholecystectomy using intraoperative specimen ultrasonography in patients with suspected early gallbladder cancer. Surg Endosc. 2016;30(10):4229–38.

- Kim S, Yoon YS, Han HS, Cho JY, Choi Y. Laparoscopic extended cholecystectomy for T3 gallbladder cancer. Surg Endosc. 2018;32(6):2984–5. https://doi.org/10.1007/s00464-017-5952-8. Epub 2017 Dec 7.
- Han HS, Yoon YS, Agarwal AK, Belli G, Itano O, Gumbs AA, Yoon DS, Kang CM, Lee SE, Wakai T, Troisi RI. Laparoscopic surgery for gallbladder cancer: an expert consensus statement. Dig Surg. 2019;36(1):1–6.
- Jang JY, Han HS, Yoon YS, Cho JY, Choi Y. Retrospective comparison of outcomes of laparoscopic and open surgery for T2 gallbladder cancer - thirteen-year experience. Surg Oncol. 2019;29:142–7. https://doi.org/10.1016/j.suronc.2019.05.007. Epub 2019 May 13.
- Yoon YS, Han HS, Agarwal A, Belli G, Itano O, Gumbs AA, Yoon DS, Kang CM, Lee SE, Wakai T, Troisi RI. Survey results of the expert meeting on laparoscopic surgery for gallbladder cancer and a review of relevant literature. Dig Surg. 2019;36(1):7–12

18.6.2 Seoul National University Hospital (SNUH), Seoul, South Korea

Jin-Young Jang and Sun-Whe Kim

- Kim SW, Her KH, Jang JY, Kim WH, Kim YT, Park YH. K-ras oncogene mutation in cancer and precancerous lesions of the gallbladder. J Surg Oncol. 2000;75(4):246–51.
- Jang JY, Kim SW, Lee SE, Hwang DW, Kim EJ, Lee JY, Kim SJ, Ryu JK, Kim YT. Differential diagnostic and staging accuracies of high resolution ultrasonography, endoscopic ultrasonography, and multidetector computed tomography for gallbladder polypoid lesions and gallbladder cancer. Ann Surg. 2009;250(6):943–9. https://doi.org/10.1097/SLA.0b013e3181b5d5fc.
- Kwon W, Jang JY, Lee SE, Hwang DW, Kim SW. Clinicopathologic features of polypoid lesions of the gallbladder and risk factors of gallbladder cancer. J Korean Med Sci. 2009;24(3):481–7. https://doi.org/10.3346/jkms.2009.24.3.481. Epub 2009 Jun 12.
- Lee SE, Jang JY, Lim CS, Kang MJ, Kim SW. Systematic review on the surgical treatment for T1 gallbladder cancer. World J Gastroenterol. 2011;17(2):174–80. https://doi.org/10.3748/wjg.v17.i2.174. Review.
- Kang MJ, Song Y, Jang JY, Han IW, Kim SW. Role of radical surgery in patients with stage IV gallbladder cancer. HPB (Oxford). 2012;14(12):805–11. https://doi.org/10.1111/j.1477-2574.2012.00544.x. Epub 2012 Aug 20.
- 1996–2010—421 operated (stage IV 94—16 surgery with curative intent—15 R0—13 recurrence, median 7 months, 1 year DFS 27%)
- Kim K, Chie EK, Jang JY, Kim SW, Han SW, Oh DY, Im SA, Kim TY, Bang YJ, Ha SW. Postoperative chemoradiotherapy for gallbladder cancer. Strahlenther Onkol. 2012;188(5):388–92. https://doi.org/10.1007/s00066-012-0074-7. Epub 2012 Mar 10.
- Lim CS, Jang JY, Lee SE, Kang MJ, Kim SW. Reappraisal of hepato-pancreato-duodenectomy as a treatment modality for bile duct and gallbladder cancer. J Gastrointest Surg. 2012;16(5):1012–8. https://doi.org/10.1007/s11605-012-1826-5. Epub 2012 Jan 24.
- Chang J, Jang JY, Lee KB, Kang MJ, Jung W, Shin YC, Kim SW. Improvement of clinical outcomes in the patients with gallbladder cancer: lessons from periodic comparison in a tertiary referral center. J Hepatobiliary Pancreat Sci. 2016;23(4):234–41. https://doi.org/10.1002/jhbp.330. Epub 2016 Mar 1.

1987–2014 692 GBC patients operated—curative resection in 59%, 5-year survival 67%

- Chang J, Jang JY, Kang MJ, Jung W, Shin YC, Kim SW. Clinicopathologic differences in patients with gallbladder cancer according to the presence of anomalous biliopancreatic junction. World J Surg. 2016;40(5):1211–7. https://doi.org/10.1007/s00268-015-3359-z.
- Jung W, Jang JY, Kang MJ, Chang YR, Shin YC, Chang J, Kim SW. Effects of surgical methods and tumor location on survival and recurrence patterns after curative resection in patients with T2 gallbladder cancer. Gut Liver. 2016;10(1):140–6. https://doi.org/10.5009/gnl15080.
- Lee H, Kwon W, Han Y, Kim JR, Kim SW, Jang JY. Optimal extent of surgery for early gallbladder cancer with regard to long-term survival: a meta-analysis. J Hepatobiliary Pancreat Sci. 2018;25(2):131–41. https://doi.org/10.1002/jhbp.521. Epub 2017 Dec 14. Review.
- Wi Y, Woo H, Won YJ, Jang JY, Shin A. Trends in gallbladder cancer incidence and survival in Korea. Cancer Res Treat. 2018;50(4):1444–51. https://doi.org/10.4143/crt.2017.279. Epub 2018 Jan 24.

18.7 United States

18.7.1 Memorial Sloan Kettering Cancer Center (MSKCC), New York USA

Leslie H. Blumgart, Yuman Fong, and William R. Jarnagin

- Fong Y, Brennan MF, Turnbull A, Colt DG, Blumgart LH. Gallbladder cancer discovered during laparoscopic surgery. Potential for iatrogenic tumor dissemination. Arch Surg. 1993;128(9):1054–6.
- Blumgart LH, Fong Y. Surgical options in the treatment of hepatic metastasis from colorectal cancer. Curr Probl Surg. 1995;32(5):333–421. Review.
- Bartlett DL, Fong Y, Fortner JG, Brennan MF, Blumgart LH. Long-term results after resection for gallbladder cancer. Implications for staging and management. Ann Surg. 1996;224(5):639–46. Review.
- Fong Y, Heffernan N, Blumgart LH. Gallbladder carcinoma discovered during laparoscopic cholecystectomy: aggressive reresection is beneficial. Cancer. 1998;83(3):423–7.
- Jarnagin WR, Burke E, Powers C, Fong Y, Blumgart LH. Intrahepatic biliary enteric bypass provides effective palliation in selected patients with malignant obstruction at the hepatic duct confluence. Am J Surg. 1998;175(6):453–60.

Segment III biliary bypass in 21 patients

- Bartlett DL. Gallbladder cancer. Semin Surg Oncol. 2000;19(2):145–55. Review.
- Fong Y, Jarnagin W, Blumgart LH. Gallbladder cancer: comparison of patients presenting initially for definitive operation with those presenting after prior noncurative intervention. Ann Surg. 2000;232(4):557–69.

Effect of prior non-curative intervention on outcome

- Weber SM, DeMatteo RP, Fong Y, Blumgart LH, Jarnagin WR. Staging laparoscopy in patients with extrahepatic biliary carcinoma. Analysis of 100 patients. Ann Surg. 2002;235(3):392–9.

Staging laparoscopy in 44 patients with GBC

- Shoup M, Fong Y. Surgical indications and extent of resection in gallbladder cancer. Surg Oncol Clin N Am. 2002;11(4):985–94. Review.
- Jarnagin WR, Ruo L, Little SA, Klimstra D, D'Angelica M, DeMatteo RP, Wagman R, Blumgart LH, Fong Y. Patterns of initial disease recurrence after resection of gallbladder carcinoma and hilar cholangiocarcinoma: implications for adjuvant therapeutic strategies. Cancer. 2003;98(8):1689–700.

1990–2001—97 resections performed in GBC—majority for incidental GBC, only one in stage III, none in stage IV—median time to disease recurrence was 11.5 months, 66% patients had recurrence 85% of the recurrences were distant (with locoregional) isolated locoregional recurrence was seen in only 15%, median overall survival was 31 months but it was only 21 months in patients with recurrence—recurrence to death interval was 9 months.

- Hawkins WG, DeMatteo RP, Jarnagin WR, Ben-Porat L, Blumgart LH, Fong Y. Jaundice predicts advanced disease and early mortality in patients with gallbladder cancer. Ann Surg Oncol. 2004;11(3):310–5.
- D'Angelica M, Martin RC II, Jarnagin WR, Fong Y, DeMatteo RP, Blumgart LH. Major hepatectomy with simultaneous pancreatectomy for advanced hepatobiliary cancer. J Am Coll Surg. 2004;198(4):570–6.

Seventeeen hepato-pancreato-duodenectomy (HPD)—only 1 for GBC

- Fong Y, Wagman L, Gonen M, Crawford J, Reed W, Swanson R, Pan C, Ritchey J, Stewart A, Choti M. Evidence-based gallbladder cancer staging: changing cancer staging by analysis of data from the National Cancer Database. Ann Surg. 2006;243(6):767–71; discussion 771–4.
- Corvera CU, Blumgart LH, Akhurst T, DeMatteo RP, D'Angelica M, Fong Y, Jarnagin WR. 18F-fluorodeoxyglucose positron emission tomography influences management decisions in patients with biliary cancer. J Am Coll Surg. 2008;206(1):57–65. Epub 2007 Oct 1.
- Duffy A, Capanu M, Abou-Alfa GK, Huitzil D, Jarnagin W, Fong Y, D'Angelica M, Dematteo RP, Blumgart LH, O'Reilly EM. Gallbladder cancer (GBC): 10-year experience at Memorial Sloan-Kettering Cancer Centre (MSKCC). J Surg Oncol. 2008;98(7):485–9. https://doi.org/10.1002/jso.21141.

1995–2005—435 GBCs were treated—159 (37%) had stage IV disease, 206 (47%) were incidental GBC—136/206 (66%) incidental GBCs were reexplored—residual disease was found on histology in 101/136 (74%). R0 resection was achieved in 49 and R1/R2 resection in 52—no residual disease in 35 (26%)—Median survival for incidental GBC was 16 months—if no residual disease was found it was 72 months; in presence of residual disease, it was 19 months after R0 resection and 13 months after R1/R2 resection.

- D'Angelica M, Dalal KM, DeMatteo RP, Fong Y, Blumgart LH, Jarnagin WR. Analysis of the extent of resection for adenocarcinoma of the gallbladder. Ann Surg Oncol. 2009;16(4):806–16. https://doi.org/10.1245/s10434-008-0189-3. Epub 2008 Nov 5.

1990–2002 long-term follow up (median 58 months) in 104 patients who underwent resection, higher (41% vs. 19%) morbidity after major hepatectomy ($n = 36$) and CBD excision ($n = 68$); 5-year disease specific survival (DSS) was 42% ($n = 68$).

- Jayaraman S, Jarnagin WR. Management of gallbladder cancer. Gastroenterol Clin North Am. 2010;39(2):331–42, x. https://doi.org/10.1016/j.gtc.2010.02.006. Review.
- Butte JM, Gönen M, Allen PJ, D'Angelica MI, Kingham TP, Fong Y, Dematteo RP, Blumgart L, Jarnagin WR. The role of laparoscopic staging in patients with incidental gallbladder cancer. HPB (Oxford). 2011;13(7):463–72. https://doi.org/10.1111/j.1477-2574.2011.00325.x. Epub 2011 Jun 7.
- Butte JM, Matsuo K, Gönen M, D'Angelica MI, Waugh E, Allen PJ, Fong Y, DeMatteo RP, Blumgart L, Endo I, De La Fuente H, Jarnagin WR. Gallbladder cancer: differences in presentation, surgical treatment, and survival in patients treated at centers in three countries. J Am Coll Surg. 2011;212(1):50–61. https://doi.org/10.1016/j.jamcollsurg.2010.09.009. Epub 2010 Nov 12.

- Ito H, Ito K, D'Angelica M, Gonen M, Klimstra D, Allen P, DeMatteo RP, Fong Y, Blumgart LH, Jarnagin WR. Accurate staging for gallbladder cancer: implications for surgical therapy and pathological assessment. Ann Surg. 2011;254(2):320–5. https://doi.org/10.1097/SLA.0b013e31822238d8.
- Maker AV, Butte JM, Oxenberg J, Kuk D, Gonen M, Fong Y, Dematteo RP, D'Angelica MI, Allen PJ, Jarnagin WR. Is port site resection necessary in the surgical management of gallbladder cancer? Ann Surg Oncol. 2012;19(2):409–17. https://doi.org/10.1245/s10434-011-1850-9. Epub 2011 Jun 23.
- Butte JM, Torres J, Veras EF, Matsuo K, Gönen M, D'Angelica MI, Waugh E, Meneses M, Inayama Y, Fong Y, Dematteo RP, De La Fuente H, Endo I, Klimstra DS, Jarnagin WR. Regional differences in gallbladder cancer pathogenesis: insights from a comparison of cell cycle-regulatory, PI3K, and pro-angiogenic protein expression. Ann Surg Oncol. 2013;20(5):1470–81. https://doi.org/10.1245/s10434-012-2761-0. Epub 2012 Dec 1.
- Kelly KJ, Dukleska K, Kuk D, Kingham TP, D'Angelica MI, DeMatteo RP, Allen PJ, Jarnagin WR, Fong Y. Prognostic significance of the highest peripancreatic lymph node in biliary tract adenocarcinoma. Ann Surg Oncol. 2014;21(3):979–85. https://doi.org/10.1245/s10434-013-3352-4. Epub 2013 Nov 9.
- Leung U, Pandit-Taskar N, Corvera CU, D'Angelica MI, Allen PJ, Kingham TP, DeMatteo RP, JarnaginWR, Fong Y. Impact of pre-operative positron emission tomography in gallbladder cancer. HPB (Oxford). 2014;16(11):1023–30. https://doi.org/10.1111/hpb.12282. Epub 2014 Jun 4.
- Butte JM, Kingham TP, Gönen M, D'Angelica MI, Allen PJ, Fong Y, DeMatteo RP, Jarnagin WR. Residual disease predicts outcomes after definitive resection for incidental gallbladder cancer. J Am Coll Surg. 2014;219(3):416–29. https://doi.org/10.1016/j.jamcollsurg.2014.01.069. Epub 2014 May 16.
- Creasy JM, Goldman DA, Dudeja V, Lowery MA, Cercek A, Balachandran VP, Allen PJ, DeMatteo RP, Kingham TP, D'Angelica MI, Jarnagin WR. Systemic chemotherapy combined with resection for locally advanced gallbladder carcinoma: surgical and survival outcomes. J Am Coll Surg. 2017;224(5):906–16. https://doi.org/10.1016/j.jamcollsurg.2016.12.058. Epub 2017 Feb 13.
- Creasy JM, Goldman DA, Gonen M, Dudeja V, Askan G, Basturk O, Balachandran VP, Allen PJ, DeMatteo RP, D'Angelica MI, Jarnagin WR, Peter Kingham T. Predicting residual disease in incidental gallbladder cancer: risk stratification for modified treatment strategies. J Gastrointest Surg. 2017;21(8):1254–61. https://doi.org/10.1007/s11605-017-3436-8. Epub 2017 May 8.
- Creasy JM, Goldman DA, Gonen M, Dudeja V, O'Reilly EM, Abou-Alfa GK, Cercek A, Harding JJ, Balachandran VP, Drebin JA, Allen PJ, Kingham TP, D'Angelica MI, Jarnagin WR. Evolution of surgical management of gallbladder carcinoma and impact on outcome: results from two decades at a single-institution. HPB (Oxford). 2019. pii: S1365-182X(19)30496-4. https://doi.org/10.1016/j.hpb.2019.03.370. [Epub ahead of print].

1992–2015—675 patients with GBC evaluated—437 operated—complete resection in 255 (59%)—fewer bile duct resection BDR and major hepatectomy, more neoadjuvant and adjuvant chemotherapy

- Cherkassky L, Jarnagin W. Selecting treatment sequence for patients with incidental gallbladder cancer: a neoadjuvant approach versus upfront surgery. Updates Surg. 2019;71(2):217–25. https://doi.org/10.1007/s13304-019-00670-z. Epub 2019 Jun 28.

18.8 India

18.8.1 Historical Publications

- Prakash A, Sharma LK, Pandit PN. Primary carcinoma of the gall bladder. Br J Surg. 1975;62:33–6.

All India Institute of Medical Sciences (AIIMS), New Delhi (north India) 1959–1974—100 patients operated—cholecystectomy 38 (12 with liver wedge, 6 with hepatic flexure), bypass 10, biopsy only 52—12% mortality—15 survived for 1 year, 3 for 3 years and 2 for 5 years

- Gupta S, Udupa KN, Gupta S. Primary carcinoma of the gall bladder: a review of 328 cases. J Surg Oncol. 1980;14:35–44.

Institute of Medical Sciences (IMS), Banaras Hindu University (BHU), Varanasi (north India)

Three hundred and twenty-eight cases of GBC managed at a university hospital in Varanasi in North India over 10 years (1967–1976)—they constituted 2.9% of all cancers and 31.8% of all GI cancers. Cholecystectomy was done in 42 (all of these had GS and probably had incidental GBC) 5 year survival was a mere 1.8%

- Talwar BL, Kanta C, Gupta NM. Biliary carcinoma: an analysis of 209 personal cases. Indian J Cancer. 1983;20:241–6.

Postgraduate Institute of Medical Education and Research (PGIMER), Chandigarh (north India)

Six hundred and fifty patients with biliary carcinoma were seen (1964–1979)—details of 209 patients treated in one unit were provided. Rescetional surgery could be performed in only 22 (11%) patients. Out of 103 patients with GBC who were followed up, after discharge from the hospital, 98 died within 6 months, 4 died after 12–18 months only 1 died after 2½ years. The 5 patients who lived beyond 6 months were incidental GBC.

- Shukla VK, Khandelwal C, Roy SK, Vaidya MP. Primary carcinoma of the gall bladder. J Surg Oncol. 1985;28:32–5.

Institute of Medical Sciences (IMS), Banaras Hindu University (BHU), Varanasi (north India)—1963–1979—631 patients—315 histologically confirmed—150 operated—cholecystectomy 20, bypass 25—only 2 survived 5 years

- Chattopadhyay TK, Kumar A, Kapoor VK, Sharma LK, Kapur MM, Kapur BM, Dhawan IK. Carcinoma of the gall bladder—can we do anything? Postgrad Med J. 1988;64(754):593–5.

All India Institute of Medical Sciences (AIIMS), New Delhi - 143 cases seen over 5 years - >60% had jaundice - only 42 could be operated - cholecystectomy in 11 + adjacent organ resection in 4 - mortality of surgery 18%

18.8.2 GB Pant Hospital (GBPH), New Delhi India

Anil K. Agarwal

- Agarwal AK, Mandal S, Singh S, Bhojwani R, Sakhuja P, Uppal R. Biliary obstruction in gall bladder cancer is not sine qua non of inoperability. Ann Surg Oncol. 2007;14(10):2831–7.
- Agarwal AK, Mandal S, Singh S, Sakhuja P, Puri S. Gallbladder cancer with duodenal infiltration: is it still resectable? J Gastrointest Surg. 2007;11(12):1722–7. Epub 2007 Sep 29.
- Agarwal AK, Kalayarasan R, Singh S, Javed A, Sakhuja P. All cholecystectomy specimens must be sent for histopathology to detect inapparent gallbladder cancer. HPB (Oxford). 2012;14(4):269–73. https://doi.org/10.1111/j.1477-2574.2012.00443.x. Epub 2012 Feb 26.
- Agarwal AK, Kalayarasan R, Javed A, Gupta N, Nag HH. The role of staging laparoscopy in primary gall bladder cancer—an analysis of 409 patients: a prospective study to evaluate the role of staging laparoscopy in the management of gallbladder cancer. Ann Surg. 2013;258(2):318–23. https://doi.org/10.1097/SLA.0b013e318271497e.
- Agarwal AK, Kalayarasan R, Javed A, Sakhuja P. Mass-forming xanthogranulomatous cholecystitis masquerading as gallbladder cancer. J Gastrointest Surg. 2013;17(7):1257–64. https://doi.org/10.1007/s11605-013-2209-2. Epub 2013 Apr 25.

- Kalayarasan R, Javed A, Puri AS, Puri SK, Sakhuja P, Agarwal AK. A prospective analysis of the preoperative assessment of duodenal involvement in gallbladder cancer. HPB (Oxford). 2013;15(3):203–9. https://doi.org/10.1111/j.1477-2574.2012.00539.x. Epub 2012 Aug 1.
- Agarwal AK, Kalayarasan R, Javed A, Sakhuja P. Role of routine 16b1 lymph node biopsy in the management of gallbladder cancer: an analysis. HPB (Oxford). 2014;16(3):229–34. https://doi.org/10.1111/hpb.12127. Epub 2013 Jul 22.
- Agarwal AK, Javed A, Raja K, Sakhuja P. Surgical techniques in the management of primary gall bladder cancer. In: Agarwal A, Fong Y, editors. Carcinoma of the gall bladder. New Delhi: Elsevier; 2014. p. 106–29.

2006–2012—569 operated—327 curative resections—CRAO in 113 (one organ 49, more organs 64) CBD excision 75, gastroduodenal sleeve resection ($n = 27$, distal gastrectomy proximal duodenectomy $n = 36$) wedge resection of pancreas $n = 7$, HPD $n = 6$, sleeve/segmental colonic resection $n = 25$, right hemicolectomy $n = 8$

- Agarwal AK, Javed A, Kalayarasan R, Sakhuja P. Minimally invasive versus the conventional open surgical approach of a radical cholecystectomy for gallbladder cancer: a retrospective comparative study. HPB (Oxford). 2015;17(6):536–41. https://doi.org/10.1111/hpb.12406. Epub 2015 Feb 28.
- Mishra PK, Saluja SS, Prithiviraj N, Varshney V, Goel N, Patil N. Predictors of curative resection and long term survival of gallbladder cancer - a retrospective analysis. Am J Surg. 2017;214(2):278–86. https://doi.org/10.1016/j.amjsurg.2017.02.006. Epub 2017 Feb 9.
- Han HS, Yoon YS, Agarwal AK, Belli G, Itano O, Gumbs AA, Yoon DS, Kang CM, Lee SE, Wakai T, Troisi RI. Laparoscopic surgery for gallbladder cancer: an expert consensus statement. Dig Surg. 2019;36(1):1–6. https://doi.org/10.1159/000486207. Epub 2018 Jan 16.

Consensus statement for laparoscopic management of gallbladder cancer

- Nag HH, Raj P, Sisodia K. The technique of laparoscopic hepatic bisegmentectomy with regional lymphadenectomy for gallbladder cancer. J Minim Access Surg. 2018;14(2):124–9. https://doi.org/10.4103/jmas.JMAS_181_16.
- Nag HH, Sachan A, Nekarakanti PK. Laparoscopic versus open extended cholecystectomy with bi-segmentectomy (s4b and s5) in patients with gallbladder cancer. J Minim Access Surg. 2019. https://doi.org/10.4103/jmas.JMAS_98_19. [Epub ahead of print].

18.8.3 Institute of Medical Sciences (IMS), Banaras Hindu University (BHU), Varanasi India

Vinod K. Shukla and Manoj Pandey

- Shukla VK, Khandelwal C, Roy SK, Vaidya MP. Primary carcinoma of the gall bladder: a review of a 16-year period at the University Hospital. J Surg Oncol. 1985;28(1):32–5.
- Shukla VK, Tiwari SC, Roy SK. Biliary bile acids in cholelithiasis and carcinoma of the gall bladder. Eur J Cancer Prev. 1993;2(2):155–60.
- Shukla VK, Shukla PK, Pandey M, Rao BR, Roy SK. Lipid peroxidation product in bile from patients with carcinoma of the gallbladder: a preliminary study. J Surg Oncol. 1994;56(4):258–62.
- Pandey M, Vishwakarma RA, Khatri AK, Roy SK, Shukla VK. Bile, bacteria, and gallbladder carcinogenesis. J Surg Oncol. 1995;58(4):282–3.
- Pandey M, Khatri AK, Dubey SS, Gautam A, Shukla VK. Erythrocyte membrane fatty acid profile in patients with primary carcinoma of the gallbladder. J Surg Oncol. 1995;59(1):31–4.

- Pandey M, Gautam A, Shukla VK. ABO and Rh blood groups in patients with cholelithiasis and carcinoma of the gall bladder. BMJ. 1995;310(6995):1639.
- Singh H, Pandey M, Shukla VK. Salmonella carrier state, chronic bacterial infection and gallbladder carcinogenesis. Eur J Cancer Prev. 1996;5(2):144.
- Nath G, Singh H, Shukla VK. Chronic typhoid carriage and carcinoma of the gallbladder. Eur J Cancer Prev. 1997;6(6):557–9.
- Shukla VK, Pandey M, Kumar M, Sood BP, Gupta A, Aryya NC, Shukla RC, Verma DN. Ultrasound-guided fine needle aspiration cytology of malignant gallbladder masses. Acta Cytol. 1997;41(6):1654–8.
- Dixit VK, Prakash A, Gupta A, Pandey M, Gautam A, Kumar M, Shukla VK. Xanthogranulomatous cholecystitis. Dig Dis Sci. 1998;43(5):940–2.
- Shukla VK, Aryya NC, Pitale A, Pandey M, Dixit VK, Reddy CD, Gautam A. Metallothionein expression in carcinoma of the gallbladder. Histopathology. 1998;33(2):154–7.
- Shukla VK, Prakash A, Tripathi BD, Reddy DC, Singh S. Biliary heavy metal concentrations in carcinoma of the gall bladder: case-control study. BMJ. 1998;317(7168):1288–9.
- Pandey M, Sood BP, Shukla RC, Aryya NC, Singh S, Shukla VK. Carcinoma of the gallbladder: role of sonography in diagnosis and staging. J Clin Ultrasound. 2000;28(5):227–32.
- Pandey M, Shukla VK. Fatty acids, biliary bile acids, lipid peroxidation products and gallbladder carcinogenesis. Eur J Cancer Prev. 2000;9(3):165–71.
- Pandey M, Shukla VK, Singh S, Roy SK, Rao BR. Biliary lipid peroxidation products in gallbladder cancer: increased peroxidation or biliary stasis? Eur J Cancer Prev. 2000;9(6):417–22.
- Shukla VK, Singh H, Pandey M, Upadhyay SK, Nath G. Carcinoma of the gallbladder—is it a sequel of typhoid? Dig Dis Sci. 2000;45(5):900–3.
- Dixit VK, Singh S, Shukla VK. Aetiopathogenesis of carcinoma gallbladder. Trop Gastroenterol. 2001;22(2):103–6. Review.
- Pandey M, Pathak AK, Gautam A, Aryya NC, Shukla VK. Carcinoma of the gallbladder: a retrospective review of 99 cases. Dig Dis Sci. 2001;46(6):1145–51.
- Shukla VK, Rastogi AN, Adukia TK, Raizada RB, Reddy DC, Singh S. Organochlorine pesticides in carcinoma of the gallbladder: a case-control study. Eur J Cancer Prev. 2001;10(2):153–6.
- Pandey M, Shukla VK. Diet and gallbladder cancer: a case-control study. Eur J Cancer Prev. 2002;11(4):365–8.
- Pradhan S, Shukla VK, Agrawal S, Dixit VK, Sharma OP. Sonographic and colour doppler morphology in carcinoma gallbladder. Indian J Cancer. 2002;39(4):143–8.
- Pandey M, Sharma LB, Singh S, Shukla VK. Erythrocyte membrane fatty acid profile and saturation index in gallbladder carcinogenesis: a case-control study. World J Surg Oncol. 2003;1(1):5.
- Pandey M, Sharma LB, Shukla VK. Cytochrome P-450 expression and lipid peroxidation in gallbladder cancer. J Surg Oncol. 2003;82(3):180–3.
- Pandey M, Shukla VK. Lifestyle, parity, menstrual and reproductive factors and risk of gallbladder cancer. Eur J Cancer Prev. 2003;12(4):269–72.
- Shukla VK, Adukia TK, Singh SP, Mishra CP, Mishra RN. Micronutrients, antioxidants, and carcinoma of the gallbladder. J Surg Oncol. 2003;84(1):31–5.
- Doval DC, Sekhon JS, Gupta SK, Fuloria J, Shukla VK, Gupta S, Awasthy BS. A phase II study of gemcitabine and cisplatin in chemotherapy-naive, unresectable gall bladder cancer. Br J Cancer. 2004;90(8):1516–20.
- Shukla VK, Prakash A, Chauhan VS, Singh S, Puneet. Biliary nitrate and risk of carcinoma of the gallbladder. Eur J Cancer Prev. 2004;13(4):355–6.
- Gupta SK, Ansari MA, Shukla VK. What makes the Gangetic belt a fertile ground for

gallbladder cancers? J Surg Oncol. 2005;91(2):143–4.

- Gupta SK, Singh SP, Shukla VK. Copper, zinc, and Cu/Zn ratio in carcinoma of the gallbladder. J Surg Oncol. 2005;91(3):204–8.
- Puneet, Ragini R, Gupta SK, Singh S, Shukla VK. Management of polypoidal lesions of gallbladder in laparoscopic era. Trop Gastroenterol. 2005;26(4):205–10. Review.
- Shukla VK, Chauhan VS, Kumar M. Telomerase activation—one step on the road to carcinoma of the gall bladder. Anticancer Res. 2006;26(6C):4761–6.
- Shukla VK, Gurubachan, Sharma D, Dixit VK, Usha. Diagnostic value of serum CA242, CA 19-9, CA 15-3 and CA 125 in patients with carcinoma of the gallbladder. Trop Gastroenterol. 2006;27(4):160–5.
- Sharma V, Chauhan VS, Nath G, Kumar A, Shukla VK. Role of bile bacteria in gallbladder carcinoma. Hepatogastroenterology. 2007;54(78):1622–5.
- Nath G, Singh YK, Kumar K, Gulati AK, Shukla VK, Khanna AK, Tripathi SK, Jain AK, Kumar M, Singh TB. Association of carcinoma of the gallbladder with typhoid carriage in a typhoid endemic area using nested PCR. J Infect Dev Ctries. 2008;2(4):302–7.
- Shukla VK, Chauhan VS, Mishra RN, Basu S. Lifestyle, reproductive factors and risk of gallbladder cancer. Singapore Med J. 2008;49(11):912–5.
- Shukla VK, Goel S, Trigun SK, Sharma D. Electrophoretic pattern of proteins in carcinoma of the gallbladder. Eur J Cancer Prev. 2008;17(1):9–12.
- Tewari M, Kumar V, Mishra RR, Kumar M, Shukla HS. Is there a role for cholecystectomy in gallbladder carcinoma discovered to be unresectable for cure at laparotomy? World J Surg. 2008;32(12):2683–7. https://doi.org/10.1007/s00268-008-9763-x.
- Shukla VK, Tandon A, Ratha BK, Sharma D, Singh TB, Basu S. Arginase activity in carcinoma of the gallbladder: a pilot study. Eur J Cancer Prev. 2009;18(3):199–202. https://doi.org/10.1097/CEJ.0b013e32832405eb.
- Mishra RR, Tewari M, Shukla HS. Helicobacter species and pathogenesis of gallbladder cancer. Hepatobiliary Pancreat Dis Int. 2010;9:129–34.
- Nath G, Gulati AK, Shukla VK. Role of bacteria in carcinogenesis, with special reference to carcinoma of the gallbladder. World J Gastroenterol. 2010;16(43):5395–404.
- Pandey M, Mishra RR, Dixit R, et al. Helicobacter bilis in human gallbladder cancer: results of a case-control study and a meta-analysis. Asian Pac J Cancer Prev. 2010;11(2):343–7.
- Basu S, Priya R, Singh TB, Srivastava P, Mishra PK, Shukla VK. Role of nicotine in gallbladder carcinoma: a preliminary report. J Dig Dis. 2012;13(10):536–40. https://doi.org/10.1111/j.1751-2980.2012.00623.x.
- Dixit R, Kumar P, Tripathi R, Basu S, Mishra R, Shukla VK. Chromosomal structural analysis in carcinoma of the gallbladder. World J Surg Oncol. 2012;10:198. https://doi.org/10.1186/1477-7819-10-198.
- Dwivedi AN, Pandey M, Shukla RC, Shukla VK, Gaharwar S, Maurya BN. Biological behavior and disease pattern of carcinoma gallbladder shown on 64-slice CT scanner: a hospital-based retrospective observational study and our experience. Indian J Cancer. 2012;49(3):303–8. https://doi.org/10.4103/0019-509X.104496.
- Shukla VK, das PC, Dixit R, Bhartiya SK, Basu S, Raman MJ. Study of AP endonuclease (APEX1/REF1), a DNA repair enzyme, in gallbladder carcinoma. Anticancer Res. 2012;32(4):1489–92.
- Basu S, Singh MK, Singh TB, Bhartiya SK, Singh SP, Shukla VK. Heavy and trace metals in carcinoma of the gallbladder. World J Surg. 2013;37(11):2641–6. https://doi.org/10.1007/s00268-013-2164-9.
- Dixit R, Srivastava P, Basu S, Srivastava P, Mishra PK, Shukla VK. Association of mustard oil as cooking media with carcinoma of the gallbladder. J Gastrointest Cancer. 2013;44(2):177–81. https://doi.org/10.1007/s12029-012-9458-2.

- Maurya SK, Tewari M, Sharma B, Shukla HS. Expression of procaspase 3 and activated caspase 3 and its relevance in hormone-responsive gallbladder carcinoma chemotherapy. Korean J Intern Med. 2013;28(5):573–8. https://doi.org/10.3904/kjim.2013.28.5.573. Epub 2013 Aug 14.
- Tewari M, Agarwal A, Mishra RR, Meena RN, Shukla HS. Epigenetic changes in carcinogenesis of gallbladder. Indian J Surg Oncol. 2013;4(4):356–61. https://doi.org/10.1007/s13193-013-0240-0. Epub 2013 Apr 4. Review.
- Scanu T, Spaapen RM, Bakker JM, Pratap CB, Wu LE, Hofland I, Broeks A, Shukla VK, Kumar M, Janssen H, Song JY, Neefjes-Borst EA, te Riele H, Holden DW, Nath G, Neefjes J. Salmonella manipulation of host signaling pathways provokes cellular transformation associated with gallbladder carcinoma. Cell Host Microbe. 2015;17(6):763–74. https://doi.org/10.1016/j.chom.2015.05.002. Epub 2015 May 28.
- Shukla HS, Sirohi B, Behari A, Sharma A, Majumdar J, Ganguly M, Tewari M, Kumar S, Saini S, Sahni P, Singh T, Kapoor VK, Sucharita V, Kaur T, Shukla DK, Rath GK. Indian Council of Medical Research consensus document for the management of gall bladder cancer. Indian J Med Paediatr Oncol. 2015;36(2):79–84. https://doi.org/10.4103/0971-5851.158829.
- Dixit R, Singh G, Pandey M, Basu S, Bhartiya SK, Singh KK, Shukla VK. Association of methylenetetrahydrafolate reductase gene polymorphism (MTHFR) in patients with gallbladder cancer. J Gastrointest Cancer. 2016;47(1):55–60. https://doi.org/10.1007/s12029-015-9794-0.
- Tewari M, Kumar S, Shukla S, Shukla HS. Analysis of wedge resection of gallbladder bed and lymphadenectomy on adequate oncologic clearance for gallbladder cancer. Indian J Cancer. 2016;53(4):552–7. https://doi.org/10.4103/ijc.IJC_88_17.
- Dixit R, Pandey M, Tripathi SK, Dwivedi AN, Shukla VK. Comparative analysis of mutational profile of sonic hedgehog gene in gallbladder cancer. Dig Dis Sci. 2017;62(3):708–14. https://doi.org/10.1007/s10620-016-4438-1. Epub 2017 Jan 5.
- Dixit R, Raza M, Kumar M, Basu S, Shukla VK. Expression analysis of Survivin and XIAP in gallbladder cancer: a case-control study in Indo-Gangetic plain. J Gastrointest Cancer. 2018;49(4):487–92. https://doi.org/10.1007/s12029-017-0008-9.
- Kumar M, Shukla VK, Misra PK, Raman MJ. Dysregulated expression and subcellular localization of base excision repair (BER) pathway enzymes in gallbladder cancer. Int J Mol Cell Med. 2018;7(2):119–32. https://doi.org/10.22088/IJMCM.BUMS.7.2.119. Epub 2018 Aug 18.

18.8.4 Tata Memorial Hospital (TMH), Mumbai India

Parul J. Shukla and Mahesh Goel

- Shukla PJ, Barreto SG, Arya S, Shrikhande SV, Hawaldar R, Purandare N, Rangarajan V. Does PET-CT scan have a role prior to radical re-resection for incidental gallbladder cancer? HPB (Oxford). 2008;10(6):439–45. https://doi.org/10.1080/13651820802286910.
- Shukla PJ, Barreto G, Kakade A, Shrikhande SV. Revision surgery for incidental gallbladder cancer: factors influencing operability and further evidence for T1b tumours. HPB (Oxford). 2008;10(1):43–7. https://doi.org/10.1080/13651820701867794.
- Shukla PJ, Neve R, Barreto SG, Hawaldar R, Nadkarni MS, Mohandas KM, Shrikhande SV. A new scoring system for gallbladder cancer (aiding treatment algorithm): an analysis of 335 patients. Ann Surg Oncol. 2008;15(11):3132–7. https://doi.org/10.1245/s10434-008-9917-y. Epub 2008 May 6.
- Barreto SG, Haga H, Shukla PJ. Hormones and gallbladder cancer in women. Indian J Gastroenterol. 2009;28(4):126–30. https://doi.org/10.1007/s12664-009-0046-8. Epub 2009 Nov 24.

- Shukla PJ, Barreto SG. Systematic review: should routine resection of the extra-hepatic bile duct be performed in gallbladder cancer? Saudi J Gastroenterol. 2010;16(3):161–7. https://doi.org/10.4103/1319-3767.65184. Review.
- Sirohi B, Mitra A, Jagannath P, Singh A, Ramadvar M, Kulkarni S, Goel M, Shrikhande SV. Neoadjuvant chemotherapy in patients with locally advanced gallbladder cancer. Future Oncol. 2015;11(10):1501–9. https://doi.org/10.2217/fon.14.308.
- Goel M, Tamhankar A, Rangarajan V, Patkar S, Ramadwar M, Shrikhande SV. Role of PET CT scan in redefining treatment of incidental gall bladder carcinoma. J Surg Oncol. 2016;113(6):652–658. https://doi.org/10.1002/jso.24198.
- Patil RS, Shah SU, Shrikhande SV, Goel M, Dikshit RP, Chiplunkar SV. IL17 producing γδT cells induce angiogenesis and are associated with poor survival in gallbladder cancer patients. Int J Cancer. 2016;139(4):869–81. https://doi.org/10.1002/ijc.30134.
- Engineer R, Goel M, Chopra S, et al. Neoadjuvant chemoradiation followed by surgery for locally advanced gallbladder cancers: a new paradigm. Ann Surg Oncol. 2016;23(9):3009–15. https://doi.org/10.1245/s10434-016-5197-0.
- Ramaswamy A, Ostwal V, Pande N, et al. Second-line palliative chemotherapy in advanced gall bladder cancer, CAP-IRI: safe and effective option. J Gastrointest Cancer. 2016;47(3):305–12. https://doi.org/10.1007/s12029-016-9828-2.
- Ostwal V, Pinninti R, Ramaswamy A, et al. Treatment of advanced Gall bladder cancer in the real world-can continuation chemotherapy improve outcomes?. J Gastrointest Oncol. 2017;8(2):368–76. https://doi.org/10.21037/jgo.2017.03.08.
- Patkar S, Ostwal V, Ramaswamy A, et al. Emerging role of multimodality treatment in gall bladder cancer: outcomes following 510 consecutive resections in a tertiary referral center. J Surg Oncol. 2018;117(3):372–9. https://doi.org/10.1002/jso.24837t.
- Barreto SG, Shukla PJ. Predicting resectability in gallbladder cancer: the Tata Memorial Hospital Staging System. J Gastrointest Surg. 2017;21(11):1969–70. https://doi.org/10.1007/s11605-017-3535-6. Epub 2017 Aug 15.
- Patkar S, Shinde RS, Kurunkar SR, et al. Radiological diagnosis alone risks overtreatment of benign disease in suspected gallbladder cancer: a word of caution in an era of radical surgery. Indian J Cancer. 2017;54(4):681–4. https://doi.org/10.4103/ijc.IJC_516_17.
- Kanetkar AV, Patkar S, Khobragade KH, Ostwal V, Ramaswamy A, Goel M. Neuroendocrine carcinoma of gallbladder: a step beyond palliative therapy, experience of 25 cases. J Gastrointest Cancer. 2019;50(2):298–303. https://doi.org/10.1007/s12029-018-0070-y.
- Ostwal V, Swami R, Patkar S, et al. Gemcitabine-cisplatin (GC) as adjuvant chemotherapy in resected stage II and stage III gallbladder cancers (GBC): a potential way forward. Med Oncol. 2018;35(4):57. Published 2018 Mar 21. https://doi.org/10.1007/s12032-018-1115-6.
- Chaudhari VA, Ostwal V, Patkar S, et al. Outcome of neoadjuvant chemotherapy in "locally advanced/borderline resectable" gallbladder cancer: the need to define indications. HPB (Oxford). 2018;20(9):841–7. https://doi.org/10.1016/j.hpb.2018.03.008.
- Barreto SG, Dutt A, Sirohi B, Shrikhande SV. Gallbladder cancer: a journey of a thousand steps. Future Oncol. 2018;14(13):1299–1306. https://doi.org/10.2217/fon-2017-0576. Epub 2018 May 3.
- Agarwala V, Ramaswamy A, Dsouza S, et al. Resection of isolated port site metastasis in gall bladder cancers-careful selection and perioperative systemic therapy may improve outcomes. Indian J Surg Oncol. 2018;9(3):427–31. https://doi.org/10.1007/s13193-018-0809-8.
- Kattepur AK, Patkar S, Goel M, Ramaswamy A, Ostwal V. Role of adjuvant chemotherapy in resected T2N0 gall bladder cancer. J Gastrointest Surg. 2019;23(11):2232–8. https://doi.org/10.1007/s11605-019-04104-4.

- Goel M, Khobragade K, Patkar S, Kanetkar A, Kurunkar S. Robotic surgery for gallbladder cancer: operative technique and early outcomes. J Surg Oncol. 2019;119(7):958–63. https://doi.org/10.1002/jso.25422.
- Engineer R, Patkar S, Lewis SC, et al. A phase III randomised clinical trial of perioperative therapy (neoadjuvant chemotherapy versus chemoradiotherapy) in locally advanced gallbladder cancers (POLCAGB): study protocol. BMJ Open. 2019;9(6):e028147. Published 2019 Jun 27. https://doi.org/10.1136/bmjopen-2018-028147.
- Acharya MR, Patkar S, Parray A, Goel M. Management of gallbladder cancer in India. Chin Clin Oncol. 2019;8(4):35. https://doi.org/10.21037/cco.2019.07.03.
- Patkar S, Patil V, Acharya MR, Kurunkar S, Goel M. Achieving margin negative resection-doing less is justified: oncological outcomes of wedge excision of liver in gallbladder cancer (GBC) surgery. Chin Clin Oncol. 2019;8(4):38. https://doi.org/10.21037/cco.2019.07.0734.
- Goel M, Kurunkar SR, Kanetkar A, Patkar S. Outcome of robot-assisted radical cholecystectomy in a high-volume tertiary cancer center in India. J Laparoendosc Adv Surg Tech Part B Videoscop. 2019;29(3):vor.2018.0539. Published 2019 Oct 17. https://doi.org/10.1089/vor.2018.0539.
- Patkar S, Chaturvedi A, Goel M, Rangarajan V, Sharma A, Engineer R. Role of positron emission tomography-contrast enhanced computed tomography in locally advanced gallbladder cancer. J Hepatobiliary Pancreat Sci. 2020;27(4):164–70. https://doi.org/10.1002/jhbp.712.
- Jearth V, Patil P, Patkar S, et al. Immunoglobulin G4-related cholecystitis mimicking a locally advanced gallbladder cancer-a case report and review of literature [published online ahead of print, 2020 Jun 28]. Clin J Gastroenterol. 2020. https://doi.org/10.1007/s12328-020-01168-7.
- Mhatre S, Rajaraman P, Chatterjee N, et al. Mustard oil consumption, cooking method, diet and gallbladder cancer risk in high- and low-risk regions of India. Int J Cancer. 2020;147(6):1621–8. https://doi.org/10.1002/ijc.32952.

18.8.5 Sanjay Gandhi Post-Graduate Institute of Medical Sciences (SGPGIMS), Lucknow India

Vinay K. Kapoor and Anu Behari

- https://expertscape.com/ex/gallbladder+neoplasms/p/earth
- SGPGIMS Lucknow India is ranked at no. 7 in the list of global institutions based on articles published since 2010; Balraj Mittal (Medical Genetics) and the Author (VKK) are in the list of top 10 global experts. Balraj Mittal has published a large number of research and review articles on the molecular biology of GBC.

- Sikora SS, Kapoor R, Pradeep R, Kapoor VK, Saxena R, Kaushik SP. Palliative surgical treatment of malignant obstructive jaundice. Eur J Surg Oncol. 1994;20(5):580–4.
- Pradeep R, Kaushik SP, Sikora SS, Bhattacharya BN, Pandey CM, Kapoor VK. Predictors of survival in patients with carcinoma of the gallbladder. Cancer. 1995;76(7):1145–9.
- Kapoor VK, Pradeep R, Haribhakti SP, Singh V, Sikora SS, Saxena R, Kaushik SP. Intrahepatic segment III cholangiojejunostomy in advanced carcinoma of the gallbladder. Br J Surg. 1996;83(12):1709–11.
- Kapoor VK, Pradeep R, Haribhakti SP, Sikora SS, Kaushik SP. Early carcinoma of the gallbladder: an elusive disease. J Surg Oncol. 1996;62(4):284–7.
- Kumar A, Krishnani N, Saxena R, Kapoor VK, Kaushik SP. Xanthogranulomatous cholecystitis. Indian J Gastroenterol. 1996;15(4):122–5.
- Haribhakti SP, Kapoor VK, Gujral RB, Kaushik SP. Staging of carcinoma of the gallbladder—an ultrasonographic evaluation. Hepatogastroenterology. 1997;44(17):1240–5.

- Haribhakti SP, Awasthi S, Pradeep R, Kapoor VK, Kaushik SP. Carcinoma gallbladder: atypical presentations and unusual associations. Trop Gastroenterol. 1997;18(1):32–4.
- Kapoor VK, Benjamin IS. Biliary malignancies. In: Pitt HA, editors. Bailliere's clinical gastroenterology: the biliary tract. London: Bailliere Tindall; 1997. p. 801–36.
- Kapoor VK, Aretxabala X de. Gall bladder cancer. Cancer J. 1997;10:73–4.
- Kaushik SP, Kapoor VK, Haribhakti SP. Carcinoma gall bladder. In: Chattopadhyay TK, editor. GI surgery annual. Vol. 4. New Delhi: Indian Association of Surgical Gastroenterology; 1997. p. 87–101.
- Kapoor VK, Sonawane RN, Haribhakti SP, Sikora SS, Saxena R, Kaushik SP. Gall bladder cancer: proposal for a modification of the TNM classification. Eur J Surg Oncol. 1998;24(6):487–91. Review.
- Kapoor VK, Benjamin IS. Resectional surgery for gall bladder cancer. Br J Surg. 1998;85:145–6.
- Kapoor VK, Benjamin IS. Gallbladder and biliary tract tumours. In: Badellino F, Gipponi M, editors. Flow charts for diagnosis and staging of cancers in developed and developing countries. Geneva: International Union Against Cancer (UICC); 1998. p. 90–103.
- Singh B, Kapoor VK, Sikora SS, Kalawat TC, Das BK, Kaushik SP. Malignant gastroparesis and outlet obstruction in carcinoma gall bladder. Trop Gastroenterol. 1998;19(1):37–9.
- Behari A, Sikora SS, Kapoor VK. Carcinoma of the gall bladder. In: Gupta RL, editor. Recent advances in surgery. Vol. 7. New Delhi: Jaypee Brothers; 1999. p. 188–209.
- Kapoor VK. Gall bladder cancer - Editor's choice. Hepato-Gastroenterology. 1999;46: 1592–4.
- Kaushik SP, Kapoor VK. The challenge of gall bladder cancer. Hepato-Gastroenterology. 1999;46:1527–8.
- Sikora SS, Kapoor VK. Bypass for malignant duodenal obstruction. Indian J Gastroenterol. 1999;18:99–100.
- Ghosh M, Kawamoto T, Koike N, Fukao K, Yoshida S, Kashiwagi H, Kapoor VK, Agarwal S, Krishnani N, Uchida K, Miwa M, Todoroki T. Cyclooxygenase expression in the gallbladder. Int J Mol Med. 2000;6(5):527–32.
- Behari A, Sikora SS, Kapoor VK. Extended cholecystectomy. In: Kaushik SP, editor. Operative procedures in surgical gastroenterology. Vol 1. New Delhi: Jaypee Brothers; 2001. p. 64–8.
- Behari A, Sikora SS, Kapoor VK. Segment III cholangiojejunostomy. In: Kaushik SP, editor. Operative procedures in surgical gastroenterology. Vol 1. New Delhi: Jaypee Brothers; 2001. p. 83–9.
- Kapoor VK. Incidental gall bladder cancer. Am J Gastroenterol. 2001;96:627–9.
- Kapoor VK, McMichael AJ. Gall bladder cancer – leave no stones unturned. Indian J Surg. 2002;64:29–30.
- Behari A, Sikora SS, Wagholikar GD, Kumar A, Saxena R, Kapoor VK. Long term survival after extended resections in patients with gallbladder cancer. J Am Coll Surg. 2003;196(1):82–8.
- Kapoor VK, McMichael AJ. Gallbladder cancer: an 'Indian' disease. Natl Med J India. 2003;16(4):209–13.
- Singh MK, Pandey UB, Ghoshal UC, Srivenu I, Kapoor VK, Choudhuri G, Mittal B. Apolipoprotein B-100 XbaI gene polymorphism in gallbladder cancer. Hum Genet. 2004;114(3):280–3. Epub 2003 Nov 14.
- Singh MK, Chetri K, Pandey UB, Kapoor VK, Mittal B, Choudhuri G. Mutational spectrum of K-ras oncogene among Indian patients with gallbladder cancer. J Gastroenterol Hepatol. 2004;19(8):916–21.
- Srikanth G, Kumar A, Khare R, Siddappa L, Gupta A, Sikora SS, Saxena R, Kapoor VK. Should laparoscopic cholecystectomy be performed in patients with thick-walled gallbladder? J Hepatobiliary Pancreat Surg. 2004;11(1):40–4.
- Wagholikar GD, Behari A, Kapoor VK. Surgery for early gall bladder cancer. In: Pandey M, Shukla VK, editors. Gallbladder cancer. New Delhi: Jaypee Brothers; 2004. p. 109–21.
- Agrawal S, Sonawane RN, Behari A, Kumar A, Sikora SS, Saxena R, Kapoor

VK. Laparoscopic staging in gallbladder cancer. Dig Surg. 2005;22(6):440–5. Epub 2006 Feb 10.
- Ghosh M, Kamma H, Kawamoto T, Koike N, Miwa M, Kapoor VK, Krishnani N, Agrawal S, Ohkohchi N, Todoroki T. MUC 1 core protein as a marker of gallbladder malignancy. Eur J Surg Oncol. 2005;31(8):891–6.
- Rao RV, Kumar A, Sikora SS, Saxena R, Kapoor VK. Xanthogranulomatous cholecystitis: differentiation from associated gall bladder carcinoma. Trop Gastroenterol. 2005;26(1):31–3.
- Agrawal S, Kapoor VK. Thick walled gall bladder. Natl Med J India. 2006;19:37–8.
- Balachandran P, Agarwal S, Krishnani N, Pandey CM, Kumar A, Sikora SS, Saxena R, Kapoor VK. Predictors of long-term survival in patients with gallbladder cancer. J Gastrointest Surg. 2006;10(6):848–54.
- Gowda GA, Somashekar BS, Ijare OB, Sharma A, Kapoor VK, Khetrapal CL. One-step analysis of major bile components in human bile using 1H NMR spectroscopy. Lipids. 2006;41(6):577–89.
- Kapoor VK. Gall bladder cancer – a global perspective. J Surg Oncol. 2006;93:607–9.
- Kapoor VK. Cholecystectomy in patients with asymptomatic gallstones to prevent gall bladder cancer—the case against. Indian J Gastroenterol. 2006;25(3):152–4.
- Prasad TL, Kumar A, Sikora SS, Saxena R, Kapoor VK. Mirizzi syndrome and gallbladder cancer. J Hepatobiliary Pancreat Surg. 2006;13(4):323–6.
- Behari A, Kapoor VK. Extended cholecystectomy for gall bladder cancer. In: Chattopadhyay TK, editor. GI surgery annual. New Delhi: Indian Association of Surgical Gastroenterology; 2007;14(Suppl):41–4.
- Kapoor VK. Gall bladder cancer – the Indian perspective. Ann Nat Acad Med Sci (India). 2007;43:47–53.
- Kapoor VK. Advanced gallbladder cancer: Indian “middle path”. J Hepatobiliary Pancreat Surg. 2007;14(4):366–73. Epub 2007 Jul 30.
- Behari A, Kapoor VK. Gall bladder cancer and cholangiocarcinoma. In Tandon BN, editor. Tropical hepatogastroenterology. New Delhi: Elsevier; 2008. p. 485–513.
- Kapoor VK. Gall bladder cancer – a challenge in India too. World Gastroenterol News. 2008;2:24.
- Krishna RP, Kumar A, Singh RK, Sikora S, Saxena R, Kapoor VK. Xanthogranulomatous inflammatory strictures of extrahepatic biliary tract: presentation and surgical management. J Gastrointest Surg. 2008;12(5):836–41. https://doi.org/10.1007/s11605-008-0478-y. Epub 2008 Feb 12.
- Sharma A, Behari A, Sikora SS, Kumar A, Saxena R, Kapoor VK. Post-cholecystectomy biliary strictures: not always benign. J Gastroenterol Hepatol. 2008;23(7 Pt 2):e63–6. Epub 2007 Jul 20.
- Srivastava M, Sharma A, Kapoor VK, Nagana Gowda GA. Stones from cancerous and benign gallbladders are different: a proton nuclear magnetic resonance spectroscopy study. Hepatol Res. 2008;38(10):997–1005. https://doi.org/10.1111/j.1872-034X.2008.00356.x. Epub 2008 May 27.
- Jayalakshmi K, Sonkar K, Behari A, Kapoor VK, Sinha N. Solid state (13)C NMR analysis of human gallstones from cancer and benign gall bladder diseases. Solid State Nucl Magn Reson. 2009;36(1):60–5. https://doi.org/10.1016/j.ssnmr.2009.06.001. Epub 2009 Jun 16.
- Kapoor VK. An Indian meets the American Indians. Natl Med J India. 2009;22:204-5.
- Priya TP, Kapoor VK, Krishnani N, Agrawal V, Agarwal S. Fragile histidine triad (FHIT) gene and its association with p53 protein expression in the progression of gall bladder cancer. Cancer Invest. 2009;27(7):764–73. https://doi.org/10.1080/07357900802711304.
- Agrawal V, Goel A, Krishnani N, Pandey R, Agrawal S, Kapoor VK. p53, carcinoembryonic antigen and carbohydrate antigen 19.9 expression in gall bladder cancer, precursor epithelial lesions and xanthogranulomatous cholecystitis. J Postgrad Med. 2010;56(4):262–6. https://doi.org/10.4103/0022-3859.70933.
- Behari A, Kapoor VK. Does gallbladder cancer divide India? Indian J Gastroenterol.

2010;29(1):3–7. https://doi.org/10.1007/s12664-010-0008-1.

- Priya TP, Kapoor VK, Krishnani N, Agrawal V, Agrawal S. Role of E-cadherin gene in gall bladder cancer and its precursor lesions. Virchows Arch. 2010;456(5):507–14. https://doi.org/10.1007/s00428-010-0908-6. Epub 2010 Apr 8.
- Yusuf A, Kapoor VK, Abdullah KO, et al. Modification and implementation of NCCN Hepato-biliary cancer guidelines in the Middle East and North African Region. J NCCN. 2010;8(Suppl 3):S36–40.
- Behari A, Kapoor VK. Asymptomatic gallstones (AsGS) - to treat or not to? Indian J Surg. 2012;74(1):4–12. https://doi.org/10.1007/s12262-011-0376-5. Epub 2011 Dec 3.
- Kumari N, Kapoor VK, Krishnani N, Kumar K, Baitha DK. Role of C-erbB2 expression in gallbladder cancer. Indian J Pathol Microbiol. 2012;55(1):75–9. https://doi.org/10.4103/0377-4929.94862.
- Behari A, Kapoor VK. Incidental gall bladder cancer. Adv Surg. 2013;47:227–49. Review.
- Kapoor VK. Gall stone disease: a heavier burden in India! World Gastroenterol News. 2013;18:15.
- Mishra K, Behari A, Kapoor VK, Khan MS, Prakash S, Agrawal S. Vascular endothelial growth factor single-nucleotide polymorphism in gallbladder cancer. J Gastroenterol Hepatol. 2013;28(10):1678–85. https://doi.org/10.1111/jgh.12343.
- Pottakkat B, Kapoor A, Prakash A, Singh RK, Behari A, Kumar A, Kapoor VK, Saxena R. Evaluation of a prospective surgical strategy of extended resection to achieve R0 status in gall bladder cancer. J Gastrointest Cancer. 2013;44(1):33–40. https://doi.org/10.1007/s12029-012-9432-z.
- Behari A, Singh MK, Kapoor VK. Molecular biology of gall bladder cancer. In: Agarwal A, Fong Y, editors. Carcinoma of the gall bladder. New Delhi: Elsevier; 2014. p. 15–31.
- Behari A, Kapoor VK. Gall bladder cancer. In: Fong Y, Dong JH, editors. Hepato-biliary cancer. Shelton: PMPH; 2014. p. 61–88.
- Kumari N, Agrawal V, Behari A, Singh MK, Kapoor VK. Etiopathogenesis of gall bladder cancer. In: Agarwal A, Fong Y, editors. Carcinoma of the gall bladder. New Delhi: Elsevier; 2014. p. 1–14.
- Kumari N, Corless CL, Warrick A, Beadling C, Nelson D, Neff T, Krishnani N, Kapoor VK. Mutation profiling in gallbladder cancer in Indian population. Indian J Pathol Microbiol. 2014;57(1):9–12. https://doi.org/10.4103/0377-4929.130849.
- Prasadbabu TLVD, Behari A, Kapoor VK. Gall bladder cancer. In: Haribhakti SP, editor. Clinical GI surgery. Hyderabad: Paras; 2014. p. 968–74.
- Agrawal S, Gupta PK, Rastogi N, Lawrence A, Kumari N, Das KJ, Saxena R. Outcomes of adjuvant chemoradiation and predictors of survival after extended cholecystectomy in gall bladder carcinoma: a single institution experience from an endemic region. J Gastrointest Cancer. 2015;46(1):48–53. https://doi.org/10.1007/s12029-014-9676-x.
- Kapoor VK. Gallbladder neck cancer and perihilar cholangiocarcinoma - siblings, cousins or look alikes? Korean J Hepatobiliary Pancreat Surg. 2015;19(2):86–8. https://doi.org/10.14701/kjhbps.2015.19.2.86. Epub 2015 May 31.
- Kapoor VK. Gall bladder cancer: what needs to be done in India? In: Gandhi V, Mehta K, Grover R, Pathak S, Aggarwal BB, editors. Multi-targeted approach to treatment of cancer. Switzerland: Springer; 2015. p. 179–87.
- Kapoor VK. Gall bladder cancer and jaundice – the yellow signal. Clin Med Rev Oncol. 2015;5:1–3.
- Kapoor VK. Is gall bladder cancer a bad cancer per se? World J Gastrointest Surg. 2015;7(7):107–9. https://doi.org/10.4240/wjgs.v7.i7.107.
- Mishra K, Behari A, Kapoor VK, Khan MS, Prakash S, Agrawal S. Platelet derived growth factor receptor and human epidermal growth factor receptor (HER2) polymorphism in gall bladder cancer. Asian Pac J Cancer Prev. 2015;16(14):5647–54.
- Shukla HS, Sirohi B, Behari A, Sharma A, Majumdar J, Ganguly M, Tewari M, Kumar S,

Saini S, Sahni P, Singh T, Kapoor VK, Sucharita V, Kaur T, Shukla DK, Rath GK. Indian Council of Medical Research consensus document for the management of gall bladder cancer. Indian J Med Paediatr Oncol. 2015;36(2):79–84. https://doi.org/10.4103/0971-5851.158829.
- Kumar A, Senthil G, Prakash A, Behari A, Singh RK, Kapoor VK, Saxena R. Mirizzi's syndrome: lessons learnt from 169 patients at a single center. Korean J Hepatobiliary Pancreat Surg. 2016;20(1):17–22. https://doi.org/10.14701/kjhbps.2016.20.1.17. Epub 2016 Feb 19.
- Agrawal S, Mohan L, Mourya C, Neyaz Z, Saxena R. Radiological downstaging with neoadjuvant therapy in unresectable gall bladder cancer cases. Asian Pac J Cancer Prev. 2016;17(4):2137–40.
- Behari A, Kapoor VK. Gall bladder cancer – is the stage set? Yet! J Gastrointest Cancer Stromal Tumors. 2016;1:1000107.
- Ikoma T, Kapoor VK, Behari A, Mishra K, Tsuchiya Y, Asai T, Endoh K, Okano K, Nakamura K. Lack of an apparent association between mycotoxin concentrations in red chili peppers and incidence of gallbladder cancer in India: an ecological study. Asian Pac J Cancer Prev. 2016;17(7):3499–503.
- Kapoor VK, Singh R, Behari A, Sharma S, Kumar A, Prakash A, Singh RK, Kumar A, Saxena R. Anticipatory extended cholecystectomy: the 'Lucknow' approach for thick walled gall bladder with low suspicion of cancer. Chin Clin Oncol. 2016;5(1):8. https://doi.org/10.3978/j.issn.2304-3865.2016.02.07.
- Sharma RK, Sonkar K, Sinha N, Rebala P, Albani AE, Behari A, Reddy DN, Farooqui A, Kapoor VK. Gallstones: a worldwide multifaceted disease and its correlations with gallbladder carcinoma. PLoS One. 2016;11(11):e0166351. https://doi.org/10.1371/journal.pone.0166351. eCollection 2016.
- Zuo M, Rashid A, Wang Y, Jain A, Li D, Behari A, Kapoor VK, Koay EJ, Chang P, Vauthey JN, Li Y, Espinoza JA, Roa JC, Javle M. RNA sequencing-based analysis of gallbladder cancer reveals the importance of the liver X receptor and lipid metabolism in gallbladder cancer. Oncotarget. 2016;7(23):35302–12. https://doi.org/10.18632/oncotarget.9181.
- Kapoor VK, Behari A. Surgical procedures for gall bladder cancer. BAOJ Cancer Res Ther. 2017;3:037.
- Sharma RK, Mishra K, Farooqui A, Behari A, Kapoor VK, Sinha N. ^{1}H nuclear magnetic resonance (NMR)-based serum metabolomics of human gallbladder inflammation. Inflamm Res. 2017;66(1):97–105. https://doi.org/10.1007/s00011-016-0998-y. Epub 2016 Oct 21.
- Agrawal S, Lawrence A, Saxena R. Does CA 19-9 have prognostic relevance in gallbladder carcinoma (GBC)? J Gastrointest Cancer. 2018;49(2):144–9. https://doi.org/10.1007/s12029-016-9914-5.
- Behari A, Kapoor VK. Gall Bladder Cancer with jaundice: the unscaled frontier. In: Sahni P, Pal S, editors. GI surgery annual. New Delhi: Springer; 2018. p. 119–30.
- Singh MK, Kapoor VK. Gallbladder cancer and aflatoxin: do we have sufficient evidence? Gastroenterology. 2018;154(1):259–60. https://doi.org/10.1053/j.gastro.2017.09.053. Epub 2017 Nov 23.
- Tsuchiya Y, Mishra K, Kapoor VK, Vishwakarma R, Behari A, Ikoma T, Asai T, Endoh K, Nakamura K. Plasma Helicobacter pylori antibody titers and Helicobacter pylori infection positivity rates in patients with gallbladder cancer or cholelithiasis: a hospital-based case-control study. Asian Pac J Cancer Prev. 2018;19(7):1911–5.
- Asai T, Tsuchiya Y, Mishra K, Behari A, Shukla P, Ikoma T, Kapoor VK, Nakamura K. Carcinogen metabolism pathway and tumor suppressor gene polymorphisms and gallbladder cancer risk in North Indians: a hospital-based case-control study. Asian Pac J Cancer Prev. 2019;20(12):3643–7.
- Dutta U, Bush N, Kalsi D, Popli P, Kapoor VK. Epidemiology of gallbladder cancer in India. Chin Clin Oncol. 2019;8(4):33. https://doi.org/10.21037/cco.2019.08.03.

- Pandey P, Bajpai P, Siddiqui MH, Sayyed U, Tiwari R, Shekh R, Mishra K, Kapoor VK. Elucidation of the chemopreventive role of stigmasterol against Jab1 in gall bladder carcinoma. Endocr Metab Immune Disord Drug Targets. 2019;19(6):826–37. https://doi.org/10.2174/1871530319666190206124120.
- Pandey P, Siddiqui MH, Behari A, Kapoor VK, Mishra K, Sayyed U, Tiwari RK, Shekh R, Bajpai P. Jab1-siRNA induces cell growth inhibition and cell cycle arrest in gall bladder cancer cells via targeting Jab1 signalosome. Anticancer Agents Med Chem. 2019. https://doi.org/10.2174/1871520619666190725122400. [Epub ahead of print].
- Mishra K, Behari A, Shukla P, Tsuchiya Y, Endoh K, Asai T, Ikoma T, Nakamura K, Kapoor VK. Risk factors for gallbladder cancer development in Northern India: a gallstones-matched, case–control study. Indian J Med Res. Accepted.

Postface

Gall bladder cancer (GBC) is an important cancer for a very large population of people in south Asia (India, Pakistan, Nepal, and Bangladesh), east Asia (Japan, Korea, and China), and central and south America (Chile and Bolivia). Not much is known and not much effort is going on to know about GBC, primarily because GBC is a "non-western" cancer (Kodama and Kodama 1994); much more remains to be found about it. Following are some of the suggested areas of work/research in GBC

1. Multi-institutional large, collaborative databases, and GBC registries—hospital, city, state, and country based, in high GBC incidence areas
2. Biobanks of biomaterial, e.g., tissue, blood, bile, stones (Fig. PF.1), urine, saliva, etc. from patients with GBC, chronic cholecystitis (CC), xantho-granulomatous cholecystitis (XGC), and normal controls
3. Natural history (in terms of the risk of development of GBC) of asymptomatic gallstones (GS) in high GBC incidence areas/populations—is it different from that in low GBC incidence areas?
4. Preventive cholecystectomy for asymptomatic GS—the incidence of preneoplastic lesions in presence of asymptomatic GS
5. Are there any serum-based tumor markers or biomarkers which can be used for screening and early diagnosis of GBC, especially in persons with asymptomatic GS?
6. Are GBC stones different from benign stones? Are GBC stones in high GBC incidence areas different from those in low GBC incidence areas?
7. Do high GBC incidence populations have a genetic predisposition to develop GBC?
8. Is non-stone GBC (seen more frequently in Japan and Korea) different from stone-associated GBC (seen more frequently in India and Chile)?
9. Descriptive and etiological epidemiology to identify risk factors for GBC
10. Role of positron emission tomography (PET) in staging of obvious as well as incidental GBC
11. Extent of liver resection, whether liver wedge or segments IVB + V, in early GBC
12. Role of neoadjuvant, adjuvant, and targeted therapy in resectable as well as advanced (locoregional and metastatic) GBC

I sincerely hope that this monograph, with commentaries by GBC experts from all continents and corners of the globe, will make the current generation of clinicians and scientists ponder over the unanswered questions related to GBC and will stimulate at least some of them to pick up some of these as the areas of their research interest so that some of the many unanswered questions related to GBC are answered (in my lifetime, at least!). The Author (VKK) will be happy to guide and advise young researchers to write such research proposals. It is also hoped that funding agencies, both international and national (in high GBC incidence countries), will allocate more funds for research on GBC.

V. K. Kapoor (ed.), *A Pictorial Treatise on Gall Bladder Cancer*,
https://doi.org/10.1007/978-981-15-5289-2

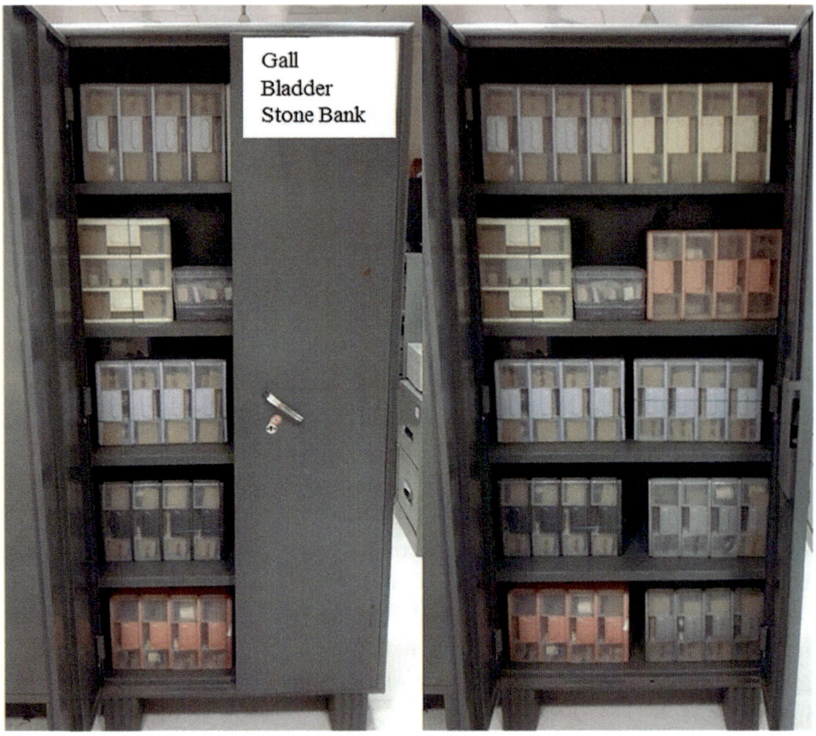

Fig. PF.1 Gall Stone 'Bank' at the Sanjay Gandhi Post-Graduate Institute of Medical Sciences (SGPGIMS), Lucknow India containing hundreds of stones from patients with gall bladder cancer (GBC), chronic cholecystitis (CC) and xantho-granulomatous cholecystitis (XGC). In addition, the Author (VKK) and his colleagues have a huge clinical database and a large biobank of tissue, paraffin blocks, slides, blood, bile, etc. of patients with GBC, CC and XGC which he will be happy to share with a young researcher wanting to use them for looking into various aspects of GBC

GBC is an "orphan" cancer (Roa et al. 2016, Nemunaitis et al. 2018)—it needs to be adopted by "foster parents" in India, Chile, Japan, and Korea! GBC has been a "forgotten" global cancer (Abou-Alfa 2019)—let us not further ignore it. In our publication (Chattopadhyay et al. 1988) in the Postgraduate Medical Journal (1988;64:593–5) (Fig. PF.2) more than three decades ago, we had posed a question "Carcinoma of the gall bladder—can we do anything?" I have made a humble beginning in the form of this Treatise on gall bladder cancer - *a bad cancer per se* (Kapoor 2015) (Fig. PF.3).

Vinay K. Kapoor
vkkapoor.india@gmail.com

Postgraduate Medical Journal (1988) **64**, 593–595

Carcinoma of the gall bladder – can we do anything?

T.K. Chattopadhyay, A. Kumar, V.K. Kapoor, L.K. Sharma, M.M. Kapur, B.M.L. Kapur and I.K. Dhawan

Department of Surgery, All India Institute of Medical Sciences, Ansari Nagar, New Delhi-110029, India.

Summary: A retrospective review of 143 cases of carcinoma of the gall bladder is presented. The disease was more common in females in the 5th and 6th decades. Pain, anorexia, weight loss and jaundice were the common presenting symptoms, and hepatomegaly and palpable gall bladder the common signs. Laboratory and radiological investigations were merely confirmatory as the diagnosis in a majority of the cases was clinically obvious. Aspiration cytology and laparoscopic biopsy were of help in obtaining histological diagnosis. Only 47 patients were considered fit enough to undergo laparotomy. In a majority of these patients biopsy alone was possible while palliative procedures were performed in the others. The operative mortality was 18% even in this selected group of patients, due to the poor general condition and the advanced stage of the disease at the time of diagnosis. Curative resection may be possible and long term survival is expected in incidentally found carcinoma at cholecystectomy. The only hope lies in prevention by prompt treatment of patients with benign biliary disease.

Fig. PF.2 Sadly, the question posed by the Author (VKK) and his colleagues more than three decades ago about gall bladder cancer remains unanswered even today

WJGS *World Journal of Gastrointestinal Surgery*

Submit a Manuscript: http://www.wjgnet.com/esps/
Help Desk: http://www.wjgnet.com/esps/helpdesk.aspx
DOI: 10.4240/wjgs.v7.i7.107

World J Gastrointest Surg 2015 July 27; 7(7): 107-109
ISSN 1948-9366 (online)

EDITORIAL

Is gall bladder cancer a bad cancer *per se*?

Vinay K Kapoor

Vinay K Kapoor, Surgical Gastroenterology, Sanjay Gandhi Post-graduate Institute of Medical Sciences, Lucknow 226014, Uttar Pradesh, India

hepato-pancreato-duodenectomy. Mortality of surgical procedures, when performed for GBC, is higher than when performed for other cancers. Survival in GBC, even after R0 resection, is poor. There is no proven role

Fig. PF.3 Fig. PF.3 This Treatise is a small contribution by the Author (VKK) toward the management of gall bladder cancer – *a bad cancer per se*

References

- Abou-Alfa GK. Gallbladder cancer, a forgotten global cancer problem. Chin Clin Oncol. 2019;8(4):30. https://doi.org/10.21037/cco.2019.07.11. Epub 2019 Aug 5.
- Chattopadhyay TK, Kumar A, Kapoor VK, Sharma LK, Kapur MM, Kapur BM, Dhawan IK. Carcinoma of the gall bladder—can we do anything? Postgrad Med J. 1988;64(754):593–5.
- Kapoor VK. Is gall bladder cancer a bad cancer per se? World J Gastrointest Surg. 2015;7(7): 107–9. https://doi.org/10.4240/wjgs.v7.i7.107.
- Kodama M, Kodama T. Epidemiological peculiarities of cancers of the gall-bladder and larynx that distinguish them from other human neoplasias. Anticancer Res. 1994;14(5B):2205–14.
- Nemunaitis JM, Brown-Glabeman U, Soares H, Belmonte J, Liem B, Nir I, Phuoc V, Gullapalli RR. Gallbladder cancer: review of a rare orphan gastrointestinal cancer with a focus on populations of New Mexico. BMC Cancer. 2018;18(1):665. https://doi.org/10.1186/s12885-018-4575-3. Review.
- Roa I, Garcia H, Game A, de Toro G, de Aretxabala X, Javle M. Somatic mutations of PI3K in early and advanced gallbladder cancer: additional options for an orphan cancer. J Mol Diagn. 2016;18(3):388–94. https://doi.org/10.1016/j.jmoldx.2015.12.003. Epub 2016 Mar 3.

Index

V. K. Kapoor (ed.), *A Pictorial Treatise on Gall Bladder Cancer*,
https://doi.org/10.1007/978-981-15-5289-2

GPSR Compliance

The European Union's (EU) General Product Safety Regulation (GPSR) is a set of rules that requires consumer products to be safe and our obligations to ensure this.

If you have any concerns about our products, you can contact us on ProductSafety@springernature.com

In case Publisher is established outside the EU, the EU authorized representative is:

Springer Nature Customer Service Center GmbH
Europaplatz 3
69115 Heidelberg, Germany

Batch number: 10731395

Printed by Printforce, the Netherlands